Instructor's Resource Manual

DAVI-ELLEN CHABNER, BA, MAT

The Language of Medicine

TENTH EDITION

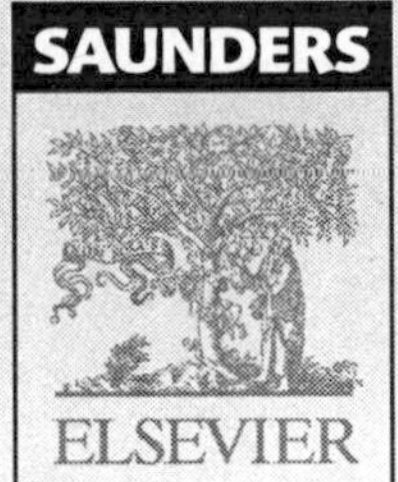

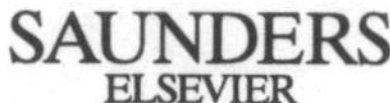

SAUNDERS
ELSEVIER

3251 Riverport Lane
Maryland Heights, Missouri 63043

INSTRUCTOR'S RESOURCE MANUAL FOR THE LANGUAGE OF MEDICINE, TENTH EDITION ISBN: 978-1-4557-5833-3

ISBN: 978-1-4557-5833-3

Content Strategist: Linda Woodard
Senior Content Development Specialist: Luke Held
Publishing Services Manager: Julie Eddy
Project Manager: Jan Waters
Senior Designer: Ellen Zanolle

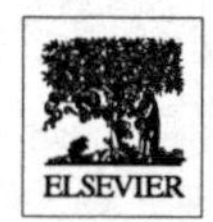

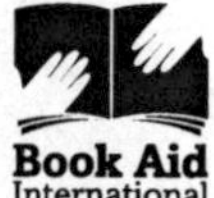

Transferred to Digital Printing in 2013

CONTENTS

INTRODUCTION

How to Use the Textbook and Instructor's Manual

I have prepared this teaching manual for instructors who will be using *The Language of Medicine*, 10th edition, with their medical terminology classes. The manual includes information about the organization of the textbook, sample course plans, classroom methods with practical suggestions for use of the text, quizzes and other materials pertinent to teaching each chapter, description of ancillary products (electronic resources on Evolve, instant translator, and online testbank), examples of practical applications (medical language in context) for use in class, suggestions for classroom activities and methods of other teachers, medical terminology humor, references and resources for supplemental materials, and transparency masters for use with overhead projectors. The organization of the textbook is as follows:

Chapters 1–4

Introductory chapters:

1. Basic Word Structure
2. Terms Pertaining to the Body as a Whole
3. Suffixes
4. Prefixes

These introductory chapters provide a foundation for the study of medical terminology. They teach students to divide words into component parts, recognize basic combining forms, suffixes, and prefixes, and know their meanings. In addition, students gain an understanding of the organization and complexity of the body and become familiar with the location and function of major body organs.

Chapter 1 should be taught first because it is a basic introduction to medical terminology and word analysis. I teach Chapters 2, 3, and 4 in that sequence, but other teachers have commented that they prefer to teach 3 and 4 and then follow with Chapter 2. The text is designed to be flexible so that you can experiment and teach the chapters in your own style.

Each of Chapters 1–4 contains a terminology list with examples of combining forms, suffixes, and prefixes. I use these lists in class to teach the medical terms. For your reference, the meanings of these terms are provided in the Answers to Combining Forms and Terminology sections included in this manual with all the materials for teaching each chapter.

Notice the Practical Applications feature in Chapters 1–4. I find that students enjoy testing their knowledge on these matching activities, and it is a good opportunity to expand their knowledge with related terms and concepts.

Exercises and **Answers** are found at the end of each text chapter. The answers are purposely placed directly after the questions so that students can check their responses easily. The exercises are not designed as tests, but rather as study aids. Students should be reminded to check their answers carefully so that they can benefit from the explanations in the answers sections.

Each chapter also contains a **Pronunciation List**. The Pronunciation List includes terms that are introduced in the chapter. In class, I use the list as an oral exercise and review before the chapter quiz. Students pronounce a term and then give its meaning. At home, students can write the term next to its pronunciation. The more times students write out words and their meanings, the easier it will be for them to learn the material. This is a workbook and students should be encouraged to use it in that manner. Don't forget to tell your students about a portable audio companion I have created called iTerms. Each term from the Pronunciation of Terms list in each chapter is pronounced and defined in iTerms. Students can purchase iTerms at www.elsevierhealth.com. Instructors can obtain access to iTerms by contacting their Elsevier representative.

A **Review Sheet** at the end of each chapter lists the combining forms, suffixes, and prefixes used in the chapter. Students in my classes write the meanings of all terms and check their answers with the Glossary of Terms list at the end of the text. I emphasize the writing of terms, over and over again, as the key to study. At times, I will use a blank review sheet as a quiz so that students know exactly what they should study. Students may find it helpful to copy these review sheets and complete them multiple times.

Chapters 5–18

These chapters explore the terminology of body systems. Once the chapters 1-4 have been completed, the body systems chapters can be presented in any order. The format of these chapters follows a specific pattern that you may find useful to follow in teaching:

Introduction: gives an overview of the function of the system.

Anatomy: presents the organs of the system and their locations and functions. Students label simple anatomical diagrams following the directions in the text, and in class, I teach the anatomical terms directly from the diagrams. Students tell me that the **flow diagrams** are especially helpful in study as they review and illustrate the relationship between individual organs within a body system.

Vocabulary: You may use this section as a review of terms previously taught in the anatomy section or as reference for anatomical terms. I ask students to cover the side of the page with the meanings and see if they can explain, in their own words, each term as we examine the list in class.

Terminology: This includes pertinent combining forms and illustrations of their use in medical words. I do this list in class with students by asking them to say the word and give its meaning. I have provided the meanings for your reference in each chapter section of this manual. Students can find meanings for these terms on my website (http://evolve.elsevier.com/Chabner/language/).

Pathology: These are often more difficult words to divide into parts. As we go over each term in class, I have a student read the paragraph explaining the etiology and treatment of the disease condition so that she or he gains experience in reading terms in a sentence context. This also helps in pronunciation of terms. I will often ask a student to explain the meaning of the sentence in her or his own words. This section contains more difficult words that can be a challenge to divide into component parts. As we go over each term in class, I often use the accompanying paragraphs to help students understand the pathological conditions. Notice that in order not to overwhelm the student with too much detail, I have put the essential information in boldface type. Terms are arranged alphabetically, often anatomically, and by category for easy study and reference.

Clinical Procedures, Laboratory Tests, and Abbreviations: This section can be taught in class or used as a reference for students, depending on the amount of time available. Often, clinical procedures are divided into diagnostic and treatment sections.

Practical Applications: These are short examples of how the medical language is used in context. They include actual medical reports, x-ray reports, autopsies, drug descriptions, case studies, and laboratory records. Use these as short exercises in oral reading or as an interesting supplement to the study of the terms in the chapter. Additional Practical Applications are included for every chapter in this manual with questions for material in the text and manual. These questions should help you engage students in dialogue and understanding terms in context. Use these short cases and paragraphs with the **Medical Forms** section as examples of how medical terms are used in the "real world." I hope that you will communicate any interesting way you use these forms via my e-mail address, daviellenchabner@gmail.com.

Chapters 19–22

These chapters on specialized areas of medicine (Cancer Medicine, Radiology and Nuclear Medicine, Pharmacology, and Psychiatry) continue the basic format of the systems chapters. Many students who do not study these chapters in class find that they can study them on their own and use them as reference for questions that may arise in their work situations.

Glossary and Appendices

The **Glossary** contains a full listing of abbreviations, which should be of practical use, and a Medical Word Parts—English list of all combining forms, suffixes, and prefixes used in the text. An English—Medical Word Parts list follows and includes each English term with its medical counterpart. In this section, I have added when to use a combining form when there are two or more for a particular organ (i.e., nephr/o and ren/o). Again: let me know (daviellenchabner@gmail.com) if this helps and communicate your own suggestions as well.

There are four **Appendices.**

- **Appendix I** contains information about forming plurals from singular nouns and gives examples of each.
- **Appendix II** is a list of commonly encountered abbreviations, acronyms, eponyms, and symbols.
- **Appendix III** presents normal laboratory values for blood cells and substances in serum and gives the implications for disease when the values are either too low or too high.
- **Appendix IV** is an alphabetized list of commonly prescribed drugs and their uses. I hope this will be a useful reference for allied health workers, both on the job and in understanding their own health issues.

Proposals for Courses

The design of *The Language of Medicine* is flexible so that it can be used in courses of varying lengths. An example of a typical two-semester syllabus follows:

Outline for First-Semester Course (16 weeks, 3 hours a week, 48 hours)

Week 1	Basic Word Structure	Chapter 1
Week 2	Terms Pertaining to the Body as a Whole	Chapter 2
Week 3	Suffixes	Chapter 3
Week 4	Prefixes	Chapter 4
Week 5	Digestive System	Chapter 5
Week 6	Additional Suffixes and Digestive System Terminology	Chapter 6

MIDTERM EXAMINATION

Week 7	Urinary System	Chapter 7
Week 8	Female Reproductive System	Chapter 8
Week 9	Male Reproductive System	Chapter 9
Week 10	Nervous System	Chapter 10
Week 11	Nervous System	
Week 12	Cardiovascular System	Chapter 11
Week 13	Cardiovascular System	
Week 14	Respiratory System	Chapter 12
Week 15	Respiratory System	
Week 16	Review	

FINAL EXAMINATION

Outline for Second-Semester Course (16 weeks, 3 hours a week, 48 hours)

Week 1	Blood System	Chapter 13
Week 2	Lymphatic and Immune Systems	Chapter 14
Week 3	Musculoskeletal System	Chapter 15
Week 4	Musculoskeletal System	
Week 5	Skin	Chapter 16
Week 6	Sense Organs: The Eye and the Ear	Chapter 17
Week 7	Endocrine System	Chapter 18
Week 8	Endocrine System	

MIDTERM EXAMINATION

Week 9	Cancer Medicine (Oncology)	Chapter 19
Week 10	Radiology and Nuclear Medicine	Chapter 20
Week 11	Radiology and Nuclear Medicine	
Week 12	Pharmacology	Chapter 21
Week 13	Pharmacology	
Week 14	Psychiatry	Chapter 22
Week 15	Psychiatry	
Week 16	Review	

FINAL EXAMINATION

Another example of a course structure was suggested to me by Susan Webb, a medical terminology instructor on Vancouver Island, British Columbia. She teaches a 12-week, 5-hours-a-week (two 2½ hour sessions), 60-hour course. Here is the syllabus for her course:

Week 1	Basic Word Structure	Chapter 1
Week 1	Terms Pertaining to the Body as a Whole	Chapter 2
Week 2	Suffixes	Chapter 3

Week 2	Prefixes	Chapter 4
Week 3	Additional Suffixes and Digestive System Terminology	Chapters 5 and 6
Week 3	Urinary System	Chapter 7
Week 4	Female Reproductive System	Chapter 8
Week 4	Male Reproductive System	Chapter 9
Week 5	Nervous System	Chapter 10
Week 5	Cardiovascular System	Chapter 11
Week 6	Respiratory System	Chapter 12
Week 6	REVIEW	Chapters 1–12
Week 7	Blood System and Review	Chapter 13
Week 7	Lymphatic and Immune Systems	Chapter 14
Week 8	Musculoskeletal System	Chapter 15
Week 8	Skin	Chapter 16
Week 9	Sense Organs: The Eye and the Ear	Chapter 17
Week 9	Endocrine System	Chapter 18
Week 10	Cancer Medicine (Oncology)	Chapter 19
Week 10	Radiology and Nuclear Medicine	Chapter 20
Week 11	Pharmacology	Chapter 21
Week 11	Psychiatry	Chapter 22
Week 12	REVIEW	Chapters 13–22
Week 12	FINAL EXAMINATION	

It may not be possible to cover all the material in your proposed time frame. You must gauge your pace to the ability of the students to absorb the material. My philosophy is to teach less and do it well, rather than rush through the material. You and your students are the best judges of how much of the book you will be able to cover. Students can always study chapters on their own and use as reference the chapters that are not taught.

Classroom Methods

While your teaching style will be characteristically your own, you may find the following ideas helpful:

- Use the method of *inquiry* and *discussion*, in conjunction with lecture. Encourage student participation by asking *why* and *how* questions. The goal is to relate medical terms to the functioning and structure of the body, thereby putting the terms in their proper context. *What* is an erythrocyte? *How* does it function? *What* enables it to carry oxygen? *Why* do body cells need oxygen? *What* is anemia? *Why* is supplemental iron necessary in some forms of the condition?
- Use of inquiry makes you aware of whether your students are "with you." If the class is open to questions and discussion, you will know if the material is being understood. Don't rush through the chapters just to meet a pre-designated schedule. The quantity of terms learned should be secondary to a thorough understanding of the meaning of the words.

- Use analogies and examples to illustrate the structure and functioning of parts of the body. For instance, you might compare the pericardium and peritoneum to sheets of polyethylene wrap, enveloping important organs such as the heart and abdominal viscera. Or neutrophils, monocytes, and lymphocytes can be described as the combat forces in your body, fighting against bacterial invasion. The relationship between air sacs (alveoli) and lung capillaries resembles balloons surrounded by fishnetting. Relating the numerous prefixes to familiar words is also helpful. Sub-and exo-, for example, can be associated with words like submarine, subway, exit, and exile. I have included such memory tips in the Answers to Combining Forms and Terminology sections in this manual.
- Give real-life examples of disease processes and procedures. Sometimes, relating the details of an actual medical situation helps fix the concepts and terminology in a student's mind. Personally, I am not shy about telling my classes about my recent colonoscopy or my daughter's experience (I was there, too) of an amniocentesis. You must be careful about getting carried away along this route, so use your and your students' experiences judiciously.
- Use of a medical dictionary and/or dental dictionary is essential. This will enable students to see how many different terms can be made using a single combining form with several different suffixes. Encyclopedic dictionaries give more than simple definitions of terms. They explain disease processes and give information about symptoms and treatments. Students should also be encouraged to use a dictionary when exploring the meanings of terms in the Combining Forms and Terminology sections of the text. Personally, I like *Miller-Keane Encyclopedia & Dictionary of Medicine, Nursing, & Allied Health* (7th edition) for excellent explanations of terms and *Mosby's Dictionary of Medicine, Nursing & Health Professions* (8th edition) for good images to illustrate terminology.
- Encourage good study skills. The more times students write out words, over and over again, the faster and better they will learn them. Listing difficult words in a separate notebook, making a file system of flash cards (medical term or word part on one side with its meaning on the other), testing and retesting themselves by covering one and then the other side of review sheets, and writing meanings and terms are all necessary to retention of the language. Some teachers encourage the use of a study buddy. Working together and testing each other is a good idea.
- Encourage use of online resources such as emedicine.com from WebMD, medlinehealthplus.com from NIH, and mayoclinic.com.
- Use visual aids. PowerPoint slides found on the Evolve website in the back of this Instructor's Resource Manual can be used during class discussion or made into quizzes and tests. Each illustration in the book is included. I have a collection of models (skeleton, female pelvis, heart, kidney) that I bring into class to illustrate anatomy. I also share my brother's gallstones, my chest x-ray (when I had pneumonia), a bone marrow biopsy needle (my daughter was a medical student), and assorted other visual aids that are enormously helpful for students to see terminology in action. Over the years I have collected old anatomical prints that are interesting to students as well.
- Give quizzes often. The tests motivate students to study and give the student, as well as the teacher, an indication as to how learning is proceeding. Often I will allow a student to retake his or her test in order to encourage mastery of the material. In addition to quizzes, I give frequent spelling tests. Students write words that I pronounce aloud. On other occasions I ask students to spell terms that are dictated and then we go over the terms and their meanings

as a review of the -vocabulary or combining forms and terminology lists. In the chapter sections of this manual, I have provided several different types of quizzes for use in classes. These quizzes are:

1. **Multiple Choice Quiz**. These are easy to grade, but may not be as comprehensive as other types of tests with more and different types of questions.
2. **Exercise Quiz**. These are taken from exercises at the end of each chapter; my students find this helpful in knowing exactly what to study.
3. **Dictation and Comprehension Quiz**. I use this type of quiz often to quickly test spelling and understanding of terms after each chapter. I may also add short answer questions depending on what I have covered in each chapter.
4. **Spelling Quiz**. These contain misspellings as well as the correct spelling. Some teachers like this, others do not. I am including them for those instructors who find them useful.
5. **Pronunciation Quiz**. These are based on the terms in the Pronunciation of Terms list in each chapter. Students indicate the accented syllable in a term, match terms with their meanings, and complete the spelling of a term from its definition.
6. **Diagram Quiz**. Each of these quizzes contains a diagram from one of the systems chapters, with a list of terms. Students are asked to complete the labeling of the diagram with the given terms. I often use flow diagrams (with labels removed) and ask students to complete them as a quiz.
7. **Vocabulary Quiz**. These are based on the terms in the vocabulary section in each chapter.
8. **Review Sheet Quiz**. These quizzes are based on the terms presented in the Review Sheets throughout the text.
9. **Abbreviations Quiz**. These ask students to spell out each abbreviation and match it with an associated sentence that helps the student understand the meaning of the abbreviation.
10. **Crossword Puzzle Quiz**. These were created by Susan Webb of Vancouver Island, who designed them for her medical terminology classes. Her students complete them in class as a review before their regular quiz.
11. **Practical Applications Quiz**. These are short paragraphs with multiple choice questions. You may use them for extra credit or for discussion in class after completing each chapter.
12. **Pathology Quiz**. These are based on the terms in the Pathology section in each chapter.
13. **Terminology Quiz**. These quizzes ask students to build terms from word parts in each chapter.
14. **Medical Scramble**. These fun exercises ask students to unscramble medical terms.
15. **NEW! Flow Chart Quiz**. These ask students to list the sequence of certain body systems and processes.

- Evaluate your teaching experience and your methods after each course is completed. Ask students to give a written critique of the course. You might ask students questions such as "What helped most?" "What helped least?" "Was the pace too fast or too slow?" "Was the course relevant to your needs?"

Ancillary Products: Evolve Resources, Instant Translator, Instructor's Resource Manual

Student Evolve Resources

Complimentary access to the online student resources on the Evolve website is included with purchase of each new copy of *The Language of Medicine,* 10th edition. These resources contain activities and information that will reinforce the medical terminology taught in each chapter of the book. The purpose of the student resources is to allow students to use their newly acquired knowledge of terminology in a way that is both fun and informative. A wide array of features—full-color images and photographs, video clips, animations, games, an assortment of interactive activities including case reports, vignettes, spelling bees, explanations of answers and hints to help students find correct responses—are made available in an attractive, easy-to-use format. In addition, pronunciation of all terms on the Pronunciation of Terms lists in every chapter is provided so that students have easy access to how each term sounds. Furthermore, the student resources contain a glossary with definitions of all word parts, a glossary of additional images, and the answers to the Pronunciation of Terms lists.

When using the resources students should see (by testing themselves) how much they have already learned and at the same time acquire new knowledge from the interactive program. Thus, the resources are specifically tailored to work chapter by chapter with *The Language of Medicine* as an invaluable study aid.

Instant Translator

The *Medical Language Instant Translator*, 5th edition (for sale separately), will help students while learning medical terminology and provide quick access to useful medically related information as a professional resource. It is a convenient, pocket-sized book containing the following features:

- Instructions on **how to analyze medical terms**
- **Word parts glossary** (medical terms to English and English to medical terms)
- Commonly used **abbreviations** and **symbols**
- Frequently encountered **acronyms** and their meanings
- Section on **eponyms**
- **Professional designations** and their meanings
- How to form **plurals** of medical terms
- Common **hematological reference values** and their implications
- Explanations of familiar **diagnostic tests and procedures**
- The top 100 principal **diagnoses** and associated **procedures**
- Major **Diagnostic Categories** and **Diagnosis-Related Groups (DRGs)**
- The **top 100 prescription drugs** (and what they treat)
- **Classes of drugs** with examples in each class
- **Surgical terminology** easy-reference list that provides quick access to surgical terms
- Listing of **complementary and alternative medicine terms**
- **Common medical terminology mistakes** that alert students to potential errors
- **Diagrams** of body systems figures and an index to reference each body part
- **Medical records** reference terms

I hope that this handy reference book will help medical terminology students decipher new terms and medical information with ease.

Testbank and Image Collection

An Instructor's Electronic Resource is available to complement this tenth edition. The test bank is accessible from the Instructor-secured EVOLVE site, with questions to use in creating exams for your students. This electronic test bank will allow you to create your own quizzes, tests, and exams very easily. The questions are grouped together by subject matter in accordance with the chapters in *The Language of Medicine*. To create a test, you can either select each question one-by-one or have the program select them randomly. If desired, you can also edit questions or add your own. An instructor's "answer key" will print out with each test you generate to make grading that much easier.

Furthermore, the student resources on the Evolve website contain an electronic image collection of all illustrations and most photographs from *The Language of Medicine* 10th edition, as well as the images in Power Point. I have provided these images both with and without the labels so you can use them in a variety of ways.

Please note:

You will notice the continued practice in *The Language of Medicine*, 10th edition, that the possessive form with eponyms is dropped throughout. While the possessive form with eponyms still remains acceptable, this text responds to a growing trend in medicine (i.e., Down syndrome, Tourette syndrome, Apgar score) as well as to a need for clarity and consistency.* Since medical dictionaries, wordbooks, and style manuals vary, the situation is often confusing for students and professionals. If you are uncomfortable with this change in tradition, you may advise your students to continue to be guided by sources such as Dorland's Dictionary or an appropriate medical or hospital reference.

*According to AHDI, when the noun is dropped (and implied), the possessive should be retained (i.e., "The patient was seen for Alzheimer's.").

Chapter 1

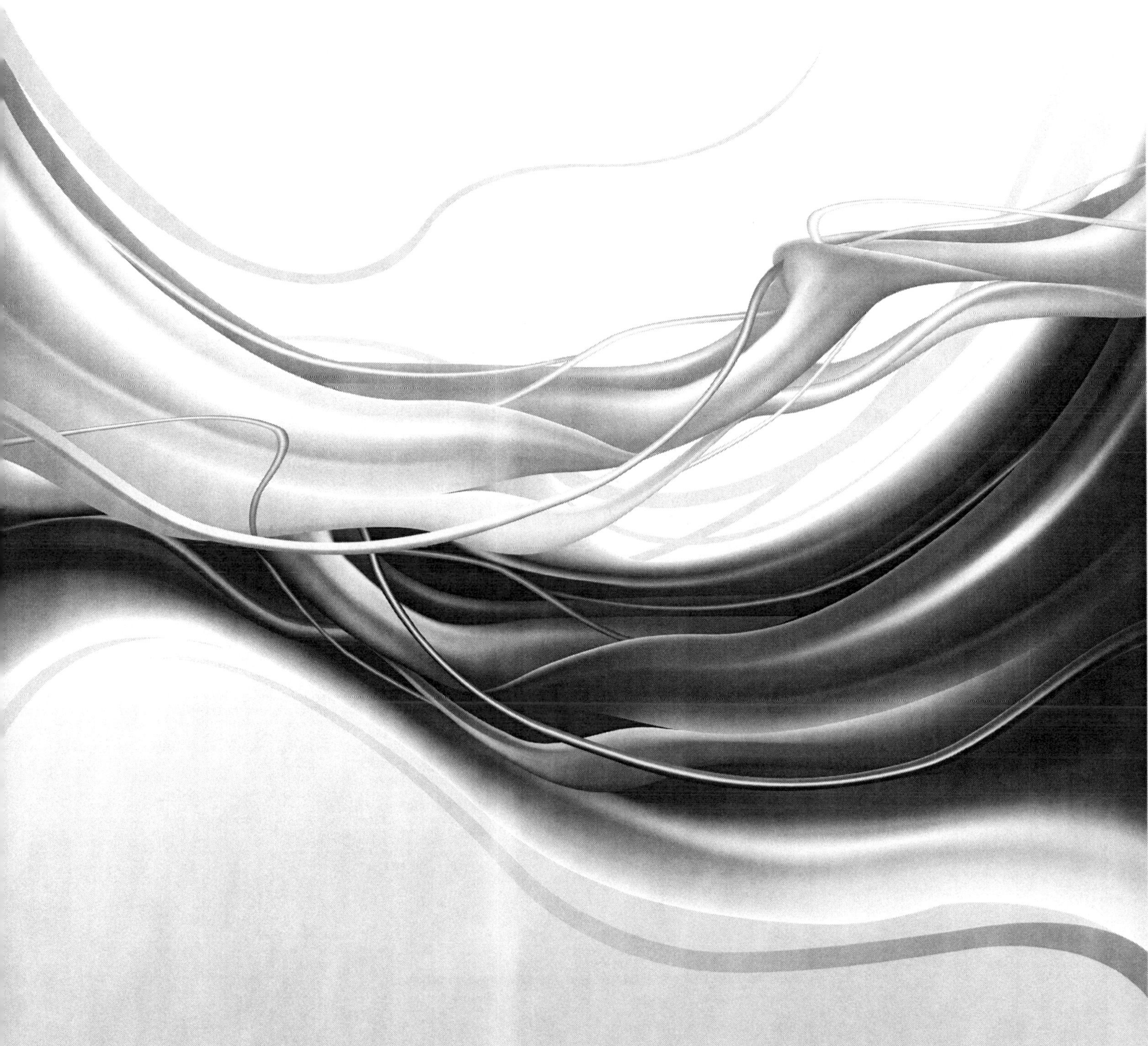

Chapter One
MULTIPLE CHOICE QUIZ

Name: ______________________

In the box write the letter of the choice that is the definition of the term or best answers the question. There is only one correct answer for each question.

1. Gastrectomy: ☐
- A. Gastric resection
- B. Intestinal incision
- C. Tumor of the stomach
- D. Incision of the stomach
- E. Resection of the intestine

2. Osteitis: ☐
- A. Incision of a bone
- B. Removal of a bone
- C. Incision of a joint
- D. Inflammation of a joint
- E. Inflammation of a bone

3. Cystoscopy: ☐
- A. Study of cells
- B. Visual examination of cells
- C. Removal of a sac of fluid
- D. Removal of the urinary bladder
- E. Visual examination of the urinary bladder

4. Hepatoma: ☐
- A. Incision of the kidney
- B. Tumor of the liver
- C. Blood mass
- D. Inflammation of the liver
- E. Red blood cell

5. Which of the following is not an endocrine gland? ☐
- A. Thyroid gland
- B. Adrenal gland
- C. Ovary
- D. Mammary gland
- E. Pituitary gland

6. Iatrogenic: ☐
- A. Pertaining to produced by treatment
- B. Produced by the mind
- C. Cancer producing
- D. Pertaining to producing a tumor
- E. Cutting into a tumor

7. Electroencephalogram: ☐
- A. Record of electricity in the brain
- B. Record of electricity in the heart
- C. X-ray of the brain
- D. Record of sound waves in the brain
- E. X-ray of the heart and brain

8. Diagnosis: ☐
- A. Is made after the prognosis
- B. Is a guess as to a patient's condition
- C. Is a prediction of the course of treatment
- D. Is made on the basis of complete knowledge about a patient's condition
- E. Is a treatment of a patient

9. Cancerous tumor: ☐
- A. Hematoma
- B. Adenoma
- C. Carcinoma
- D. Carcinogenic
- E. Neurotomy

10. Microscopic examination of living tissue: ☐
- A. Incision
- B. Pathology
- C. Biopsy
- D. Autopsy
- E. Resection

11. Pertaining to the largest part of the brain: ☐
- A. Cerebral
- B. Cephalic
- C. Renal
- D. Cardiac
- E. Neural

12. Removal of a gland: ☐
- A. Gastrotomy
- B. Gastric
- C. Hepatic resection
- D. Nephric section
- E. Adenectomy

13. Decrease in numbers of red blood cells or hemoglobin within red blood cells: ....

A. Anemia
B. Erythrocytosis
C. Thrombocytosis
D. Leukemia
E. Leukocytosis

14. Pathologist: ....

A. One who examines x-rays
B. One who operates on the urinary tract
C. One who performs autopsies and reads biopsies
D. One who operates on the kidney
E. One who treats diseases with chemicals

15. Pain in a joint: ....

A. Ostealgia
B. Arthritis
C. Osteoarthritis
D. Arthroalgia
E. Arthralgia

16. Increase in numbers of malignant white blood cells: ....

A. Leukocytosis
B. Leukemia
C. Erythremia
D. Thrombocytosis
E. Erythrocytosis

17. Instrument to view the eye: ....

A. Ophthalmoscopy
B. Opthalmoscope
C. Opthalmology
D. Ophthalmoscope
E. Opthalmoscopy

18. A platelet: ....

A. Hematoma
B. Thrombosis
C. Leukocyte
D. Thrombocyte
E. Erythrocyte

19. Abnormal condition of the mind: ....

A. Physchosis
B. Psychosis
C. Psychogenic
D. Encephalopathy
E. Adenoma

20. Inflammation of the nose: ....

A. Arthrosis
B. Hepatitis
C. Nephritis
D. Dermatosis
E. Rhinitis

21. Study of cells: ....

A. Pathology
B. Cytology
C. Cystology
D. Dermatology
E. Urology

22. Pertaining to through the liver: ....

A. Subrenal
B. Transdermal
C. Transhepatic
D. Subhepatic
E. Hepatoma

23. Abnormal condition of the kidney: ....

A. Neurologic
B. Neuralgia
C. Nephrotomy
D. Neural
E. Nephrosis

24. Incision of a bone: ....

A. Sarcoma
B. Pathogenic
C. Osteotomy
D. Ostectomy
E. Endoscopy

25. High level of sugar in the blood: ....

A. Hematoma
B. Hypodermic
C. Hypoglycemia
D. Hyperglycemia
E. Hypogastric

Chapter One
EXERCISE QUIZ

Name: ______________________________

A. Give meanings for the following combining forms:

1. arthr/o ______________________
2. cyst/o ______________________
3. encephal/o ______________________
4. aden/o ______________________
5. cyt/o ______________________
6. carcin/o ______________________

B. Give meanings for the following suffixes:

7. -gram ______________________
8. -itis ______________________
9. -opsy ______________________
10. -oma ______________________
11. -scopy ______________________
12. -logy ______________________

C. Using slashes, divide the following terms into parts and give the meaning of the entire term:

13. cerebral ______________________________
14. electrocardiogram ______________________________
15. dermatitis ______________________________
16. cephalic ______________________________

D. Complete the medical term from its meaning given below:

17. red blood cell: ______________ cyte
18. mass of blood: ______________ oma
19. white blood cell: ______________ cyte
20. pain of nerves: neur ______________

E. Underline the suffix in each term and give the meaning of the entire term:

21. nephrectomy ______________________
22. osteotomy ______________________
23. oncology ______________________
24. renal ______________________
25. psychosis ______________________
26. carcinogenic ______________________

F. Give the meanings for the following prefixes:

27. hyper- ______________________
28. peri- ______________________
29. epi- ______________________
30. trans- ______________________
31. hypo- ______________________
32. dia- ______________________

G. Underline the prefix and give the meaning of the entire term:

33. subhepatic ______________________________
34. hyperglycemia ______________________________
35. pericardium ______________________________
36. resection ______________________________
37. prognosis ______________________________
38. hypodermic ______________________________

H. Match the English term in Column I with its combining form in Column II:

Column I English Term	Column II Combining Form
39. kidney ____________	onc/o
40. disease ____________	ophthalm/o
41. eye ____________	oste/o
42. nose ____________	path/o
43. flesh ____________	psych/o
44. bone ____________	radi/o
45. mind ____________	ren/o
46. tumor ____________	rhin/o
47. clotting ____________	sarc/o
48. urinary tract ____________	sect/o
49. x-rays ____________	thromb/o
50. to cut ____________	ur/o

Chapter One

DICTATION AND COMPREHENSION QUIZ

Name: ______________________________

A. Dictation of Terms

1.	______________________________	11.	______________________________
2.	______________________________	12.	______________________________
3.	______________________________	13.	______________________________
4.	______________________________	14.	______________________________
5.	______________________________	15.	______________________________
6.	______________________________	16.	______________________________
7.	______________________________	17.	______________________________
8.	______________________________	18.	______________________________
9.	______________________________	19.	______________________________
10.	______________________________	20.	______________________________

B. Comprehension of Terms: Match number of the above term with its meaning below.

______ Pain of nerves
______ Inflammation of bone
______ Prediction about the outcome of treatment
______ Microscopic examination of living tissue
______ Blood cell that carries oxygen
______ Physician who specializes in drug treatment of cancerous tumors
______ Disease of a gland
______ Resection of a kidney
______ A platelet
______ Process of visual examination of the urinary bladder
______ Pertaining to an abnormal condition produced by a treatment
______ Incision of the stomach
______ Pertaining to producing cancer
______ An instrument to visually examine the eye
______ High blood sugar: diabetes mellitus
______ A physician who examines dead bodies to determine the cause of death
______ Pain of a joint
______ Mass or collection of blood
______ Slight increase in numbers of white blood cells as response to infection
______ Increase in abnormal, immature white blood cells; a malignant condition

Chapter One
SPELLING QUIZ

Name: ______________________

A. Circle the term that is spelled correctly and write its meaning in the space provided:

1.	luekocyte	leukocyte ______________
2.	neuralgia	nueralgia ______________
3.	biospy	biopsy ______________
4.	gynocology	gynecology ______________
5.	erythrocyte	erthyrocyte ______________
6.	opthalmoscopy	ophthalmoscopy ______________
7.	pathogenic	pathojenic ______________
8.	thrombocyte	thrombocyt ______________
9.	sacroma	sarcoma ______________
10.	psychology	physcology ______________

B. Circle the term that is spelled correctly. The meaning of each term is given.

11.	resection of a nerve	neruotomy	neurectomy	neurotomy
12.	pertaining to produced by treatment........	iatrogenic	iatragenic	itarogenic
13.	pertaining to the brain.............................	cerebrol	serebral	cerebral
14.	cancerous tumor	carcinoma	carsinoma	karsinoma
15.	collection of blood....................................	hepatoma	hematoma	hepitoma
16.	high blood sugar.......................................	hypoglycemia	hyperglicemia	hyperglycemia
17.	membrane surrounding the heart...........	perycardium	pericardium	pericardum
18.	instrument to examine within.................	endoscope	endoskope	endoscopy
19.	disease of the intestines............................	entrapathy	interopathy	enteropathy
20.	inflammation of the urinary bladder	cytitis	cystitis	sistitis

Chapter One

PRONUNCIATION QUIZ

Name: ______________________________

A. Underline the accented syllable in the following terms (for example: a<u>ne</u>mia, diag<u>no</u>sis, <u>en</u>docrine):

1. arthrotomy
2. cystoscopy
3. gastrectomy
4. endocrinology
5. neuralgia
6. pericarditis
7. ophthalmoscope
8. hepatoma
9. retrogastric
10. cytology

B. Match the term in Column I with its meaning in Column II:

Column I		Column II
1. encephalopathy	_______	A. Low levels of blood sugar
2. carcinogenic	_______	B. Treatment of the mind
3. oncology	_______	C. Study of tumors
4. dermatosis	_______	D. Excision of the stomach
5. psychiatry	_______	E. Pertaining to producing cancer
6. leukemia	_______	F. Abnormal condition (slight increase) of white blood cells
7. hypoglycemia	_______	G. Brain disease
8. iatrogenic	_______	H. Abnormal condition of the skin
9. gastric resection	_______	I. Cancerous condition of white blood cells
10. leukocytosis	_______	J. Pertaining to produced by treatment

C. Complete the following medical terms:

1. pro ______________________ Prediction about the outcome of a disease; "before knowledge."
2. ______________________ itis Inflammation of the kidney.
3. patho ______________________ Pertaining to producing disease.
4. ______________________ ology Study of women and female diseases.
5. electro ______________________ Record of electricity in the brain.
6. thrombocyt ______________________ Abnormal condition of clotting cells.
7. bi ______________________ Examination of living tissue under a microscope.
8. ______________________ al Pertaining to the largest part of the brain.
9. ______________________ oma Tumor of a gland (benign).
10. ______________________ arthritis Inflammation of bone and joint.

Chapter One
REVIEW SHEET QUIZ

Name: ______________________________

A. Give meanings for the following combining forms:

1. cephal/o ____________________
2. cerebr/o ____________________
3. cyt/o ____________________
4. encephal/o ____________________
5. enter/o ____________________
6. hepat/o ____________________
7. ped/o ____________________
8. ren/o ____________________
9. ur/o ____________________
10. cis/o ____________________

B. Give combining forms for the following meanings:

1. heart ____________________
2. skin ____________________
3. sugar ____________________
4. woman, female ____________________
5. x-rays ____________________
6. mind ____________________
7. nose ____________________
8. flesh ____________________

C. Give meanings for the following suffixes and prefixes

1. hypo-____________________
2. dia- ____________________
3. -scopy ____________________
4. -gram ____________________
5. -globin ____________________
6. trans- ____________________
7. sub- ____________________
8. retro- ____________________
9. epi- ____________________
10. end-, endo- ____________________

Chapter One

MEDICAL SCRAMBLE

Name: ______________________________

Unscramble the letters to form medical terms from the clues. Use the letters in squares to complete the bonus term.

1. *Clue:* Complete knowledge of a patient's condition

   ___ ☐ ___ ___ ___ ___ ___ ___ ___ S I G O A D S N I

2. *Clue:* Outermost layer of skin

   ☐ ___ ___ ___ ___ ___ ___ ___ ___ S R E M E I D P I

3. *Clue:* Collection of blood below the skin

   ___ ___ ☐ ___ ___ ___ ___ ☐ M A T E H O A M

4. *Clue:* Pertaining to treatment of the mind

   ___ ___ ___ ___ ___ ___ ☐ ___ ___ ___ ___ I C A I T S H Y R P C

5. *Clue:* Study of malignant tumors

   ___ ☐ ___ ___ ___ ___ ___ ___ O C L O Y G N O

BONUS TERM: *Clue:* A condition marked by deficiency of hemoglobin or decreased erythrocytes.

☐ ☐ ☐ ☐ ☐ ☐

Chapter One

CROSSWORD PUZZLE

Name: ______________________________

Fill in the crossword puzzle below using the clues listed underneath it.

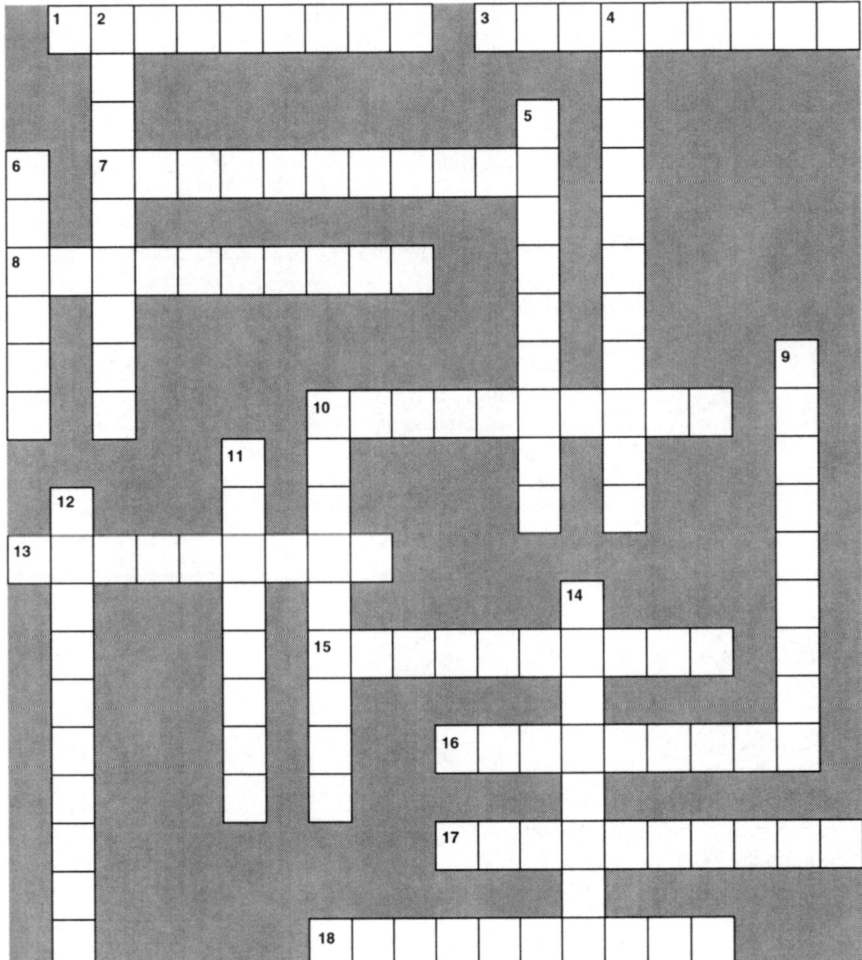

Across Clues

1. Process of cutting back (removal).
3. Complete knowledge.
7. Red blood cell.
8. Pertaining to above the stomach.
10. Study of women's diseases.
13. White blood cell.
15. Pertaining to produced by treatment.
16. Inflammation of the liver.
17. Pertaining to under the skin.
18. Pertaining to below the liver.

Down Clues

2. Inflammation of the small intestine.
4. Removal of the stomach.
5. Study of nerves.
6. Blood condition of low numbers of erythrocytes or deficient hemoglobin in the red blood cell.
9. Before knowledge (prediction about the outcome of treatment).
10. Inflammation of the stomach.
11. Process to cut into a part of the body.
12. Study of the kidney.
14. Mass of blood under the skin.

Chapter One
ANSWERS TO THE QUIZZES

Multiple Choice Quiz

1. A
2. E
3. E
4. B
5. D
6. A
7. A
8. D
9. C
10. C
11. A
12. E
13. A
14. C
15. E
16. B
17. D
18. D
19. B
20. E
21. B
22. C
23. E
24. C
25. D

Exercise Quiz

A

1. joint
2. urinary bladder
3. brain
4. gland
5. cell
6. cancer

B

7. record
8. inflammation
9. to view
10. tumor
11. process of visual examination
12. study of

C

13. cerebr/al—pertaining to the cerebrum (largest part of the brain)
14. electr/o/cardi/o/gram—record of the electricity in the heart
15. dermat/itis—inflammation of the skin
16. cephal/ic—pertaining to the head

D

17. erythrocyte
18. hematoma
19. leukocyte
20. neuralgia

E

21. nephrectomy—removal of the kidney
22. osteotomy—incision of a bone
23. oncology—study of tumors (cancerous)
24. renal—pertaining to the kidney
25. psychosis—abnormal condition of the mind
26. carcinogenic—pertaining to producing cancer

F

27. excessive; above
28. surrounding
29. above
30. across; through
31. below; deficient
32. through; complete

G

33. subhepatic—pertaining to below the liver
34. hyperglycemia—excessive blood sugar
35. pericardium—membrane surrounding the heart
36. resection—process of cutting back (removal)
37. prognosis—prediction about the outcome of treatment
38. hypodermic—pertaining to under the skin

H

39. ren/o
40. path/o
41. ophthalm/o
42. rhin/o
43. sarc/o
44. oste/o
45. psych/o
46. onc/o
47. thromb/o
48. ur/o
49. radi/o
50. sect/o

Dictation and Comprehension Quiz

A

1. adenopathy
2. arthralgia
3. biopsy
4. carcinogenic
5. cystoscopy
6. erythrocyte
7. gastrotomy
8. hematoma
9. hyperglycemia
10. iatrogenic
11. leukemia
12. leukocytosis
13. nephrectomy
14. neuralgia
15. oncologist
16. ophthalmoscope
17. osteitis
18. pathologist
19. prognosis
20. thrombocyte

B

14 Pain of nerves
17 Inflammation of bone
19 Prediction about the outcome of treatment
3 Microscopic examination of living tissue
6 Blood cell that carries oxygen
15 Physician who specializes in drug treatment of cancerous tumors
1 Disease of a gland
13 Resection of a kidney
20 A platelet
5 Process of visual examination of the urinary bladder
10 Pertaining to an abnormal condition produced by a treatment
7 Incision of the stomach
4 Pertaining to producing cancer
16 An instrument to visually examine the eye
9 High blood sugar: diabetes mellitus
18 A physician who examines dead bodies to determine the cause of death
2 Pain of a joint
8 Mass or collection of blood
12 Slight increase in numbers of white blood cells as response to infection
11 Increase in abnormal, immature white blood cells; a malignant condition

Spelling Quiz

A

1. leukocyte—white blood cell
2. neuralgia—pain of nerves

3. biopsy—view (microscopic) of living tissue
4. gynecology—study of female diseases
5. erythrocyte—red blood cell
6. ophthalmoscopy—visual examination of the eye
7. pathogenic—pertaining to producing disease
8. thrombocyte—clotting cell (platelet)
9. sarcoma—tumor of flesh tissue (malignant)
10. psychology—study of the mind

B

11. neurectomy
12. iatrogenic
13. cerebral
14. carcinoma
15. hematoma
16. hyperglycemia
17. pericardium
18. endoscope
19. enteropathy
20. cystitis

Pronunciation Quiz

A

1. arthrotomy
2. cystoscopy
3. gastrectomy
4. endocrinology
5. neuralgia
6. pericarditis
7. ophthalmoscope
8. hepatoma
9. retrogastric
10. cytology

B

1. G
2. E
3. C
4. H
5. B
6. I
7. A
8. J
9. D
10. F

C

1. prognosis
2. nephritis
3. pathogenic
4. gynecology
5. electroencephalogram
6. thrombocytosis
7. biopsy
8. cerebral
9. adenoma
10. osteoarthritis

Review Sheet Quiz

A

1. head
2. cerebrum (largest part of the brain)
3. cell
4. brain
5. intestine (usually small intestine)
6. liver
7. child
8. kidney
9. urine, urinary tract
10. to cut

B

1. cardi/o
2. derm/o, dermat/o
3. glyc/o
4. gynec/o
5. radi/o
6. psych/o
7. rhin/o
8. sarc/o

C

1. deficient, below, under, less than normal
2. through, complete
3. process of visually examining (with an endoscope)
4. record
5. protein
6. across, through
7. below, under
8. behind
9. above, upon
10. within

Medical Scramble

1. DIAGNOSIS
2. EPIDERMIS
3. HEMATOMA
4. PSYCHIATRIC
5. ONCOLOGY

BONUS TERM: ANEMIA

Crossword Puzzle

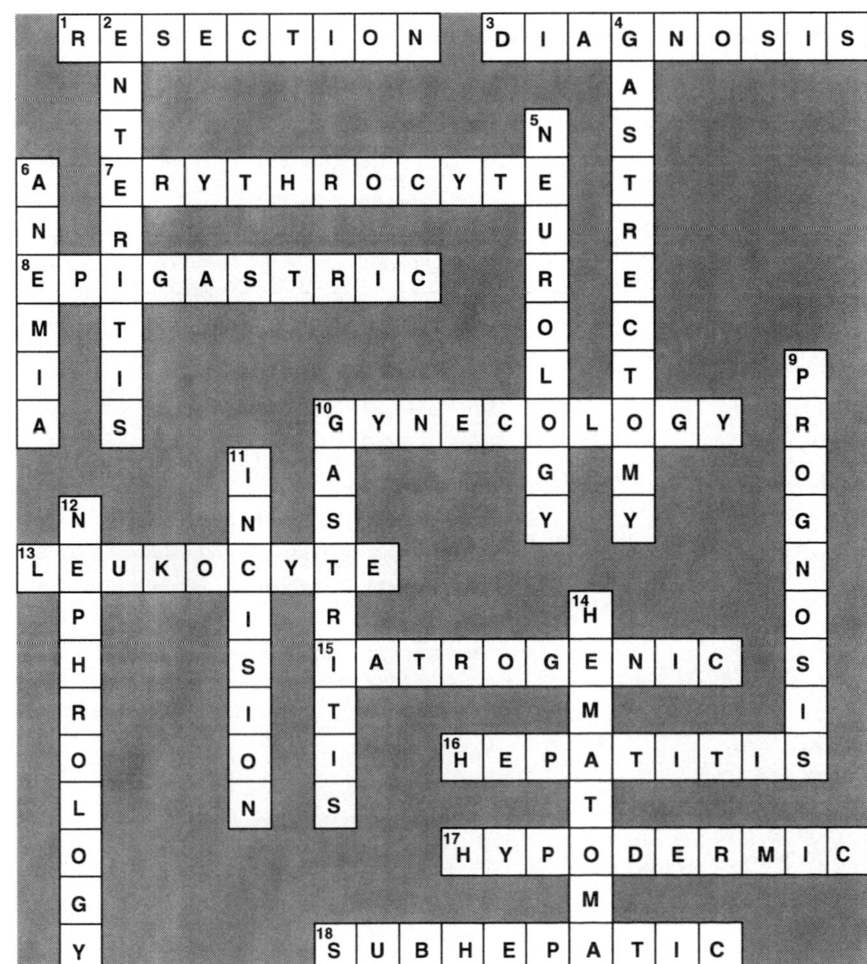

Chapter One

Answers to Combining Forms and Terminology Sections

(textbook pages 6–14)

Terminology	Meaning
adenoma	Tumor of a gland.
adenitis	Inflammation of a gland.
arthritis	Inflammation of a joint.
biology	Study of life.
biopsy	Removal of living tissue and examination under a microscope.
carcinoma	Cancerous tumor.
cardiology	Study of the heart.
cephalic	Pertaining to the head.
cerebral	Pertaining to the brain.
incision	Process of cutting into. *Scissors cut.*
excision	Process of cutting out.
endocrine glands	Glands that secrete hormones within the body.
cystoscopy	Process of visual examination of the urinary bladder.
cytology	Study of cells.
dermatitis	Inflammation of the skin.
hypodermic	Pertaining to under the skin.
electrocardiogram	Record of the electricity in the heart.
electroencephalogram	Record of the electricity of the brain.
enteritis	Inflammation of the intestines.
erythrocyte	A red blood cell.
gastrectomy	Removal of the stomach.
gastrotomy	Incision of the stomach.
diagnosis	State of complete knowledge; information gathered about a patient's illness (dia- = complete; gnos/o = knowledge; -sis = state of).
prognosis	State of before knowledge; prediction about the outcome of an illness. *An agnostic is a person who professes no (a-) knowledge of God.*
hyperglycemia	Condition of increased blood sugar.
gynecology	Study of females and female diseases.
hematology	Study of blood.
hematoma	Collection (mass) of blood.
hemoglobin	Blood protein found in red blood cells. Hemoglobin carries oxygen to the cells from the lungs and carbon dioxide away from cells to the lungs.
hepatitis	Inflammation of the liver.
iatrogenic	Pertaining to being produced by treatment. *A rash occurring after treatment with a drug, such as penicillin, is an iatrogenic condition. A related term, nosocomial, refers to any infection acquired in a hospital (nos/o means disease and -comial comes from the Greek "I take care of").*
leukocyte	White blood cell.
dermatology	Study of skin.
nephritis	Inflammation of the kidney.
nephrology	Study of the kidney.
neurology	Study of nerves.
oncology	Study of tumors.
oncologist	Specialist in the study of tumors.

ophthalmoscope	Instrument for visual examination of the eye. *Proper pronunciation* helps in the spelling of this term. The initial syllable is pronounced *"off"* and is spelled *"oph"*.
osteitis	Inflammation of bone.
osteoarthritis	Inflammation of bone and joints (actually degeneration of joint tissue).
pathology	Study of disease.
pathologist	One who studies diseases, performs autopsies, and examines biopsy samples.
pediatric	Pertaining to treatment of children.
psychology	Study of the mind.
psychiatrist	Specialist in the treatment of the mind.
radiology	Study of x-rays.
renal	Pertaining to the kidney. *Ren/o* (Latin) is used with *-al* (Latin), and *nephr/o* (Greek) is used with *-ic* (Greek).
rhinitis	Inflammation of the nose.
sarcoma	Tumor of flesh tissue (cancerous tumor of connective tissues, such as bone, muscle, cartilage, fat). *Sarcasm is an utterance intended to "cut into the flesh" and a sarcophagus is a box or container (Egyptian coffin) intended to "swallow flesh."* Phag/o means to eat or swallow.
resection	Process of cutting out; removal.
thrombocyte	A clotting cell.
urology	Study of the urinary tract.
cardiac	Pertaining to the heart.
neural	Pertaining to nerves.
arthralgia	Pain of a joint.
neuralgia	Nerve pain.
erythrocyte	Red blood cell.
nephrectomy	Removal (resection) of a kidney.
leukemia	Blood condition of white cells; malignant (cancerous) condition.
carcinogenic	Pertaining to producing cancer. *From the Greek gennao meaning "I produce." Other words to help remember -genic are gene and genesis.*
pathogenic	Pertaining to producing disease.
iatrogenic	Pertaining to produced by treatment (physician).
hemoglobin	Literally, blood (hem/o) protein (-globin). Hemoglobin is a protein found in red blood cells. It helps erythrocytes carry oxygen.
electroencephalogram	Record of the electricity in the brain.
gastric	Pertaining to the stomach.
neurologic	Pertaining to the study of nerves.
excision	Process of cutting out; removal.
ophthalmologist	Specialist in the study of diagnosing and treating disorders of the eye.
cystitis	Inflammation of the urinary bladder.
endocrinology	Study of the endocrine glands.
hepatoma	Tumor (malignant) of the liver.
biopsy	Process of viewing life; removal of living tissue for microscopic examination.
nephrosis	Abnormal condition of the kidney.
leukocytosis	Abnormal condition (slight increase) of normal white blood cells.
enteropathy	Disease of the intestines.
adenopathy	Disease of glands.
endoscope	Instrument to visually examine within (the body).
endoscopy	Process of visually examining within (the body).

prognosis	State of before knowledge; prediction about the outcome of treatment.
osteotomy	Incision of a bone.
gastroenterology	Process of study of the stomach and intestines.
anemia	A decrease in erythrocytes or hemoglobin.
autopsy	"Self-view"—examination of a dead body, understand its function.
diagnosis	State of complete knowledge; information gathered about a patient's illness.
endoscopy	Process of visually examining within (the body).
endocrinologist	One who specializes in endocrine glands.
epigastric	Pertaining to above the stomach.
epidermis	Outer layer of skin; above the dermis layer.
excision	Process of cutting out; to resection.
exocrine glands	Glands that secrete chemicals to the outside of the body.
hyperthyroidism	Condition of too much secretion of hormone (thyroxine) from the thyroid gland.
hypogastric	Pertaining to below the stomach.
hypoglycemia	Condition of low blood sugar.
incision	Process of cutting into; to section.
pericardium	Structure (membrane) surrounding the heart.
prostate gland	Exocrine gland in front of (before) the urinary bladder in males.
resection	Removal; excision. *From the Latin "resecare" meaning "to cut back, trim or curtail." Thus a resection is an operation wherein an organ is "cut back" or removed.*
retrocardiac	Pertaining to behind the heart.
subhepatic	Pertaining to below the liver.
transhepatic	Pertaining to across or through the liver.

Chapter 2

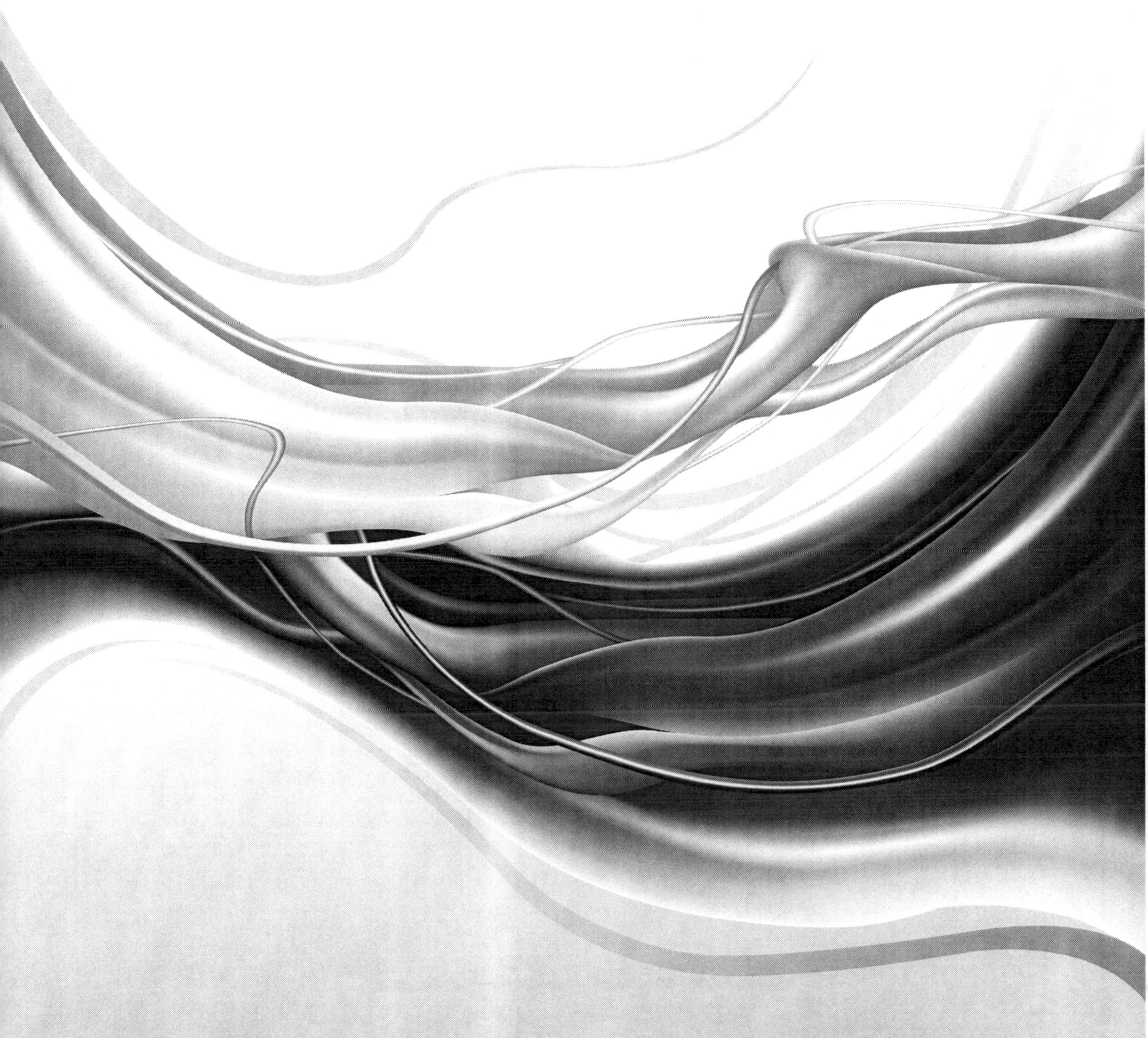

Chapter Two

MULTIPLE CHOICE QUIZ

Name: ______________________

In the box write the letter of the choice that is the definition of the term or best answers the question. There is only one correct answer for each question.

1. The process by which food is burned to release energy: ☐
A. Nuclear energy
B. Anabolism
C. Phagocytosis
D. Catabolism
E. Protein synthesis

2. Part of the cell where formation of proteins occurs: ☐
A. Genes
B. Chromosomes
C. Endoplasmic reticulum
D. Cartilage
E. Cell membrane

3. Sum of the chemical processes in a cell: ☐
A. Anabolism
B. Metabolism
C. Protein synthesis
D. Catabolism
E. A and C

4. Picture of nuclear structures arranged in numerical order: ☐
A. Biopsy
B. X-ray
C. Electroencephalogram
D. Sonogram
E. Karyotype

5. Part of a cell where catabolism primarily occurs: ☐
A. Cell membrane
B. Nucleus
C. Mitochondria
D. Genes
E. Endoplasmic reticulum

6. Allows materials to pass into and out of the cell: ☐
A. Cytoplasm
B. Cell membrane
C. Chromosomes
D. Mitochondria
E. Nucleus

7. Genes are composed of: ☐
A. Chromosomes
B. Ribosomes
C. Hemoglobin
D. Deoxyribonucleic acid (DNA)
E. Mitochondria

8. Muscular wall separating the abdominal and thoracic cavities: ☐
A. Mediastinum
B. Diaphragm
C. Pleura
D. Pericardium
E. Peritoneum

9. The space in the chest between the lungs is the: ☐
A. Peritoneum
B. Esophagus
C. Pleural cavity
D. Mediastinum
E. Retroperitoneal space

10. Adipose means pertaining to: ☐
A. Cartilage
B. Bone
C. Fat
D. Skin
E. Nervous tissue

11. Throat: ☐
A. Trachea
B. Coccyx
C. Larynx
D. Esophagus
E. Pharynx

12. Sarcoma: ☐
A. Part of the backbone
B. Flesh tumor; benign
C. Malignant tumor of flesh tissue
D. Mass of blood
E. Skin tumor of epithelial cells

13. **Craniotomy:** ....
   A. Incision of the skull
   B. Pertaining to the skull
   C. Pertaining to the brain
   D. Incision of the chest
   E. Pertaining to the head

14. **A histologist studies:** ....
   A. Drugs
   B. X-rays
   C. Tissues
   D. The backbone
   E. The spinal cord

15. **An epithelial cell is a(an):** ....
   A. Skin cell
   B. Nerve cell
   C. Fat cell
   D. Organ
   E. Muscle cell

16. **The pleural cavity is the:** ....
   A. Space within the abdomen
   B. Space within the backbones
   C. Space surrounding the hip
   D. Space between the membranes around the lungs
   E. Space within the skull

17. **Viscera:** ....
   A. Cells in the blood
   B. Internal organs
   C. Parts of cells
   D. Cavities of the body
   E. Tissues composed of cartilage

18. **The pituitary gland is in which body cavity?** ....
   A. Cranial
   B. Spinal
   C. Pelvic
   D. Abdominal
   E. Thoracic

19. **Voice box:** ....
   A. Bronchial tube
   B. Pharynx
   C. Esophagus
   D. Larynx
   E. Tongue

20. **The tailbone is the:** ....
   A. Sacrum
   B. Cervix
   C. Ilium
   D. Coccyx
   E. Cranium

21. **Supine means:** ....
   A. Lying on the back
   B. Conducting toward a structure
   C. In front of the body
   D. Lying on the belly
   E. Pertaining to the side

22. **The upper lateral regions of the abdomen, beneath the ribs, are the:** ....
   A. Hypogastric regions
   B. Inguinal regions
   C. Lumbar regions
   D. Umbilical regions
   E. Hypochondriac regions

23. **The RUQ contains the:** ....
   A. Liver
   B. Appendix
   C. Lung
   D. Spleen
   E. Heart

24. **Pertaining to a plane that divides the body into right and left portions:** ....
   A. Coronal
   B. Transverse
   C. Frontal
   D. Sagittal
   E. Distal

25. **A disk is:** ....
   A. Part of the hip bone
   B. A piece of cartilage between backbones
   C. A piece of bony tissue connecting the joints in the back
   D. An abnormal structure in the back
   E. A pad of fatty tissue between backbones

Chapter Two
EXERCISE QUIZ

Name: ______________________________

A. *Use medical terms to complete the following sentences:*

1. Control center of the cell, containing chromosomes ______________________________
2. The process of building up proteins in a cell is called ______________________________
3. The total of the chemical processes in a cell is known as ______________________________
4. A scientist who studies tissues is called a(an) ______________________________
5. Regions of DNA within a chromosome ______________________________

B. *Match the part of the body listed with its description below:*

adipose tissue	pharynx	ureter
cartilage	pleura	urethra
larynx	trachea	

6. throat ______________________________
7. collection of fat cells ______________________________
8. windpipe ______________________________
9. tube from the kidney to the urinary bladder ______________________________
10. voice box ______________________________
11. membrane surrounding the lungs ______________________________
12. flexible connective tissue at joints ______________________________
13. tube from the urinary bladder to the outside of the body ______________________________

C. *Name the five cavities of the body:*

14. cavity surrounded by the skull ______________________________
15. cavity in the chest surrounded by ribs ______________________________
16. cavity surrounded by the hip bone ______________________________
17. cavity surrounded by the backbones ______________________________
18. cavity below the chest containing digestive organs ______________________________

D. *Name the five divisions of the back:*

19. region of the neck ____________________
20. region of the chest ____________________
21. region of the waist ____________________
22. region of the sacrum ____________________
23. region of the tailbone ____________________

E. Give opposites of the following terms:

24. deep ______________________
25. proximal ______________________
26. supine ______________________
27. dorsal ______________________

F. Select from the following to complete the sentences below:

distal	lateral	sagittal	transverse
inferior (caudal)	proximal	superior	vertebra

28. The left lung lies ______________________ to the heart.
29. The ______________________ end of the humerus is at the shoulder.
30. The liver lies ______________________ to the intestines.
31. A backbone is called a (an)______________________.
32. The ______________________ end of the thigh bone (femur) joins with the kneecap.
33. The ______________________ plane divides the body into upper and lower portions.
34. The ______________________ plane divides the body into right and left portions.
35. The diaphragm lies ______________________ to the organs in the thoracic cavity.

G. Give meanings for the following terms:

36. craniotomy ______________________
37. epigastric ______________________
38. chondroma ______________________
39. umbilical ______________________
40. posterior ______________________
41. intervertebral ______________________

H. Complete each term from its meaning:

42. Space between the lungs: media ______________________
43. Endocrine gland at the base of the brain: ______________________ ary gland
44. Sausage-shaped cellular structures in which catabolism takes place: mito ______________________
45. Pertaining to skin (surface) cells: epi ______________________
46. Tumor of flesh tissue (malignant): ______________________ oma
47. Pertaining to internal organs: ______________________ al
48. Picture of the chromosomes in the cell nucleus: ______________________ type

I. Give meanings for the following abbreviations:

49. RUQ ______________________
50. L5-S1 ______________________

Chapter Two

DICTATION AND COMPREHENSION QUIZ

Name: ______________________

A. *Dictation of Terms*

1. ______________________ 11. ______________________
2. ______________________ 12. ______________________
3. ______________________ 13. ______________________
4. ______________________ 14. ______________________
5. ______________________ 15. ______________________
6. ______________________ 16. ______________________
7. ______________________ 17. ______________________
8. ______________________ 18. ______________________
9. ______________________ 19. ______________________
10. ______________________ 20. ______________________

B. *Comprehension of Terms: Match number of the above term with its meaning below.*

______ Incision of the skull
______ Pertaining to the groin
______ Malignant tumor of connective tissue
______ Picture (photograph) of nuclear structures
______ Pertaining to internal organs
______ Study of tissues
______ Secretory organ in the neck
______ Flexible connective tissue at joints
______ Divides the body horizontally
______ Tube from the urinary bladder to the outside of the body
______ Cytoplasmic structures where catabolism takes place
______ Throat
______ Divides the body vertically into right and left parts
______ Secretory organ at the base of the brain
______ Voice box
______ Pertaining to the navel
______ Pertaining to the windpipe
______ Pertaining to fat tissue
______ Line external body surface and internal surface of organs
______ Rod-shaped nuclear structures

Chapter Two
SPELLING QUIZ

Name: ______________________________

A. Circle the term that is spelled correctly and write its meaning in the space provided (optional).

1.	abdomin	abdomen ______________________
2.	cartiledge	cartilage ______________________
3.	chromosome	chromosone ______________________
4.	diaphram	diaphragm ______________________
5.	saggital	sagittal ______________________
6.	larynx	larnyx ______________________
7.	cervecal	cervical ______________________
8.	chrondroma	chondroma ______________________
9.	nucleus	neucleus ______________________
10.	traychea	trachea ______________________

B. Circle the term that is spelled correctly. The meaning of the term is given.

11.	internal organs	viscera	vicsera	vissera
12.	malignant tumor of flesh (connective tissue)....................................	sacroma	sarcoma	sarkoma
13.	pertaining to the chest	thoracic	thorasic	thoroacic
14.	lying on the back	surpine	supin	supine
15.	pertaining to the abdomen........................	abdominel	abdominal	abdomineal
16.	picture (photograph) of the chromosomes in the nucleus...	karyotype	karryotype	kariotype
17.	double-folded membrane surrounding the lungs	pleura	ploora	plura
18.	space between the lungs...........................	mediastinim	mediastinam	mediastinum
19.	pertaining to skin (surface) cells	epitheleal	epithelial	epithelal
20.	endocrine gland at the base of the brain	pitiutary	pituitary	pituitery

Chapter Two
PRONUNCIATION QUIZ

Name: ______________________________

A. *Underline the accented syllable in the following terms (for example: a<u>ne</u>mia, diag<u>no</u>sis, <u>en</u>docrine):*

1. cephalic
2. posterior
3. proximal
4. thoracotomy
5. hypochondriac
6. cranial
7. catabolism
8. chondrosarcoma
9. pharynx
10. viscera

B. *Match the term in Column I with its meaning in Column II:*

Column I		Column II
1. karyotype	_______	A. A backbone
2. epithelium	_______	B. The voice box
3. cartilage	_______	C. Skin cells
4. anabolism	_______	D. Vertical plane dividing the body into a right and a left portion
5. diaphragm	_______	E. The throat
6. vertebra	_______	F. Classification of chromosomes
7. sagittal	_______	G. Lying on one's back
8. supine	_______	H. Muscle dividing the thoracic and abdominal cavities
9. mitochondria	_______	I. Connective tissue at the joints
10. larynx	_______	J. Lying on one's belly
		K. Structures in a cell where food is burned to produce energy
		L. Building-up process in a cell; proteins are synthesized for use in the body

C. *Complete the following terms from their definitions:*

1. ______________________ gland	Endocrine gland at the base of the brain
2. ______________________ ology	Study of tissues
3. ______________________ al	Pertaining to the navel
4. ______________________ eal	Pertaining to the tailbone
5. ______________________ gland	Endocrine gland in front of the trachea
6. media ______________________	Central cavity in the chest

7. ______________________vertebral Pertaining to between the backbones

8. ______________________ tomy Incision of the skull

9. ______________________ somes Bodies in the nucleus of a cell; contain DNA

10. peri______________________ Membrane surrounding the abdominal cavity

Chapter Two
DIAGRAM QUIZ 1

Name: ______________________

Label the diagram below using the terms listed below:

BODY CAVITIES

Abdominal
Cranial
Pelvic
Spinal
Thoracic

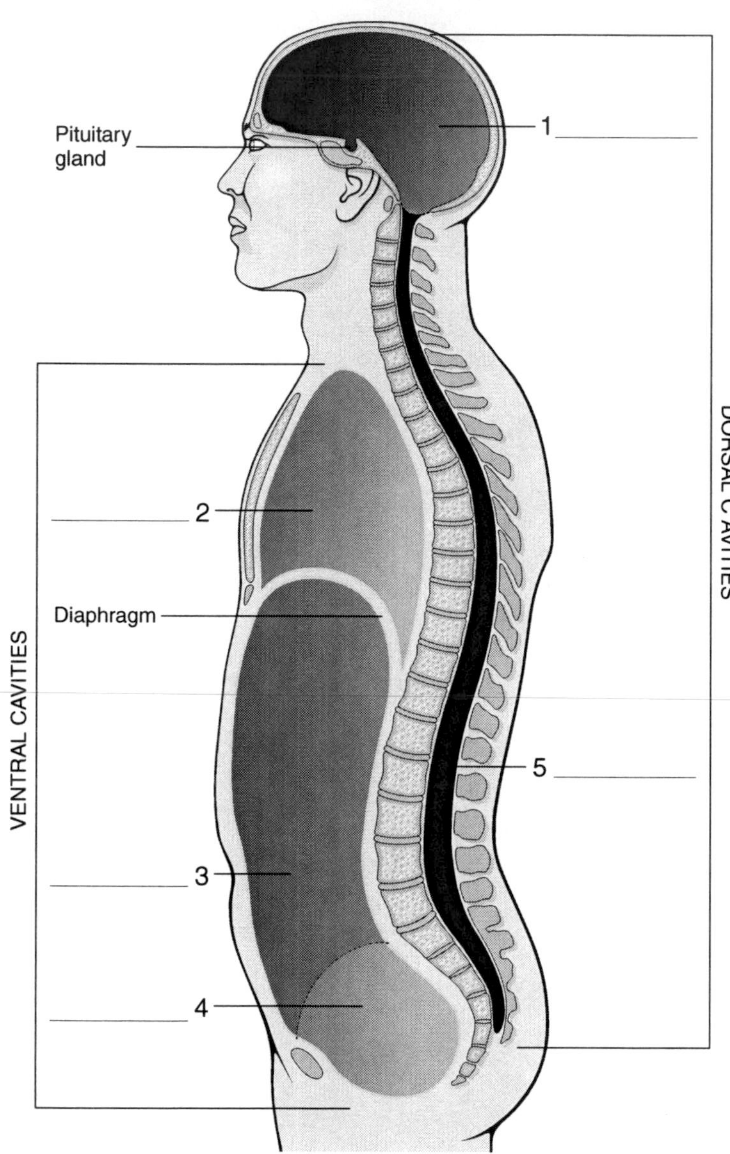

Chapter Two

DIAGRAM QUIZ 2

Name: ______________________________

Label the diagram using the terms listed.

Cervical
Coccygeal
Lumbar
Sacral
Thoracic

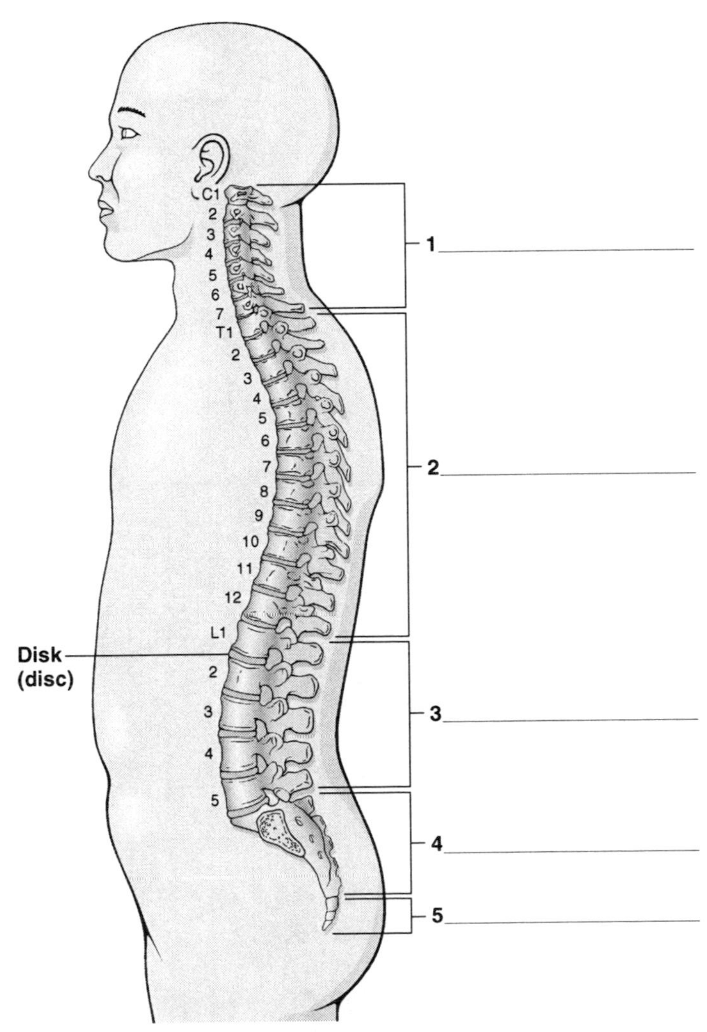

Chapter Two
DIAGRAM QUIZ 3

Name: ______________________

Label the diagram using the terms listed.

Anterior (ventral)	Lateral	Proximal
Distal	Medial	Superficial
Deep	Posterior (dorsal)	Superior
Inferior	Prone	Supine

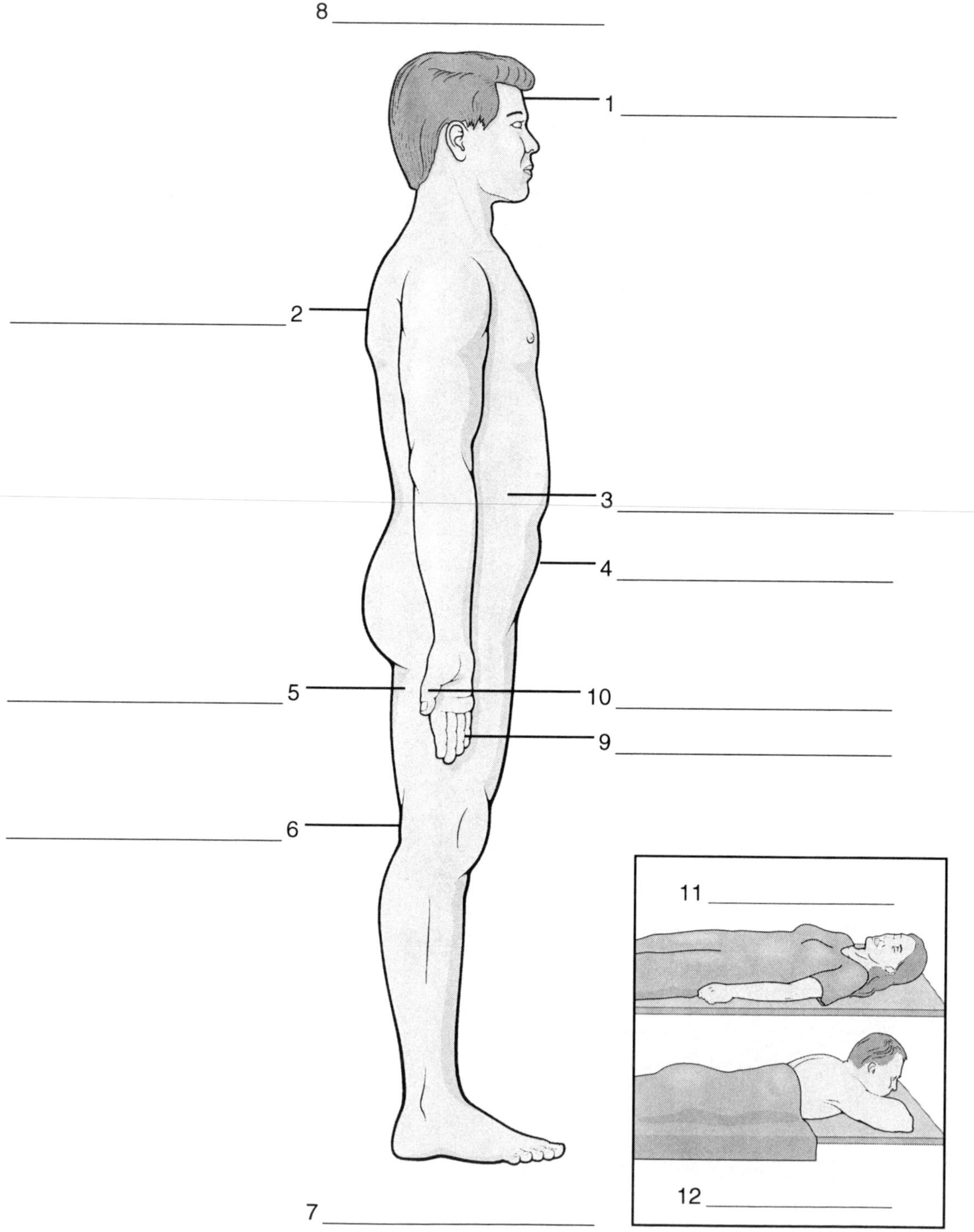

Chapter Two
REVIEW SHEET QUIZ

Name: ______________________

A. Give meanings for the following combining forms:

1. crani/o ______________
2. cervic/o ______________
3. sacr/o ______________
4. trache/o ______________
5. inguin/o ______________
6. viscer/o ______________
7. sarc/o ______________
8. chondr/o ______________
9. thorac/o ______________
10. hist/o ______________

B. Give meanings for the following word parts:

1. inter- ______________
2. hypo- ______________
3. ana- ______________
4. -ose ______________
5. -eal ______________
6. epi- ______________
7. -ectomy ______________
8. kary/o ______________
9. -tomy ______________

C. Name the 5 divisions of the spinal column:

1. C1-C7 ______________
2. T1-T12 ______________
3. L1-L5 ______________
4. S1-S5 ______________
5. Tailbone region ______________

D. Name the plane of the body described below:

1. Horizontal plane dividing the body into superior and inferior parts: ______________
2. Vertical plane dividing the body into right and left parts: ______________
3. Vertical plane dividing the body into anterior and posterior parts: ______________

E. Give the positional or directional term:

1. on the surface of the body ______________
2. lying on the back ______________
3. below another structure ______________

4. pertaining to the side ______________________________

5. pertaining to the middle ______________________________

6. lying on the belly ______________________________

7. above another structure ______________________________

8. near the point of attachment to the trunk or near the beginning of a structure ______________

9. away from the surface of the body ______________________________

10. far from the point of attachment to the trunk or far from the beginning of a structure __________

F. Give the name of the structure or space described below:

1. double-folded membrane surrounding abdominal viscera ______________________________

2. a backbone ______________________________

3. membrane surrounding the lungs ______________________________

4. pad of cartilage between each backbone ______________________________

5. space between the lungs containing the heart, trachea, aorta ______________________________

Chapter Two
MEDICAL SCRAMBLE

Name: ______________________________

Unscramble the letters to form medical terms from the clues. Use the letters in the squares to complete the bonus term.

1. *Clue:* Endocrine gland in the neck

   ___ ___ ☐ ___ ___ ☐ ___ RYDIHOT

2. *Clue:* Control center of a cell

   ___ ___ ___ ___ ___ ☐ ___ LUSNECU

3. *Clue:* Internal organs

   ___ ☐ ___ ___ ___ ___ ___ ACSRVEI

4. *Clue:* Windpipe

   ☐ ___ ___ ___ ___ ___ ☐ AHCRATE

5. *Clue:* Tube connecting the kidneys and urinary bladder

   ___ ___ ___ ☐ ___ ___ TRUERE

6. *Clue:* The double-layered membrane surrounding the lung

   ☐ ___ ___ ___ ☐ ___ AUPELR

BONUS TERM: *Clue:* The gland at the base of the brain that secretes growth hormone, thyroid-stimulating hormone, and hormones that affect the ovaries and testes.

☐ ☐ ☐ ☐ ☐ ☐ ☐ ☐ ☐

Chapter Two
CROSSWORD PUZZLE

Name: ______________________________

Fill in the crossword puzzle below using the clues listed underneath it.

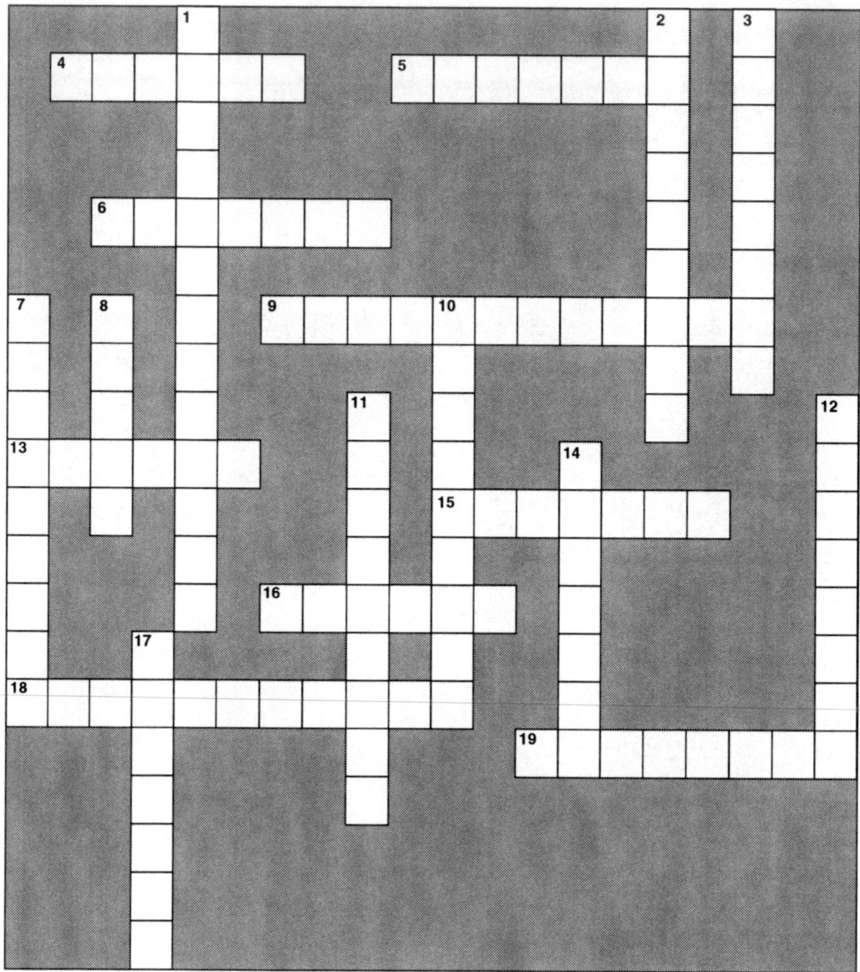

Across Clues

4. Voice box.
5. Collection of fat cells.
6. Control center of a cell.
9. Structures in cytoplasm where food is burned to release energy.
13. A double-layered membrane surrounding each lung.
15. Throat.
16. Loin (waist) region.
18. Area between the lungs.
19. Vertical plane dividing body into right and left sides.

Down Clues

1. Upper right and left regions beneath the ribs.
2. Backbones.
3. Lower right and left regions near the groin.
7. Muscle separating the abdominal and thoracic cavities.
8. Regions of DNA within each chromosome.
10. All the material that is outside the nucleus yet within the cell membrane.
11. Body cavity of the stomach, small and large intestines, spleen, liver, gallbladder, and pancreas.
12. Bones and joints; musculo______system.
14. Tube from the urinary bladder to the outside of the body.
17. Internal organs.

Chapter Two
ANSWERS TO THE QUIZZES

Multiple Choice Quiz

1. D
2. C
3. B
4. E
5. C
6. B
7. D
8. B
9. D
10. C
11. E
12. C
13. A
14. C
15. A
16. D
17. B
18. A
19. D
20. D
21. A
22. E
23. A
24. D
25. B

Exercise Quiz

A

1. nucleus
2. anabolism
3. metabolism
4. histologist
5. genes

B

6. pharynx
7. adipose tissue
8. trachea
9. ureter
10. larynx
11. pleura
12. cartilage
13. urethra

C

14. cranial
15. thoracic
16. pelvic
17. spinal
18. abdominal

D

19. cervical
20. thoracic
21. lumbar
22. sacral
23. coccygeal

E

24. superficial
25. distal
26. prone
27. ventral (anterior)

F

28. lateral
29. proximal
30. superior
31. vertebra
32. distal
33. transverse
34. sagittal
35. inferior (caudal)

G

36. incision of the skull
37. pertaining to above the stomach
38. tumor of cartilage (benign)
39. pertaining to the navel
40. pertaining to the back
41. pertaining to between vertebrae

H

42. mediastinum
43. pituitary
44. mitochondria
45. epithelial
46. sarcoma
47. visceral
48. karyotype

I

49. right upper quadrant (of the abdomen)
50. between the 5th lumbar and the 1st sacral vertebrae

Dictation and Comprehension Quiz

A

1. adipose
2. cartilage
3. chondrosarcoma
4. chromosomes
5. craniotomy
6. epithelial cells
7. histology
8. inguinal
9. karyotype
10. larynx
11. mitochondria
12. pharynx
13. pituitary gland
14. sagittal plane
15. thyroid gland
16. tracheal
17. transverse plane
18. umbilical
19. urethra
20. visceral

B

5 Incision of the skull
8 Pertaining to the groin
3 Malignant tumor of connective (flesh) tissue
9 Picture of nuclear structures
20 Pertaining to internal organs
7 Study of tissues
15 Secretory organ in the neck
2 Flexible connective tissue at joints
17 Divides the body horizontally
19 Tube from the urinary bladder to the outside of the body
11 Cytoplasmic structures where catabolism takes place
12 Throat
14 Divides the body vertically into right and left parts
13 Secretory organ at the base of the brain
10 Voice box
18 Pertaining to the navel
16 Pertaining to the windpipe
1 Pertaining to fat tissue
6 Line external body surface and internal surface of organs
4 Rod-shaped nuclear structures

Spelling Quiz

A

1. abdomen—area under the chest containing the stomach, intestines, liver, gallbladder
2. cartilage—flexible connective tissue between joints
3. chromosome—contains genetic material in nucleus of a cell
4. diaphragm—muscular wall separating the chest and abdomen
5. sagittal—vertical plane dividing the body into right and left portions
6. larynx—voice box
7. cervical—pertaining to the neck
8. chondroma—tumor of cartilage (benign)

9. nucleus—control center of the cell
10. trachea—windpipe

B

11. viscera
12. sarcoma
13. thoracic
14. supine
15. abdominal
16. karyotype
17. pleura
18. mediastinum
19. epithelial
20. pituitary

Pronunciation Quiz

A

1. cephalic
2. posterior
3. proximal
4. thoracotomy
5. hypochondriac
6. cranial
7. catabolism
8. chondrosarcoma
9. pharynx
10. viscera

B

1. F
2. C
3. I
4. L
5. H
6. A
7. D
8. G
9. K
10. B

C

1. pituitary
2. histology
3. umbilical
4. coccygeal
5. thyroid
6. mediastinum
7. intervertebral
8. craniotomy
9. chromosomes
10. peritoneum

Diagram Quiz 1

1. Cranial
2. Thoracic
3. Abdominal
4. Pelvic
5. Spinal

Diagram Quiz 2

1. Anterior (ventral)
2. Posterior (dorsal)
3. Deep
4. Superficial
5. Proximal
6. Distal
7. Inferior
8. Superior
9. Medial
10. Lateral
11. Supine
12. Prone

Diagram Quiz 3

1. Cervical
2. Thoracic
3. Lumbar
4. Sacral
5. Coccygeal

Review Sheet Quiz

A

1. skull
2. neck
3. sacrum
4. trachea, windpipe
5. groin
6. internal organs
7. flesh
8. cartilage
9. chest
10. tissue

B

1. between
2. below
3. up
4. pertaining to, full of
5. pertaining to
6. above
7. removal, excision, resection
8. picture, classification
9. cut into, incision, section

C

1. cervical
2. thoracic
3. lumbar
4. sacral
5. coccygeal

D

1. transverse, axial
2. sagittal, lateral
3. frontal, coronal

E

1. superficial
2. supine
3. inferior, caudalv
4. lateral
5. medial
6. prone
7. superior, cephalic
8. proximal
9. deep
10. distal

F

1. peritoneum
2. vertebra
3. pleura
4. disk
5. mediastinum

Medical Scramble

1. THYROID
2. NUCLEUS
3. VISCERA
4. TRACHEA
5. URETER
6. PLEURA

BONUS TERM: PITUITARY

Crossword Puzzle

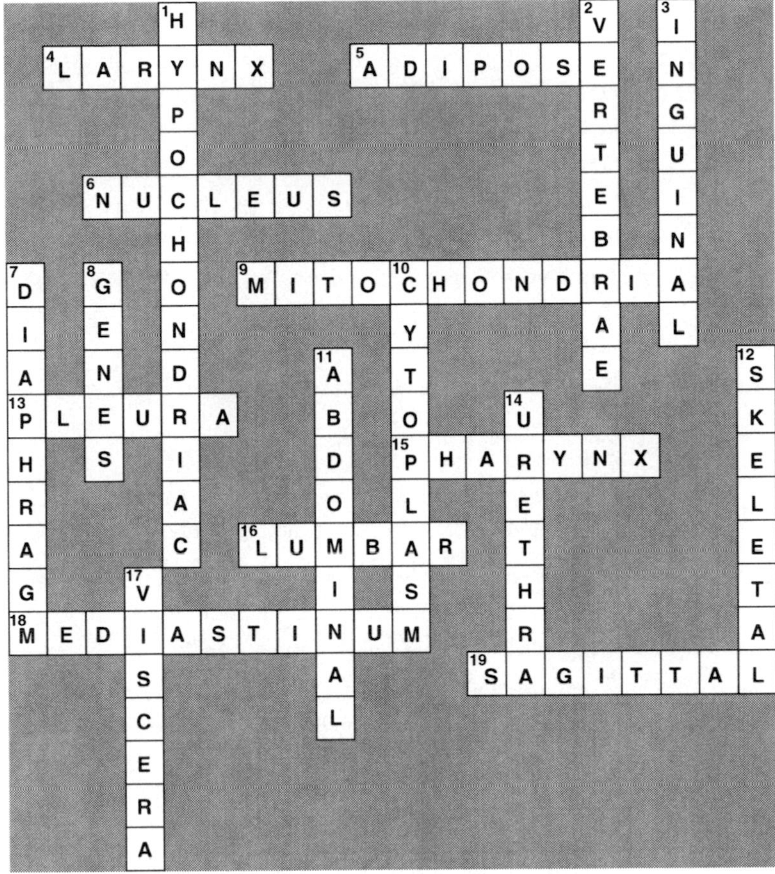

Chapter Two
Answers to Terminology Section

(textbook pages 50–53)

Terminology	Meaning
abdominal	Pertaining to the abdomen.
adipose	Pertaining to fat.
anterior	Pertaining to the front.
anabolism	Process of casting up (building-up or synthesizing process in a cell).
cervical	Pertaining to the neck.
chondroma	Tumor of cartilage.
chondrosarcoma	Flesh tumor (malignant) of cartilage (tissue). All sarcomas are malignant (cancerous) tumors.
chromosomes	"Color bodies"; contain genetic material and are located in the nucleus of cell.
coccygeal	Pertaining to the tailbone.
craniotomy	Incision of the skull.
cytoplasm	Contents (formation) of the cell (apart from the nucleus and cell membrane).
distal	Pertaining to far (from the beginning of a structure).
dorsal	Pertaining to the back.
histology	Study of tissues.
iliac	Pertaining to the ilium.
inguinal	Pertaining to the groin.
karyotype	Picture (classification) of the nucleus (and its chromosomes).
lateral	Pertaining to the side.
lumbosacral	Pertaining to the lumbar and sacral regions.
medial	Pertaining to the middle.
nucleic	Pertaining to the nucleus.
pelvic	Pertaining to the pelvis (bones in the region of the hip).
posterior	Pertaining to the back, behind.
proximal	Pertaining to near the beginning of a structure.
sacral	Pertaining to the sacrum (lower back).
sarcoma	Tumor (malignant) of flesh tissue .
spinal	Pertaining to the spine, backbone.
epithelial cell	Cell covering the surface of the skin and inner lining of body cavities and tubes.
thoracic	Pertaining to the chest.
thoracotomy	Incision of the chest.
tracheal	Pertaining to the windpipe.
umbilical	Pertaining to the navel.
ventral	Pertaining to the belly side of the body.
vertebral	Pertaining to vertebrae.
visceral	Pertaining to internal organs.
anabolic	Pertaining to casting up; building up substances (proteins) in the cell.
catabolism	Process of casting down; breaking down material in the cell to release energy.
epigastric	Pertaining to above the stomach.
hypochondriac region	Pertaining to under the rib cartilages (area of the abdomen).
intervertebral	Pertaining to between the vertebrae.
metabolism	State of building up (anabolism) and breaking down (catabolism); processes in a cell.

Chapter 3

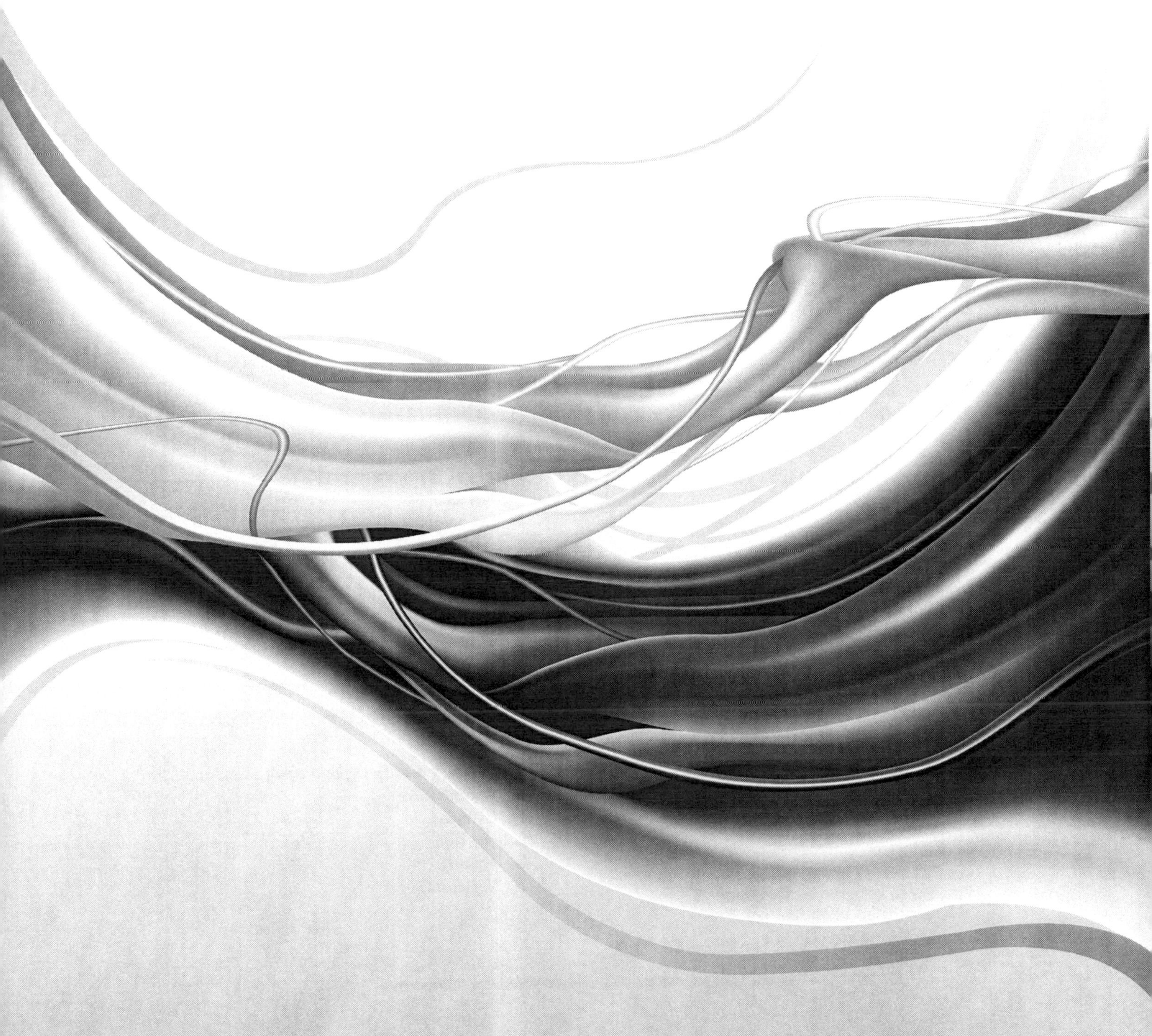

Chapter Three

MULTIPLE CHOICE QUIZ

Name: ______________________

In the box write the letter of the choice that is the definition of the term or best answers the question. There is only one correct answer for each question.

1. **Amniocentesis:** ☐
   A. Incision of the abdomen
   B. Paracentesis
   C. Surgical puncture to remove fluid from the abdomen
   D. Puncture of the chest region
   E. Surgical puncture to remove fluid from the sac around the embryo

2. **Inflammation of lymph tissue in the throat:** ☐
   A. Bronchitis
   B. Laryngitis
   C. Pharyngeal
   D. Tonsilitis
   E. Tonsillitis

3. **Prolapse:** ☐
   A. -pathy
   B. -ptosis
   C. -trophy
   D. -plasty
   E. -plasm

4. **Blood is held back from an area:** ☐
   A. Thrombocyte
   B. Anemia
   C. Ischemia
   D. Hematoma
   E. Hemolysis

5. **Death:** ☐
   A. Neur/o
   B. Nephr/o
   C. Neutr/o
   D. Nucle/o
   E. Necr/o

6. **Acromegaly:** ☐
   A. Exocrine disorder of bone enlargement
   B. Enlargement of extremities after puberty due to pituitary gland problem
   C. Abnormal growth of bones before puberty
   D. Endocrine gland problem in young children
   E. Fear of extremities (heights)

7. **Pain in the ear:** ☐
   A. Pleurodynia
   B. Otitis
   C. Otalgia
   D. Osteitis
   E. Neuralgia

8. **Continuing over a long period** ☐
   A. Chronic
   B. Acute
   C. Chromic
   D. Relapse
   E. Remission

9. **Small artery** ☐
   A. Capillary
   B. Arteriole
   C. Venule
   D. Lymph vessel
   E. Blood vessel leading from the heart

10. **Instrument to visually examine:** ☐
    A. -scope
    B. -scopy
    C. -opsy
    D. -stasis
    E. -tomy

11. **Hernia of the urinary bladder:** ☐
    A. Rectocele
    B. Inguinal hernia
    C. Hiatal hernia
    D. Rectalgia
    E. Cystocele

12. **Tumor of bone marrow (cancerous):** ☐
    A. Myosarcoma
    B. Multiple myeloma
    C. Osteogenic sarcoma
    D. Adenocarcinoma
    E. Metastasis

13. **Inflammation of the spinal cord:** ☐
    A. Encephalitis
    B. Osteitis
    C. Myelitis
    D. Myoma
    E. Vertebral

14. **Berry-shaped (spheroidal) bacteria:** ....
A. Staphyl/o
B. Pneum/o
C. -cele
D. Strept/o
E. -cocci

15. **Neutrophil:** ....
A. Lymphocyte
B. Polymorphonuclear leukocyte
C. Monocyte
D. Mononuclear agranulocyte
E. Platelet

16. **Instrument to record:** ....
A. -gram
B. -scopy
C. -scope
D. -graph
E. -graphy

17. **Resembling:** ....
A. -osis
B. -eal
C. lith/o
D. -oid
E. -ic

18. **An eosinophil is a(an):** ....
A. Erythrocyte
B. Leukocyte
C. Mononuclear cell
D. Platelet
E. Lymphocyte

19. **Removal of the voice box:** ....
A. Larnygectomy
B. Pharyngotomy
C. Pharynostomy
D. Laryngectomy
E. Trachectomy

20. **Angioplasty means:** ....
A. Pertaining to fat
B. Fear of extremities
C. Therapy with chemicals
D. Surgical puncture of a blood vessel
E. Surgical repair of a blood vessel

21. **A blood cell that produces antibodies:** ....
A. Erythrocyte
B. Platelet
C. Lymphocyte
D. Monocyte
E. Basophil

22. **Opposite of -malacia is:** ....
A. -megaly
B. -sclerosis
C. -emia
D. -plasia
E. -lysis

23. **Excessive development:** ....
A. Hypoplasia
B. Dystrophy
C. Achondroplasia
D. Morphology
E. Hypertrophy

24. **Treatment:** ....
A. -therapy
B. -genic
C. -plasty
D. -osis
E. -stasis

25. **Surgical creation of a permanent opening to the outside of the body:** .....
A. -stomy
B. -tomy
C. -ectomy
D. -plasty
E. -scopy

Chapter Three
EXERCISE QUIZ

Name: ______________________________

A. Give the meanings for the following suffixes:

1. -cele ______________________________
2. -coccus ______________________________
3. -centesis ______________________________
4. -genesis ______________________________
5. -graphy______________________________
6. -emia ______________________________

B. Using the following combining forms and your knowledge of suffixes, build the following medical terms:

amni/o	cyst/o	laryng/o	myel/o	thorac/o
angi/o	isch/o	my/o	staphyl/o	

7. inflammation of the spinal cord ______________________________
8. process of recording blood vessels ______________________________
9. pain of a muscle ______________________________
10. surgical puncture to remove fluid from the chest ______________________________
11. berry-shaped (spheroidal) bacteria in clusters ______________________________
12. resection of the voice box ______________________________
13. to hold back blood from cells ______________________________
14. hernia of the urinary bladder ______________________________

C. Match the following terms that describe blood cells with their meanings below:

eosinophil	lymphocyte	neutrophil
erythrocyte	monocyte	thrombocyte

15. a clotting cell; platelet ______________________________
16. a red blood cell ______________________________
17. a granulocytic white blood cell that destroys cells by engulfing and digesting them; polymorphonuclear leukocyte ______________________________
18. a mononuclear leukocyte that is a phagocyte ______________________________
19. a mononuclear leukocyte that destroys foreign cells by making antibodies ______________________________
20. a leukocyte whose granules turn red with stain and whose numbers are elevated in allergic reactions ______________________________

D. Give the meanings for the following suffixes:

21. -lysis ______________________
22. -pathy ______________________
23. -penia ______________________
24. -malacia ______________________
25. -megaly ______________________
26. -phobia______________________
27. -plasty ______________________
28. -stasis ______________________
29. -plasia ______________________
30. -sclerosis ______________________

E. Using the following combining forms and your knowledge of suffixes, build medical terms:

acr/o	cardi/o	morph/o	myel/o
blephar/o	chondr/o	my/o	sarc/o

31. fear of heights (extremities) ______________________
32. flesh (malignant) tumor of muscle ______________________
33. study of the shape (of cells) ______________________
34. inflammation of an eyelid ______________________
35. softening of cartilage ______________________
36. tumor of bone marrow ______________________
37. disease of heart muscle ______________________

F. Give meanings for the following suffixes:

38. -ptosis ______________________
39. -stomy ______________________
40. -tomy ______________________
41. -ule ______________________
42. -genic ______________________
43. -trophy______________________
44. -oid______________________
45. -ole______________________
46. -opsy______________________
47. -ectomy ______________________

G. Underline the suffix in the following terms and give the meaning of each term:

48. pulmonary ______________________
49. necrotic ______________________
50. inguinal ______________________

Chapter Three
DICTATION AND COMPREHENSION QUIZ

Name: ______________________

A. Dictation of Terms

1. ______________	11. ______________
2. ______________	12. ______________
3. ______________	13. ______________
4. ______________	14. ______________
5. ______________	15. ______________
6. ______________	16. ______________
7. ______________	17. ______________
8. ______________	18. ______________
9. ______________	19. ______________
10. ______________	20. ______________

B. Comprehension of Terms: Match number of the above term with its meaning below.

_______ Pertaining to the groin
_______ Prolapse of an eyelid
_______ Disease of heart muscle
_______ Resection of a breast
_______ Ear pain
_______ Pertaining to the voice box
_______ Formation of blood vessels
_______ Pertaining to the membrane surrounding the abdomen
_______ Destruction of blood (RBCs)
_______ Incision of the abdomen
_______ Spread of a malignant tumor
_______ Holding back blood from tissues
_______ Fear of heights
_______ New opening of the windpipe to the outside of body
_______ Abnormal condition of death of cells
_______ Hernia of the urinary bladder
_______ Record of the electricity in the brain
_______ Deficiency of clotting cells (platelets)
_______ Removal of living tissue and examination under a microscope
_______ Abnormal condition of fluid (water) in the kidney

Chapter Three
SPELLING QUIZ

Name: ______________________________

A. Circle the term that is spelled correctly and write its meaning in the space provided:

1.	pericardeum	pericardium ______________________
2.	arteriosclerosis	arteriosklerosis ______________________
3.	myleitis	myleitis ______________________
4.	hepatomeagaly	hepatomegaly ______________________
5.	trachostomy	tracheostomy ______________________
6.	tonsillitis	tonsilitis ______________________
7.	abdominocentesis	adbominocentesis ______________________
8.	ploorodinia	pleurodynia ______________________
9.	ophthalmology	opthalmology ______________________
10.	staphylococci	staphlococci ______________________

B. Circle the term that is spelled correctly. The meaning of each term is given:

11.	beyond control (spread of a cancerous tumor)	metastesis	metastasis	metastatis
12.	pertaining to the voice box	larnygeal	laryngeal	laryngel
13.	condition (disease) of the lung	pneumonia	pneumoneia	pnuemonia
14.	hernia of the urinary bladder	cytocele	cystocele	cystosele
15.	deficiency in white blood cells	leukopenia	luekopenia	lucopinea
16.	excessive development	hypertropy	hypertrophy	hypertrofe
17.	pertaining to the groin	inguinal	ingiuinal	ingwanal
18.	clotting cell	platelete	platlet	platelet
19.	incision of a vein	pilbotomy	phlebotomy	plebotomy
20.	small vein	venule	vanule	venuel

Chapter Three
PRONUNCIATION QUIZ

Name: ______________________

A. Underline the accented syllable in the following terms (for example: anemia, diagnosis, endocrine):

1. arteriole
2. hypertrophy
3. osteomalacia
4. necrosis
5. carcinogenesis
6. laparoscopy
7. arteriosclerosis
8. thrombocytopenia
9. abdominocentesis
10. hydrotherapy

B. Match the suffix in Column I with its meaning in Column II:

Column I		Column II
1. -malacia	________	A. Prolapse
2. -phobia	________	B. Surgical repair
3. -plasia	________	C. Nourishment or development
4. -ptosis	________	D. Fear
5. -pathy	________	E. Blood condition
6. -plasty	________	F. Formation
7. -emia	________	G. Enlargement
8. -penia	________	H. Softening
9. -trophy	________	I. Disease condition
10. -megaly	________	J. Deficiency

C. Complete the following terms from their definitions:

1. ____________________ oma — Tumor of bone marrow.
2. ____________________ cocci — Berry-shaped (spheroidal) bacteria in twisted chains.
3. ____________________ cele — Hernia of the urinary bladder.
4. colo ____________________ — New opening from the colon to the outside of the body.
5. staphylo____________________ — Berry-shaped (spheroidal) bacteria in clusters.
6. ____________________ phobia — Fear of heights.
7. ____________________ ology — Study of the eye.
8. ____________________ ule — Small vein.
9. arterio ____________________ — Hardening of arteries.
10. hemo ____________________ — Destruction of blood.

Chapter Three
REVIEW SHEET QUIZ

Name: ______________________________

A. Give meanings for the following noun suffixes:

1. -centesis ____________________
2. -dynia ____________________
3. -stasis ____________________
4. -plasty ____________________
5. -genesis ____________________
6. -cyte ____________________
7. -penia ____________________
8. -trophy ____________________
9. -emia ____________________
10. -graphy ____________________

B. Give the suffixes for the following meanings:

1. instrument to visually examine _____
2. fear ____________________
3. enlargement ____________________
4. prolapse ____________________
5. separation, destruction ____________
6. softening ____________________
7. incision ____________________
8. treatment ____________________
9. excision ____________________
10. new opening ____________________

C. Give meanings for the following combining forms:

1. chondr/o ____________________
2. lapar/o ____________________
3. inguin/o ____________________
4. axill/o ____________________
5. blephar/o ____________________
6. mamm/o ____________________
7. angi/o ____________________
8. cyst/o ____________________
9. isch/o ____________________
10. adip/o ____________________

D. Give the combining forms for the following meanings:

1. liver ____________________
2. muscle ____________________
3. ear ____________________
4. tonsil ____________________
5. shape ____________________
6. lung ____________________

Chapter Three
MEDICAL SCRAMBLE

Name: ______________________________

Unscramble the letters to form suffixes from the clues. Use the letters in squares to complete the bonus term.

1. *Clue:* Surgical puncture to remove fluid

   –☐ ___ ☐ ___ ___ ___ ___ ___ ESTICESN

2. *Clue:* Hardening

   –___ ___ ___ ___ ___ ☐ ___ ___ ___ LSOSSECRI

3. *Clue:* Treatment

   –___ ___ ☐ ☐ ___ ___ ___ RHPEYAT

4. *Clue:* Softening

   –☐ ___ ___ ___ ___ ☐ ___ ACLAMAI

5. *Clue:* Surgical repair

   –☐ ___ ___ ___ ☐ ___ YSLTAP

6. *Clue:* Development

   –___ ___ ☐ ___ ___ ___ HYPTOR

7. *Clue:* Enlargement

   –___ ___ ___ ___ ___ ☐ AGYMLE

8. *Clue:* Excision

   –___ ___ ☐ ☐ ___ ___ MCYOET

9. *Clue:* Pain

   –___ ___ ___ ___ ☐ IGLAA

10. *Clue:* Fear

    –___ ☐ ___ ☐ ___ ___ AIBHPO

BONUS TERM: ***Clue:*** Deficiency of platelets

☐ ☐ ☐ ☐ ☐ ☐ ☐ ☐ ☐ ☐ ☐ ☐ ☐ ☐ ☐ ☐

Chapter Three
CROSSWORD PUZZLE

Name: ____________________

Fill in the crossword puzzle below using the clues listed underneath it.

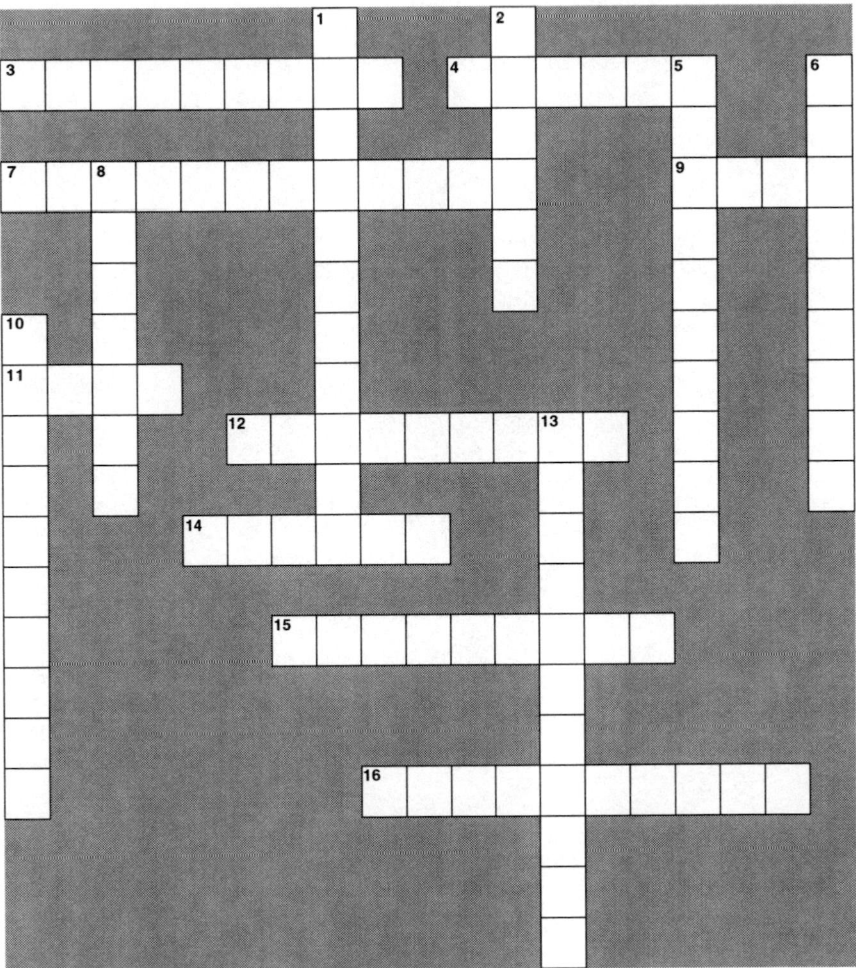

Across Clues

3. -malacia
4. -gram
7. -itis
9. -phobia
11. -algia
12. -therapy
14. -ule
15. -osis (abnormal____________)
16. -oid

Down Clues

1. -megaly
2. -cele
5. -penia
6. -sclerosis
8. -genesis
10. -ist
13. -trophy

Chapter Three
ANSWERS TO THE QUIZZES

Multiple Choice Quiz

1. E
2. E
3. B
4. C
5. E
6. B
7. C
8. A
9. B
10. A
11. E
12. B
13. D
14. E
15. B
16. D
17. D
18. B
19. D
20. E
21. C
22. B
23. E
24. A
25. A

Exercise Quiz

A

1. hernia
2. berry-shaped bacterium
3. surgical puncture to remove fluid
4. formation
5. process of recording
6. blood condition

B

7. myelitis
8. angiography
9. myalgia
10. thoracentesis
11. staphylococci
12. laryngectomy
13. ischemia
14. cystocele

C

15. thrombocyte
16. erythrocyte
17. neutrophil
18. monocyte
19. lymphocyte
20. eosinophil

D

21. separation, destruction
22. disease condition
23. deficiency
24. softening
25. enlargement
26. fear
27. surgical repair
28. stop; control
29. formation
30. hardening

E

31. acrophobia
32. myosarcoma
33. morphology
34. blepharitis
35. chondromalacia
36. myeloma
37. cardiomyopathy

F

38. prolapse
39. new opening
40. incision
41. small; little
42. pertaining to producing
43. nourishment; development
44. resembling
45. small; little
46. to view
47. removal

G

48. pulmon<u>ary</u>—pertaining to the lungs
49. necro<u>tic</u>—pertaining to death
50. inguin<u>al</u>—pertaining to the groin

Dictation and Comprehension Quiz

A

1. acrophobia
2. angiogenesis
3. biopsy
4. blepharoptosis
5. cardiomyopathy
6. cystocele
7. electroencephalogram
8. hemolysis
9. hydronephrosis
10. inguinal
11. ischemia
12. laparotomy
13. laryngeal
14. mastectomy
15. metastasis
16. necrosis
17. otalgia
18. peritoneal
19. thrombocytopenia
20. tracheostomy

B

10 Pertaining to the groin
4 Prolapse of an eyelid
5 Disease of heart muscle
14 Resection of a breast
17 Ear pain
13 Pertaining to the voice box
2 Formation of blood vessels
18 Pertaining to the membrane surrounding the abdomen
8 Destruction of blood (RBCs)
12 Incision of the abdomen
15 Spread of a malignant tumor
11 Holding back blood from tissues
1 Fear of heights
20 New opening of the windpipe to the outside of body
16 Abnormal condition of death of cells
6 Hernia of the urinary bladder
7 Record of the electricity in the brain
19 Deficiency of clotting cells (platelets)
3 Removal of living tissue and examination under a microscope
9 Abnormal condition of fluid (water) in the kidney

Spelling Quiz

A

1. pericardium—lining (membrane) surrounding the heart
2. arteriosclerosis—hardening of arteries
3. myelitis—inflammation of the spinal cord
4. hepatomegaly—enlargement of the liver
5. tracheostomy—new opening of the trachea to the outside of the body
6. tonsillitis—inflammation of the tonsils
7. abdominocentesis—surgical puncture to remove fluid from the abdomen (paracentesis)
8. pleurodynia—pain of the pleura (chest wall muscles)

9. ophthalmology—study of the eyes
10. staphylococci—berry-shaped bacteria in clusters

B

11. metastasis
12. laryngeal
13. pneumonia
14. cystocele
15. leukopenia
16. hypertrophy
17. inguinal
18. platelet
19. phlebotomy
20. venule

Pronunciation Quiz

A

1. arteriole
2. hypertrophy
3. osteomalacia
4. necrosis
5. carcinogenesis
6. laparoscopy
7. arteriosclerosis
8. thrombocytopenia
9. abdominocentesis
10. hydrotherapy

B

1. H
2. D
3. F
4. A
5. I
6. B
7. E
8. J
9. C
10. G

C

1. myeloma
2. streptococci
3. cystocele
4. colostomy
5. staphylococci
6. acrophobia
7. ophthalmology
8. venule
9. arteriosclerosis
10. hemolysis

Review Sheet Quiz

A

1. surgical procedure to remove fluid
2. pain
3. stopping; controlling
4. surgical repair
5. condition of producing; forming
6. cell
7. deficiency
8. development, nourishment
9. blood condition
10. process of recording

B

1. -scope
2. -phobia
3. -megaly
4. -ptosis
5. -lysis
6. -malacia
7. -tomy
8. -therapy
9. -ectomy
10. -stomy

C

1. cartilage
2. abdomen
3. groin
4. armpit
5. eyelid
6. breast
7. blood vessel
8. urinary bladder
9. to hold back
10. fat

D

1. hepat/o
2. my/o
3. ot/o
4. tonsill/o
5. morph/o
6. pulmon/o

Medical Scramble

1. -CENTESIS
2. -SCLEROSIS
3. -THERAPY
4. -MALACIA
5. -PLASTY
6. -TROPHY
7. -MEGALY
8. -ECTOMY
9. -ALGIA
10. -PHOBIA

BONUS TERM: THROMBOCYTOPENIA

Crossword Puzzle

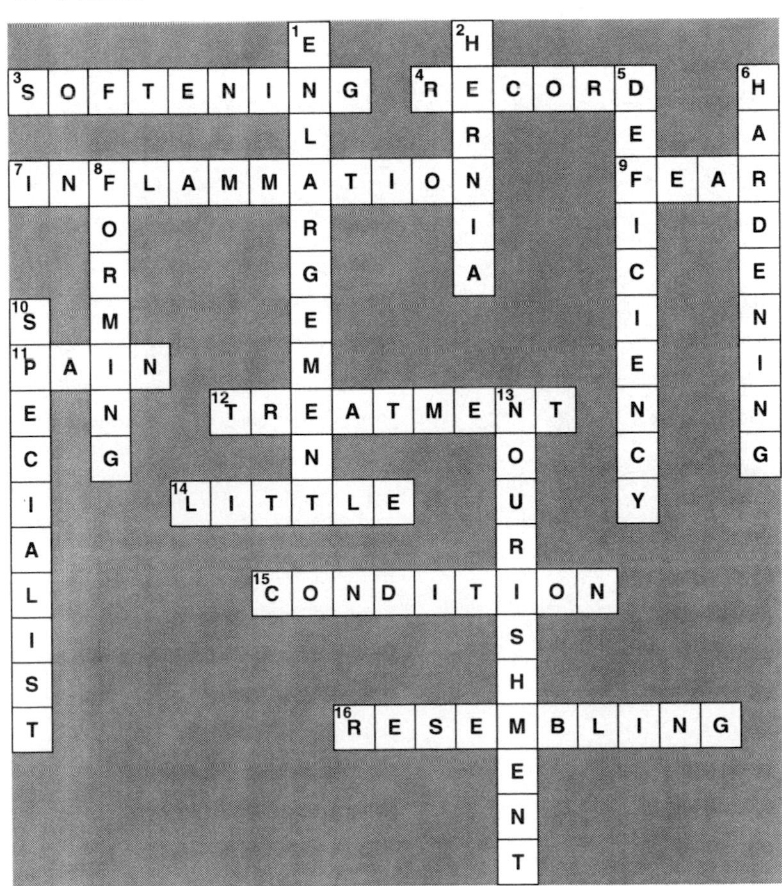

Chapter Three

Answers to Terminology Section

(textbook pages 74–83)

Terminology	Meaning
arthralgia	Pain in a joint.
otalgia	Pain in the ear.
neuralgia	Pain of nerves.
myalgia	Pain of muscles.
rectocele	Hernia of the rectum.
cystocele	Hernia of the urinary bladder.
thoracentesis	Surgical puncture to remove fluid from the chest.
amniocentesis	Surgical puncture of the amnion.
abdominocentesis	Surgical puncture of the abdomen.
streptococcus	Berry-shaped (spheroidal) bacterium found in twisted chains.
staphylococci	Berry-shaped (spheroidal) bacteria in clusters.
erythrocyte	Red blood cell.
leukocyte	White blood cell.
thrombocyte	Clotting cell.
pleurodynia	Pain in the chest wall muscles that is aggravated by breathing (literally: pain of the pleura).
laryngectomy	Removal of the larynx.
mastectomy	Removal of a breast.
anemia	Decrease in erythrocytes or hemoglobin.
ischemia	To hold back blood from an area of the body.
carcinogenesis	Condition of producing cancer.
pathogenesis	Condition of producing disease.
angiogenesis	Formation of blood vessels.
electroencephalogram	Record of the electricity in the brain.
myelitis	Inflammation of the spinal cord.
mammogram	Record (x-ray) of the breast.
electroencephalograph	Instrument for recording the electricity in the brain.
electroencephalography	Process of recording the electricity in the brain.
angiography	Process of recording (x-ray imaging) blood vessels.
bronchitis	Inflammation of the bronchi.
tonsillitis	Inflammation of the tonsils.
thrombophlebitis	Inflammation of a vein with clot formation.
ophthalmology	Study of the eye.
morphology	Study of shape or form.
hemolysis	Destruction of blood (breakdown of red blood cells with release of hemoglobin).
osteomalacia	Softening of bone.
chondromalacia	Softening of cartilage.
acromegaly	Enlargement of extremities.
splenomegaly	Enlargement of the spleen.
myoma	Tumor (benign) of muscle.

myosarcoma	Tumor (malignant) of muscle—a type of flesh (sarc/o) tissue.
multiple myeloma	Tumor (malignant) of bone marrow.
hematoma	Collection of blood; a bruise.
biopsy	To view life; microscopic examination of living tissue.
necrosis	Condition of death (of cells).
necropsy	Autopsy or postmortem examination.
hydronephrosis	Abnormal condition of water (found) in the kidney.
leukocytosis	Abnormal condition (slight increase in numbers) of normal white blood cells.
cardiomyopathy	Disease of heart muscle.
erythropenia	Deficiency of red blood cells.
neutropenia	Deficiency in neutrophils.
thrombocytopenia	Deficiency of clotting cells.
acrophobia	Fear of heights.
agoraphobia	Fear of being in open, crowded spaces (marketplace).
achondroplasia	No (improper) development of cartilage.
angioplasty	Surgical repair of blood vessels.
blepharoptosis	Prolapse, sagging of an eyelid.
arteriosclerosis	Hardening of arteries.
laparoscope	Instrument to visually examine the abdomen.
laparoscopy	Process of visual examination of the abdomen.
metastasis	Beyond control; spreading of a cancerous tumor.
hemostasis	Stopping the flow of blood (naturally by clotting or artificially by compression).
colostomy	New opening of the colon (to the outside of the body).
tracheostomy	New opening of the windpipe (to the outside of the body).
hydrotherapy	Treatment with water.
chemotherapy	Treatment with drugs.
radiotherapy	Treatment with x-rays.
laparotomy	Incision into the abdomen. *Often referred to as a "lap," this exploratory procedure is performed under general anesthesia.*
phlebotomy	Incision of a vein.
tracheotomy	Incision of the trachea.
hypertrophy	Excessive development. *Memory Tip: You can earn a trophy for a new stage in development!*
atrophy	No development; wasting away of tissue.
radiographer	One who records x-rays; radiologic technologist—a professional who, under the supervision of a physician, operates radiologic equipment and assists radiologists.
leukemia	Condition of increase in white blood cells (malignancy).
pneumonia	Condition (abnormal) of lungs.
nephrologist	Specialist in the study of the kidney.
arteriole	Small artery.
venule	Small vein.
pericardium	Structure surrounding the heart.
mucus	Sticky secretion from mucous membrane.
esophagus	Muscular tube carrying food from the throat to the stomach.

nephropathy	Disease of the kidney.
cardiac	Pertaining to the heart.
peritoneal	Pertaining to the peritoneum.
inguinal	Pertaining to the groin.
pleural	Pertaining to the pleura.
tonsillar	Pertaining to tonsils.
pulmonary	Pertaining to the lungs.
axillary	Pertaining to the armpit.
laryngeal	Pertaining to the voice box.
carcinogenic	Pertaining to producing cancer.
osteogenic	Pertaining to produced within bone.
chronic	Long-term; over a long period.
pathologic	Pertaining to the study of disease.
adenoids	Collections of lymphatic tissue resembling (-oid) glands (-aden) in the throat, near the nose.
mucoid	Resembling mucus.
adipose	Pertaining to fat.
mucous membrane	A lining that secretes mucus.
necrotic	Pertaining to death (of cells).

Chapter 4

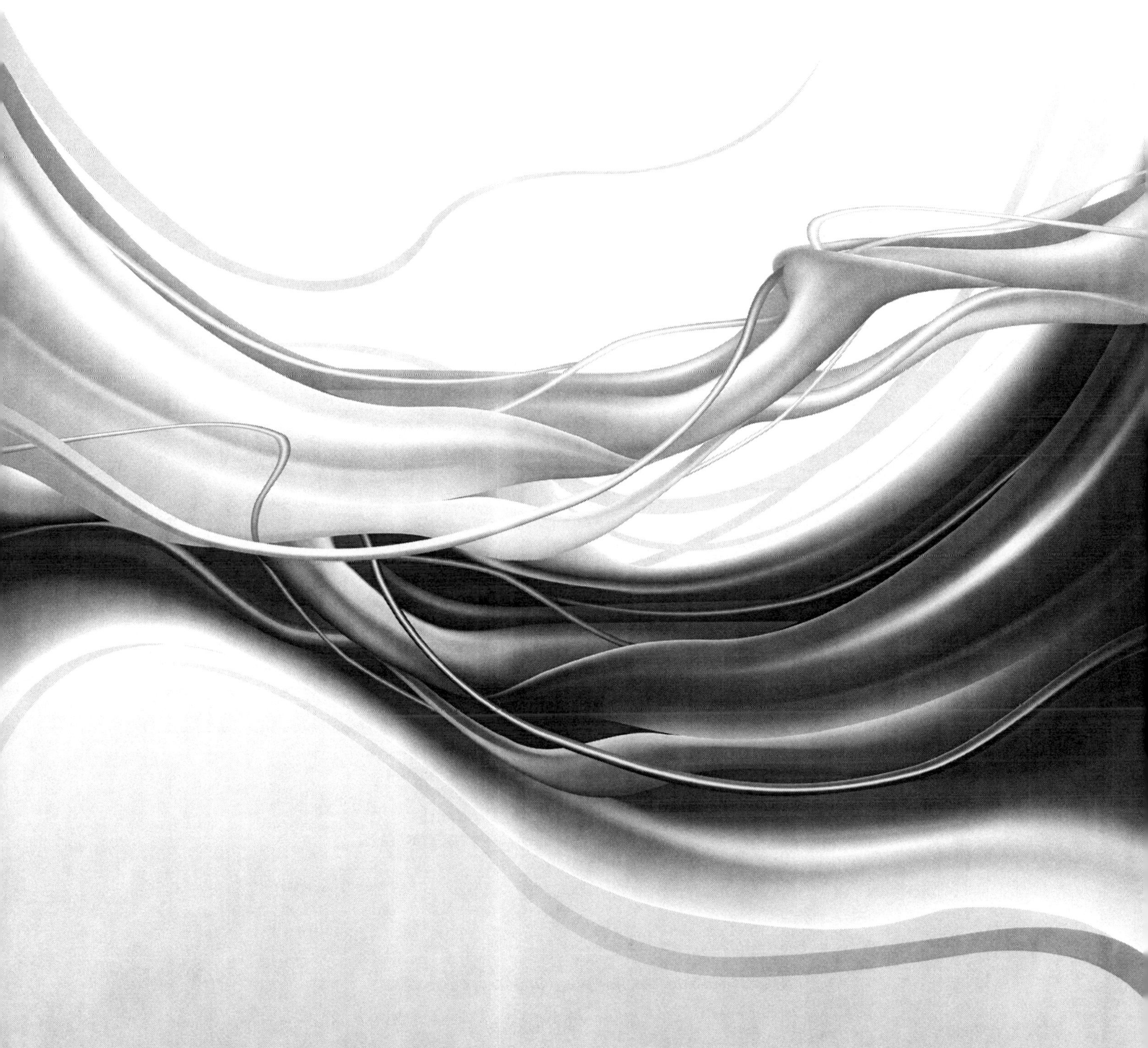

Chapter Four
MULTIPLE CHOICE QUIZ

Name: ______________________

In the box write the letter of the choice that is the definition of the term or best answers the question. There is only one correct answer for each question.

1. **Pertaining to between the ribs:** .... ☐
   A. Intracostal
   B. Infracostal
   C. Costochondral
   D. Mediastinal
   E. Intercostal

2. **Pertaining to the opposite side:** .... ☐
   A. Bilateral
   B. Contralateral
   C. Unilateral
   D. Contraindication
   E. Ipsilateral

3. **Protrusion of an eyeball:** .... ☐
   A. Cystocele
   B. Inguinal hernia
   C. Exopthalmos
   D. Ectopic
   E. Exophthalmos

4. **A congenital anomaly:** .... ☐
   A. Cerebral ischemia
   B. Prosthesis
   C. Hemiglossectomy
   D. Syndactyly
   E. Acromegaly

5. **Symbiosis:** .... ☐
   A. Parasitism is an example
   B. Symmetrical organs
   C. Biopsy
   D. Group of symptoms
   E. Prolapse of the uterus

6. **Signs and symptoms precede an illness:** .... ☐
   A. Apnea
   B. Syndrome
   C. Euphoria
   D. Prodrome
   E. Prognosis

7. **Before meals:** .... ☐
   A. Prenatal
   B. Anti cibum
   C. Postpartum
   D. Antenatal
   E. Ante cibum

8. **Antibodies:** .... ☐
   A. Bacteria
   B. Protein substances made by leukocytes
   C. Phagocytes
   D. Produced by erythrocytes to fight disease
   E. Antibiotics

9. **Symphysis:** .... ☐
   A. Bifurcation
   B. Symptoms occur together
   C. Living organisms grow together for mutual benefit
   D. Bones grow together, as in the pelvis
   E. Synthesis of substances

10. **Ultrasonography:** .... ☐
    A. X-ray recording of sound waves
    B. Amniocentesis
    C. Sound waves and echoes are used to create an image
    D. Radioactive material is injected and sound waves are recorded
    E. Abdominal x-ray recording

11. **Metamorphosis:** .... ☐
    A. Paralysis of limbs
    B. Spread of a cancerous growth
    C. Precancerous
    D. Change in shape or form
    E. After death

12. **Hypertrophy:** .... ☐
    A. Underdeveloped
    B. Poor development
    C. Increase in cell size; increased development
    D. Increase in cell numbers
    E. Newborn

13. **Excessive sugar in the blood:** .... ☐
    A. Hypodermic
    B. Hypoglycemia
    C. Glycosuria
    D. Hematuria
    E. Hyperglycemia

14. **Retroperitoneal:** ☐
   A. Region of the stomach
   B. Within the chest
   C. Behind the abdomen
   D. Within the abdomen
   E. Below the pelvis

15. **Antigens:** ☐
   A. Streptococci
   B. Antibiotics
   C. Antitoxins
   D. Produced by antibodies
   E. Penicillins

16. **Return of disease symptoms:** ☐
   A. Prolapse
   B. Relapse
   C. Syndrome
   D. Prodrome
   E. Remission

17. **Dia-:** ☐
   A. Flow
   B. Down, lack of
   C. Complete, through
   D. Against
   E. Near

18. **Abductor muscle:** ☐
   A. Bending forward
   B. Located proximally
   C. Pertains to both sides
   D. Carries a limb toward the body
   E. Carries a limb away from the body

19. **Dyspnea:** ☐
   A. Abnormal formation
   B. Difficult breathing
   C. Not able to sleep
   D. Condition of lack of water
   E. Not able to breathe

20. **Brady-:** ☐
   A. Fast
   B. Bad
   C. Short
   D. Slow
   E. Large

21. **Located on the dorsal side of an endocrine gland in the neck:** ☐
   A. Pituitary gland
   B. Parathyroid glands
   C. Adrenal glands
   D. Mammary glands
   E. Salivary glands

22. **Recombinant DNA:** ☐
   A. Pregnancy that is out of place
   B. Artificial kidney machine
   C. Backward development
   D. Antibodies are made against normal tissue
   E. Gene from one organism is inserted into another organism

23. **Tachycardia:** ☐
   A. Bad, painful swallowing
   B. Inability to swallow
   C. Near the windpipe
   D. Rapid breathing
   E. Rapid heartbeat

24. **Epithelium:** ☐
   A. Surface cells that line internal organs and are found in the skin
   B. Membrane surrounding bone
   C. Connective tissue that binds muscles to bones
   D. Adipose tissue
   E. Above the stomach

25. **Percutaneous:** ☐
   A. Within a vein
   B. Through a vein
   C. Through the skin
   D. Surrounding cartilage
   E. Surrounding a bone

Chapter Four
EXERCISE QUIZ

Name: ______________________

A. Give meanings for the following prefixes:

1. ante- ______________________
2. anti- ______________________
3. ana- ______________________
4. brady- ______________________
5. con- ______________________
6. contra- ______________________
7. bi- ______________________
8. ad- ______________________
9. dys- ______________________
10. dia- ______________________

B. Match the following terms with their meanings below:

anoxia	antisepsis	congenital anomaly
anteflexion	apnea	contralateral
antepartum	bilateral	ipsilateral

11. against infection ______________________
12. not breathing ______________________
13. before birth ______________________
14. condition of no oxygen ______________________
15. irregularity at birth ______________________
16. pertaining to opposite side ______________________

C. Give meanings of the following prefixes:

17. epi- ______________________
18. eu- ______________________
19. intra- ______________________
20. de- ______________________
21. inter- ______________________
22. hypo- ______________________
23. hyper- ______________________
24. mal- ______________________

D. Complete the following terms by supplying the word part that is called for:

25. pregnancy that is out of place: ______________________topic
26. good feeling (well-being): ______________________ phoria
27. condition of abnormal formation (of cells): dys ______________________
28. pertaining to within the windpipe: endo ______________________
29. pertaining to below the ribs: infra ______________________
30. blood condition of less than normal sugar: ______________________ glycemia

E. Match the following terms with their meanings below:

dialysis	exophthalmos	malignant	metastasis	ptosis
diarrhea	malaise	metamorphosis	pancytopenia	

31. condition of change of shape or form ______
32. vague feeling of bodily discomfort ______
33. deficiency of all blood cells ______
34. separation of wastes from the blood ______
35. spread of a cancerous tumor to a secondary organ or tissue ______
36. eyeballs that bulge outward ______

F. Give meanings for the following prefixes:

37. peri-______
38. poly- ______
39. per- ______
40. syn- ______
41. neo- ______
42. meta- ______
43. para-______
44. post-______

G. Underline the prefix and give the meaning of the entire term:

45. retroperitoneal ______
46. transurethral ______
47. subcutaneous ______
48. tachypnea ______
49. unilateral ______
50. prosthesis ______

H. Match the terms with their meanings below:

neoplasm	parathyroid	relapse	syndactyly
paralysis	prodrome	remission	syndrome

51. loss of movement in muscles ______
52. signs and symptoms that appear before an illness ______
53. symptoms lessen ______
54. disease or symptoms return ______
55. webbed fingers or toes ______
56. new growth (tumor) ______

Chapter Four

DICTATION AND COMPREHENSION QUIZ

Name: ______________________

A. Dictation of Terms

1. ______________________ 11. ______________________
2. ______________________ 12. ______________________
3. ______________________ 13. ______________________
4. ______________________ 14. ______________________
5. ______________________ 15. ______________________
6. ______________________ 16. ______________________
7. ______________________ 17. ______________________
8. ______________________ 18. ______________________
9. ______________________ 19. ______________________
10. ______________________ 20. ______________________

B. Comprehension of Terms: Match number of the above term with its meaning below.

______ Pertaining to below a rib
______ New growth (tumor)
______ Membrane surrounding a bone
______ Condition of slow heartbeat
______ Pertaining to under the skin
______ Condition of deficiency of all (blood cells)
______ Carrying away from (the body)
______ Two endocrine glands each above a kidney
______ Condition of "no" oxygen (deficiency)
______ Pertaining to through the tube leading from the bladder to the outside of the body
______ A substance that acts against a poison
______ Pertaining to within the windpipe
______ Rapid breathing
______ Pertaining to the opposite side
______ Four endocrine glands in the neck region
______ Feeling of well-being
______ Removal of half of the tongue
______ Pertaining to between the ribs
______ Harmless, noncancerous
______ Pertaining to behind the membrane surrounding the abdominal organs

Chapter Four
SPELLING QUIZ

Name: ______________________________

A. Circle the term that is spelled correctly and write its meaning in the space provided:

1.	neonatal	neonatel	______________________
2.	postmortum	postmortem	______________________
3.	metastasis	metastesis	______________________
4.	symdrone	syndrome	______________________
5.	biforcation	bifurcation	______________________
6.	antebody	antibody	______________________
7.	antibiotic	antebiotic	______________________
8.	diarrhea	diarhhea	______________________
9.	symbiosis	symbyosis	______________________
10.	benign	beningn	______________________

B. Circle the term that is spelled correctly. The meaning of each term is given.

11.	slow heartbeat	bradicardia	bradycardia	bradicardea
12.	both sides	bilateral	bilaterel	bilataral
13.	lack of water	dehydrashun	dehidration	dehydration
14.	without oxygen	anoxia	aoxyia	anocksia
15.	against infection	antesepsis	antisepsis	antisespsis
16.	before birth	antipartum	antipartem	antepartum
17.	not breathing	apnea	aphnea	afpnea
18.	foreign substance	antigene	antigen	antegen
19.	feeling of well being	euforia	uforea	euphoria
20.	through the skin	pericutaneus	percutaneous	percutanous

Chapter Four
PRONUNCIATION QUIZ

Name: ______________________

A. Underline the accented syllable in the following terms (for example: a<u>ne</u>mia, diag<u>no</u>sis, <u>en</u>docrine):

1. symbiosis
2. endotracheal
3. metamorphosis
4. congenital anomaly
5. hyperplasia
6. symphysis
7. polyneuritis
8. antitoxin
9. malaise
10. bifurcation

B. Match the prefix in Column I with its meaning in Column II:

Column I		Column II
1. inter-	________	A. Together; with
2. intra-	________	B. Toward
3. infra-	________	C. Away from
4. contra-	________	D. Within
5. ad-	________	E. Surrounding
6. para-	________	F. Below
7. peri-	________	G. Above
8. per-	________	H. Against
9. syn-	________	I. Before
10. pro-	________	J. Between
		K. Abnormal; near, beside
		L. Through

C. Complete the following terms from their definitions:

1. ______________________ natal — Pertaining to after birth.
2. ______________________ cardia — Slow heart rate.
3. ec______________________ — Out of place.
4. inter ______________________ — Pertaining to between the ribs.
5. ______________________ cytopenia — Deficiency in all (blood) cells.
6. ______________________ glycemia — Condition of increased blood sugar.
7. supra ______________________ — Pertaining to above the kidney.
8. ______________________ plasia — Bad (abnormal) formation.
9. ______________________ partum — Before birth.
10. re ______________________ — Return of disease symptoms.

Chapter Four
REVIEW SHEET QUIZ

Name: ______________________

A. Give meanings for the following prefixes:

1. ab- ______________
2. ante- ______________
3. cata- ______________
4. contra- ______________
5. epi- ______________
6. eu- ______________
7. hyper- ______________
8. hypo- ______________
9. poly- ______________
10. post- ______________
11. syn-, sym- ______________
12. retro- ______________
13. supra- ______________
14. intra- ______________
15. endo- ______________

B. Give prefixes for the following meanings:

1. two ______________
2. no, not, without ______________
3. all ______________
4. new ______________
5. surrounding ______________
6. half ______________
7. between ______________
8. small ______________
9. fast ______________
10. false ______________

C. Give meanings for the following prefixes:

1. dys- ______________
2. dia- ______________
3. brady- ______________
4. pro- ______________
5. ultra- ______________
6. con- ______________
7. mal- ______________
8. meta- ______________
9. para- ______________
10. anti- ______________

D. Give meanings for the following combining forms and suffixes:

1. necr/o ______________
2. carp/o ______________
3. gloss/o ______________
4. seps/o ______________
5. cost/o ______________
6. -rrhea ______________
7. -plasa ______________
8. -pnea ______________
9. -partum ______________
10. -trophy ______________

Chapter Four

MEDICAL SCRAMBLE

Name: ______________________________

Unscramble the letters to form a medical term from the clues. Use the letters in squares to complete the bonus term.

1. *Clue:* Bodily discomfort

☐ ___ ___ ___ ___ ☐ ___ I S A M E L A

2. *Clue:* Well-being

☐ ___ ___ ___ ☐ ___ ___ ___ R H U A E P O I

3. *Clue:* Difficult breathing

☐ ☐ ___ ___ ☐ ___ ___ N A Y D E P S

4. *Clue:* Loss of movement

___ ___ ☐ ___ ___ ___ ☐ ___ ___ Y S A L S A I P R

BONUS TERM: *Clue:* Examples are carpal tunnel, Down, Reye, and toxic shock.

☐ ☐ ☐ ☐ ☐ ☐ ☐ ☐ ☐

Chapter Four
CROSSWORD PUZZLE

Name: ______________________

Fill in the crossword puzzle below using the clues listed underneath it.

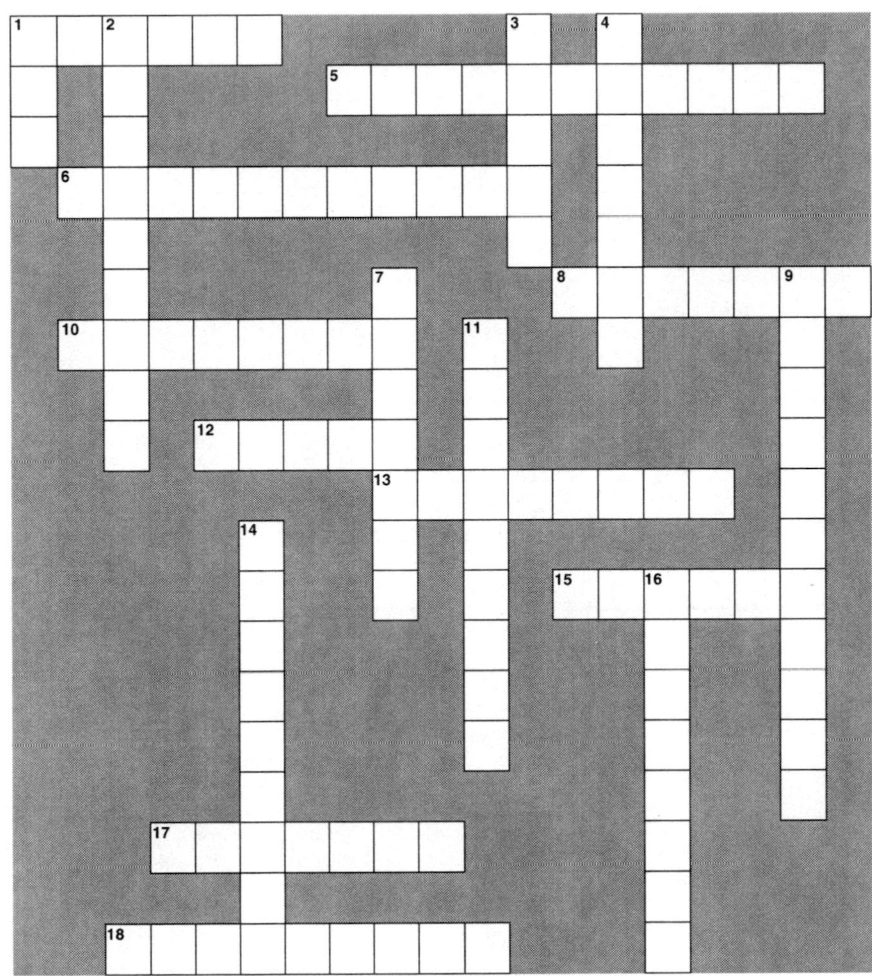

Across Clues

1. thyr/o (Greek, *thyreus*) means _____.
5. -trophy means development and _____.
6. -plasia means formation and _____.
8. contra- means opposite and _____.
10. trache/o means _____.
12. morph/o means form or _____.
13. para- means near, beside and _____.
15. intra- means in or _____.
17. dactyl/o means toes or _____.
18. -rrhea means flow or _____.

Down Clues

1. -ptosis means prolapse or to _____.
2. seps/o means _____.
3. -partum means _____.
4. trans- means across or _____.
7. infra- means below or _____.
9. peri- means _____.
11. furc/o means forking or _____.
14. -blast means immature or _____.
16. con- means with or _____.

Chapter Four
ANSWERS TO THE QUIZZES

Multiple Choice Quiz

1. E
2. B
3. E
4. D
5. A
6. D
7. E
8. B
9. D
10. C
11. D
12. C
13. E
14. C
15. A
16. B
17. C
18. E
19. B
20. D
21. B
22. E
23. E
24. A
25. C

Exercise Quiz

A

1. before
2. against
3. up
4. slow
5. together; with
6. against; opposite
7. two
8. toward
9. bad, painful, difficult
10. complete; through

B

11. antisepsis
12. apnea
13. antepartum
14. anoxia
15. congenital anomaly
16. contralateral

C

17. above
18. good, normal
19. within
20. lack of, down
21. between
22. under, deficient
23. above, excessive
24. bad

D

25. ectopic
26. euphoria
27. dysplasia
28. endotracheal
29. infracostal
30. hypoglycemia

E

31. metamorphosis
32. malaise
33. pancytopenia
34. dialysis
35. metastasis
36. exophthalmos

F

37. surrounding
38. many, much
39. through
40. together, with
41. new
42. beyond; change
43. near, beside, abnormal
44. after, behind

G

45. retroperitoneal—pertaining to behind the abdominal membrane
46. transurethral—pertaining to across or through the urethra
47. subcutaneous—pertaining to under the skin
48. tachypnea—fast or rapid breathing
49. unilateral—pertaining to one side
50. prosthesis—artificial limb or part of the body (literally, to put or place forward)

H

51. paralysis
52. prodrome
53. remission
54. relapse
55. syndactyly
56. neoplasm

Dictation and Comprehension Quiz

A

1. abduction
2. adrenal
3. anoxia
4. antitoxin
5. benign
6. bradycardia
7. contralateral
8. endotracheal
9. euphoria
10. hemiglossectomy
11. hypodermic
12. infracostal
13. intercostal
14. neoplasm
15. pancytopenia
16. parathyroid
17. periosteum
18. retroperitoneal
19. tachypnea
20. transurethral

B

12 Pertaining to below a rib
14 New growth (tumor)
17 Membrane surrounding a bone
6 Condition of slow heartbeat
11 Pertaining to under the skin
15 Condition of deficiency of all (blood cells)
1 Carrying away from (the body)
2 Two endocrine glands each above a kidney
3 Condition of "no" oxygen (deficiency)
20 Pertaining to through the tube leading from the bladder to the outside of the body
4 A substance that works against a poison
8 Pertaining to within the windpipe
19 Rapid breathing
7 Pertaining to the opposite side
16 Four endocrine glands in the neck region
9 Feeling of well-being
10 Removal of half of the tongue
13 Pertaining to between the ribs
5 Harmless, noncancerous
18 Pertaining to behind the membrane surrounding the abdominal organs

Spelling Quiz

A

1. neonatal—newborn
2. postmortem—after death
3. metastasis—beyond control (spread of tumor)

4. syndrome—symptoms that occur together
5. bifurcation—branching into two
6. antibody—protein made by leukocytes to fight infection
7. antibiotic—substance against germ life
8. diarrhea—complete discharge (from colon)
9. symbiosis—living together for mutual benefit
10. benign—harmless; not cancerous

B

11. bradycardia
12. bilateral
13. dehydration
14. anoxia
15. antisepsis
16. antepartum
17. apnea
18. antigen
19. euphoria
20. percutaneous

Pronunciation Quiz

A

1. symbiosis
2. endotracheal
3. metamorphosis
4. congenital anomaly
5. hyperplasia
6. symphysis
7. polyneuritis
8. antitoxin
9. malaise
10. bifurcation

B

1. J
2. D
3. F
4. H
5. B
6. K
7. E
8. L
9. A
10. I

C

1. postnatal
2. bradycardia
3. ectopic
4. intercostal
5. pancytopenia
6. hyperglycemia
7. suprarenal
8. dysplasia
9. antepartum
10. relapse

Review Sheet Quiz

A

1. away from
2. before
3. down
4. against, opposite
5. upon, on, above
6. good, normal
7. excessive, above
8. deficient, under
9. many, much
10. after, behind
11. together, with
12. behind, backward
13. above, upper
14. into, within
15. in, within

B

1. bi-
2. a-, an-
3. pan-
4. neo-
5. peri-
6. hemi-
7. inter-
8. micro-
9. tachy-
10. pseudo-

C

1. bad, painful, difficult, abnormal
2. through, complete
3. slow
4. before, forward
5. beyond, excess
6. with, together
7. bad
8. beyond, change
9. abnormal, beside, near
10. against

D

1. death
2. wrist bones, carpals
3. tongue
4. infection
5. ribs
6. flow, discharge
7. development, formation
8. breathing
9. birth, labor
10. nourishment, development

Medical Scramble

1. MALAISE
2. EUPHORIA
3. DYSPNEA
4. PARALYSIS

BONUS TERM: SYNDROMES

Crossword Puzzle

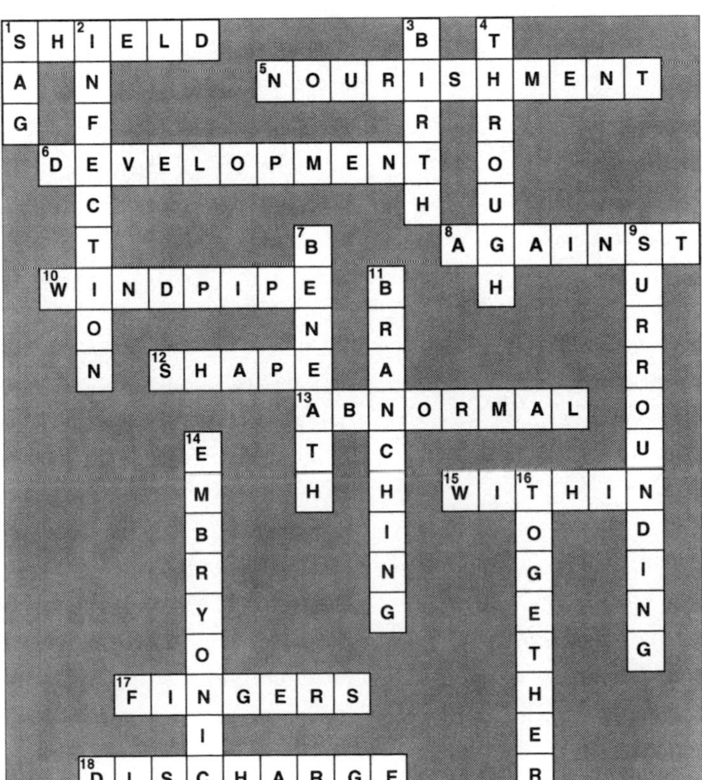

Chapter Four
Answers to Terminology Section

(textbook pages 109–118)

Terminology	Meaning
apnea	Not breathing.
anoxia	Without oxygen (decrease in tissues).
abnormal	Pertaining to away from the norm (rule); not regular.
abductor	One who (muscle which) leads away from the body. *To abduct means to carry away by force; kidnap.*
adductor	One who (muscle which) leads toward the body. *To admit means to send toward or permit entrance.*
adrenal glands	Endocrine glands located above (toward) the kidneys.
anabolism	Process of casting (building) up materials (proteins) within cells.
analysis	To separate (apart). *Psychoanalysis is a psychiatric treatment that explores the mind. Urinalysis (urin/o + [an]alysis) is a laboratory examination of urine to aid in diagnosis.*
ante cibum	Before meals.
anteflexion	Bending forward.
antepartum	Before birth.
antisepsis	Condition against infection.
antibiotic	Pertaining to against life (germ life).
antibody	Protein substance made in the body to destroy foreign antigens.
antigen	A substance (usually foreign) that stimulates the production of antibodies.
antitoxin	A substance (antibody) produced in response to and capable of neutralizing a toxin (such as those causing diphtheria or tetanus). *Antivenin contains antitoxin specific for an animal or insect venom.*
autoimmune disease	A condition related to making antibodies (immune substances) against one's own (auto-) cells and tissues.
bifurcation	Forking (branching) into two; as the trachea bifurcates into two individual tubes.
bilateral	Pertaining to two sides.
bradycardia	Condition of slow heartbeat.
catabolism	Process of casting down materials (sugar) to release energy in cells.
congenital anomaly	Irregularity at birth.
connective	To tie (bind) together. *A conference (fer-means to carry or bring) is where people gather together or meet.*
contraindication	To point out against; as reasons why a drug should not be taken.
contralateral	Pertaining to the opposite side. *Ipsilateral means pertaining to the same side.*
dehydration	Condition of lack of water.
diameter	To measure through; as the diameter of a circle.
diarrhea	To flow through; water is not properly absorbed through the walls of the colon.
dialysis	Complete separation; two types are hemodialysis and peritoneal dialysis.
dyspnea	Difficult breathing.
dysplasia	Abnormal ("bad") development or formation.
ectopic pregnancy	Pregnancy out of the normal place (usually in the fallopian tubes).
endocardium	Inner lining (membrane) of the heart.
endoscope	Instrument to view within the body; gastroscope, bronchoscope, laparoscope.
endotracheal	Pertaining to within the trachea.
epithelium	Skin cell; *literally, "upon a nipple."*

euphoria	Good feeling, "high." *A eulogy is a speech saying good things about a person after his/her death.*
euthyroid	Normal thyroid function.
exophthalmos	Eyeballs that protrude.
hemiglossectomy	Removal of half the tongue.
hyperglycemia	Increase in blood sugar.
hyperplasia	Condition of increased formation (increase in number of cells).
hypertrophy	Increase in development; increase in size of cells.
hypodermic injection	Use of a needle and syringe to force liquid under the skin.
hypoglycemia	Decrease in blood sugar.
insomniac	Pertaining to inability to sleep.
incision	Process of cutting into; sectioning.
infracostal	Pertaining to below ribs.
intercostal	Pertaining to between the ribs.
intravenous	Pertaining to within a vein.
macrocephaly	Pertaining to an enlarged head; a congenital anomaly.
malignant	Harmful, bad; cancerous condition.
malaise	Feeling of discomfort; "bad feeling."
metacarpal bones	Five hand bones (beyond the wrist).
metamorphosis	Condition of change of shape or form. *A worm-like larva undergoes a change in shape to become a butterfly. This is an example of metamorphosis.*
metastasis	Beyond control; spreading of a malignant tumor.
microscope	Instrument to view small objects.
neonatal	Pertaining to a newborn (infant).
neoplasm	New growth; new formation (tumor).
pancytopenia	Condition of decrease in all cells (blood cells).
paralysis	Abnormal destruction (of nerves) leading to loss of muscle function.
parathyroid glands	Endocrine glands located near (on the dorsal side of) the thyroid gland. *A paramedic works beside and assists a doctor; also called an emergency medical technician (EMT). A parasite (-site means grain or food) is an organism that feeds and lives on or within another organism. Lice, ticks, and fleas are examples of parasites.*
percutaneous	Pertaining to through the skin.
pericardium	Membrane surrounding the heart.
periosteum	Membrane surrounding the bone.
polymorphonuclear	Pertaining to a many-shaped nucleus; a type of white blood cell.
polyneuritis	Inflammation of many nerves.
postmortem	After death.
postpartum	After childbirth; this most often refers to the mother.
precancerous	Pertaining to before cancer; a lesion that may become cancerous.
prenatal	Pertaining to before birth.
prodrome	Signs and symptoms that appear before the onset of a more severe illness.
prolapse	Sliding forward or downward.
prosthesis	Artificial limb or part of the body (literally, to put or place forward)
relapse	A sliding back; recurrence of symptoms of disease.
remission	To send back; disappearance of symptoms of disease.
recombinant DNA	Inserting a gene (region of DNA) from one organism into the DNA of another organism.
retroperitoneal	Pertaining to behind the peritoneum.

retroflexion	Bending backward.
subcutaneous	Pertaining to under the skin.
suprapubic	Pertaining to above the pubic bone (part of the pelvis).
syndactyly	Condition of webbed (held together) fingers or toes; a congenital anomaly.
synthesis	To put or place together, as in protein synthesis or photosynthesis.
syndrome	A group of symptoms that run (occur) together. *In synchrony means timed (chron/o) together.*
symbiosis	Condition or state of "life together"; two organisms living together for mutual benefit or not (parasitism).
symmetry	State of "measurement together"; equality of parts; mirror images.
symphysis	To grow together; bones that grow together at the joint.
tachypnea	Rapid breathing.
transfusion	To pour across, as in transferring blood from one person to another.
transurethral	Pertaining to through the urethra.
ultrasonography	Process of recording ultrasound (beyond the normal range) waves.
unilateral	Pertaining to one side.

Chapter 5

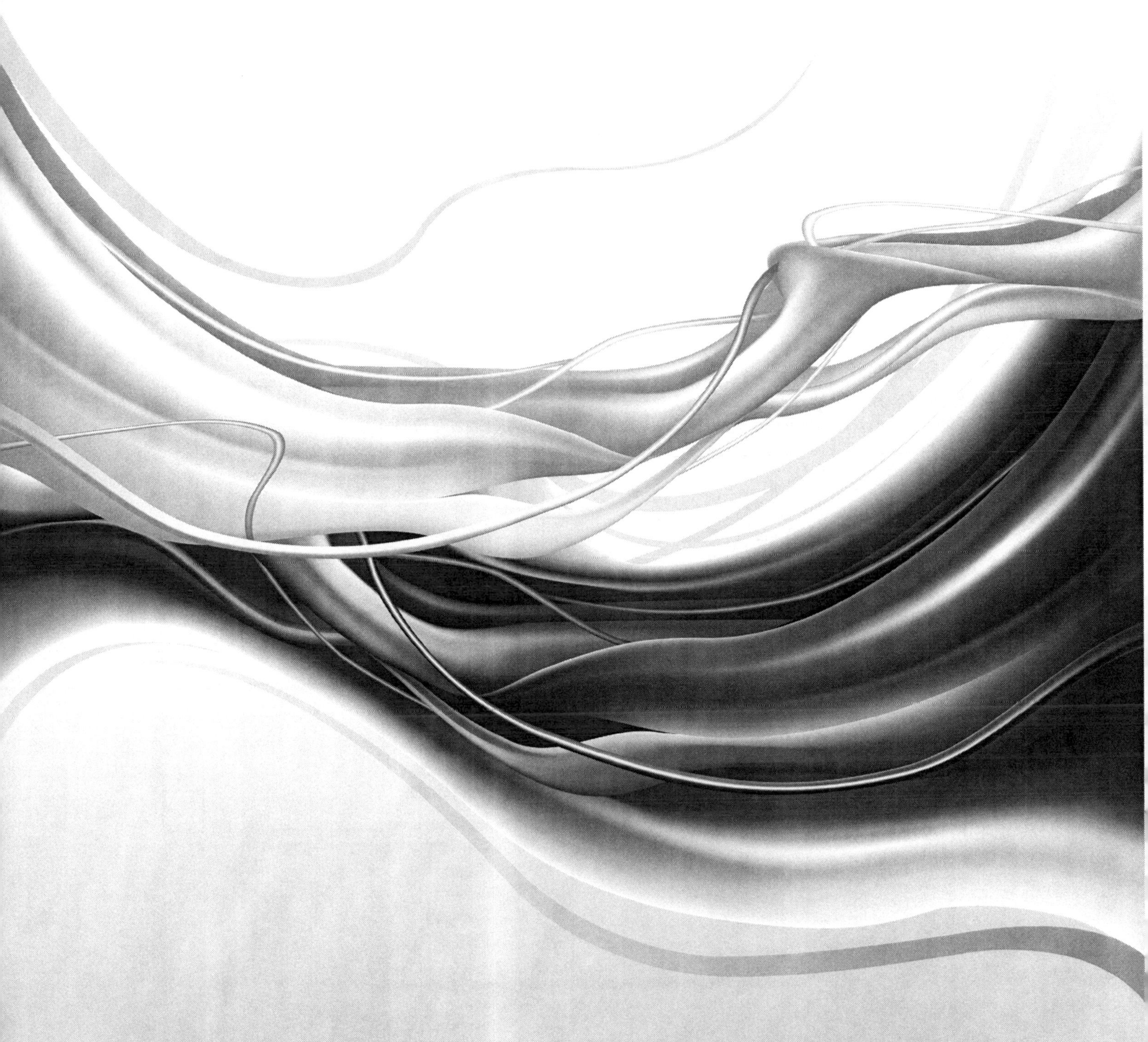

Chapter Five
MULTIPLE CHOICE QUIZ

Name: ______________________________

In the box write the letter of the choice that is the definition of the term or best answers the question. There is only one correct answer for each question.

1. The combining form of the first part of the large intestine is: ☐
A. Ile/o
B. Jejun/o
C. Ili/o
D. Duoden/o
E. Cec/o

2. Pertaining to the abdomen: ☐
A. Gastric
B. Celiac
C. Colonic
D. Pelvic
E. Esophageal

3. Muscular wave-like movement to transport food through the digestive system: ☐
A. Mastication
B. Regurgitation
C. Emulsification
D. Peristalsis
E. Anastomosis

4. Part of the tooth that contains a rich supply of nerves and blood vessels: ☐
A. Enamel
B. Dentin
C. Pulp
D. Cementum
E. Periodontal membrane

5. Gingiv/o means: ☐
A. Tooth
B. Stomach
C. Intestine
D. Chest
E. Gums

6. Buccal means: ☐
A. Pertaining to the cheek
B. Petaining to the soft palate
C. Pertaining to the tongue
D. Pertaining to the teeth
E. Pertaining to the throat

7. High blood levels of a pigment released by the liver with bile: ☐
A. Cholecystitis
B. Hypoglycemia
C. Hyperbilirubinemia
D. Hematoma
E. Steatorrhea

8. Carries bile into the duodenum: ☐
A. Cystic duct
B. Portal vein
C. Lymph duct
D. Hepatic duct
E. Common bile duct

9. Enzyme to digest starch: ☐
A. Lipase
B. Amylase
C. Glucose
D. Bile
E. Amino acid

10. Chronic inflammation of the intestinal tract: ☐
A. Crohn disease
B. Colonic polyps
C. Irritable bowel syndrome
D. Dysentery
E. Achalasia

11. Ring of muscles: ☐
A. Uvula
B. Rugae
C. Papillae
D. Myoma
E. Sphincter

12. Specialist in gums: ☐
A. Endodontist
B. Periodontist
C. Orthodontist
D. Pedodontist
E. Proctologist

13. Stomat/o means: ☐
A. Roof of the mouth
B. Mouth
C. Cheek
D. Stomach
E. Tongue

14. Cheil/o means the same as:................
A. Lingu/o
B. Gingiv/o
C. Gloss/o
D. Palat/o
E. Labi/o

15. Stone in a salivary gland: ....
A. Lithiasis
B. Cholecystolithiasis
C. Adenolithiasis
D. Sialadenolithiasis
E. Renal calculus

16. Membrane that connects parts of small intestine:.................................
A. Anastomosis
B. Ileum
C. Mesentery
D. Appendix
E. Pylorus

17. New opening from the large bowel to the surface of the body: ....
A. Jejunostomy
B. Jejunotomy
C. Enterostomy
D. Colostomy
E. Duodenotomy

18. Fats are improperly digested and appear in the feces:............................
A. Adipose
B. Steatorrhea
C. Lipase
D. Lipolysis
E. Glycogenolysis

19. Lack of appetite: ....
A. Anorexia
B. Aphthous stomatitis
C. Leukoplakia
D. Postprandial
E. Achlorhydria

20. Another term for jaundice:.................
A. Achalasia
B. Icterus
C. Hypobilirubinemia
D. Gallstones
E. Melena

21. Esophageal varices are:......................
A. Hernias around the opening of the stomach
B. Hemorrhoids
C. Perianal fistulae
D. Polyps
E. Swollen, twisted veins

22. Abnormal side pockets in a hollow organ, such as the intestine: ....
A. Caries
B. Ulcers
C. Dysentery
D. Diverticula
E. Ascites

23. Telescoping of the intestine: ....
A. Volvulus
B. Anal fistula
C. Intussusception
D. Ileus
E. Hiatal hernia

24. Difficulty in swallowing: ....
A. Regurgitation
B. Flatus
C. Nausea
D. Eructation
E. Dysphagia

25. White plaques on the mucosa of the mouth: ....
A. Herpetic stomatitis
B. Aphthous stomatitis
C. Oral leukoplakia
D. Rectocele
E. Melena

Chapter Five
VOCABULARY QUIZ

(textbook pages 150-153)

Name: ______________________

A. Match the following terms with their meanings:

absorption	bilirubin	emulsification
amino acids	defecation	enamel
amylase	deglutition	fatty acids
bile	dentin	glucose

1. Swallowing ______________________
2. Pigment released by the liver in bile ______________________
3. Substances produced when proteins are digested ______________________
4. Major tissue composing teeth ______________________
5. Removal of waste material from the body ______________________
6. Passage of materials through villi into the blood ______________________
7. Enzyme secreted by the pancreas to digest starch ______________________
8. Hard, outermost layer of a tooth ______________________
9. Process of breaking up large fat globules ______________________
10. Simple sugar ______________________
11. Digestive juice made by the liver and stored in the gallbladder ______________________
12. Substances produced when fats are digested ______________________

B. Match the following terms with their meanings:

feces	insulin	parotid gland
glycogen	lipase	peristalsis
hydrochloric acid	LES	portal vein
incisor	palate	protease

1. Contractions of the gastrointestinal tubes ______________________
2. Pancreatic enzyme necessary to digest fats ______________________
3. Starch; stored sugar ______________________
4. Solid wastes; stools ______________________
5. Roof of the mouth ______________________
6. Blood vessel bringing blood to the liver ______________________
7. Chemical produced by the stomach to aid digestion ______________________
8. Hormone produced by the pancreas ______________________

9. One of four front teeth ______________________
10. Enzyme that digests proteins ______________________
11. Ring of muscles between the esophagus and stomach ______________________
12. Secretes enzymes into the mouth ______________________

C. Match the following terms with their meanings:

mastication	pyloric sphincter	uvula
papillae	rugae	villi
pulp	triglycerides	

1. Soft tissue hanging from the soft palate ______________________
2. Microscopic projections in the walls of the small intestine ______________________
3. Ring of muscles at the distal region of the stomach ______________________
4. Small elevations on the tongue ______________________
5. Chewing ______________________
6. Ridges on the hard palate and wall of the stomach ______________________
7. Soft tissue within a tooth ______________________
8. Large fat molecules ______________________

Chapter Five
TERMINOLOGY QUIZ

(textbook pages 153–158)

Name: ______________________________

A. Match the following terms with their meanings below:

buccal mucosa	cheilosis	colonoscopy	perianal
cecal	cholecystectomy	colostomy	
celiac	choledochotomy	dentibuccal	

1. Abnormal condition of the lip ______________________________
2. Pertaining to surrounding the anus ______________________________
3. Removal of the gallbladder ______________________________
4. Pertaining to the belly or abdomen ______________________________
5. New opening of the colon to the outside of the body ______________________________
6. Pertaining to the teeth and cheek ______________________________
7. Visual examination of the colon ______________________________
8. Incision of the common bile duct ______________________________
9. Mucous membrane lining of the cheek ______________________________
10. Pertaining to the first part of the large intestine ______________________________

B. Build medical terms from the following meanings:

1. Inflammation of the appendix ______________________________
2. Pertaining to the face ______________________________
3. Inflammation of gums ______________________________
4. Pertaining to the large intestine ______________________________
5. Tumor of the liver ______________________________
6. Inflammation of the small and large intestine ______________________________
7. Removal of the appendix ______________________________
8. New opening of the stomach to the outside of the body ______________________________
9. Pertaining to the tube leading from the throat to the stomach ______________________________
10. Pertaining to the first part of the small intestine ______________________________

C. Match the following terms with their meanings below:

choledochojejunostomy	labial	palatoplasty	submandibular
enteroenterostomy	laparoscopy	parenteral	
ileostomy	mesentery	sublingual	

1. Pertaining to under the tongue ______
2. Membrane that holds the intestines together ______
3. Pertaining to under the lower jaw ______
4. Visual examination of the abdomen ______
5. New opening between two previously unconnected parts of the small intestine (an anastomosis) ______
6. Pertaining to the lip ______
7. Surgical repair of the roof of the mouth ______
8. Pertaining to apart from the intestine (such as IV delivery of nutrients and drugs) ______
9. New opening between the common bile duct and the second part of the small intestine (an anastomosis) ______
10. New opening of the third part of the small intestine to the outside of the body ______

D. Build medical terms from the following meanings:

1. Enlargement of the liver ______
2. Inflammation of the third part of the small intestine ______
3. New opening between the stomach and the jejunum ______
4. Specialist in straightening teeth ______
5. Specialist in gums ______
6. Specialist in root canal therapy ("within a tooth") ______
7. Inflammation of the pancreas ______
8. Inflammation of the lining surrounding abdominal organs ______
9. Pertaining to the throat ______
10. Specialist in the anal and rectal region ______
11. Discharge of pus (from gums) ______

E. Match the following terms with their meanings below:

biliary	palatopharyngoplasty	sialadenectomy	uvulectomy
cholelithiasis	pyloroplasty	sigmoidoscopy	
lithogenesis	rectocele	stomatitis	

1. Removal of the soft tissue hanging from the palate ____________________
2. Visual examination of the lower part of the large intestine ____________________
3. Hernia of the rectum ____________________
4. Abnormal condition of gallstones ____________________
5. Inflammation of the mouth ____________________
6. Surgical repair of the roof of the mouth and the throat ____________________
7. Formation of a stone (calculus) ____________________
8. Pertaining to bile ____________________
9. Surgical repair of the sphincter between the stomach and intestine ____________________
10. Removal of a salivary gland ____________________

F. Give medical terms for the following meanings:

1. Enzyme that digests starch ____________________
2. High blood sugar ____________________
3. Excess bilirubin in the blood ____________________
4. Tumor of fat (benign) ____________________
5. Enzyme that digests protein ____________________
6. Lack of hydrochloric acid ____________________
7. Salivary (gland) stone ____________________
8. Production of new sugar ____________________
9. Enzyme that digests fat ____________________
10. Condition of stones in the common bile duct ____________________
11. Pertaining to after meals ____________________
12. Discharge of fats (in feces) ____________________

Chapter Five

PATHOLOGY QUIZ

Name: ______________________________

A. Match the following pathologic signs and symptoms with their meanings below:

anorexia
ascites
borborygmus
constipation
diarrhea
dysphagia
eructation
flatus
hematochezia
jaundice (icterus)
melena
nausea
steatorrhea

1. Passage of bright red fresh blood from the rectum ______________________________
2. Gas expelled from the stomach through the mouth ______________________________
3. Lack of appetite ______________________________
4. Gas expelled through the anus ______________________________
5. Fat in the feces ______________________________
6. Unpleasant sensation in the stomach associated with tendency to vomit ______________
7. Yellow-orange skin and whites of the eyes ______________________________
8. Abnormal accumulation of fluid in the abdomen ______________________________
9. Difficulty in swallowing ______________________________
10. Frequent passage of loose, watery stools ______________________________
11. Rumbling noise produced by the movement of gas or fluid through the gastrointestinal tract ______________________________
12. Difficulty in passing stools ______________________________
13. Black tarry stools ______________________________

B. Match the following pathologic conditions with their explanations below:

aphthous stomatitis
anal fistula
colonic polyps
colorectal cancer
Crohn disease (Crohn's)
dental caries
diverticulosis
dysentery
esophageal cancer
esophageal varices
gastric cancer
gastroesophageal reflux disease

1. Malignant tumor of the stomach ______________________________
2. Swollen, varicose veins at the lower end of the esophagus ______________________________
3. Benign growths protruding from the mouth mucous membrane of the large intestine ______________

4. Inflammation of the mouth with small, painful ulcers ______________________
5. Tooth decay ______________________
6. Abnormal tube-like passageway near the anus ______________________
7. Adenocarcinoma of the colon or rectum or both ______________________
8. Abnormal outpouchings in the intestinal wall ______________________
9. Chronic inflammation of the intestinal tract (such as ileum and colon) ______________________
10. Painful, inflamed intestines ______________________
11. Solids and fluids return to the mouth from the stomach ______________________
12. Malignant tumor of the esophagus ______________________

C. Match the following pathologic conditions with their explanations below:

hemorrhoids
hernia
herpetic stomatitis
ileus
intussusception
irritable bowel syndrome
oral leukoplakia
peptic ulcer
periodontal disease
ulcerative colitis
volvulus

1. Telescoping of the intestine ______________________
2. Chronic inflammation of the colon with destruction of its inner surface ______________________
3. Inflammation and degeneration of gums, teeth, and surrounding bone ______________________
4. Twisting of the intestine on itself ______________________
5. White plaques or patches on the mucosa of the mouth ______________________
6. Group of gastrointestinal symptoms associated with stress and tension ______________________
7. Loss of peristalsis with resulting obstruction of the intestines ______________________
8. Protrusion of an organ or body part through the muscle normally containing it ______________________
9. Open sore in the lining of the stomach or duodenum ______________________
10. Swollen, twisted varicose veins in the region of the rectum ______________________
11. Inflammation of the mouth caused by infection with the herpesvirus ______________________

D. Name the pathologic conditions from their descriptions below:

1. Degeneration of liver tissue as the result of chronic alcoholism or viral hepatitis ______________________
2. Inflammation of the liver caused by a virus ______________________
3. Abnormal condition of stones in the gallbladder ______________________
4. Malignant tumor of the pancreas ______________________
5. Inflammation of the pancreas ______________________

Chapter Five

EXERCISE QUIZ

Name: ______________________

A. Match the following digestive system structures with their meanings.

cecum	duodenum	gallbladder	pancreas
colon	esophagus	ileum	pharynx

1. Third part of the small intestine ______________________
2. Organ under the stomach; produces insulin and enzymes ______________________
3. First part of the large intestine ______________________
4. Small sac under the liver; stores bile ______________________
5. Tube connecting the throat to the stomach ______________________
6. Large intestine ______________________
7. First part of the small intestine ______________________
8. Throat ______________________

B. Complete the following:

9. lapar/o and celi/o both mean ______________________
10. gloss/o and lingu/o both mean ______________________
11. or/o and stomat/o both mean ______________________
12. labi/o and cheil/o both mean ______________________

C. Build medical terms:

13. Enlargement of the liver ______________________
14. Study of the cause (of disease) ______________________
15. Incision of the common bile duct ______________________
16. Surgical repair of the roof of the mouth ______________________
17. After meals ______________________
18. New opening between the common bile duct and the jejunum ______________________

D. Build medical terms to describe the following inflammations:

19. Inflammation of the appendix ______________________
20. Inflammation of the membrane around the abdomen ______________________
21. Inflammation of the large intestine ______________________

22. Inflammation of the gallbladder ____________________

23. Inflammation of a salivary gland ____________________

24. Inflammation of the small and large intestines ____________________

25. Inflammation of the liver ____________________

26. Inflammation of the pancreas ____________________

27. Inflammation of the mouth ____________________

28. Inflammation of the gums ____________________

29. Inflammation of the third part of the small intestine ____________________

E. Match the following pathologic diagnoses with their definitions:

cholecystolithiasis	dysentery	ileus	ulcerative colitis
cirrhosis	hemorrhoids	irritable bowel syndrome	
diverticula	hepatitis	ulcer	

30. Swollen, twisted veins in the rectal region ____________________

31. Chronic liver disease resulting from alcoholism and malnutrition ____________________

32. Failure of peristalsis ____________________

33. Calculi in the sac that stores bile ____________________

34. Sore or lesion of the mucous membrane in the stomach or duodenum ____________________

35. Painful, inflamed intestines often caused by bacterial infection ____________________

36. Inflammation of the liver caused by type A, type B, or type C virus ____________________

37. Chronic inflammation of the large bowel with ulcers ____________________

38. Abnormal side pockets in the intestinal wall ____________________

39. Group of gastrointestinal symptoms associated with stress, but without inflammation of the intestines ____________________

F. Give the names of the following gastrointestinal symptoms from their descriptions:

40. Lack of appetite ____________________

41. Bright, fresh red blood in stools ____________________

42. Abnormal accumulation of fluid in the abdomen ____________________

43. Loose, watery stools ____________________

44. Gas expelled through the anus ____________________

45. Discharge of fat in the feces ____________________

G. Complete the spelling of the medical terms below:

46. Black, dark brown tarry stools: mel ______________________________

47. Membrane that holds the intestines together: mes ______________________________

48. Pertaining to under the tongue: sub ______________________________

49. High levels of pigment in the blood (jaundice): hyper ______________________________

50. New connection between two previously unconnected tubes: ana ______________________________

Chapter Five

DICTATION AND COMPREHENSION QUIZ: VOCABULARY

Name: ______________________

A. Dictation of Terms

1.	______________________	11.	______________________
2.	______________________	12.	______________________
3.	______________________	13.	______________________
4.	______________________	14.	______________________
5.	______________________	15.	______________________
6.	______________________	16.	______________________
7.	______________________	17.	______________________
8.	______________________	18.	______________________
9.	______________________	19.	______________________
10.	______________________	20.	______________________

B. Comprehension of Terms: Match number of the above term with its meaning below.

_______ Physical process of breaking down large fat globules into smaller parts
_______ Salivary gland near the ear
_______ Swallowing
_______ Small substances that are produced when proteins are digested
_______ Pigment released by the liver in bile
_______ Soft inner tissue within a tooth containing nerves and blood vessels
_______ Microscopic projections in the walls of the small intestine
_______ Rhythm-like contractions of the tubes of the alimentary tract
_______ Hormone produced by the endocrine cells of the pancreas
_______ This tube carries bile from the liver and gallbladder into the duodenum
_______ Small nipple-like elevations on the tongue
_______ Soft tissue hanging from the roof of the mouth
_______ An enzyme that digests starch
_______ Chewing
_______ Simple sugar
_______ Substance produced by the stomach and necessary for digestion of foods
_______ Solid wastes; stools
_______ Pancreatic enzyme necessary to digest fats
_______ Ring of muscle at the distal region of the stomach
_______ Large fat molecules

Chapter Five

DICTATION AND COMPREHENSION QUIZ: PATHOLOGIC SYMPTOMS

Name: ____________________

A. Dictation of Terms

1.	____________________	7.	____________________
2.	____________________	8.	____________________
3.	____________________	9.	____________________
4.	____________________	10.	____________________
5.	____________________	11.	____________________
6.	____________________	12.	____________________

B. Comprehension of Terms: Match number of the above term with its meaning below.

______ Feces containing fat
______ Unpleasant sensation from the stomach with tendency to vomit
______ Gas expelled through the anus
______ Lack of appetite
______ Bright red fresh blood from the rectum
______ Difficult, delayed elimination of feces
______ Black tarry stools; feces containing blood
______ Yellow-orange skin; icterus
______ Rumbling or gurgling noises produced by the movement of gas or fluid
______ Difficulty in swallowing
______ Loose, liquid stools
______ Abnormal accumulation of fluid in the peritoneal cavity

Chapter Five

DICTATION AND COMPREHENSION QUIZ: PATHOLOGIC CONDITIONS

Name: ____________________

A. Dictation of Terms

1. ____________________ 11. ____________________
2. ____________________ 12. ____________________
3. ____________________ 13. ____________________
4. ____________________ 14. ____________________
5. ____________________ 15. ____________________
6. ____________________ 16. ____________________
7. ____________________ 17. ____________________
8. ____________________ 18. ____________________
9. ____________________ 19. ____________________
10. ____________________ 20. ____________________

B. Comprehension of Terms: Match number of the above term with its meaning below.

______ Inflammation and degeneration of gums
______ Twisting of the intestine upon itself
______ Small benign growths protruding from the mucous membrane of the large bowel
______ Telescoping of the intestines
______ Solids and fluids return to the mouth from the stomach
______ Gallbladder calculi
______ Inflammation of the liver; viral etiology
______ Chronic liver disease; etiology is often alcoholism and malnutrition
______ Sore or lesion of the mucous membrane of the first part of the small intestine
______ Abnormal tube-like passageway in the distal end of the alimentary tract
______ Painful inflamed intestines; etiology is often bacterial
______ Swollen, tortuous veins in the distal portion of the tube connecting the throat and stomach
______ Inflammation of a gland behind the stomach; cysts may form
______ Inflammation of small side pockets in the intestinal wall
______ Chronic inflammation of the large bowel with open sores of mucous membrane
______ Chronic inflammation of the intestinal tract (terminal ileum)
______ Failure of peristalsis
______ Failure of the LES muscle to relax
______ Inflammation of the mouth with open sores
______ Tooth decay

Chapter Five
SPELLING QUIZ

Name: ______________________________

A. Circle the term that is spelled correctly and write its meaning in the space provided:

1. pancreatitis — pancreasitis ______________________________
2. anal fistula — anal fistulla ______________________________
3. dental karies — dental caries ______________________________
4. cholitis — colitis ______________________________
5. ileus — ilius ______________________________
6. assites — ascites ______________________________
7. melana — melena ______________________________
8. polyposis — poliposis ______________________________
9. dysentery — dysentary ______________________________
10. anarexia — anorexia ______________________________

B. Circle the term that is spelled correctly. The meaning of each term is given.

11. membrane connecting the intestines	mesentary	mezentary	mesentery
12. gallbladder resection	cholocystectomy	cholecystectomy	colecystectomy
13. twisting of the intestine	vulvulus	volvulus	vulvulos
14. chronic intestinal inflammation	Chron disease	Chrohn disease	Crohn disease
15. pertaining to bile	billiary	biliary	billiery
16. yellow coloration of the skin	jaundice	jaundise	jawndice
17. salivary gland near the ear	perotid gland	parrotid gland	parotid gland
18. failure of muscles in the lower esophagus to relax	achalsia	achalasia	acalasia
19. nutrition is given other than through the intestine	parenteral	perinteral	perenteral
20. new opening between two previously unconnected tubes	anastomosis	anastomosus	anastamosis

Chapter Five
PRONUNCIATION QUIZ

Name: ______________________________

A. Underline the accented syllable in the following words:

1. aphthous stomatitis
2. dysentery
3. choledocholithiasis
4. leukoplakia
5. esophageal varices
6. pyloric sphincter
7. biliary
8. cheilitis
9. diverticula
10. volvulus

B. Match the term in Column I with its meaning in Column II:

Column I		Column II
1. jejunum	_______	A. Collection of fluid in the abdominal cavity
2. pharynx	_______	B. First part of the small intestine
3. sigmoid colon	_______	C. First part of the colon
4. duodenum	_______	D. The throat
5. uvula	_______	E. After meals
6. amylase	_______	F. Enzyme to digest starch
7. cecum	_______	G. Second part of the small intestine
8. ascites	_______	H. Soft tissue hanging from the roof of the mouth
9. intussusception	_______	I. Telescoping of the intestines
10. postprandial	_______	J. S-shaped portion of the large bowel

C. Complete the following terms from their definitions:

1. ______________________ itis — Inflammation of the pancreas.
2. ______________________ ectomy — Removal of the gallbladder.
3. an ______________________ — Loss of appetite.
4. ______________________ itis — Inflammation of the third part of the small intestine.
5. ______________________ lithiasis — Abnormal condition of salivary stones.
6. enteric ana ______________________ — New opening between two previously unconnected parts of the intestine.
7. ______________________ plasty — Surgical repair of roof of the mouth.
8. ______________________ logist — One who studies the anus and rectum.
9. gluco ______________________ — Formation of new sugar from fats and protein.
10. peri ______________________ — Muscular wave-like movement of digestive tract walls.

Chapter Five

DIAGRAM QUIZ 1

Name: ______________________________

Label the diagram below using the structures listed. In addition, select the combining form(s) for each structure.

STRUCTURES

cheeks
gums
hard palate
lips
soft palate
teeth
tongue
tonsils
uvula

COMBINING FORMS
(Note: Some structures have more than one combining form. One combining form is used for two structures listed on the diagram)

bucc/o
cheil/o
dent/i
gingiv/o
gloss/o
labi/o
lingu/o
odont/o
palat/o
tonsill/o
uvul/o

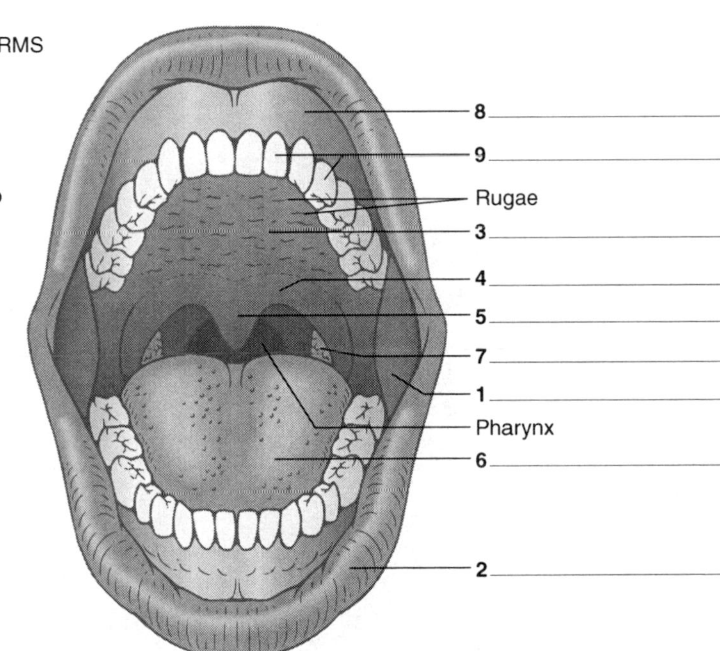

Chapter Five
DIAGRAM QUIZ 2

Name: ______________________

Label the diagram below using the terms listed below:

Anus	Descending colon	Ileum	Rectum
Appendix	Duodenum	Jejunum	Sigmoid colon
Ascending colon	Esophagus	Liver	Stomach
Cecum	Gallbladder	Pancreas	Transverse colon

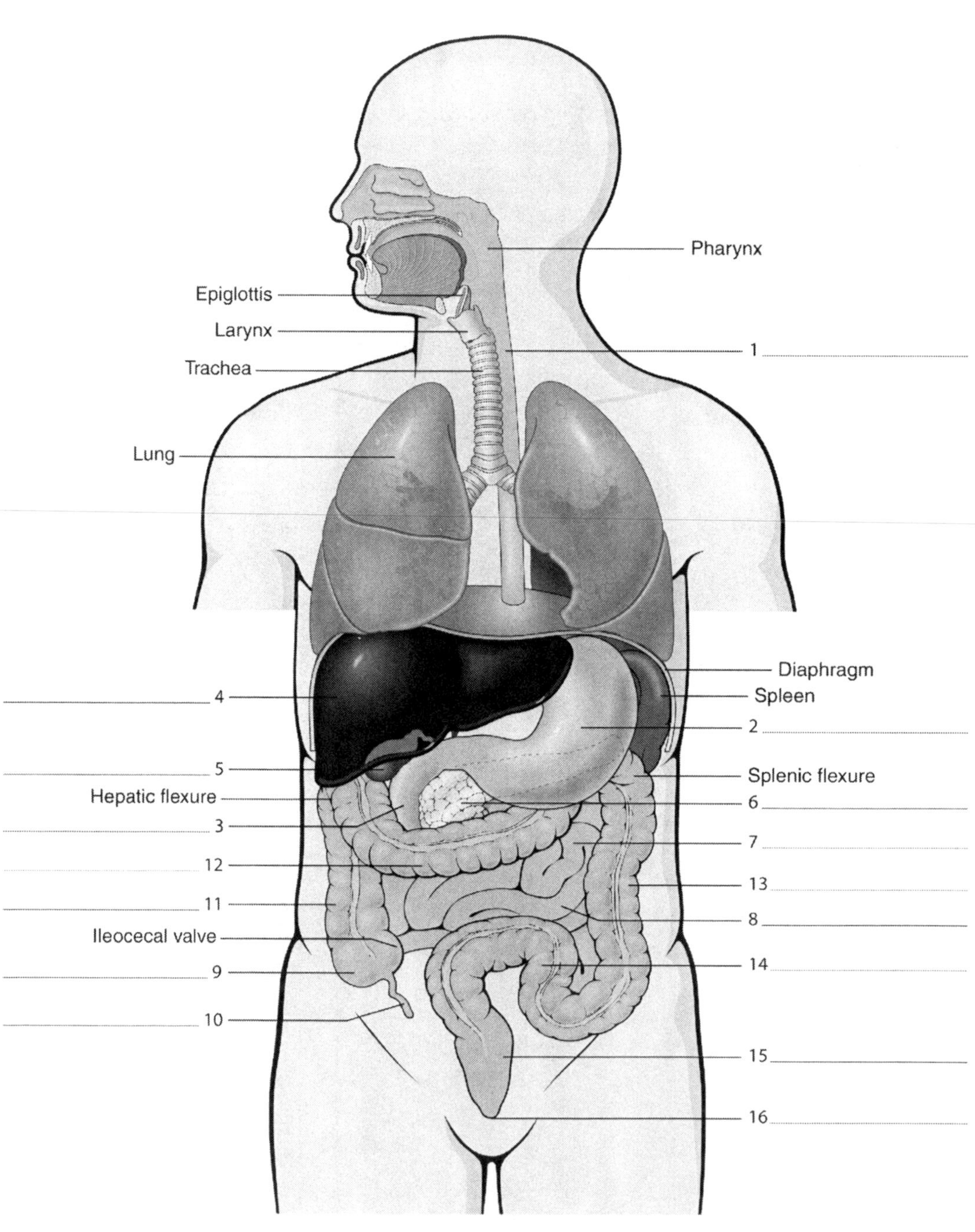

Chapter Five
DIAGRAM QUIZ 3

Name: ______________________________

Label the diagram using the terms listed below:

Common bile duct	Gallbladder	Pancreatic duct
Duodenum	Liver	Pancreas

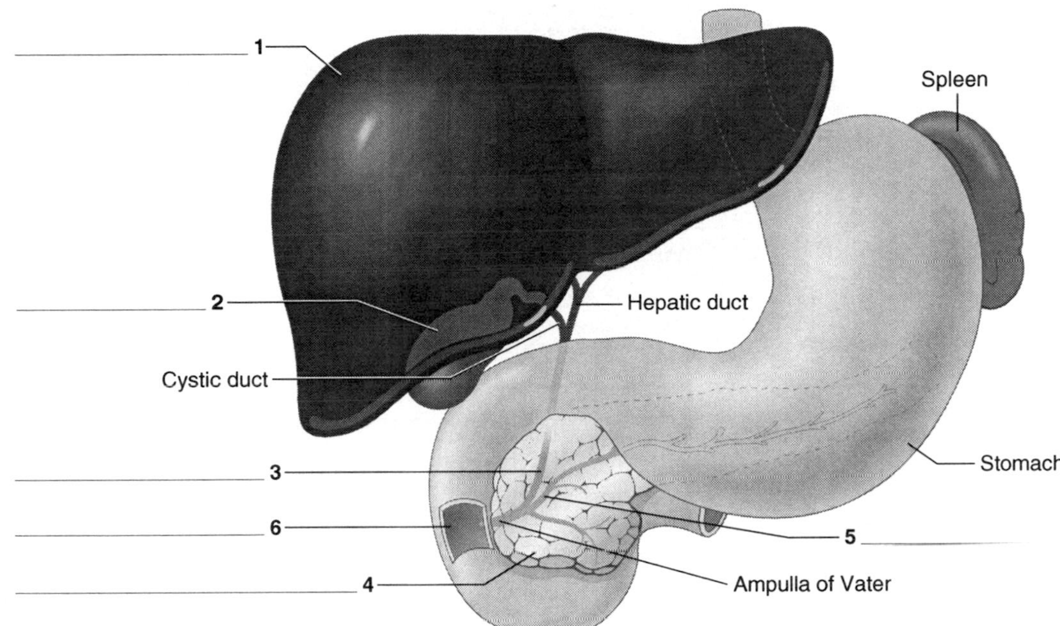

Chapter Five
FLOW CHART QUIZ

Name: ______________________________

Complete the following flow chart using the terms listed below:

anus
ascending colon
cecum
descending colon
duodenum
esophagus
gallbladder
ileum
jejunum
liver
oral cavity
pancreas
pharynx
rectum
salivary glands
sigmoid colon
stomach
transverse colon

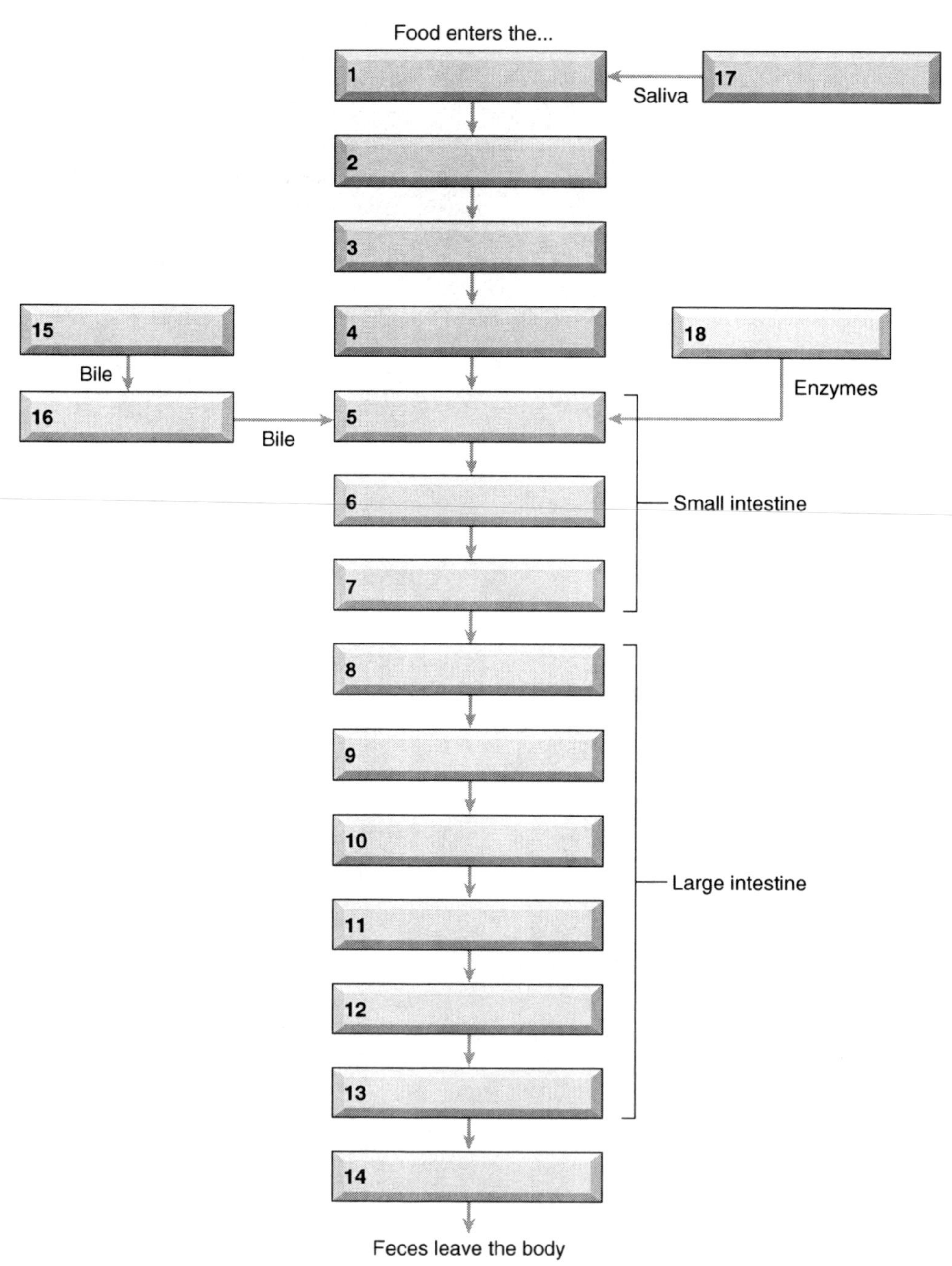

Chapter Five
MEDICAL SCRAMBLE

Name: ______________________________

Unscramble the letters to form suffixes from the clues. Use the letters in squares to complete the bonus term.

1. *Clue:* Yellow discoloration of skin

   ___ ___ ___ ☐ ___ ___ ___ ___ I C N A J U E D

2. *Clue:* Discharge of watery waste from colon

   ___ ☐ ___ ___ ___ ___ ___ ☐ A E R D H R A I

3. *Clue:* Fluid-filled enlargement of the abdomen

   ☐ ☐ ___ ___ ☐ ___ ☐ T A S S E I C

4. *Clue:* Rumbling, gurgling sounds from the GI tract

   ___ ☐ ___ ___ ___ ☐ ___ ___ ☐ ___ ☐ Y R O M O S G B R U B

BONUS TERM: *Clue:* Surgical reconnection of gastrointestinal organs.

☐ ☐ ☐ ☐ ☐ ☐ ☐ ☐ ☐ ☐ ☐

Chapter Five
CROSSWORD PUZZLE

Name: ______________________________

Fill in the crossword puzzle below using the clues listed underneath it.

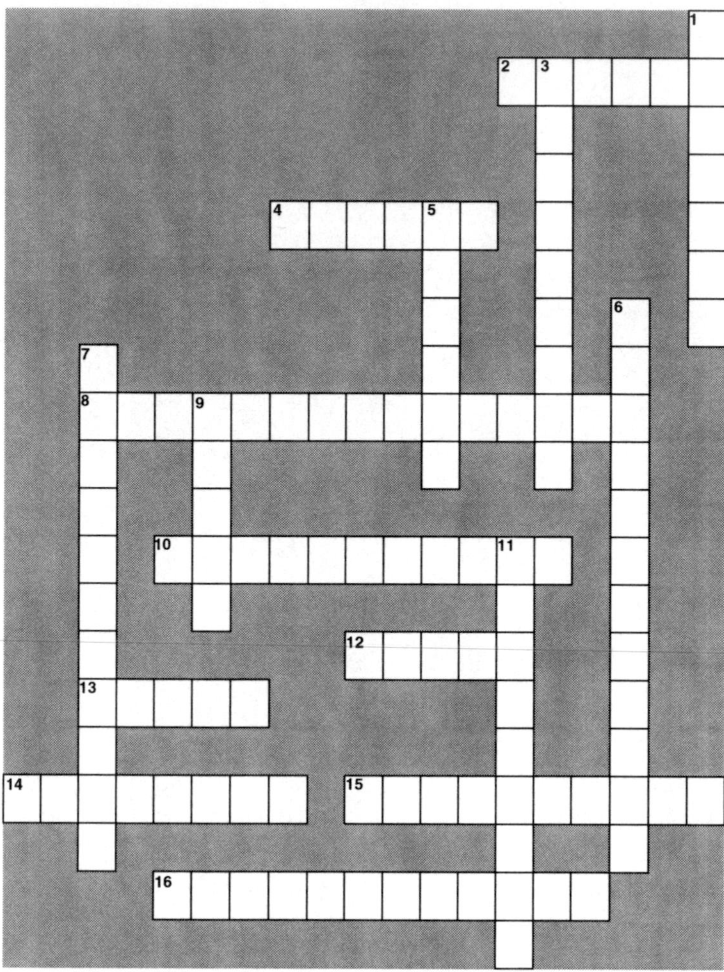

Across Clues

2. Decay.
4. Feces containing dark tarry blood.
8. Telescoping of the intestines.
10. Swollen, twisted, varicose veins in the rectal region.
12. Failure of peristalsis.
13. Chronic inflammation of the terminal ileum is called _____________ disease.
14. Twisting of the intestine upon itself.
15. Belching or raising gas from the stomach.
16. Lack of hydrochloric acid in the stomach.

Down Clues

1. Abnormal accumulation of fluid in the abdomen.
3. Failure of the muscles of the lower esophagus to relax during swallowing.
5. Unpleasant sensation from the stomach with a tendency to vomit.
6. Inflammation of the pancreas.
7. Abnormal side pockets in the intestinal wall.
9. Open sore or lesion of skin tissue.
11. Painful, inflamed intestines.

Chapter Five
ANSWERS TO THE QUIZZES

Multiple Choice Quiz

1. E
2. B
3. D
4. C
5. E
6. A
7. C
8. E
9. B
10. A
11. E
12. B
13. B
14. E
15. D
16. C
17. D
18. B
19. A
20. B
21. E
22. D
23. C
24. E
25. C

Vocabulary Quiz

A

1. deglutition
2. bilirubin
3. amino acids
4. dentin
5. defecation
6. absorption
7. amylase
8. enamel
9. emulsification
10. glucose
11. bile
12. fatty acids

B

1. peristalsis
2. lipase
3. glycogen
4. feces
5. palate
6. portal vein
7. hydrochloric acid
8. insulin
9. incisor
10. protease
11. LES
12. parotid gland

C

1. uvula
2. villi
3. pyloric sphincter
4. papillae
5. mastication
6. rugae
7. pulp
8. triglycerides

Terminology Quiz

A

1. cheilosis
2. perianal
3. cholecystectomy
4. celiac
5. colostomy
6. dentibuccal
7. colonoscopy
8. choledochotomy
9. buccal mucosa
10. cecal

B

1. appendicitis
2. facial
3. gingivitis
4. colonic
5. hepatoma
6. enterocolitis
7. appendectomy
8. gastrostomy
9. esophageal
10. duodenal

C

1. sublingual
2. mesentery
3. submandibular
4. laparoscopy
5. enteroenterostomy
6. labial
7. palatoplasty
8. parenteral
9. choledochojejunostomy
10. ileostomy

D

1. hepatomegaly
2. ileitis
3. gastrojejunostomy
4. orthodontist
5. periodontist
6. endodontist
7. pancreatitis
8. peritonitis
9. pharyngeal
10. proctologist
11. pyorrhea

E

1. uvulectomy
2. sigmoidoscopy
3. rectocele
4. cholecystolithiasis
5. stomatitis
6. palatopharyngoplasty
7. lithogenesis
8. biliary
9. pyloroplasty
10. sialadenectomy

F

1. amylase
2. hyperglycemia
3. hyperbilirubinemia
4. lipoma
5. protease
6. achlorhydria
7. sialolith
8. gluconeogenesis
9. lipase
10. choledocholithiasis
11. postprandial
12. steatorrhea

Pathology Quiz

A

1. hematochezia
2. eructation
3. anorexia
4. flatus
5. steatorrhea
6. nausea
7. jaundice (icterus)
8. ascites
9. dysphagia
10. diarrhea
11. borborygmus
12. constipation
13. melena

B

1. gastric cancer
2. esophageal varices
3. colonic polyps
4. aphthous stomatitis
5. dental caries
6. anal fistula
7. colorectal cancer
8. diverticulosis
9. Crohn disease (Crohn's)
10. dysentery
11. gastroesophageal reflux disease
12. esophageal cancer

C

1. intussusception
2. ulcerative colitis
3. periodontal disease
4. volvulus
5. oral leukoplakia
6. irritable bowel syndrome
7. ileus
8. hernia
9. peptic ulcer
10. hemorrhoids
11. herpetic stomatitis

D

1. cirrhosis
2. hepatitis
3. cholecystolithiasis
4. pancreatic cancer
5. pancreatitis

Exercise Quiz

A

1. ileum
2. pancreas
3. cecum
4. gallbladder
5. esophagus
6. colon
7. duodenum
8. pharynx

B

9. abdomen
10. tongue
11. mouth
12. lip

C

13. hepatomegaly
14. etiology
15. choledochotomy
16. palatoplasty
17. postprandial
18. choledochojejunostomy

D

19. appendicitis
20. peritonitis
21. colitis
22. cholecystitis
23. sialadenitis
24. enterocolitis
25. hepatitis
26. pancreatitis
27. stomatitis
28. gingivitis
29. ileitis

E

30. hemorrhoids
31. cirrhosis
32. ileus
33. cholecystolithiasis
34. ulcer
35. dysentery
36. hepatitis
37. ulcerative colitis
38. diverticula
39. irritable bowel syndrome

F

40. anorexia
41. hematochezia
42. ascites
43. diarrhea
44. flatus
45. steatorrhea

G

46. melena
47. mesentery
48. sublingual
49. hyperbilirubinemia
50. anastomosis

Dictation and Comprehension Quiz: Vocabulary

A

1. amino acids
2. amylase
3. bilirubin
4. common bile duct
5. deglutition
6. emulsification
7. feces
8. glucose
9. hydrochloric acid
10. insulin
11. lipase
12. mastication
13. papillae
14. parotid
15. peristalsis
16. pulp
17. pyloric sphincter
18. triglycerides
19. uvula
20. villi

B

6 Physical process of breaking down large fat globules into smaller parts
14 Salivary gland near the ear
5 Swallowing
1 Small substances that are produced when proteins are digested
3 Pigment released by the liver in bile
16 Soft inner tissue within a tooth containing nerves and blood vessels
20 Microscopic projections in the walls of the small intestine
15 Rhythm-like contractions of the tubes of the alimentary tract
10 Hormone produced by the endocrine cells of the pancreas
4 This tube carries bile from the liver and gallbladder into the duodenum
13 Small nipple-like elevations on the tongue
19 Soft tissue hanging from the roof of the mouth
2 An enzyme to digest starch
12 Chewing
8 Simple sugar
9 Substance produced by the stomach and necessary for digestion of foods
7 Solid wastes; stools
11 Pancreatic enzyme necessary to digest fats
17 Ring of muscle at the distal region of the stomach
18 Large fat molecules

Dictation and Comprehension Quiz: Pathologic Symptoms

A

1. anorexia
2. ascites
3. borborygmus
4. constipation
5. diarrhea
6. dysphagia
7. flatus
8. hematochezia
9. jaundice
10. melena
11. nausea
12. steatorrhea

B

12 Feces containing fat
11 Unpleasant sensation from the stomach with tendency to vomit
7 Gas expelled through the anus
1 Lack of appetite
8 Bright red fresh blood from the rectum
4 Difficult, delayed elimination of feces
10 Black tarry stools; feces containing blood
9 Yellow-orange skin; icterus
3 Rumbling or gurgling noises produced by the movement of gas or fluid
6 Difficulty in swallowing
5 Loose, liquid stools
2 Abnormal accumulation of fluid in the peritoneal cavity

Dictation and Comprehension Quiz: Pathologic Conditions

A

1. achalasia
2. anal fistula
3. aphthous stomatitis
4. cholecystolithiasis
5. cirrhosis
6. colonic polyps
7. Crohn disease
8. dental caries
9. diverticulitis
10. peptic ulcer
11. dysentery
12. esophageal varices
13. gastroesophageal reflux disease
14. hepatitis
15. ileus
16. intussusception
17. pancreatitis
18. periodontal disease
19. ulcerative colitis
20. volvulus

B

18 Inflammation and degeneration of gums
20 Twisting of the intestine upon itself
6 Small benign growths protruding from the mucous membrane of the large bowel
16 Telescoping of the intestines
13 Solids and fluids return to the mouth from the stomach
4 Gallbladder calculi
14 Inflammation of the liver; viral etiology
5 Chronic liver disease; etiology is often alcoholism and malnutrition
10 Sore or lesion of the mucous membrane of the first part of the small intestine
2 Abnormal tube-like passageway in the distal end of the alimentary tract
11 Painful inflamed intestines; etiology is often bacterial
12 Swollen, tortuous veins in the distal portion of the tube connecting the throat and stomach
17 Inflammation of a gland behind the stomach; cysts may form
9 Inflammation of small side pockets in the intestinal wall
19 Chronic inflammation of the large bowel with open sores of mucous membrane
7 Chronic inflammation of the intestinal tract (terminal ileum)
15 Failure of peristalsis
1 Failure of the LES muscle to relax
3 Inflammation of the mouth with open sores
8 Tooth decay

Spelling Quiz

A

1. pancreatitis—inflammation of the pancreas
2. anal fistula—abnormal tube-like opening in the anus
3. dental caries—tooth decay
4. colitis—inflammation of the colon
5. ileus—intestinal obstruction
6. ascites—abnormal collection of fluid in the abdomen
7. melena—dark tarry blood in the feces
8. polyposis—abnormal condition of polyps (small growths)
9. dysentery—abnormal, painful intestines
10. anorexia—loss of appetite

B

11. mesentery
12. cholecystectomy
13. volvulus
14. Crohn disease
15. biliary
16. jaundice
17. parotid gland
18. achalasia
19. parenteral
20. anastomosis

Pronunciation Quiz

A

1. aphthous stomatitis
2. dysentery
3. choledocholithiasis
4. leukoplakia
5. esophageal varices
6. pyloric sphincter
7. biliary
8. cheilitis
9. diverticula
10. volvulus

B

1. G
2. D
3. J
4. B
5. H
6. F
7. C
8. A
9. I
10. E

C

1. pancreatitis
2. cholecystectomy
3. anorexia
4. ileitis
5. sialolithiasis
6. enteric anastomosis
7. palatoplasty
8. proctologist
9. gluconeogenesis
10. peristalsis

Diagram Quiz 1

1.	cheeks	bucc/o
2.	lips	cheil/o, labi/o
3.	hard palate	palat/o
4.	soft palate	palat/o
5.	uvula	uvul/o
6.	tongue	gloss/o, lingu/o
7.	tonsils	tonsill/o
8.	gums	gingiv/o
9.	teeth	dent/i, odont/o

Diagram Quiz 2

1. Esophagus
2. Stomach
3. Duodenum
4. Liver
5. Gallbladder
6. Pancreas
7. Jejunum
8. Ileum
9. Cecum
10. Appendix
11. Ascending colon
12. Transverse colon
13. Descending colon
14. Sigmoid colon
15. Rectum
16. Anus

Diagram Quiz 3

1. liver
2. gallbladder
3. common bile duct
4. pancreas
5. pancreatic duct
6. duodenum

FLOW CHART QUIZ

1. oral cavity
2. pharynx
3. esophagus
4. stomach
5. duodenum
6. jejunum
7. ileum
8. cecum
9. ascending colon
10. transverse colon
11. descending colon
12. sigmoid colon
13. rectum
14. anus
15. liver
16. gallbladder
17. salivary glands
18. pancreas

Medical Scramble

1. JAUNDICE
2. DIARRHEA
3. ASCITES
4. BORBORYGMUS

BONUS TERM: ANASTOMOSIS

Crossword Puzzle

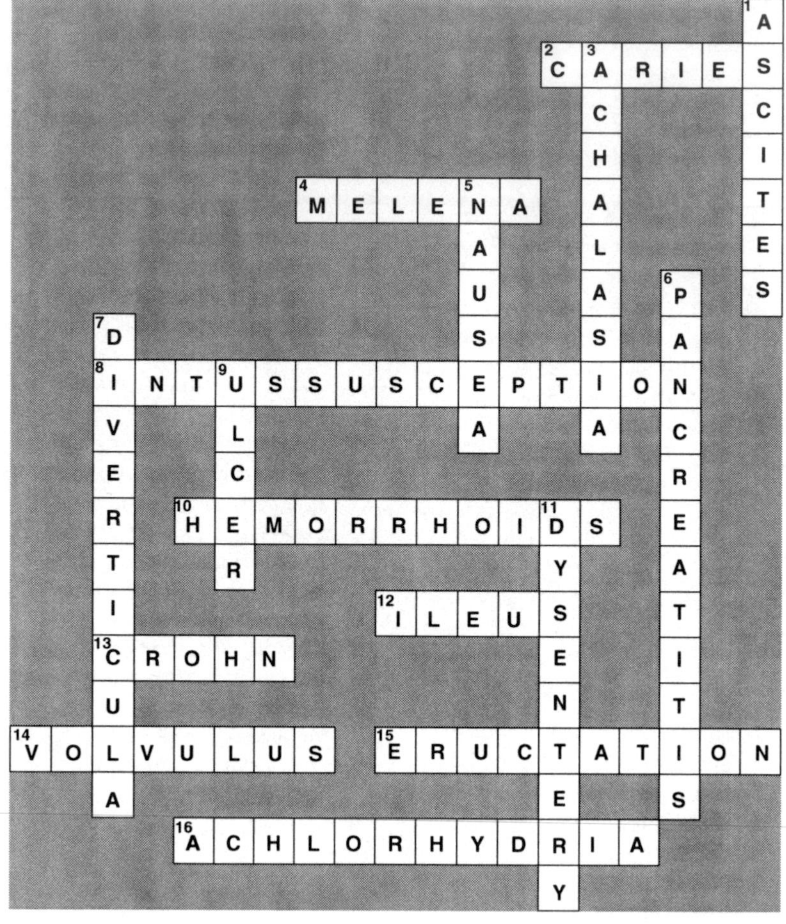

Chapter Five

Answers to Terminology Section

(textbook pages 153–158)

Terminology	Meaning
Parts of the Body	
perianal	Pertaining to surrounding the anus.
appendectomy	Removal (resection) of the appendix.
appendicitis	Inflammation of the appendix.
buccal mucosa	The mucous membrane (mucosa) lining the cheek.
cecal	Pertaining to the cecum.
celiac	Pertaining to the abdomen.
cheilosis	Abnormal condition of the lips.
cholecystectomy	Removal of the gallbladder.
choledochotomy	Incision of the common bile duct.
colostomy	New opening of the colon to the outside of the body.
colonic	Pertaining to the colon.
colonoscopy	Process of visual examination of the colon.
dentibuccal	Pertaining to tooth and cheek.
duodenal	Pertaining to the duodenum (first part of the small intestine).
enterocolitis	Inflammation of the small and large intestines.
enteroenterostomy	New opening between two previously unconnected parts of the small intestine.
mesentery	Membrane that holds the intestines together (literally, middle of the intestines).
parenteral	Pertaining to apart from the intestines (refers to delivery of substances any way other than through the digestive tract).
esophageal	Pertaining to the esophagus.
facial	Pertaining to the face.
gastrostomy	New opening into the stomach through the abdominal wall. This may be necessary to introduce food into the stomach.
gingivitis	Inflammation of the gums.
hypoglossal	Pertaining to under the tongue.
hepatoma	Tumor (malignant) of the liver; hepatocellular carcinoma.
hepatomegaly	Enlargement of the liver.
ileocecal sphincter	Pertaining to the ring of muscles between the ileum and the cecum.
ileitis	Inflammation of the ileum.
ileostomy	New opening of the ileum to the outside of the body.
choledochojejunostomy	New opening between the common bile duct and the jejunum; anastomosis.
gastrojejunostomy	New opening between the stomach and the jejunum; anastomosis.
labial	Pertaining to the lip.
laparoscopy	Visual examination of the abdomen.
sublingual	Pertaining to under the tongue.
submandibular	Pertaining to under the lower jaw.
orthodontist	Dentist specializing in straightening teeth.
periodontist	Dentist specializing in gums.
endodontist	Dentist specializing in operating within the tooth (root canal specialist).
oral	Pertaining to the mouth.
palatoplasty	Surgical repair of the palate.

pancreatitis	Inflammation of the pancreas.
peritonitis	Inflammation of the peritoneum.
pharyngeal	Pertaining to the throat.
palatopharyngoplasty	Surgical repair of the palate and throat.
proctologist	Specialist in the anus and rectum.
pyloroplasty	Surgical repair of the pyloric sphincter.
rectocele	Hernia of the rectum.
sialadenitis	Inflammation of salivary glands.
sigmoidoscopy	Visual examination of the sigmoid colon.
stomatitis	Inflammation of the mouth.
uvulectomy	Removal of the uvula.

Substances

amylase	Enzyme that digests starch.
biliary	Pertaining to bile.
hyperbilirubinemia	Excess bilirubin in the blood; jaundice.
cholelithiasis	Abnormal condition of gallstones.
achlorhydria	Lack of hydrochloric acid.
gluconeogenesis	Production of new sugar from proteins and fats (by the liver).
hyperglycemia	High blood sugar.
glycogenolysis	Breakdown of glycogen to form sugar (glucose).
lipoma	Tumor of fat (benign).
lithogenesis	Formation of a stone (calculus).
protease	Enzyme that digests protein.
pyorrhea	Discharge of pus from gums.
sialolith	Salivary (gland) stone.
steatorrhea	Discharge of fats (in feces).

Suffixes

lipase	Enzyme to digest fats.
hematochezia	Bright red blood in the feces.
choledocholithiasis	Condition of stones in the common bile duct.
postprandial	Pertaining to after meals.

Chapter 6

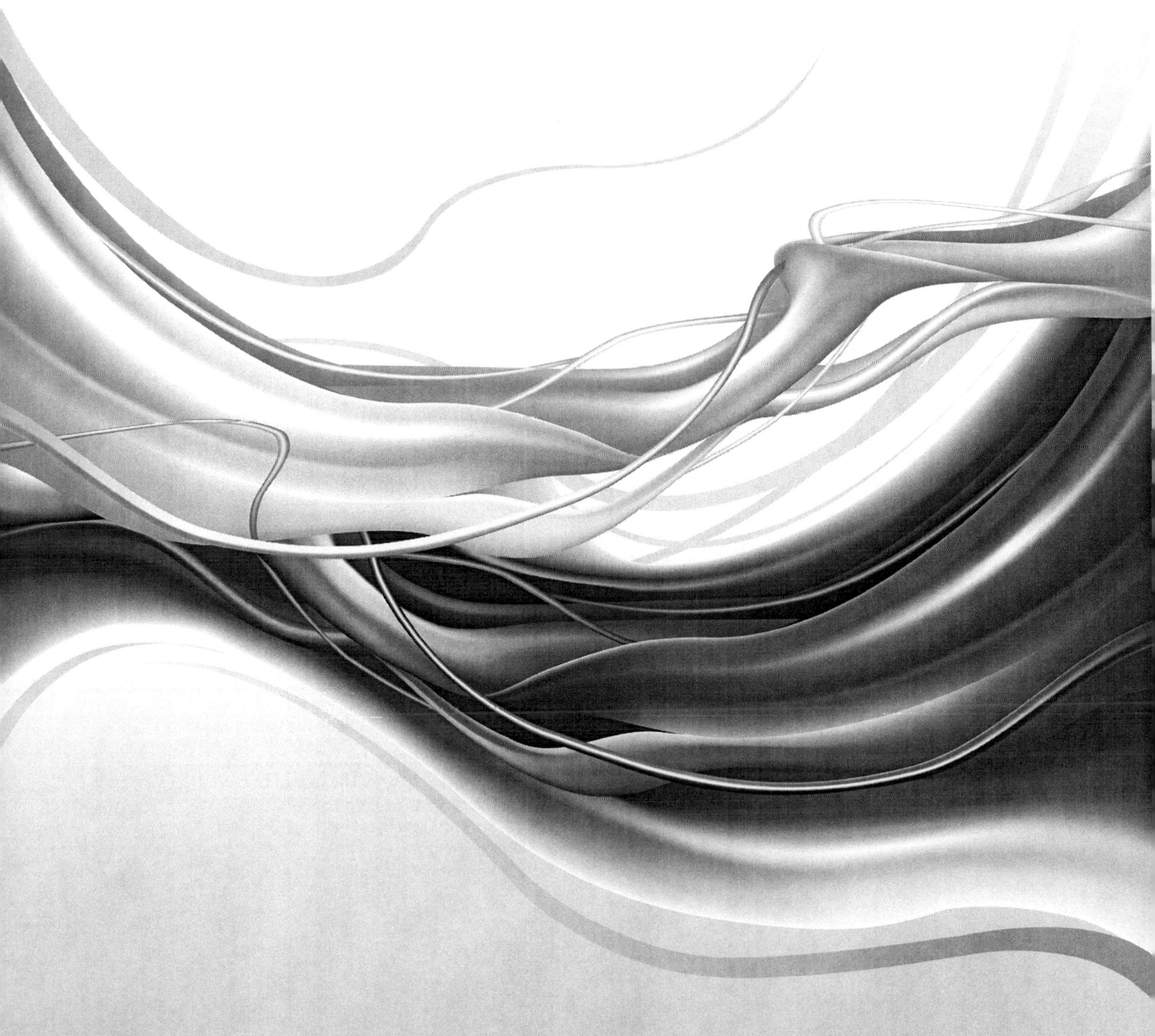

Chapter Six
MULTIPLE CHOICE QUIZ

Name: ______________________

In the box write the letter of the choice that is the definition of the term or best answers the question. There is only one correct answer for each question.

1. Spitting up blood from the respiratory tract and lungs: ....
A. Hyperemesis
B. Hematemesis
C. Hemorrhage
D. Hemoptysis
E. Hemolysis

2. Suture: ....
A. -rrhapy
B. -rrhagia
C. -ectasis
D. -stasis
E. -rrhaphy

3. New opening between two parts of the jejunum: ....
A. Jejunojejunostomy
B. Duodenostomy
C. Duodenojejunostomy
D. Jejunostomy
E. Jejunocecal anastomosis

4. Dilation of a bile vessel: ....
A. Cholecystolithiasis
B. Cholangitis
C. Cholangiography
D. Cholangiectasis
E. Choledocholithiasis

5. Difficult digestion: ....
A. Deglutition
B. Dysphagia
C. Aphagia
D. Polyphagia
E. Dyspepsia

6. Pyloric stenosis: ....
A. Gastric ulcer
B. Narrowing of the opening between the stomach and intestine
C. Hiatal hernia
D. Cardiospasm
E. Achalasia

7. Which test would tell the presence of melena? ....
A. Barium enema
B. Upper GI series
C. Stool culture
D. Stool guaiac
E. Abdominal ultrasonography

8. A stomach ulcer would most likely be detected by which of the following tests? ....
A. Cholecystography
B. Serum hepatitis B surface antigen
C. Intravenous cholangiogram
D. Gastroscopy
E. Colonoscopy

9. Esophageal atresia: ....
A. New opening of the esophagus into the stomach
B. Esophagus is dilated
C. Esophageal sphincter will not relax
D. Esophagus does not open to the stomach at birth
E. Twisted veins around the esophagus

10. Bursting forth of blood from the spleen: ....
A. Spleenorrhagia
B. Splenorrhagia
C. Splenomegaly
D. Spleenomegaly
E. Spleenectasis

11. Lipase is: ....
A. An enzyme that digests starch
B. An enzyme that digests protein
C. An enzyme that digests fat
D. A breakdown product of fat digestion
E. A hormone secreted by the pancreas

12. Palatoplasty: ....
A. Surgical repair of the roof of the mouth
B. Overgrowth of gum tissue
C. Surgical repair of the tongue
D. Cleft palate
E. Prolapse of the palate

13. **Which test is NOT a liver function test?** ....
   A. Serum bilirubin
   B. ALP (alkaline phosphatase)
   C. Endoscopic retrograde cholangiopancreatography (ERCP)
   D. AST
   E. ALT

14. **Which test would demonstrate choledocholithiasis?** ....
   A. Transhepatic cholangiography
   B. Barium enema
   C. Gastric intubation
   D. Upper GI series
   E. Gastric endoscopy

15. **Opposite of -ectasis:** ....
   A. -stenosis
   B. -ptysis
   C. -spasm
   D. -stasis
   E. -lysis

16. **Flow, discharge:** ....
   A. -ptysis
   B. -emesis
   C. -rrhaphy
   D. -rrhea
   E. -phagia

17. **Anastomosis:** ....
   A. Ileostomy
   B. Duodenorrhaphy
   C. Cholecystojejunostomy
   D. Colostomy
   E. Gingivectomy

18. **Common bile duct:** ....
   A. Cholecyst/o
   B. Celi/o
   C. Cholelith/o
   D. Choledoch/o
   E. Cheil/o

19. **Surgical repair of eyelid:** ....
   A. Abdominoplasty
   B. Blepharoplasty
   C. Blepharoptosis
   D. Rectocele
   E. Herniorrhaphy

20. **Surgical puncture to remove fluid from the abdomen:** ....
   A. Cholestasis
   B. Dyspepsia
   C. Hemostasis
   D. Ascites
   E. Paracentesis

21. **Twisting of part of the intestine upon itself:** ....
   A. Proctosigmoidoscopy
   B. Cecal volvulus
   C. Pyloric stenosis
   D. Biliary atresia
   E. Rectal stenosis

22. **Periodontal procedure:** ....
   A. Glossotomy
   B. Glycolysis
   C. Gingivectomy
   D. Biliary lithotripsy
   E. Cheilostomatoplasty

23. **Discharge of blood from the stomach:** ....
   A. Diarrhea
   B. Herniorrhaphy
   C. Hemoptysis
   D. Gastrorrhagia
   E. Steatorrhea

24. **Visual examination of the abdomen:** ....
   A. Laparoscopy
   B. Colonoscopy
   C. Liver scan
   D. Colectomy
   E. Enterorrhaphy

25. **Salivary stones:** ....
   A. Lithotripsy
   B. Cholecystolithiasis
   C. Sialolithiasis
   D. Renal calculi
   E. Nephroptosis

Chapter Six
SUFFIXES AND TERMINOLOGY QUIZ

Name: ______________________________

A. *Choose from the following meanings, and write each next to the suffix below:*

bursting forth of blood
digestion
eating, swallowing
flow, discharge
involuntary contraction of muscles
opening
spitting
stopping, controlling
stretching, dilation, widening
surgical repair
suture
tightening, narrowing, stricture
vomiting

1. -spasm ______________________________
2. -stenosis ______________________________
3. -emesis ______________________________
4. -phagia ______________________________
5. -ectasis, -ectasia ______________________________
6. -pepsia ______________________________
7. -rrhea ______________________________
8. -rrhaphy ______________________________
9. -rrhage, -rrhagia ______________________________
10. -plasty ______________________________
11. -ptysis ______________________________
12. -tresia ______________________________
13. -stasis ______________________________

B. *Match the following medical terms with their meanings below:*

buccal
cecal volvulus
celiac disease
cheilosis
cholelithiasis
cholangitis
cholecystectomy
choledochal
colectomy
colonoscopy
dentalgia
duodenal

1. Excision of the large intestine ______________________________
2. Abnormal condition of lips ______________________________
3. Pertaining to the first portion of the small intestine ______________________________

4. Pertaining to the common bile duct ____________________
5. Inflammation of bile vessels ____________________
6. Autoimmune condition in which villi in the small intestine are damaged ____________________
7. Pertaining to the cheek ____________________
8. Visual examination of the large intestine ____________________
9. Abnormal condition of gallstones ____________________
10. Excision of the gallbladder ____________________
11. Tooth pain ____________________
12. Twisting of the first portion of the large intestine ____________________

C. Match the following medical terms with their meanings below:

cholecystojejunostomy
esophageal atresia
gastroenteritis
gastrojejunostomy
gastrostomy
gingivectomy
glossectomy
gluconeogenesis
hepatomegaly
herniorrhaphy
ileostomy
labiodental

1. Suture of a hernia ____________________
2. New opening of the stomach to the outside of the body ____________________
3. Production of new sugar (by liver cells) ____________________
4. Enlargement of the liver ____________________
5. New opening of the stomach and second part of the small intestine (an anastomosis) ____________________
6. No opening of the esophagus to the stomach (congenital anomaly) ____________________
7. Inflammation of the stomach and small intestine ____________________
8. New opening of the third part of the small intestine to the outside of the body ____________________
9. Removal of gum tissue ____________________
10. New opening of the gallbladder and the second part of the small intestine (an anastomosis) ____________________
11. Pertaining to the lip and tooth (surface of the tooth facing the lip) ____________________
12. Excision of the tongue ____________________

D. Match the following medical terms with their meanings below:

cholecystolithiasis
lipase
oropharynx
palatoplasty
pancreatoduodenectomy
periodontal membrane
proctosigmoidoscopy
pyloric stenosis
sialadenectomy
splenic flexure
steatorrhea
sublingual

1. Surgical repair of the palate ______________________
2. Narrowing of the distal gastric sphincter ______________________
3. Visual examination of the rectum and the anus ______________________
4. Enzyme that digests fat ______________________
5. Tissue surrounding a tooth ______________________
6. Removal of the pancreas and first part of the small intestine ______________________
7. Bending of the intestine in the area of the spleen ______________________
8. Abnormal condition of stones in the gallbladder ______________________
9. Discharge of fat (in feces) ______________________
10. Removal of a salivary gland ______________________
11. Pertaining to under the tongue ______________________
12. Region of the throat near the mouth ______________________

E. Match the following laboratory tests and clinical procedures with the phrases below:

abdominal ultrasonography
CT scan
ERCP
gastric bypass
GI endoscopy
laparoscopy
liver function tests
lower GI series
MRI
nasogastric intubation
paracentesis
stool culture
stool guaiac
upper GI series

1. Visual examination of the abdomen with an endoscope inserted through a small incision ______________________
2. Sound waves beamed into the abdomen produce an image of abdominal viscera ______________________
3. Contrast medium is injected via catheter through the mouth to bile ducts and x-ray images are produced ______________________
4. Test to detect microorganisms in feces ______________________
5. Series of x-ray images are taken in multiple views (especially in cross-section) ______________________

6. Test to detect occult blood in feces ______________________________
7. Barium enema ______________________________
8. Serum tests for enzymes and bilirubin ______________________________
9. Magnetic waves produce images of organs and tissues in all three planes of the body ______________________________
10. Bariatric surgery for weight loss ______________________________
11. Surgical puncture to remove fluid from the abdomen ______________________________
12. Sigmoidoscopy and esophagoduodenoscopy are examples ______________________________
13. Insertion of a tube through the nose and into the stomach ______________________________
14. Barium swallow and small bowel follow-through are examples of this type of diagnostic procedure ______________________________

Chapter Six
EXERCISE QUIZ

Name: ______________________

A. Give the meanings for the following suffixes:

1. -pepsia ______________
2. -ptysis ______________
3. -emesis ______________
4. -rrhagia ______________
5. -phagia ______________
6. -plasty ______________
7. -rrhaphy ______________
8. -ectasis ______________
9. -stenosis ______________
10. -stasis ______________
11. -lysis ______________
12. -rrhea ______________

B. Give meanings for the following terms:

13. polyphagia ______________
14. dyspepsia ______________
15. esophageal atresia ______________

C. Match the following surgical procedures with their meanings below:

blepharoplasty
cecostomy
cholecystectomy
gastroduodenal anastomosis
gingivectomy
herniorrhaphy
paracentesis
sphincterotomy

16. surgical repair of the eyelid ______________
17. incision of a ring of muscles ______________
18. removal of the gallbladder ______________
19. suture of a weakened muscular wall ______________
20. new surgical connection between the stomach and the first part of the small intestine ______________
21. new opening of the first part of the colon to the outside of the body ______________
22. removal of gum tissue ______________
23. surgical puncture of the abdomen for withdrawal of fluid ______________

D. Build medical terms:

24. difficult swallowing ____________________
25. pertaining to the cheek ____________________
26. enlargement of the liver ____________________
27. discharge of fat (in feces) ____________________
28. pertaining to under the tongue ____________________
29. pertaining to the common bile duct ____________________

E. Give meanings for the following terms:

30. aphthous stomatitis ____________________
31. lipase ____________________
32. cheilosis ____________________
33. sialadenectomy ____________________
34. periodontal membrane ____________________
35. colectomy ____________________

F. Match the name of the laboratory test or clinical procedure with its description:

abdominal ultrasonography	liver biopsy	serum bilirubin
barium enema	liver scan	stool culture
CT of the abdomen	nasogastric intubation	stool guaiac (Hemoccult)
endoscopic retrograde cholangiopancreatography	percutaneous transhepatic cholangiography	upper gastrointestinal series

36. tube is inserted through the nose into the stomach ____________________
37. measurement of bile pigment in the blood ____________________
38. x-ray examination of the lower gastrointestinal tract ____________________
39. test to reveal hidden blood in feces ____________________
40. sound waves are used to image abdominal organs ____________________
41. feces are placed in a growth medium for bacterial analysis ____________________
42. percutaneous removal of liver tissue followed by microscopic analysis ____________________
43. contrast material is injected through an endoscope and x-rays taken of the pancreas and bile ducts ____________________
44. radioactive material is injected and image recorded of uptake in liver cells ____________________
45. transverse x-ray pictures of abdominal organs ____________________
46. x-ray images of the esophagus, stomach, and small intestine after administering barium by mouth ____________________
47. contrast material is injected through the liver and x-rays are taken of bile vessels ____________________

Chapter Six
DICTATION AND COMPREHENSION QUIZ

Name: ______________________________

A. Dictation of Terms

1. ______________________ 11. ______________________
2. ______________________ 12. ______________________
3. ______________________ 13. ______________________
4. ______________________ 14. ______________________
5. ______________________ 15. ______________________
6. ______________________ 16. ______________________
7. ______________________ 17. ______________________
8. ______________________ 18. ______________________
9. ______________________ 19. ______________________
10. ______________________ 20. ______________________

B. Comprehension of Terms: Match number of the above term with its meaning below.

_____ Difficult digestion
_____ Vomiting blood
_____ Bursting forth of blood
_____ Gingivitis
_____ Dilation of a bile vessel
_____ Food tube is not connected to the stomach from birth
_____ Suture of an abdominal protrusion
_____ Surgical repair of the lip and mouth
_____ Removal of the large bowel
_____ Pertaining to the common bile duct
_____ Spitting up blood
_____ Pertaining to the cheek
_____ An anastomosis
_____ Difficult swallowing
_____ Removal of gum tissue
_____ Removal of the gallbladder
_____ Discharge of watery fecal material
_____ Narrowing of a ring of muscles
_____ Ulcers and inflammation of the mouth
_____ Pertaining to the tongue and throat

Chapter Six
SPELLING QUIZ

Name: ____________________

A. Circle the term that is spelled correctly and write its meaning in the space provided:

1.	herniorrhapy	herniorrhaphy ________
2.	hematemesis	hematemisis ________
3.	hemmorhage	hemorrhage ________
4.	colestasis	cholestasis ________
5.	pylorospasm	plyorspasm ________
6.	choleangiectasis	cholangiectasis ________
7.	blepharophlasty	blepharoplasty ________
8.	choleductal	choledochal ________
9.	glossotomy	glosotomy ________
10.	stenosis	stanosis ________

B. Circle the term that is spelled correctly. The meaning of each term is given.

11.	Abnormal condition of the lip.................. cheilosis	chielosis	cielosis
12.	Pertaining to the cheek............................ buckel	buckal	buccal
13.	Discharge of blood from the stomach....... gastorrhagia	gastrrhagia	gastrorrhagia
14.	Record of bile vessels................................ colangiogram	cholangiogram	choleangiogram
15.	Not open.. treesia	atresia	atrezia
16.	Spitting up blood...................................... hemmoptsyis	hemotisis	hemoptysis
17.	Enlargement of the liver .... hepatomeagaly	hepatomegaly	hepatomegely
18.	Difficult swallowing.................................. dysfagia	disphagia	dysphagia
19.	Discharge of pus .... plyorrhea	pyorrhea	pyorhea
20.	Pertaining to the abdomen .... cieliac	celiac	sealiac

Chapter Six
PRONUNCIATION QUIZ

Name: ______________________________

A. Underline the accented syllable in the following terms:

1. hemoptysis
2. gingivectomy
3. cholestasis
4. diarrhea
5. cholangiectasis
6. herniorrhaphy
7. glycolysis
8. cholecystolithiasis
9. colonoscopy
10. lipase

B. Match the term in Column I with its meaning in Column II:

Column I		Column II
1. -rrhagia	______	A. New opening
2. -rrhea	______	B. Suture
3. -tomy	______	C. Flow; discharge
4. -phagia	______	D. Narrowing
5. -plasty	______	E. Widening; dilation
6. -spasm	______	F. Discharge of blood
7. -rrhaphy	______	G. Surgical repair
8. -stenosis	______	H. Swallowing, eating
9. -stomy	______	I. Involuntary muscular contraction
10. -ectasis	______	J. Incision
		K. Removal

C. Complete the following terms from their definitions:

1. dys ______________________________ Difficult digestion.
2. dys ______________________________ Difficult swallowing.
3. hemat ____________________________ Vomiting blood.
4. gloss _____________________________ Incision of the tongue.
5. ________________________________ al Pertaining to the cheek.
6. ___________________________ orrhea Discharge of fat.
7. hepato ___________________________ Enlargement of the liver.
8. entero ___________________________ Suture of the small intestine.
9. a _________________________________ No opening.
10. a ______________________ stomatitis Inflammation of the mouth with small ulcers.

Chapter Six

REVIEW SHEET QUIZ

Name: ________________________

A. Give meanings for the following combining forms:

1. amyl/o ____________
2. an/o ____________
3. appendic/o ____________
4. bil/i ____________
5. bronch/o ____________
6. celi/o ____________
7. cheil/o ____________
8. cholangi/o ____________
9. cib/o ____________
10. col/o ____________
11. dent/i ____________
12. duoden/o ____________
13. enter/o ____________
14. esophag/o ____________
15. eti/o ____________
16. gloss/o ____________
17. glyc/o ____________
18. hem/o ____________
19. herni/o ____________
20. lapar/o ____________

B. Give combining forms for the following meanings:

1. cheek ____________
2. gallbladder ____________
3. common bile duct ____________
4. stomach ____________
5. liver ____________
6. ileum ____________
7. jejunum ____________
8. stone ____________
9. pancreas ____________
10. throat ____________

C. Give meanings for the following combining forms:

1. labi/o ____________
2. lingu/o ____________
3. lip/o ____________
4. cholangi/o ____________
5. mandibul/o ____________
6. abdomin/o ____________
7. odont/o ____________
8. py/o ____________
9. or/o ____________
10. peritone/o ____________
11. proct/o ____________
12. prote/o ____________

13. pylor/o ____________
14. rect/o ____________
15. sialaden/o ____________
16. sigmoid/o ____________
17. splen/o ____________
18. steat/o ____________
19. stomat/o ____________
20. tonsill/o ____________

D. Give meanings for the following suffixes:

1. -ase ____________
2. -centesis ____________
3. -chezia ____________
4. -ectasia ____________
5. -ectomy ____________
6. -spasm ____________
7. -emia ____________
8. -genesis ____________
9. -graphy ____________
10. -iasis ____________
11. -lysis ____________
12. -megaly ____________
13. -orexia ____________
14. -pathy ____________
15. -pepsia ____________
16. -phagia ____________
17. -plasty ____________
18. -prandial ____________
19. -ptosis ____________
20. -tresia ____________

E. Give suffixes for the following meanings:

1. bursting forth of blood ____________
2. suture ____________
3. flow, discharge ____________
4. process of visual examination ____________
5. narrowing, tightening ____________
6. new opening ____________
7. to stop, control ____________
8. incision ____________
9. spitting ____________
10. vomiting ____________

Chapter Six
MEDICAL SCRAMBLE

Name: ______________________

Unscramble the letters to form suffixes from the clues. Use the letters in the squares to complete the bonus term.

1. *Clue*: Narrowing

   – ___ ___ ___ ☐ ☐ ___ ___ ___ OTSESSNI

2. *Clue*: Bursting forth of blood

   – ☐ ___ ☐ ___ ___ ___ ___ GRAIRAH

3. *Clue*: Spitting

   – ☐ ___ ☐ ___ ___ ___ SPSTIY

4. *Clue*: Vomiting

   – ☐ ___ ___ ___ ☐ ___ SMIESE

5. *Clue*: Flow, discharge

   – ☐ ☐ ☐ ___ ___ HARER

6. *Clue*: Eating or swallowing

   – ___ ☐ ☐ ___ ___ ___ AGPAHI

BONUS TERM: ***Clue:*** This common surgical procedure fixes a bulge or protrusion

☐ ☐ ☐ ☐ ☐ ☐ ☐ ☐ ☐ ☐ ☐ ☐ ☐

Chapter Six

CROSSWORD PUZZLE

Name: ______________________

Fill in the crossword puzzle below using the clues listed underneath it.

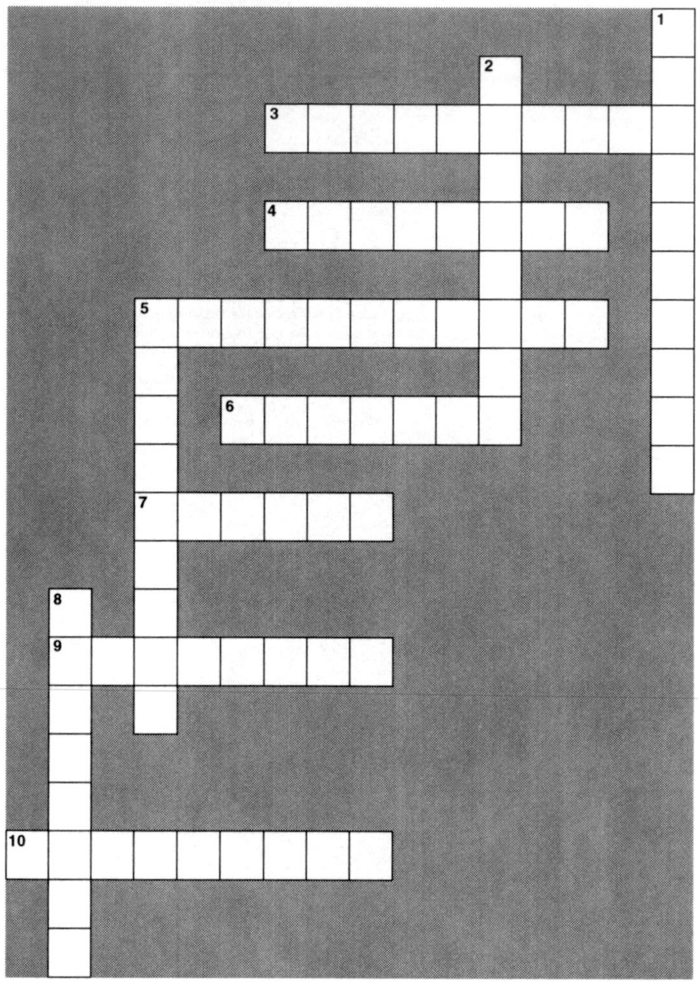

Across Clues

3. -phagia
4. -ectasis means stretching, widening, or __________.
5. -lysis means separation or __________.
6. -tresia
7. -rrhaphy
9. -ptosis means to sag or __________.
10. -rrhea means flow or __________.

Down Clues

1. -stenosis means narrowing or __________.
2. -emesis
5. -pepsia
8. -ptysis

Chapter Six

PRACTICAL APPLICATIONS

Name: ______________________________

History and Plan

cc: Leonard Smith, M.D.

Identifying Data:

This 72-year-old female presents with a biopsy proven adenocarcinoma of the sigmoid colon at 20 cm.

History of Present Illness:

The patient has been noted to have some bright red bleeding intermittently for approximately 8 months, initially presumable of a hemorrhoidal basis. She recently has had intensification of the rectal bleeding but no weight loss, anorexia, or obstructive pain. No significant diarrhea or constipation. Some low back pain, probably unrelated. Recent colonoscopy by Dr. Scoma revealed a large sessile (attached by a broad base) polyp, which was partially excised at the 20-cm level, showing infiltrating adenocarcinoma at the base. The patient is to enter the hospital at this time, after home antibiotic and mechanical bowel prep, to undergo sigmoid colectomy and possible further resection.

Questions

1. **The patient has had which of the following chronic symptoms: ....** ☐
   A. Loss of appetite
   B. Melena
   C. Hematochezia
   D. Loose stools

2. **The cause of her chronic symptom was: ....** ☐
   A. Glandular tumor of the stomach
   B. Swollen rectal veins
   C. Ulcerative colitis
   D. Malignant tumor of the colon

3. **What procedure did she have recently that diagnosed her condition? ....** ☐
   A. Visual examination of her large intestine
   B. Removal of her sigmoid colon
   C. Low anterior resection of the large intestine
   D. Hemorrhoidectomy

4. **The patient is scheduled for which of the following procedures? ....** ☐
   A. Biopsy of the sigmoid colon
   B. Excision of polyp in her colon
   C. Removal of the sigmoid colon and possible excision of additional colon tissue
   D. Removal of 20 cm of colon, including the sigmoid colon

Chapter Six
ANSWERS TO THE QUIZZES

Multiple Choice Quiz

1. D
2. E
3. A
4. D
5. E
6. B
7. D
8. D
9. D
10. B
11. C
12. A
13. C
14. A
15. A
16. D
17. C
18. D
19. B
20. E
21. B
22. C
23. D
24. A
25. C

Matching: Suffix and Terminology

A

1. involuntary contraction of muscles
2. tightening, narrowing, stricture
3. vomiting
4. eating, swallowing
5. stretching, dilation, widening
6. digestion
7. flow, discharge
8. suture
9. bursting forth of blood
10. surgical repair
11. spitting
12. opening
13. stopping, controlling

B

1. colectomy
2. cheilosis
3. duodenal
4. choledochal
5. cholangitis
6. celiac disease
7. buccal
8. colonoscopy
9. cholelithiasis
10. cholecystectomy
11. dentalgia
12. cecal volvulus

Sections C-E

C

1. herniorrhaphy
2. gastrostomy
3. gluconeogenesis
4. hepatomegaly
5. gastrojejunostomy
6. esophageal atresia
7. gastroenteritis
8. ileostomy
9. gingivectomy
10. cholecystojejunostomy
11. labiodental
12. glossectomy

D

1. palatoplasty
2. pyloric stenosis
3. proctosigmoidoscopy
4. lipase
5. periodontal membrane
6. pancreatoduodenectomy
7. splenic flexure
8. cholecystolithiasis
9. steatorrhea
10. sialadenectomy
11. sublingual
12. oropharynx

E

1. laparoscopy
2. abdominal ultrasonography
3. ERCP
4. stool culture
5. CT scan
6. stool guaiac
7. lower GI series
8. liver function tests
9. MRI
10. gastric bypass
11. paracentesis
12. GI endoscopy
13. nasogastric intubation
14. upper GI series

Exercise Quiz

A

1. digestion
2. spitting
3. vomiting
4. bursting forth of blood
5. eating, swallowing
6. surgical repair
7. suture
8. widening, dilation
9. narrowing
10. stop, control
11. separation; destruction
12. flow, discharge

B

13. excessive eating
14. difficult digestion
15. the esophagus is not open to the stomach at birth

C

16. blepharoplasty
17. sphincterotomy
18. cholecystectomy
19. herniorrhaphy
20. gastroduodenal anastomosis
21. cecostomy
22. gingivectomy
23. paracentesis

D

24. dysphagia
25. buccal
26. hepatomegaly
27. steatorrhea
28. sublingual or hypoglosssal
29. choledochal

E

30. inflammation of the mouth with small ulcers
31. enzyme to digest fat
32. abnormal condition of the lip
33. removal of a salivary gland
34. tissue surrounding a tooth
35. removal of the colon

F

36. nasogastric intubation
37. serum bilirubin
38. barium enema
39. stool guaiac
40. abdominal ultrasonography
41. stool culture
42. liver biopsy
43. endoscopic retrograde cholangiopancreatography
44. liver scan
45. CT of the abdomen
46. upper gastrointestinal series
47. percutaneous transhepatic cholangiography

Dictation and Comprehension Quiz

A

1. aphthous stomatitis
2. cholangiectasis
3. buccal
4. cheilostomatoplasty
5. cholecystectomy
6. cholecystojejunostomy
7. choledochal
8. colectomy
9. congenital esophageal atresia
10. diarrhea
11. dyspepsia
12. dysphagia
13. gingivectomy
14. glossopharyngeal
15. hematemesis
16. hemoptysis
17. herniorrhaphy
18. hemorrhage
19. pyloric stenosis
20. periodontal disease

B

11 Difficult digestion
15 Vomiting blood
18 Bursting forth of blood
20 Discharge of pus (gingivitis)
2 Dilation of a bile vessel
9 Food tube is not connected to the stomach from birth
17 Suture of an abdominal protrusion
4 Surgical repair of the lip and mouth
8 Removal of the large bowel
7 Pertaining to the common bile duct
16 Spitting up blood
3 Pertaining to the cheek
6 An anastomosis
12 Difficult swallowing
13 Removal of gum tissue
5 Removal of the gallbladder
10 Watery, loose, discharge of feces
19 Narrowing of a ring of muscles
1 Ulcers and inflammation of the mouth
14 Pertaining to the tongue and throat

Spelling Quiz

A

1. herniorrhaphy—suture (repair) of a hernia
2. hematemesis—vomiting blood
3. hemorrhage—bursting forth of blood
4. cholestasis—stoppage of flow of bile
5. pylorospasm—involuntary contraction of the pyloric sphincter
6. cholangiectasis—dilation of a bile vessel
7. blepharoplasty—surgical repair of the eyelids
8. choledochal—pertaining to the common bile duct
9. glossotomy—incision of the tongue
10. stenosis—narrowing, tightening

B

11. cheilosis
12. buccal
13. gastrorrhagia
14. cholangiogram
15. atresia
16. hemoptysis
17. hepatomegaly
18. dysphagia
19. pyorrhea
20. celiac

Pronunciation Quiz

A

1. hemoptysis
2. gingivectomy
3. cholestasis
4. diarrhea
5. cholangiectasis
6. herniorrhaphy
7. glycolysis
8. cholecystolithiasis
9. colonoscopy
10. lipase

B

1. F
2. C
3. J
4. H
5. G
6. I
7. B
8. D
9. A
10. E

C

1. dyspepsia
2. dysphagia
3. hematemesis
4. glossotomy
5. buccal
6. steatorrhea
7. hepatomegaly
8. enterorrhaphy
9. atresia
10. aphthous stomatitis

Review Sheet Quiz

A

1. starch
2. anus
3. appendix
4. bile
5. bronchial tube
6. belly, abdomen
7. lip
8. bile vessel
9. meal
10. colon
11. tooth
12. duodenum
13. intestine (usually small intestine)
14. esophagus
15. cause
16. tongue
17. sugar
18. blood
19. hernia
20. abdomen

B

1. bucc/o
2. cholecyst/o
3. choledoch/o
4. gastr/o
5. hepat/o
6. ile/o
7. jejun/o
8. lith/o
9. pancreat/o
10. pharyng/o

C

1. lip
2. tongue
3. fat
4. bile vessel
5. mandible (lower jaw bone)
6. abdominal
7. tooth

8. pus
9. mouth
10. peritoneum
11. anus and rectum
12. protein
13. pylorus or pyloric sphincter
14. rectum
15. salivary gland
16. sigmoid colon
17. spleen
18. fat
19. mouth
20. tonsils

D

1. enzyme
2. surgical puncture to remove fluid
3. defecation
4. dilation, stretching, widening
5. removal, excision, resection
6. sudden, involuntary contraction of muscles
7. blood condition
8. formation
9. process of recording
10. abnormal condition
11. breakdown, destruction
12. enlargement
13. appetite
14. disease condition
15. digestion
16. eating, swallowing
17. surgical repair
18. meal
19. drooping, sagging, prolapse
20. opening

E

1. -rrhage, -rrhagia
2. -rrhaphy
3. -rrhea
4. -scopy
5. -stenosis
6. -stomy
7. -stasis
8. -tomy
9. -ptysis
10. -emesis

Medical Scramble

1. -STENOSIS
2. -RRHAGIA
3. -PTYSIS
4. -EMESIS
5. -RRHEA
6. -PHAGIA

BONUS TERM: HERNIORRHAPHY

Crossword Puzzle

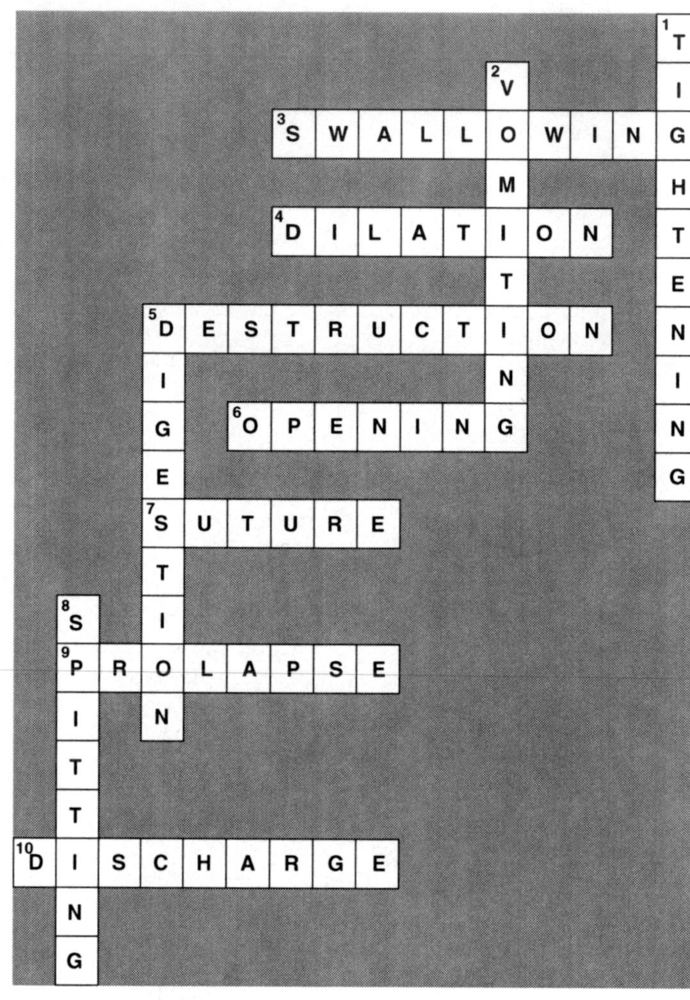

Practical Applications

1. C
2. D
3. A
4. C

Chapter Six

Answers to Terminology Section

(textbook pages 188–192)

Terminology	Meaning

Suffixes

Terminology	Meaning
cholangiectasis	Dilation of bile vessel.
hematemesis	Vomiting blood (from the digestive tract).
dyspepsia	Difficult digestion; indigestion.
polyphagia	Much (over) eating.
dysphagia	Difficult swallowing.
abdominoplasty	Surgical repair of the abdomen.
hemoptysis	Spitting up blood (from the respiratory tract).
hemorrhage	Bursting forth of blood.
gastrorrhagia	Discharge of blood from the stomach.
herniorrhaphy	Suture (repair) of a hernia.
diarrhea	Loose, watery discharge of feces.
pylorospasm	Involuntary contraction of the pyloric sphincter.
bronchospasm	Sudden, involuntary contraction of bronchial tubes (as during an asthmatic attack).
cholestasis	Stoppage of the flow of bile.
pyloric stenosis	Narrowing of the pyloric sphincter.
atresia	Not open (no opening).
esophageal atresia	No opening of the esophagus (into the stomach).
biliary atresia	No opening of the bile ducts (into the duodenum).

Combining Forms

Terminology	Meaning
buccal	Pertaining to the cheek.
cecal volvulus	Twisting of a part of the cecum upon itself.
celiac disease	Autoimmune disorder of the small intestine; villi are damaged as a result of eating gluten.
cheilosis	Abnormal condition of the lip.
cholelithiasis	Abnormal condition of gallstones.
cholangitis	Inflammation of bile vessels.
cholangiocarcinoma	Malignant tumor of bile vessel.
cholecystectomy	Removal of the gallbladder.
choledochal	Pertaining to the common bile duct.
choledochectasia	Dilation of the common bile duct.
colectomy	Removal of the colon.
colonoscopy	Visual examination of the colon.
dentalgia	Pain in a tooth.
duodenal	Pertaining to the duodenum.
gastroenteritis	Inflammation of the stomach and intestines.

esophageal atresia	Closure of the esophagus.
gastrojejunostomy	New opening between the stomach and the jejunum.
gastrostomy	New opening of the stomach to the outside of the body.
gingivectomy	Removal of gum tissue.
glossectomy	Removal of the tongue.
gluconeogenesis	Formation of new glucose (by liver cells).
glycogen	Storage form of sugar.
hepatomegaly	Enlargement of the liver.
herniorrhaphy	Suture of a hernia.
ileostomy	New opening of the ileum to the outside of the body.
cholecystojejunostomy	New opening between the gallbladder and the jejunum.
labiodental	Pertaining to the lips and teeth.
sublingual	Pertaining to under the tongue.
lipase	Enzyme to digest fat.
cholecystolithiasis	Abnormal condition of stones in the gallbladder.
periodontal membrane	Membrane surrounding a tooth.
oropharynx	The region of the throat near the mouth.
palatoplasty	Surgical repair of the palate.
pancreatic	Pertaining to the pancreas.
pancreatoduodenectomy	Removal of the pancreas and duodenum; Whipple procedure.
proctosigmoidoscopy	Visual examination of the anus and rectum.
pyloric stenosis	Narrowing of the pyloric sphincter.
rectal carcinoma	Cancer of the rectum.
sialadenectomy	Removal of a salivary gland.
splenic flexure	Area of the colon that bends downward near the spleen.
steatorrhea	Discharge of fat in feces.
aphthous stomatitis	Inflammation of the mouth with small ulcers.

Chapter 7

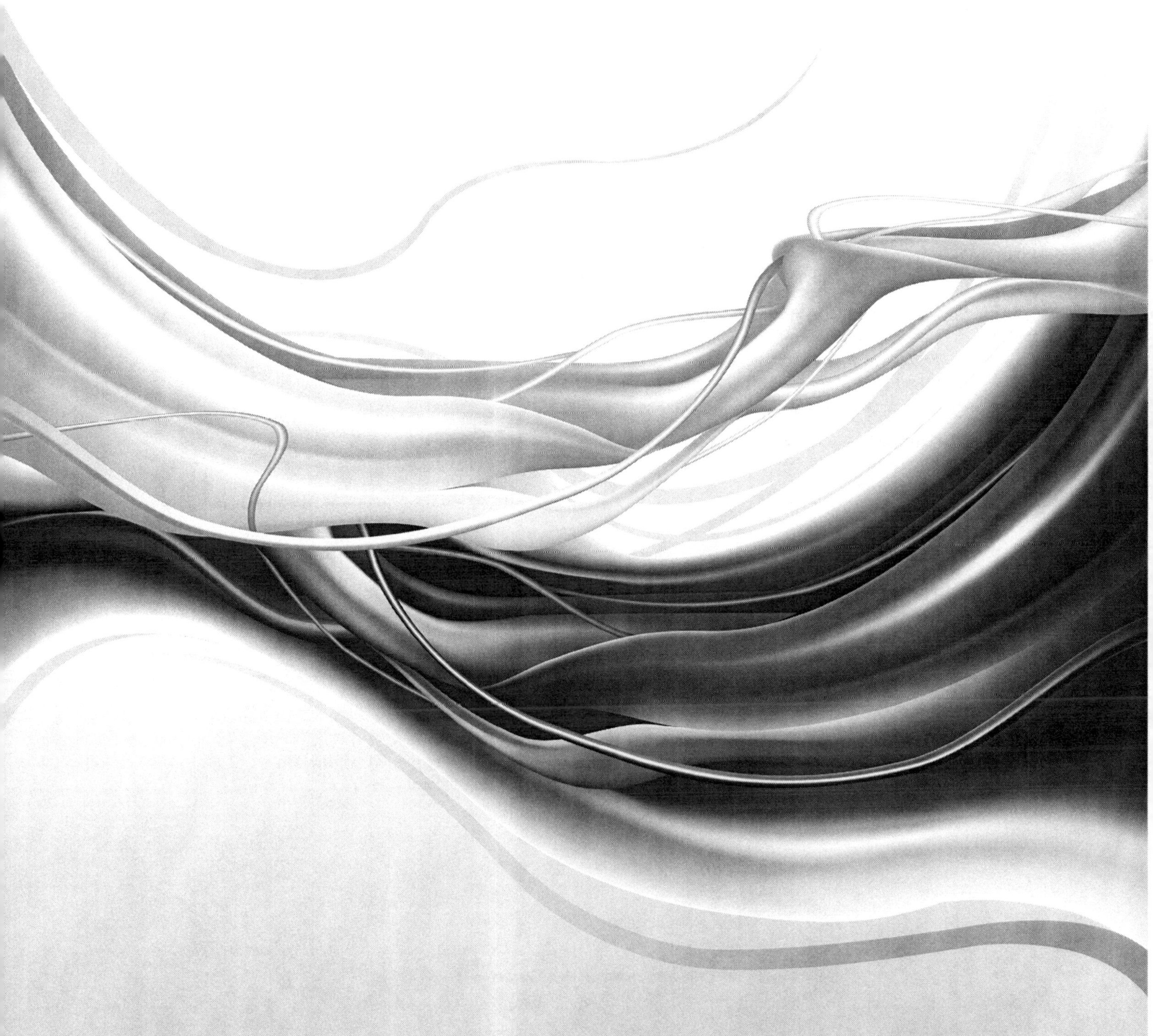

Chapter Seven

MULTIPLE CHOICE QUIZ

Name: ______________________

In the box write the letter of the choice that is the definition of the term or best answers the question. There is only one correct answer for each question.

1. **Portion of the urinary bladder:** ....
   A. Hilum
   B. Pylorus
   C. Fundus
   D. Medulla
   E. Trigone

2. **Glomerular:** ....
   A. Pertaining to a tube leading from the kidney to the bladder
   B. Pertaining to small balls of capillaries in the kidney
   C. Pertaining to a tube in the bladder
   D. Pertaining to a collecting chamber in the kidney
   E. Pertaining to the urinary bladder

3. **Meatal stenosis:** ....
   A. Enlargement of an opening
   B. Stoppage of blood flow to the kidney
   C. Incision of an opening
   D. Widening of the bladder orifice
   E. Narrowing of the urethral opening to the outside of the body

4. **Electrolyte:** ....
   A. Bilirubin
   B. Creatinine
   C. Albumin
   D. Sodium
   E. Glucose

5. **Nitrogenous waste:** ....
   A. Creatinine
   B. Fatty acid
   C. Lipid
   D. Carbon dioxide
   E. Sugar

6. **Renal pelvis:** ....
   A. nephr/o
   B. cyst/o
   C. ren/o
   D. py/o
   E. pyel/o

7. **A term that means no urine production is:** ....
   A. Diuresis
   B. Anuria
   C. Voiding
   D. Micturition
   E. Nocturia

8. **Surrounding the urinary bladder:** ....
   A. Suprarenal
   B. Infrarenal
   C. Perivisceral
   D. Perivesical
   E. Perinephric

9. **Uremia:** ....
   A. Azotemia
   B. Hematuria
   C. Dysuria
   D. Cystitis
   E. Hemorrhage

10. **X-ray of the urinary tract:** ....
    A. Renal ultrasonography
    B. KUB
    C. BUN
    D. Cystoscopy
    E. Renal dialysis

11. **Oliguria:** ....
    A. Nocturia
    B. Polyuria
    C. Scanty urination
    D. Bacteriuria
    E. Pus in the urine

12. **Diabetes insipidus is characterized by all of the following EXCEPT:** ....
    A. Polydipsia
    B. Glycosuria
    C. Polyuria
    D. Pituitary gland malfunction
    E. Insufficient ADH

13. Hernia of the tube connecting the kidney and urinary bladder:................
A. Herniorrhaphy
B. Urethrocele
C. Ureterocele
D. Urethroileostomy
E. Urethrostomy

14. Artificial kidney machine: ....
A. Renal biopsy
B. CAPD
C. Lithotripsy
D. Hemodialysis
E. Renal transplantation

15. Nephrolithotomy: ....
A. Hardening of a stone
B. Removal of the urinary bladder and kidney stones
C. Removal of the kidney and stones
D. Bladder calculi
E. Incision to remove a renal calculus

16. Protein in the urine:..........................
A. Ketonuria
B. Acetonuria
C. Hyperbilirubinemia
D. Bilirubinuria
E. Albuminuria

17. Renal abscess may lead to:.................
A. Diabetes mellitus
B. Pyuria
C. Nephroptosis
D. Ascites
E. Diabetes insipidus

18. Alkaline:...
A. Acidic
B. pH
C. Basic
D. Acetone
E. Water

19. A group of symptoms marked by edema, proteinuria, and hypoalbuminemia: ....
A. Renal ischemia
B. Essential hypertension
C. Polycystic kidney
D. Nephrotic syndrome
E. Diabetes mellitus

20. High levels of ketones in the blood can lead to:.......................................
A. High pH of urine
B. Acidosis
C. Excessive elimination of fats
D. Diabetes insipidus
E. Low specific gravity

21. Childhood renal carcinoma: ....
A. Hypernephroma
B. Polycystic kidney
C. Glomerulonephritis
D. Wilms tumor
E. Phenylketonuria

22. Urine is held in the bladder:................
A. Urinary incontinence
B. Pyuria
C. Polyuria
D. Nocturia
E. Urinary retention

23. Test that measures the amount of urea in the blood: ....
A. CT scan
B. RP
C. BUN
D. VCU
E. Creatinine clearance test

24. Nephrosclerosis:................................
A. Hardening of blood vessels in the kidney
B. Loss of protein in the urine
C. A test of kidney function
D. Prolapse of the kidney
E. Excess fluid in the kidney

25. Lithotripsy: ....
A. Renal transplant
B. Shock waves crush urinary tract stones
C. Radioscopic study
D. Panendoscopy
E. Foley catheterization

Chapter Seven
VOCABULARY QUIZ

Name: ______________________________

A. Match each vocabulary term listed with its meaning below:

arteriole	cortex	erythropoietin	glomerulus
calyx	creatinine	filtration	hilum
catheter	electrolyte	glomerular (Bowman) capsule	kidney

1. Cup-like collecting region of the renal pelvis ______________________________
2. Nitrogenous waste excreted in urine ______________________________
3. Depression in an organ where blood vessels and nerves enter and leave ______________
4. Small artery ______________________________
5. Process whereby some substances, but not all, pass through a filter ______________
6. Outer region of an organ ______________________________
7. Chemical element that carries an electrical charge ______________________________
8. Tiny ball of capillaries in the kidney ______________________________
9. Hormone secreted by the kidney to stimulate the production of red blood cells by bone marrow ______________________________
10. One of two bean-shaped organs on either side of the backbone in the lumbar region ______________________________
11. Tube for injecting or removing fluids ______________________________
12. Enclosing structure surrounding each glomerulus ______________________________

B. Match each vocabulary term listed with its meaning below:

K^+	nitrogenous waste	renal pelvis	trigone
meatus	reabsorption	renal tubules	
nephron	renal artery	renal vein	

1. Substance containing nitrogen and excreted in urine ______________________________
2. Blood vessel that carries blood to the kidney ______________________________
3. Triangular area in the urinary bladder ______________________________
4. Potassium; an electrolyte regulated by the kidney; essential for muscle and nerve function ______________________________
5. Combination of glomerulus and renal tubule where urine is formed ______________
6. Opening or canal ______________________________

7. Process whereby renal tubules return materials necessary to the body back into the blood vessel ____________________
8. Blood vessels that carries blood away from the kidney ____________________
9. Microscopic tubes in the kidney where urine is formed after filtration ____________________
10. Central collecting region in the kidney ____________________

C. *Match each vocabulary term listed with its meaning below:*

calciferol	renin	urethra
medulla	urea and uric acid	urinary bladder
Na^+	ureters	urination (voiding)

1. Hormone secreted by the kidney; raises blood pressure ____________________
2. Active form of Vitamin D; secreted by the kidney ____________________
3. Nitrogenous wastes excreted in urine ____________________
4. Hollow, muscular sac that holds and stores urine ____________________
5. Process of expelling urine ____________________
6. Tube leading from the urinary bladder to the outside of the body ____________________
7. Tubes leading from the kidneys to the urinary bladder ____________________
8. Sodium; an electrolyte regulated in the blood and urine by the kidneys ____________________
9. Inner region of an organ ____________________

Chapter Seven

TERMINOLOGY: STRUCTURES, SUBSTANCES, AND URINARY SIGNS AND SYMPTOMS QUIZ

Name: ______________________________

A. Match the following terms with their meanings below:

caliectasis	cystitis	meatal stenosis	paranephric
caliceal	cystostomy	nephropathy	
cystectomy	glomerular capsule	nephroptosis	

1. New opening of the urinary bladder to the outside of the body ______________________
2. Prolapse (dropping) of a kidney ______________________
3. Pertaining to a calyx ______________________
4. Narrowing of the opening of the urethra to the outside of the body ______________________
5. Widening, dilation of a calyx ______________________
6. Enclosing and collecting structure surrounding each glomerulus ______________________
7. Disease of a kidney ______________________
8. Removal of the urinary bladder ______________________
9. Pertaining to near the kidney ______________________
10. Inflammation of the urinary bladder ______________________

B. Compose medical terms from the meaning given below:

1. new opening of the kidney to the outside of the body ______________________
2. incision to remove a stone from the kidney ______________________
3. abnormal condition of water (fluid) in the kidney ______________________
4. incision to remove a stone from the renal pelvis ______________________
5. inflammation of the trigone ______________________
6. surgical repair of a ureter ______________________
7. new opening between the ureters and a segment of the ileum ______________________
8. inflammation of the urethra ______________________
9. surgical repair of the urethra ______________________
10. pertaining to within the urinary bladder ______________________

C. Match the following terms with their meanings below:

albuminuria	ketonuria	nocturia	renal ischemia
azotemia	ketosis (ketoacidosis)	polydipsia	urethral stricture
bacteriuria	nephrolithiasis	renal colic	vesicoureteral reflux

1. Condition of excess nitrogen in the blood ________________
2. Spasms of pain from stones in the kidney ________________
3. Condition of ketones in the blood and tissues ________________
4. Frequent, excessive urination at night ________________
5. Condition of much thirst ________________
6. Returning (backing up) of fluid from the urinary bladder to the ureters ________________
7. Protein present in the urine ________________
8. Holding back blood from the kidney ________________
9. Microorganisms in the urine ________________
10. Ketones in the urine ________________
11. Abnormal narrowing of the urethra ________________
12. Abnormal condition of kidney stones ________________

D. Compose medical terms from the meanings given below:

1. high potassium in the blood ________
2. low sodium in the blood ________
3. scanty urination ________
4. difficult, painful urination ________
5. excessive urination ________
6. pus in the urine ________
7. sugar in the urine ________
8. blood in the urine ________
9. crushing of stones ________
10. no production of urine ________

E. Match the following medical terms with their meanings below:

antidiuretic hormone	enuresis	urinary incontinence
diuresis	erythropoietin	urinary retention

1. Loss of control of the passage of urine from the bladder ________________
2. Increased excretion of urine ________________
3. Bedwetting ________________
4. Hormone produced by the kidney to increase formation of red blood cells ________________
5. Hormone that promotes the kidney to reabsorb water ________________
6. Urine is held within the bladder and not released ________________

Chapter Seven
PATHOLOGY QUIZ

Name: ______________________

A. Match the following abnormal conditions with their descriptions below:

glomerulonephritis
interstitial nephritis
nephrolithiasis
nephrotic syndrome
polycystic kidney disease
pyelonephritis

1. inflammation of the lining of the renal pelvis and renal parenchyma ______________
2. kidney stones (renal calculi) ______________
3. inflammation of the connective tissue that lies between the renal tubules ______________
4. multiple fluid-filled sacs within and on the kidney ______________
5. inflammation of the glomeruli within the kidney ______________
6. group of clinical signs and symptoms caused by excessive protein loss in urine ______________

B. From the following descriptions, name the pathologic condition:

1. high blood pressure that results from kidney disease ______________
2. cancerous tumor of the kidney in adulthood ______________
3. malignant tumor of the kidney occurring in childhood ______________
4. malignant tumor of the sac that holds urine ______________
5. high blood pressure of unknown cause ______________
6. kidneys decrease excretion of wastes due to impaired filtration function ______________
7. insulin is not secreted adequately or not used properly in the body ______________
8. antidiuretic hormone is not secreted adequately or the kidney is resistant to its effect ______________

Chapter Seven

LABORATORY TESTS AND CLINICAL PROCEDURES QUIZ

Name: ______________________________

A. Match the following with their meanings below:

creatinine clearance test	MRI urography	ultrasonography
CT urography	renal angiography	VCUG
cystoscopy	renal scan	
KUB	RP	

1. X-ray examination (with contrast) of the kidneys, ureters, and bladder ______________________
2. X-ray imaging of the renal pelvis and ureters after injection of contrast through a catheter into the urethra ______________________
3. X-ray images show multiple cross-sectional and other views of the urinary tract ______________________
4. Changing magnetic field produces images of the kidney and surrounding structures in three planes of the body ______________________
5. Measurement of the rate at which a nitrogenous waste is cleared from the blood by the kidney ______________________
6. X-ray record (with contrast) of the urinary bladder and urethra obtained while the patient is voiding ______________________
7. Image of the kidney after injecting a radioactive substance into the bloodstream ______________________
8. Direct visualization of the urethra and urinary bladder with an endoscope ______________________
9. Imaging urinary tract structures using high-frequency sound waves ______________________
10. X-ray examination (with contrast) of the blood vessels of the kidney ______________________

B. Give the names of the procedures described below:

1. Urinary tract stones are crushed ______________________
2. Separating nitrogenous wastes from the blood using an artifical kidney machine ______________________
3. Separating nitrogenous wastes from the blood using a catheter to introduce fluid into the abdominal cavity ______________________
4. Passage of a flexible, tubular instrument through the urethra into the urinary bladder ______________________
5. Dilation of narrowed areas in renal arteries ______________________
6. Surgical transfer of a kidney from a donor to a recipient ______________________
7. Removal of kidney tissue for microscopic examination ______________________

Chapter Seven

ABBREVIATIONS QUIZ

Name: ______________________________

A. On the line provided, give meanings for the following abbreviations, then write each abbreviation next to its explanation below:

1. ADH ______________________________
2. AKI ______________________________
3. BUN ______________________________
4. CAPD ______________________________
5. CrCl ______________________________
6. CRF ______________________________
7. C&S______________________________
8. Cysto ______________________________
9. GFR ______________________________
10. HD ______________________________
11. K^+ ______________________________

a. __________ Direct visualization of the urethra and urinary bladder with an endoscope

b. __________ Determines antibiotic effectiveness against bacteria

c. __________ Use of an artificial kidney machine to eliminate nitrogenous wastes from blood

d. __________ Progressive loss of kidney function

e. __________ Blood test of nitrogenous waste

f. __________ An electrolyte excreted by the kidney

g. __________ Severe damage to the kidney

h. __________ Method of dialysis by continuously inserting fluid in and out of the peritoneal cavity

i. __________ Hormone secreted by the pituitary gland and acting on the kidney to retain water

j. __________ Rate at which the glomerulus filters fluid from the body

k. __________ Rate at which creatinine is cleared from the blood by the kidney

B. *On the line provided, give meanings for the following abbreviations, then write each abbreviation next to its explanation below:*

1. ESWL ______________________________
2. KUB ______________________________
3. IVP ______________________________
4. Na^+ ______________________________
5. pH ______________________________
6. PKD ______________________________
7. RP ______________________________
8. sp gr ______________________________
9. UA ______________________________
10. UTI ______________________________
11. VCUG ______________________________

a. __________ Examination of urine to determine its contents

b. __________ An electrolyte necessary for proper functioning of muscles and nerves

c. __________ Use of ultrasonic waves to crush stones in the urinary tract

d. __________ Cysts form in and on the kidneys

e. __________ X-ray of the kidneys, ureters and bladder without contrast

f. __________ X-ray images are taken of the urethra and urinary bladder after contrast is injected through the urethra

g. __________ Bacterial infection of the urinary tract

h. __________ X-ray images are taken of the urinary tract after contrast is injected into a vein

i. __________ X-rays of the urethra and bladder are taken while a patient is voiding

j. __________ Scale to indicate the degree of acidity or alkalinity of a fluid

k. __________ Specific determination of the amount of solids in urine

Chapter Seven
EXERCISE QUIZ

Name: ______________________

A. Using the following terms, trace the path of urine formation from afferent renal arterioles to the point at which urine leaves the body:

glomerular (Bowman) capsule	renal pelvis	ureter	urinary bladder
glomerulus	renal tubule	urethra	urinary meatus

1. ______________________
2. ______________________
3. ______________________
4. ______________________
5. ______________________
6. ______________________
7. ______________________
8. ______________________

B. Give the meanings for the following medical terms:

9. caliceal ______________________
10. urinary meatal stenosis ______________________
11. creatinine ______________________
12. medullary ______________________
13. cystocele ______________________
14. vesicoureteral reflux ______________________

C. Match the following terms that pertain to urinalysis with their meanings below:

bilirubinuria	hematuria	pH	pyuria
glycosuria	ketonuria	proteinuria	sediment

15. Sugar in the urine; a symptom of diabetes mellitus ______________________
16. Color of the urine is smoky red owing to presence of blood ______________________
17. Urine is turbid (cloudy) owing to presence of WBCs and pus ______________________
18. Abnormal particles are present in urine—cells, bacteria, casts ______________________
19. Urine test that reflects the acidity or alkalinity of urine ______________________
20. Dark pigment accumulates in urine as a result of liver disease ______________________
21. High levels of acids and acetones accumulate in urine ______________________
22. Leaky glomeruli can produce this accumulation of albumin in urine ______________________

D. Give the meanings for the following terms that relate to urinary symptoms:

23. azotemia ______________________
24. polydipsia ______________________
25. nocturia ______________________
26. oliguria ______________________
27. dysuria ______________________
28. urinary retention ______________________
29. polyuria ______________________
30. anuria ______________________
31. bacteriuria ______________________
32. enuresis ______________________

E. Match the following terms with their meanings below:

abscess	edema	secondary hypertension
catheter	essential hypertension	stricture
diabetes insipidus	hypernephroma	

33. High blood pressure that is idiopathic ____________________
34. Malignant tumor of the kidney ____________________
35. High blood pressure caused by kidney disease ____________________
36. Tube for withdrawing or giving fluid____________________
37. Collection of pus ____________________
38. Swelling, fluid in tissues ____________________
39. Inadequate secretion of ADH ____________________
40. Narrowed area in a tube ____________________

F. Identify the following tests, procedures, or abbreviations:

41. C&S ____________________
42. BUN ____________________
43. cysto ____________________
44. Na^+ ____________________
45. UTI ____________________
46. MRI ____________________
47. hemodialysis ____________________
48. CAPD ____________________
49. renal biopsy ____________________
50. renal angiography ____________________

Chapter Seven

DICTATION AND COMPREHENSION QUIZ

Name: ______________________________

A. Dictation of Terms

1.	______________________	11.	______________________
2.	______________________	12.	______________________
3.	______________________	13.	______________________
4.	______________________	14.	______________________
5.	______________________	15.	______________________
6.	______________________	16.	______________________
7.	______________________	17.	______________________
8.	______________________	18.	______________________
9.	______________________	19.	______________________
10.	______________________	20.	______________________

B. Comprehension of Terms: Match number of the above term with its meaning below.

______ X-ray record of the renal pelvis and urinary tract
______ Blood is held back from the kidney
______ A tube for withdrawing and inserting fluid
______ Act of urination
______ Hormone secreted by the kidney to increase production of red blood cells
______ Narrowing of the opening of the urinary tract to the outside of the body
______ Sodium and potassium are examples
______ High blood pressure due to kidney disease
______ Swelling or fluid in tissue spaces
______ Collection of pus
______ Hardening of arterioles in the kidney
______ Visual examination of the urinary bladder
______ Protein in the urine
______ High levels of nitrogenous waste in the blood
______ Inability to hold urine in the bladder
______ A nitrogenous waste excreted in the urine
______ Renal calculi
______ Inflammation of the small balls of capillaries in the kidney
______ Blood in the urine
______ An anastomosis

Chapter Seven
SPELLING QUIZ

Name: ______________________

A. Circle the term that is spelled correctly and write its meaning in the space provided:

1. nitrogenous	nitrogenius	______
2. urinalysis	urinanalysis	______
3. meatis	meatus	______
4. dysuria	dysurea	______
5. abcess	abscess	______
6. dyalysis	dialysis	______
7. medulla	medula	______
8. pyleogram	pyelogram	______
9. vesicorectal	visicorectal	______
10. creatinine	cretatinine	______

B. Circle the term that is spelled correctly. The meaning of each term is given.

11. Swelling; fluid in tissues	ademia	edema	edemia
12. Visual examination of the bladder	sistoscopy	cystascopy	cystoscopy
13. Hardening of vessels in the kidney	nephroscherosis	nephrosclerosis	neferosclerosis
14. Protein in the urine	albuminuria	albuminurea	albumenuria
15. Stone	calkulus	calculus	calculis
16. Excessive thirst	polydipsia	polydypsia	polidipsia
17. Collecting area in the kidney	calics	kalyx	calyx
18. Inability to hold urine in bladder	incontenence	incontinence	incontinance
19. Chemical that carries an electrical charge	electrolite	electricolyte	electrolyte
20. Hormone secreted by the kidney to increase red blood cells	erithropoeitin	erythropoietin	erythropoeitin

Chapter Seven
PRONUNCIATION QUIZ

Name: ______________________________

A. Underline the accented syllables in the following terms:

1. cystourethrogram
2. meatotomy
3. edema
4. hilum
5. nephrolithotomy
6. trigone
7. urethroplasty
8. ureterocele
9. glycosuria
10. creatinine

B. Match the term in Column I with its meaning in Column II:

Column I			Column II
1. hematuria	_______	A.	Painful urination
2. diuresis	_______	B.	Bedwetting
3. abscess	_______	C.	Collection of pus
4. uremia	_______	D.	Pertaining to the outer section of an organ
5. perivesical	_______	E.	Blood in the urine
6. dysuria	_______	F.	Excessive urination
7. cortical	_______	G.	Pertaining to the inner section of an organ
8. medullary	_______	H.	Excessive urea in the bloodstream
9. renal cell carcinoma	_______	I.	Malignant tumor of the kidney
10. enuresis	_______	J.	Pertaining to surrounding the urinary bladder

C. Complete the following terms from their definitions:

1. cali ______________________ Dilation of a calyx
2. ______________________ uria Scanty urination
3. nephro ______________________ Disease of the kidney
4. bacteri ______________________ Bacteria in the urine
5. poly ______________________ Excessive thirst
6. ______________________ lithotomy Incision to remove a stone from the renal pelvis
7. ______________________ uria Protein in the urine
8. ______________________ scopy Visual examination of the urinary bladder
9. litho ______________________ Crushing of a stone
10. ______________________ uria Sugar in the urine

Chapter Seven
DIAGRAM QUIZ

Name: ______________________________

Label the diagram below using the terms listed below:

Kidney
Ureter
Urethra
Urinary bladder

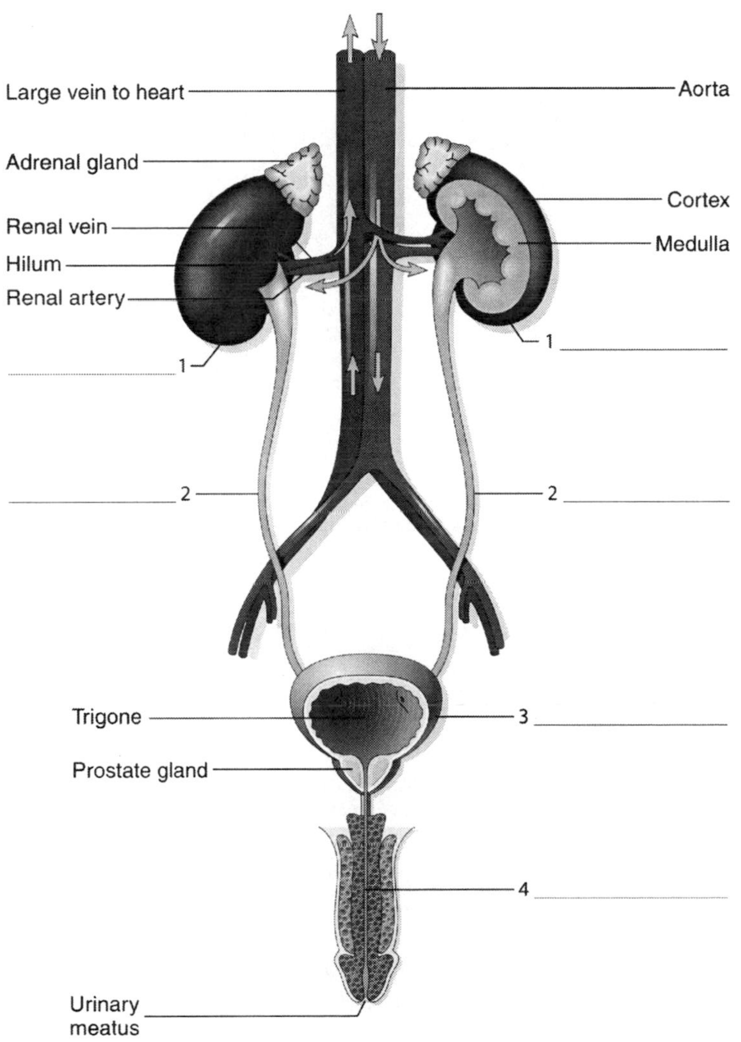

Chapter Seven
FLOW CHART QUIZ

Name: ______________________________

Label the flow chart using the terms listed below:

Bladder	Glomerular Capsule	Ureter
Bloodstream	Renal Pelvis	Urethra
Glomerulus	Renal Tubule	Urinary Meatus

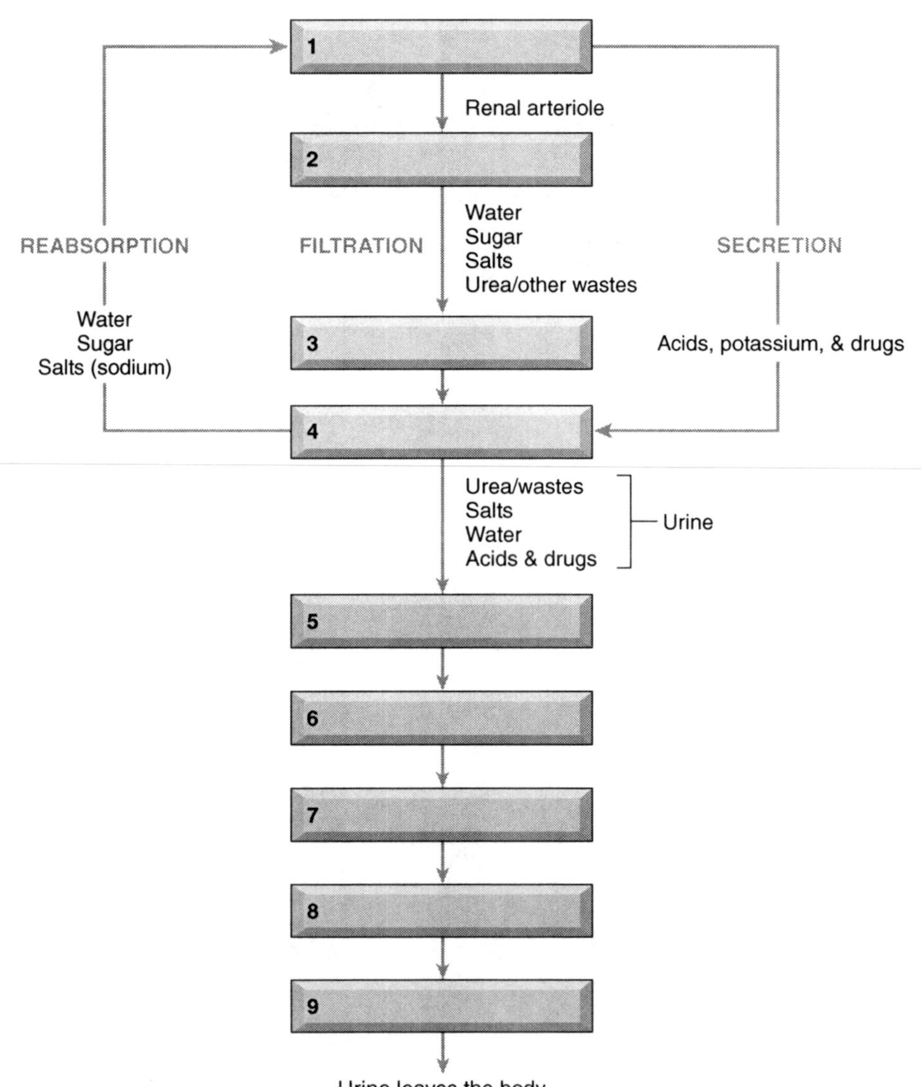

Chapter Seven
REVIEW SHEET QUIZ

Name: ______________________________

A. Give meanings for the following combining forms:

1. cyst/o ______________________
2. pyel/o ______________________
3. vesic/o ______________________
4. lith/o ______________________
5. ren/o ______________________
6. albumin/o ______________________
7. hydr/o ______________________
8. py/o ______________________
9. azot/o ______________________
10. olig/o ______________________

B. Give meanings for the following suffixes:

1. -ptosis ______________________
2. -tripsy ______________________
3. -stenosis ______________________
4. -lysis ______________________
5. -ectasis ______________________
6. -megaly ______________________
7. -poietin ______________________
8. -uria ______________________
9. -sclerosis ______________________
10. -ole ______________________

C. Give meanings for the following prefixes:

1. anti- ______________________
2. peri- ______________________
3. retro- ______________________
4. poly- ______________________
5. dys- ______________________
6. dia- ______________________
7. en- ______________________
8. a-, an- ______________________

D. Give suffixes or combining forms for the following:

1. new opening ______________________
2. incision ______________________
3. disease condition ______________________
4. removal ______________________
5. record ______________________
6. surgical repair ______________________
7. blood condition ______________________
8. thirst ______________________
9. night ______________________
10. blood vessel ______________________

Chapter Seven
MEDICAL SCRAMBLE

Name: ______________________________

Unscramble the letters to form urinary system terms from the clues. Use the letters in the squares to complete the bonus term.

1. *Clue:* Pus in the urine

   ___ ☐ ___ ☐ ___ ☐ RAPIYU

2. *Clue:* Blood in the urine

   ___ ___ ___ ___ ___ ___ ___ ☐ ___ TAMIHUERA

3. *Clue:* Sugar in the urine

   ___ ☐ ___ ___ ___ ☐ ☐ ___ ___ ___ CILASGUYRO

4. *Clue:* Protein in the urine

   ___ ___ ___ ___ ___ ___ ☐ ___ ___ ☐ ___ NLIBAIMURAU

5. *Clue:* An electrolyte

   ☐ ___ ___ ___ ___ ___ MIDOSU

BONUS TERM: *Clue:* Examination of urine to determine its contents

☐ ☐ ☐ ☐ ☐ ☐ ☐ ☐ ☐ ☐

Chapter Seven
CROSSWORD PUZZLE

Name: ______________________________

Fill in the crossword puzzle below using the clues listed underneath it.

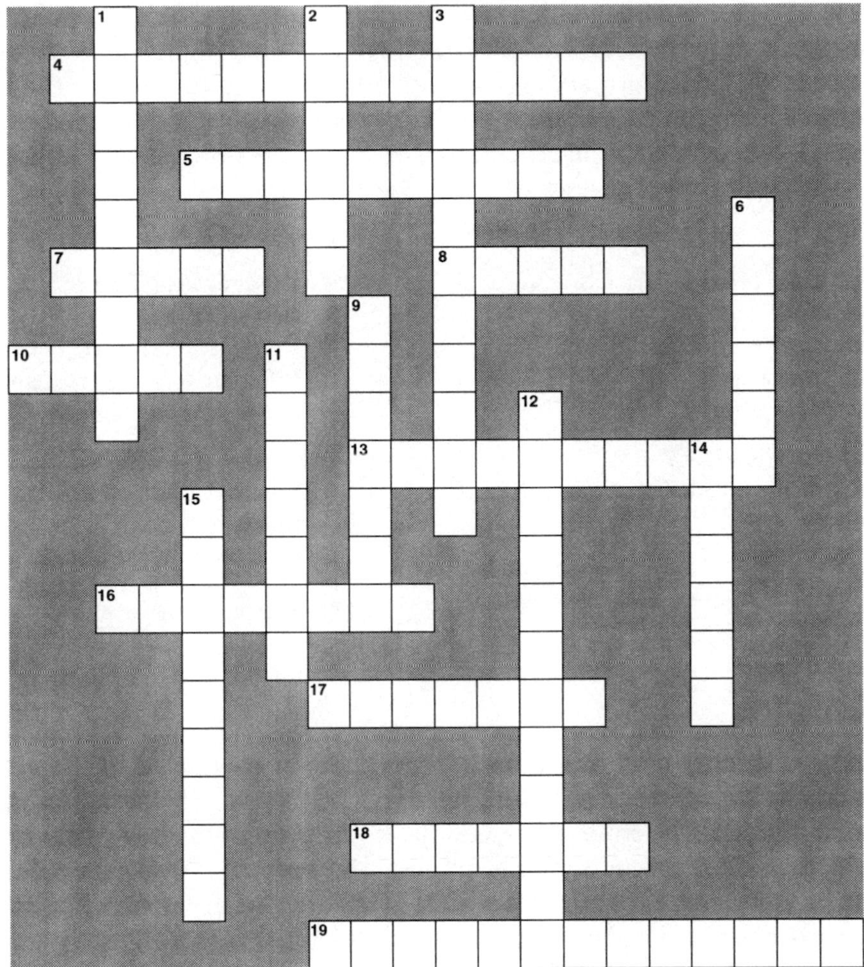

Across Clues

4. Secreted by the kidney to stimulate red blood cell production.
5. Process whereby some substances pass through the walls of a glomerulus.
7. Notch on the medial surface of the kidney where blood vessels and nerves enter and leave.
8. Substance, made in the kidney, that increases blood pressure.
10. Cup-like collecting region of the renal pelvis.
13. Tiny ball of capillaries in cortex of the kidney.
16. Tube for injecting fluids into or removing fluids from the urinary tract.
17. Tube leading from the bladder to the outside of the body.
18. Expelling urine for renal cell carcinoma.
19. Malignant tumor of the kidney: another term.

Down Clues

1. A small artery _____.
2. The outer region of the kidney is the renal _____.
3. Another term for urination.
6. Opening or canal.
9. Triangular area in the bladder where the ureters enter and urethra exits.
11. Sac that holds urine.
12. The process of accepting again or taking back; substances needed by the body pass from the renal tubules back into the bloodstream.
14. One of two tubes leading from the kidney to the urinary bladder.
15. Urine cannot leave the bladder; urinary _____.

Chapter Seven

PRACTICAL APPLICATIONS

Name: ______________________

A. Patient History

The patient is a 75-year-old male with a history of hematuria, dysuria, chronic UTIs, and benign prostatic hyperplasia. At present, he has nocturia three times per night with slow urinary stream. A CT scan showed a distended urinary bladder with large postvoid residual. In the kidney there is evidence of cortical renal cysts. Cystoscopy was performed, revealing a diverticulum of the bladder with a neoplastic lesion within the diverticulum. A biopsy was performed, and it showed ulceration and chronic cystitis, but no malignancy.

1. The patient has a history of: ☐
- A. Bladder cancer
- B. Prostate cancer
- C. Painful urination
- D. Protein in his urine

2. What x-ray test showed an abnormality of the bladder? ☐
- A. Cystoscopy
- B. Pelvic ultrasound
- C. Cystourethrogram
- D. Computed tomography

3. What is a diverticulum? ☐
- A. Neoplastic lesion
- B. Outpouching of a wall of an organ
- C. Inflammatory region of an organ
- D. Sac of fluid in an organ

4. The biopsy revealed: ☐
- A. Inflammation and defect in the bladder lining
- B. Carcinoma of the bladder
- C. Distended urinary bladder
- D. Hernia of the ureter

B. UTI in Children

The symptoms of urinary tract infections in older children are similar to those seen in adults. Cystitis manifests by suprapubic discomfort, burning, urgency, and polyuria. An upper UTI such as pyelonephritis manifests by chills, fever, and flank (the sides of the body, between the ribs and the ilium) pain. Any child previously toilet-trained who suddenly develops enuresis or daytime wetting should be evaluated. However, many UTIs in children are asymptomatic, and the younger the child, the more obscure the signs and symptoms. An infant with a UTI may present only with fever, lethargy, irritability, and/or failure to thrive.

1. A symptom of cystitis is: ☐
- A. Inability to urinate
- B. Frequent urination
- C. Chest pain
- D. Jaundice and itching

2. An example of an upper UTI is: ☐
- A. Nephrosclerosis
- B. Flank pain
- C. Lithotripsy
- D. Inflammation of the renal pelvis

3. Enuresis is: ☐
- A. Bedwetting
- B. Nocturia
- C. Anuria
- D. Strong sensation of having to urinate throughout the day

4. What type of symptoms do young children with UTIs frequently manifest? ☐
- A. Blood in the urine
- B. Protein in the urine
- C. Often no symptoms
- D. Elevated BUN

Chapter Seven
ANSWERS TO THE QUIZZES

Multiple Choice Quiz

1. E
2. B
3. E
4. D
5. A
6. E
7. B
8. D
9. A
10. B
11. C
12. B
13. C
14. D
15. E
16. E
17. B
18. C
19. D
20. B
21. D
22. E
23. C
24. A
25. B

Vocabulary Quiz

A

1. calyx
2. creatinine
3. hilum
4. arteriole
5. filtration
6. cortex
7. electrolyte
8. glomerulus
9. erythropoietin
10. kidney
11. catheter
12. glomerular (Bowman) capsule

B

1. nitrogenous waste
2. renal artery
3. trigone
4. K^+
5. nephron
6. meatus
7. reabsorption
8. renal vein
9. renal tubules
10. renal pelvis

C

1. renin
2. calciferol
3. urea and uric acid
4. urinary bladder
5. urination (voiding)
6. urethra
7. ureters
8. Na^+
9. medulla

Terminology: Structures, Substances, and Urinary Signs and Symptoms

A

1. cystostomy
2. nephroptosis
3. caliceal
4. meatal stenosis
5. caliectasis
6. glomerular capsule
7. nephropathy
8. cystectomy
9. paranephric
10. cystitis

B

1. nephrostomy
2. nephrolithotomy
3. hydronephrosis
4. pyelolithotomy
5. trigonitis
6. ureteroplasty
7. ureteroileostomy
8. urethritis
9. urethroplasty
10. intravesical

C

1. azotemia
2. renal colic
3. ketosis (ketoacidosis)
4. nocturia
5. polydipsia
6. vesicoureteral reflux
7. albuminuria
8. renal ischemia
9. bacteriuria
10. ketonuria
11. urethral stricture
12. nephrolithiasis

D

1. hyperkalemia
2. hyponatremia
3. oliguria
4. dysuria
5. polyuria
6. pyuria
7. glycosuria
8. hematuria
9. lithotripsy
10. anuria

E

1. urinary incontinence
2. diuresis
3. enuresis
4. erythropoietin
5. antidiuretic hormone
6. urinary retention

Pathology Quiz

A

1. pyelonephritis
2. nephrolithiasis
3. interstitial nephritis
4. polycystic kidney disease
5. glomerulonephritis
6. nephrotic syndrome

B

1. secondary hypertension
2. renal carcinoma
3. Wilms tumor
4. bladder cancer
5. essential hypertension
6. chronic kidney disease
7. diabetes mellitus
8. diabetes insipidus

Laboratory Tests and Clinical Procedures Quiz

A

1. KUB
2. RP
3. CT urography
4. MRI urography
5. creatinine clearance test
6. VCUG
7. renal scan
8. cystoscopy
9. ultrasonography
10. renal angiography

B

1. lithotripsy
2. hemodialysis
3. peritoneal dialysis
4. urinary catheterization
5. renal angioplasty
6. renal transplantation
7. renal biopsy

Abbreviations Quiz

A

1. antidiuretic hormone
2. acute kidney injury
3. blood urea nitrogen
4. continuous ambulatory peritoneal dialysis
5. creatinine clearance
6. chronic renal failure
7. culture and sensitivity testing
8. cystoscopy
9. estimated glomerular filtration rate
10. hemodialysis
11. potassium

a. Cysto
b. C&S
c. HD
d. CRF
e. BUN
f. K^+
g. AKI
h. CAPD
i. ADH
j. eGFR
k. CrCl

B

1. extracorporeal shock wave lithotripsy
2. kidney, ureter, and bladder
3. intravenous pyelogram
4. sodium
5. potential hydrogen
6. polycystic kidney disease
7. retrograde pyelography
8. specific gravity
9. urinalysis
10. urinary tract infection
11. voiding cystourethrogram

a. UA
b. Na^+
c. ESWL
d. PKD
e. KUB
f. RP
g. UTI
h. IVP
i. VCUG
j. pH
k. sp gr

Exercise Quiz

A

1. glomerulus
2. Bowman capsule
3. renal tubule
4. renal pelvis
5. ureter
6. urinary bladder
7. urethra
8. urinary meatus

B

9. pertaining to a calyx
10. narrowing of the opening of the urethra to the outside of the body
11. nitrogenous waste
12. pertaining to the inner section of an organ
13. hernia of the urinary bladder
14. backflow of urine from the urinary bladder to the ureter

C

15. glycosuria
16. hematuria
17. pyuria
18. sediment
19. pH
20. bilirubinuria
21. ketonuria
22. proteinuria

D

23. nitrogenous wastes in the blood
24. excessive thirst
25. frequent urination at night
26. scanty urination
27. painful urination
28. urine is held in the bladder
29. excessive urination
30. no urination
31. bacteria in the urine
32. bedwetting

E

33. essential hypertension
34. hypernephroma
35. secondary hypertension
36. catheter
37. abscess
38. edema
39. diabetes insipidus
40. stricture

F

41. culture and sensitivity
42. blood, urea, nitrogen
43. cystoscopy
44. sodium
45. urinary tract infection
46. magnetic resonance imaging
47. separation of wastes from the blood by removing the blood and filtering it through a machine
48. continuous ambulatory peritoneal dialysis
49. removal of tissue from the kidney and microscopic examination
50. x-ray record of the blood vessels in the kidney

Dictation and Comprehension Quiz

A

1. abscess
2. albuminuria
3. catheter
4. creatinine
5. cystoscopy
6. edema
7. electrolyte
8. erythropoietin
9. glomerulonephritis
10. hematuria
11. meatal stenosis
12. micturition
13. nephrolithiasis
14. nephrosclerosis
15. pyelography
16. renal ischemia
17. secondary hypertension
18. uremia
19. ureteroneocystostomy
20. urinary incontinence

B

15 X-ray record of the renal pelvis and urinary tract
16 Blood is held back from the kidney
3 A tube for withdrawing and inserting fluid
12 Act of urination
8 Hormone secreted by the kidney to increase production of red blood cells
11 Narrowing of the opening of the urinary tract to the outside of the body
7 Sodium and potassium are examples
17 High blood pressure due to kidney disease
6 Swelling or fluid in tissue spaces
1 Collection of pus
14 Hardening of arterioles in the kidney
5 Visual examination of the urinary bladder
2 Protein in the urine
18 High levels of nitrogenous waste in the blood
20 Inability to hold urine in the bladder
4 A nitrogenous waste excreted in the urine
13 Renal calculi
9 Inflammation of the small balls of capillaries in the kidney
10 Blood in the urine
19 An anastomosis

Spelling Quiz

A

1. nitrogenous—pertaining to nitrogen
2. urinalysis—examination of urine
3. meatus—opening or canal
4. dysuria—painful urination
5. abscess—collection of pus
6. dialysis—separation of wastes from blood
7. medulla—inner section of an organ
8. pyelogram—x-ray record of the renal pelvis
9. vesicorectal—pertaining to the bladder and rectum
10. creatinine—nitrogen-containing waste

B

11. edema
12. cystoscopy
13. nephrosclerosis
14. albuminuria
15. calculus
16. polydipsia
17. calyx
18. incontinence
19. electrolyte
20. erythropoietin

Pronunciation Quiz

A

1. cystourethrogram
2. meatotomy
3. edema
4. hilum
5. nephrolithotomy
6. trigone
7. urethroplasty
8. ureterocele
9. glycosuria
10. creatinine

B

1. E
2. F
3. C
4. H
5. J
6. A
7. D
8. G
9. I
10. B

C

1. caliectasis
2. oliguria
3. nephropathy
4. bacteriuria
5. polydipsia
6. pyelolithotomy
7. albuminuria; proteinuria
8. cystoscopy
9. lithotripsy
10. glycosuria

Diagram Quiz

1. Kidney
2. Ureter
3. Urinary bladder
4. Urethra

Flow Chart Quiz

1. Bloodstream
2. Glomerulus
3. Glomerular Capsule
4. Renal Tubule
5. Renal Pelvis
6. Ureter
7. Bladder
8. Urethra
9. Urinary Meatus

Review Sheet Quiz

A

1. urinary bladder
2. renal pelvis
3. urinary bladder
4. stone
5. kidney
6. protein; albumin
7. water
8. pus
9. nitrogen
10. scanty

B

1. prolapse
2. crushing
3. narrowing
4. destruction; separation
5. widening; stretching; dilation
6. enlargement
7. formation
8. urine condition
9. hardening
10. small; little

C

1. against
2. surrounding
3. back; behind
4. much; many
5. bad; painful; difficult; abnormal
6. complete; through
7. in; within
8. no; not; without

D

1. -stomy
2. -tomy
3. -pathy
4. -ectomy
5. -gram
6. -plasty
7. -emia
8. dips/o
9. noct/o
10. angi/o

Medical Scramble

1. PYURIA
2. HEMATURIA
3. GLYCOSURIA
4. ALBUMINURIA
5. SODIUM

BONUS TERM: URINALYSIS

Practical Applications

A

1. C
2. D
3. B
4. A

B

1. B
2. D
3. A
4. C

Crossword Puzzle

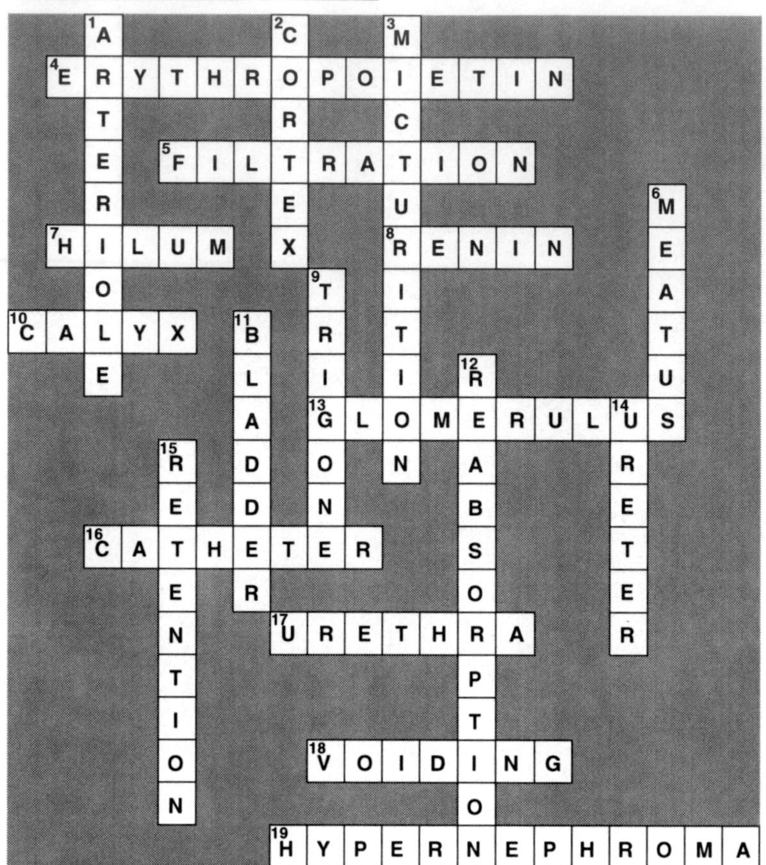

Chapter Seven

Answers to Terminology Section

(textbook pages 223–227)

Terminology	Meaning
caliectasis	Dilation of a calyx.
caliceal	Pertaining to a calyx.
cystitis	Inflammation of the urinary bladder.
cystectomy	Removal of the urinary bladder.
cystostomy	New opening of the bladder to the outside of the body.
glomerular capsule	Pertaining to the capsule surrounding each glomerulus; Bowman capsule.
meatal stenosis	Narrowing of the meatus (opening of the urethra to the outside of the body).
paranephric	Pertaining to near the kidney.
nephropathy	Disease of the kidney.
nephroptosis	Downward displacement of a kidney.
nephrolithotomy	Incision to remove a kidney stone.
hydronephrosis	Condition of excess fluid (water) in the kidney.
nephrostomy	New opening of the kidney to the outside of the body.
pyelolithotomy	Incision of the renal pelvis to remove a stone.
renal ischemia	Holding back of blood flow to the kidney.
renal colic	Kidney pain resulting from a stone in the ureter or kidney.
trigonitis	Inflammation of the trigone (area in the bladder).
ureteroplasty	Surgical repair of a ureter.
ureteroileostomy	New opening between a ureter and the ileum (for removal of urine after cystectomy).
urethritis	Inflammation of the urethra.
urethroplasty	Surgical repair of the urethra.
urethral stricture	Narrowing of the urethra.
intravesical	Pertaining to within the bladder.
vesicoureteral reflux	Backflow of urine from the bladder into the ureters.
albuminuria	Protein in the urine.
azotemia	Nitrogen (increased amounts of nitrogenous waste) in the blood.
bacteriuria	Bacteria in the urine.
polydipsia	Condition of increased thirst.
hyperkalemia	High levels of potassium in the blood.
ketosis	Abnormal condition of ketones in the blood and body tissues.
ketonuria	Ketone bodies (acids and acetone) in the urine.
nephrolithiasis	Abnormal condition of kidney stones.
hyponatremia	Low levels of sodium in the blood.
nocturia	Excessive urination at night.
oliguria	Scanty urination.
erythropoietin	Hormone secreted by the kidney to increase red blood cell formation in the bone marrow.
pyuria	Pus in the urine.
lithotripsy	Process of crushing a stone in the urinary tract.
uremia	Urea (urine) in the blood; a potentially fatal condition.
enuresis	Bedwetting (literally, "in urine").
diuresis	Condition of complete (excessive) urination.

antidiuretic hormone	Secreted by the pituitary gland and helps reabsorb water from the renal tubules back into the bloodstream.
urinary incontinence	Inability to hold urine in the bladder.
urinary retention	Inability to release urine from the bladder.
dysuria	Difficult, painful urination.
anuria	No urine is produced.
hematuria	Blood in the urine.
glycosuria	Sugar in the urine.
polyuria	Excessive urination.

Chapter 8

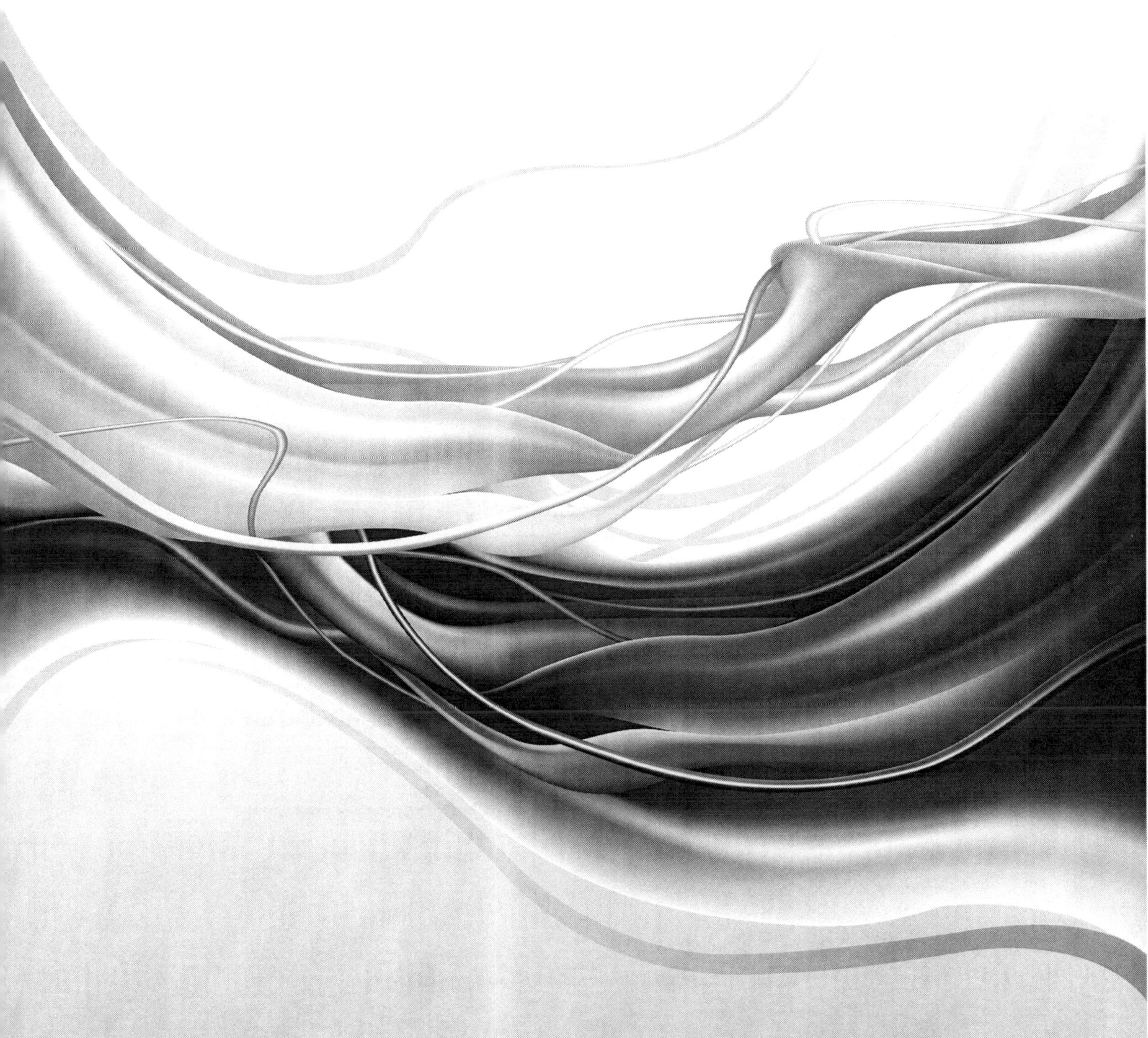

Chapter Eight
MULTIPLE CHOICE QUIZ

Name: ______________________

In the box write the letter of the choice that is the definition of the term or best answers the question. There is only one correct answer for each question.

1. **The ovum is the:** ☐
   A. Female gonad
   B. Female gamete
   C. Embryo
   D. Fertilized egg cell
   E. Fetus

2. **Pregnancy:** ☐
   A. Lactation
   B. Micturition
   C. Parturition
   D. Ovulation
   E. Gestation

3. **Area between the uterus and the rectum:** ☐
   A. Cul-de-sac
   B. Peritoneum
   C. Labia minora
   D. Clitoris
   E. Perineum

4. **Part of the perineum:** ☐
   A. Uterine cervix
   B. Fallopian tubes
   C. Labia majora
   D. Ovaries
   E. All of the above

5. **Adnexa uteri:** ☐
   A. Fetus
   B. Chorion
   C. Ovaries and fallopian tubes
   D. Bartholin glands
   E. Vagina

6. **Ovarian sac:** ☐
   A. Endometrium
   B. Corpus luteum
   C. Amnion
   D. Chorion
   E. Placenta

7. **Respiratory disorder in the neonate:** ☐
   A. Pyloric stenosis
   B. Hydrocephalus
   C. Hemolytic disease
   D. Melena
   E. Hyaline membrane disease

8. **Incision of the perineum during childbirth:** ☐
   A. Episiotomy
   B. Colpotomy
   C. Perineoplasty
   D. Laparotomy
   E. Perineorrhaphy

9. **Finger-like ends of the fallopian tubes are called:** ☐
   A. Ligaments
   B. Papillae
   C. Cysts
   D. Fimbriae
   E. Labia

10. **The study and treatment of newborns is called:** ☐
    A. Obstetrics
    B. Neonatology
    C. Gynecology
    D. Pediatrics
    E. Endocrinology

11. **Sac containing the egg is the:** ☐
    A. Corpus luteum
    B. Ovarian cyst
    C. Amnion
    D. Ovarian follicle
    E. Placenta

12. **Hormone produced by an endocrine gland located below the brain:** ☐
    A. hCG
    B. Progesterone
    C. Estrogen
    D. Follicle-stimulating hormone
    E. Erythropoietin

13. **Removal of the fallopian tubes and ovaries:** ☐
    A. Total hysterectomy
    B. Conization
    C. Bilateral salpingo-oophorectomy
    D. Salpingectomy
    E. Partial hysterectomy

14. Premature separation of placenta:.......
A. Ectopic pregnancy
B. Placenta previa
C. Abruptio placentae
D. Pseudocyesis
E. Dyspareunia

15. A woman who has had 3 miscarriages and 2 live births: ....
A. Grav. 3, para 2
B. Grav. 5, para 2
C. Grav. 2, para 3
D. Grav. 5, para 3
E. Grav. 2, para 5

16. Endometrial carcinoma may be detected by: ....
A. Cryocauterization
B. Ovarian biopsy
C. D & C
D. Cesarean section
E. Cystoscopy

17. Removal of internal and reproductive organs in the region of the hip:..........
A. Tubal ligation
B. Abortion and D & C
C. Pelvic exenteration
D. Gonadal resection
E. Bilateral oophorectomy

18. Physician's effort to turn the fetus during delivery: ....
A. Involution
B. Retroflexion
C. Retroversion
D. Cephalic version
E. Presentation

19. Gynecomastia: ....
A. Occurs after lactation in females
B. Abnormal development of breast tissue in males
C. Abnormal discharge of milk from the breast
D. Abnormal condition of pregnancy
E. Lumpectomy and chemotherapy are treatments

20. Excessive flow of blood from the uterus between menstrual periods:......
A. Menorrhea
B. Menorrhagia
C. Metrorrhagia
D. Oligomenorrhea
E. Dysmenorrhea

21. Painful labor and delivery: ....
A. Dystocia
B. Eutocia
C. Dyspareunia
D. Eclampsia
E. Endometriosis

22. Menarche: ....
A. Last menstrual period
B. First menstrual period
C. Absence of menstruation
D. Painful menstruation
E. Frequent menstrual periods

23. Ms. Sally Ping has vaginal discharge, pain in the LLQ and RLQ, dysmenorrhea, and a gonococcal infection. A likely diagnosis is: ....
A. Ovarian carcinoma
B. Choriocarcinoma
C. Fibroids
D. Pelvic inflammatory disease (PID)
E. Vulvovaginitis

24. Pieces of the inner lining of the uterus are ectopic: ....
A. Endocervicitis
B. Ectopic pregnancy
C. Endometriosis
D. Cystadenocarcinoma
E. Fibrocystic disease of the breast

25. Leukorrhea is associated with which of the following conditions?.......................................
A. Ovarian cysts
B. Menorrhagia
C. Eclampsia
D. Cervicitis
E. Oophoritis

Chapter Eight
VOCABULARY QUIZ

(textbook pages 266–268)

Name: ______________________________

A. Match the following terms with their meanings below:

adnexa uteri	cervix	corpus luteum
amnion	chorion	cul-de-sac
areola	clitoris	
Bartholin glands	coitus	

1. Lower, neck-like portion of the uterus ______________________
2. Sexual intercourse ______________________
3. Innermost membranous sac surrounding the developing fetus ______________________
4. Fallopian tubes, ovaries, and supporting ligaments ______________________
5. Region in the lower abdomen midway between the rectum and uterus ______________________
6. Empty ovarian follicle that secretes progesterone ______________________
7. Dark-pigmented area surrounding the breast nipple ______________________
8. Sensitive erectile tissue anterior to the opening of the female urethra ______________________
9. Outermost layer of two membranes surrounding the embryo ______________________
10. Small mucus-secreting glands at the vaginal orifice ______________________

B. Match the following terms with their meanings below:

embryo	fertilization	gamete
endometrium	fetus	genitalia
estrogen	fimbriae	
fallopian tube	follicle-stimulating hormone	

1. Finger or fringe-like projections at the end of the fallopian tubes ______________________
2. Hormone produced by the ovaries; promotes female secondary sex characteristics ______________________
3. Union of the sperm cell and ovum ______________________
4. Stage in prenatal development from 2 to 8 weeks ______________________
5. Reproductive organs ______________________
6. Stage in prenatal development from 8 to 39 to 40 weeks ______________________
7. Hormone secreted by the pituitary gland to stimulate maturation of the ovum ______________________
8. Inner, mucous membrane lining of the uterus ______________________
9. Male or female sexual reproductive cell; ovum and sperm ______________________
10. One of a pair of ducts through which the ovum travels to the uterus ______________________

C. Match the following terms with their meanings below:

gestation	labia	menarche
gonad	lactiferous ducts	menopause
gynecology	luteinizing hormone	
hCG	mammary papilla	

1. Tubes carrying milk within the breast ________________
2. Hormone produced by the placenta to sustain pregnancy ________________
3. Breast nipple ________________
4. Study of female reproductive organs and breast ________________
5. Lips of the vagina ________________
6. Female or male reproductive organ ________________
7. Gradual ending of menstruation ________________
8. Pituitary gland secretion; promotes ovulation ________________
9. Beginning of the first menstrual period ________________
10. Pregnancy ________________

D. Match the following terms with their meanings below:

menstruation	orifice	parturition
myometrium	ovarian follicle	perineum
neonatology	ovulation	
obstetrics	ovum	

1. Study of the care of newborns ________________
2. Mature egg cell ________________
3. Area between the anus and the vagina ________________
4. Branch of medicine concerned with pregnancy and childbirth ________________
5. Release of an egg cell from the ovary ________________
6. Muscle layer of the uterus ________________
7. An opening ________________
8. Monthly shedding of the uterine lining ________________
9. Act of giving birth ________________
10. Sac enclosing each egg cell within the ovary ________________

E. Match the following terms with their meanings below:

ovary	progesterone	vulva
pituitary gland	puberty	zygote
placenta	uterine serosa	
pregnancy	vagina	

1. Stage in prenatal development from fertilization and implantation to 2 weeks ________________
2. Outermost layer of the uterus ________________
3. Hormone produced by the corpus luteum and placenta of pregnant women ________________
4. Period of life when the ability to reproduce begins ________________
5. Vascular organ that develops in the uterine wall as communication between maternal and fetal bloodstreams ________________
6. One of a pair of female gonads; produces egg cells and hormones ________________
7. Muscular, mucosal tube extending from the uterus to the exterior of the body ________________
8. Endocrine gland at the base of the brain; secretes FSH and LH ________________
9. Condition in a female of sustaining a developing embryo/fetus in her uterus ________________
10. External female genitalia that includes labia, hymen, clitoris, and vaginal orifice ________________

Chapter Eight TERMINOLOGY QUIZ

Name: ______________________________

A. Match the following terms with their meanings below.

amniocentesis	colposcopy	episiotomy	lactation
amniotic fluid	culdocentesis	galactorrhea	
chorionic	endocervicitis	gynecomastia	

1. Pertaining to the outermost layer of the two membranes surrounding the embryo ______________________________
2. Abnormal, persistent discharge of milk from the breast ______________________________
3. Normal production of milk from the breast ______________________________
4. Inflammation of the inner lining of the cervix ______________________________
5. Incision of the perineum ______________________________
6. Enlargement of breasts in a male ______________________________
7. Visual examination of the vagina ______________________________
8. Surgical puncture to remove fluid from the amniotic cavity ______________________________
9. Surgical puncture to remove fluid from the area between the rectum and the vagina ______________________________
10. Liquid produced by the fetal membranes; surrounding the fetus throughout gestation ______________________________

B. Create a medical term from the following definitions:

1. pertaining to under the breast ______________________________
2. removal of the uterus ______________________________
3. surgical repair of the breast ______________________________
4. inflammation of the breast ______________________________
5. visual examination of the uterus ______________________________
6. removal of a breast ______________________________
7. scanty menstrual flow ______________________________
8. painful menstrual flow ______________________________
9. absence of menstrual flow ______________________________
10. abnormally heavy or long menstrual periods ______________________________

11. inflammation of the Bartholin glands ______________________

12. pain in the vulvar area ______________________

C. *Match the following terms with their meanings below.*

menometrorrhagia	myometrium	oocyte	ovum
metrorrhagia	neonatal	oogenesis	
myomectomy	obstetrics	oophorectomy	

1. Muscle layer lining the uterus ______________________
2. Mature egg cell ______________________
3. Pertaining to a newborn ______________________
4. Immature egg cell ______________________
5. Branch of medicine concerned with pregnancy and childbirth ______________________
6. Removal of an ovary ______________________
7. Formation of egg cells ______________________
8. Removal of a benign muscle tumor ______________________
9. Heavy bleeding between menses ______________________
10. Excessive uterine bleeding between and during menstrual periods ______________________

D. *Create a medical term from the following definitions:*

1. pertaining to an ovary ______________________
2. inflammation of an ovary ______________________
3. removal of a fallopian tube ______________________
4. suture of the perineum ______________________
5. pertaining to no ovulation ______________________
6. inflammation of the vagina ______________________
7. inflammation of the vulva and the vagina ______________________
8. false pregnancy ______________________
9. whitish discharge from the vagina ______________________
10. beginning of menses (first menstrual period) ______________________

E. Match the following terms with their meanings below.

cephalic version	menorrhea	primiparous	vaginal orifice
dystocia	oxytocia	pyosalpinx	
involution of the uterus	primigravida	uterine prolapse	

1. Rapid labor and birth ____________________
2. Menstrual discharge ____________________
3. A woman who is pregnant for the first time ____________________
4. Pus in a fallopian (uterine) tube ____________________
5. Falling, sagging of the uterus ____________________
6. Normal opening of the vagina to the outside of the body ____________________
7. Difficult or abnormal labor and delivery ____________________
8. Pertaining to a woman who has given birth to one baby ____________________
9. The fetus is turned so the head is closer to the cervix ____________________
10. The uterus returns to its normal, nonpregnant size ____________________

F. Create medical terms from the definitions below:

1. inflammation of the inner lining of the uterus ____________________
2. painful sexual intercourse ____________________
3. pertaining to before birth ____________________
4. pertaining to within the uterus ____________________
5. a woman who has had many births ____________________
6. a woman who has had many pregnancies ____________________
7. a woman who has had no pregnancies ____________________
8. a woman who has never given birth to a child ____________________
9. a woman who going through her first pregnancy ____________________
10. backward tilting (of the uterus) ____________________

Chapter Eight
PATHOLOGY QUIZ

Name: ______________________

A. Match the following pathologic conditions with the definitions below:

carcinoma of the cervix
cervicitis
carcinoma of the breast
carcinoma of the endometrium
endometriosis
fibroids
fibrocystic disease
ovarian carcinoma
ovarian cysts
pelvic inflammatory disease

1. Inflammation of the lower section of the uterus ______________________
2. Benign tumors in the uterus ______________________
3. Malignant tumor the breast ______________________
4. Malignant cells within the cervix ______________________
5. Tissue from the lining of the uterus is located outside of the uterus ______________________
6. Malignant tumor of the uterus ______________________
7. Collections of fluid within a sac in the ovary ______________________
8. Malignant tumor of the ovary ______________________
9. Numerous small sacs of fibrous connective tissue and fluid in the breast ______________________
10. Inflammation and infection of organs in the pelvic region ______________________

B. Using the list of terms in A, match each with descriptions below:

1. Woman notices lumpy consistency of the breast in this benign condition ______________________
2. This type of cancer is often diagnosed in an advanced stage; ascites appears as an initial sign ______________________
3. Bacterial infections (chlamydia and gonorrhea) lead to salpingitis, oophoritis, endometritis in this sexually transmitted condition ______________________
4. Dysmenorrhea, pelvic pain, infertility, and dyspareunia are symptoms as ectopic endometrial tissue blocks the lumen of the fallopian tube ______________________
5. Leiomyomas are the problem and myomectomy and hysterectomy may be indicated ______________________
6. Human papillomavirus is the cause; dysplasia and CIS are early and localized forms of the condition ______________________

7. Acutely, cervical erosion is seen; cryocauterization and antibiotic treatment may be indicated ____________________
8. Postmenopausal bleeding is the most common symptom; hysterectomy with bilateral salpingo-oophorectomy can be curative if malignancy is confined to the uterus ____________________
9. Teratomas can occur within these sacs, which are sometimes dermoid cysts ____________________
10. Invasive ductal carcinoma and lobular and medullary carcinoma are types of this condition ____________________

C. Match the following abnormal conditions with their definitions below:

abruptio placentae
Down syndrome
ectopic pregnancy
erythroblastosis fetalis
hyaline membrane disease
hydrocephalus
meconium aspiration syndrome
multiple gestations
placenta previa
preeclampsia
pyloric stenosis

1. Hemolytic disease of the newborn ____________________
2. Associated with pregnancy and marked by high blood pressure, proteinuria, headache, and edema ____________________
3. Trisomy 21 resulting in mental retardation and other abnormalities ____________________
4. Implantation of the placenta over the cervical opening in the lower region of the uterus ____________________
5. Premature separation of the implanted placenta ____________________
6. Implantation of the fertilized egg in any site other than the normal uterine location ____________________
7. Abnormal inhalation or ingestion of first stool produced by a fetus or newborn ____________________
8. Narrowing of the opening of the stomach to the duodenum in an infant ____________________
9. Abnormal accumulation of fluid in the spaces of the brain ____________________
10. More than one fetus inside the uterus during pregnancy ____________________
11. Acute lung disease commonly seen in the newborn ____________________

Chapter Eight
ABBREVIATIONS QUIZ

Name: ______________________________

A. On the line provided, give meanings for the following abbreviations, then write each abbreviation next to its explanation below:

1. AB ______________________________
2. C-section ______________________________
3. CIS ______________________________
4. CVS ______________________________
5. Cx ______________________________
6. D & C ______________________________
7. FSH ______________________________
8. G ______________________________
9. GYN ______________________________
10. hCG or HCG ______________________________

a. _______ Pituitary gland secretion that stimulates the ovaries

b. _______ Pregnancy hormone

c. _______ Lower, neck-like portion of the uterus

d. _______ Study of women and disorders of the female reproductive system

e. _______ Spontaneous or induced termination of pregnancy

f. _______ Localized cancer growth

g. _______ Sampling of placental tissue for prenatal diagnosis

h. _______ Surgical incision of the abdominal wall to deliver a fetus

i. _______ A pregnant woman

j. _______ Procedure to widen the cervix and scrap the lining of the uterus

B.

1. HDN ______________________________
2. HPV ______________________________
3. HRT ______________________________
4. HSG ______________________________
5. IUD ______________________________
6. IVF ______________________________
7. LEEP ______________________________
8. LH ______________________________

9. multip ______________________________

10. OB ______________________________

a. _______ X-ray imaging of the uterus and fallopian tubes

b. _______ Egg and sperm are united outside the body

c. _______ Use of heat to destroy tissue

d. _______ Contraceptive device

e. _______ Branch of medicine dealing with pregnancy, labor and delivery of infants

f. _______ a woman who has had more than one delivery of an infant

g. _______ Erythroblastosis fetalis; Rh factor incompatibility between the mother and fetus

h. _______ Relieves symptoms of menopause and delays development of weak bones

i. _______ Pituitary hormone stimulates the ovary to promote ovulation

j. _______ Cause of cervical cancer

C. On the line provided, give meanings for the following abbreviations, then write each abbreviation next to its explanation below:

1. Pap test ______________________________
2. PID ______________________________
3. PMS ______________________________
4. primip ______________________________
5. SNB ______________________________
6. TAH-BSO ______________________________
7. UAE ______________________________
8. VH ______________________________

a. _______ Inflammation and infection of organs in the region of the pelvis; salpingitis, oophoritis, endometritis

b. _______ Breast tenderness, irritability and depression before menstruation

c. _______ Removal of the uterus through the vagina

d. _______ Method of treating fibroids without surgery

e. _______ A woman who has given birth to one child

f. _______ Dye or radioisotope identifies the first lymph node draining the breast lymphatics and it is removed

g. _______ Microscopic examination of stained cells removed from the vagina and cervix

h. _______ Removal of uterus through an abdominal incision

Chapter Eight
EXERCISE QUIZ

Name: ______________________________

A. Match the following terms for structures or tissues with their meanings below:

amnion	clitoris	fimbriae	perineum
areola	endometrium	mammary papilla	placenta
cervix	fallopian tubes	ovaries	vulva

1. Inner lining of the uterus ______________________________
2. Nipple of the breast ______________________________
3. Innermost membrane around the developing embryo ______________________________
4. Dark-pigmented area around the breast nipple ______________________________
5. External genitalia of female (perineum, labia, hymen, clitoris) ______________________________
6. Area between the anus and vagina in females ______________________________
7. Female gonads; producing ova and hormones ______________________________
8. Blood-vessel-filled organ that develops during pregnancy ______________________________
9. Uterine tubes ______________________________
10. Organ of sensitive erectile tissue in females ______________________________
11. Finger-like ends of the fallopian tube ______________________________
12. Lower, neck-like portion of the uterus ______________________________

B. Give short answers for the following:

13. galact/o and lact/o mean ______________________________
14. colp/o and vagin/o mean ______________________________
15. oophor/o and ovari/o mean ______________________________
16. mamm/o and mast/o mean ______________________________
17. metr/o and hyster/o mean ______________________________
18. -cyesis and gravid/o mean ______________________________
19. episi/o and vulv/o mean ______________________________
20. ovul/o and o/o mean ______________________________

C. Give meanings for the following gynecologic symptoms:

21. leukorrhea ______________________
22. metrorrhagia ______________________
23. amenorrhea ______________________
24. dyspareunia ______________________
25. pyosalpinx ______________________

D. Give the medical term for the following:

26. pertaining to newborn ______________________
27. surgical puncture to remove fluid from the cul-de-sac ______________________
28. inflammation of the cervix ______________________
29. first menstrual period ______________________
30. rapid labor ______________________

E. Match the following terms with their meanings below:

abruptio placentae	cystadenocarcinoma	placenta previa
carcinoma in situ	endometrial carcinoma	preeclampsia
choriocarcinoma	endometriosis	

31. Malignant tumor of the pregnant uterus ______________________
32. Condition during pregnancy; hypertension, proteinuria, edema, and uremia ______________________
33. Malignant condition of the inner lining of the uterus ______________________
34. Malignant tumor; often of the ovary ______________________
35. Displaced placenta; implantation in lower region of uterus ______________________
36. Uterine tissue is located outside the uterus ______________________
37. Cancerous tumor cells are localized in a small area ______________________
38. Premature separation of a normally implanted placenta ______________________

F. Give the name of the test or procedure described below:

39. visual examination of the vagina ______________________
40. withdrawal of fluid by suction with a needle ______________________
41. cold temperatures are used to destroy tissue ______________________
42. cone-shaped section of the cervix is removed ______________________
43. hCG is measured in urine or blood ______________________
44. widening the cervical opening and scraping the uterine lining ______________________

G. *Give medical terms for the following.*

45. benign muscle tumors in the uterus ______________________________
46. accessory organs of the uterus ______________________________
47. ovarian hormone that sustains pregnancy ______________________________
48. removal of an ovary ______________________________
49. inflammation of the vulva and vagina ______________________________
50. reproductive organs ______________________________

Chapter Eight
DICTATION AND COMPREHENSION QUIZ: VOCABULARY AND TERMINOLOGY

Name:________________

A. Dictation of Terms

1.	________________	11.	________________
2.	________________	12.	________________
3.	________________	13.	________________
4.	________________	14.	________________
5.	________________	15.	________________
6.	________________	16.	________________
7.	________________	17.	________________
8.	________________	18.	________________
9.	________________	19.	________________
10.	________________	20.	________________

B. Comprehension of Terms: Match number of the above term with its meaning below.

______ Woman who has had more than one live birth
______ Painful sexual intercourse
______ Outermost membrane surrounding the developing embryo
______ Tissue lying between the anus and vagina
______ First menstrual period
______ Hormone secreted by the ovary during pregnancy
______ Ovary and fallopian tubes; accessory uterine structures
______ An opening
______ Pigmented area around the nipple of the breast
______ Inner lining of the uterus
______ Visual examination of the vagina
______ Practice of caring for women during pregnancy and delivering neonates
______ Pertaining to no egg production
______ Surgical puncture to remove fluid from the membrane surrounding the embryo
______ Excessive discharge of blood from the uterus (not during menstruation)
______ Pus in the fallopian tubes
______ Difficult labor and delivery
______ Removal of a breast
______ Reproductive organs
______ Female organ of sexual stimulation; located anterior to the urethra

Chapter Eight

DICTATION AND COMPREHENSION QUIZ: PATHOLOGIC CONDITIONS, CLINICAL TESTS AND PROCEDURES

Name: ______________

A. Dictation of Terms

1. ______________ 11. ______________
2. ______________ 12. ______________
3. ______________ 13. ______________
4. ______________ 14. ______________
5. ______________ 15. ______________
6. ______________ 16. ______________
7. ______________ 17. ______________
8. ______________ 18. ______________
9. ______________ 19. ______________
10. ______________ 20. ______________

B. Comprehension of Terms: Match number of the above term with its meaning below.

______ Tissue from the inner lining of the uterus is found in abnormal locations
______ Benign tumor in the uterus; fibroid
______ Visual examination of the abdomen; minimally invasive surgery
______ Examination by touch
______ Fluid is removed by a needle
______ Type of bacteria found as a common cause of pelvic inflammatory disease
______ Malignant tumor that is localized and not invasive
______ X-ray examination of the breast
______ Narrowing of the opening of the stomach to the intestine in a newborn
______ Condition during pregnancy marked by hypertension, proteinuria, and edema
______ Tying off the fallopian tubes; sterilization procedure
______ Accumulation of fluid in the spaces of the brain and can occur in a neonate
______ Widening the cervix and scraping the lining of the uterus
______ Burning tissue with chemicals or an electrically heated instrument
______ Abnormal growth of tissue in the neck of the uterus
______ Removal of an infant through an incision of the abdominal wall
______ Abnormal location of the organ connecting the infant and the mother
______ X-ray examination of the uterus and the fallopian tubes
______ Embryo is not implanted in the uterus
______ Removal of a cone-shaped section of the cervix for biopsy

Chapter Eight
SPELLING QUIZ

Name: ______________________

A. Circle the term that is spelled correctly, and write its meaning in the space provided:

1. amenorhea — amenorrhea ______________________
2. oophoritis — oopheritis ______________________
3. menarchy — menarche ______________________
4. cervisitis — cervicitis ______________________
5. areola — aereola ______________________
6. pappila — papilla ______________________
7. progesterone — progestrone ______________________
8. esterogen — estrogen ______________________
9. dialation — dilation ______________________
10. carsinoma en situ — carcinoma in situ ______________________

B. Circle the term that is spelled correctly. The meaning of each term is given.

11. Secreted by the anterior pituitary gland to promote ovulation	leutinizing hormone	luteinizing hormone	lutienizing hormone
12. Muscular tube leading from the uterus	vagina	vajina	vigina
13. Reproductive organs	genatalia	genitalia	genitailia
14. Scraping of tissue	currettage	curettage	cruettage
15. Development of female breasts in a male	gynecomastia	gynomastia	gynacomastia
16. Instrument to visually examine the tube leading from the uterus	culposcope	colposcope	coldoscope
17. Act of giving birth	parrition	parturition	partrition
18. Organ in the pregnant female's uterus that provides nourishment for the fetus	placenta	plasenta	plecenta
19. Monthly discharge of blood from the lining of the uterus	menstration	menstruation	menstrashun
20. Innermost membrane around the developing embryo	amnion	amneoin	amneon

Chapter Eight
PRONUNCIATION QUIZ

Name: ______________________________

A. Underline the accented syllables in the following terms:

1. fimbriae	4. menarche	7. perineum	10. endometriosis
2. genitalia	5. gravida	8. areola	
3. primipara	6. pelvimetry	9. gamete	

B. Match the term in Column I with its meaning in Column II:

Column I		Column II
1. gestation	_______	A. Fluid accumulation in the head
2. cauterization	_______	B. Period of pregnancy
3. dilation	_______	C. Scraping to remove tissue
4. coitus	_______	D. Sexual intercourse
5. parturition	_______	E. Burning to remove tissue
6. hydrocephalus	_______	F. Hormone necessary during pregnancy
7. progesterone	_______	G. Widening
8. curettage	_______	H. To examine by touch
9. palpation	_______	I. Act of giving birth
10. menstruation	_______	J. Monthly discharge of blood and cells from the uterus

C. Complete the following terms from their definitions:

1. pyo______________________________	Pus in the fallopian tubes.
2. ______________________________orrhea	Lack of menstrual flow.
3. ______________________________oscopy	Process of visually examining the vagina.
4. ______________________________plasty	Surgical repair of the breast.
5. ______________________________para	A woman who has never borne a child.
6. ______________________________ ectomy	Removal of an ovary.
7. ______________________________ ectomy	Removal of the uterus.
8. dys______________________________	Difficult labor and delivery.
9. pseudo______________________________	False pregnancy.
10. perine ______________________________	Suture of the perineum.

Chapter Eight
DIAGRAM QUIZ 1

Name: ______________________________

Label the diagram below using the terms listed below:

Bartholin glands
Clitoris
Cul-de-sac
Fallopian tube
Ovary
Perineum
Uterus
Vagina

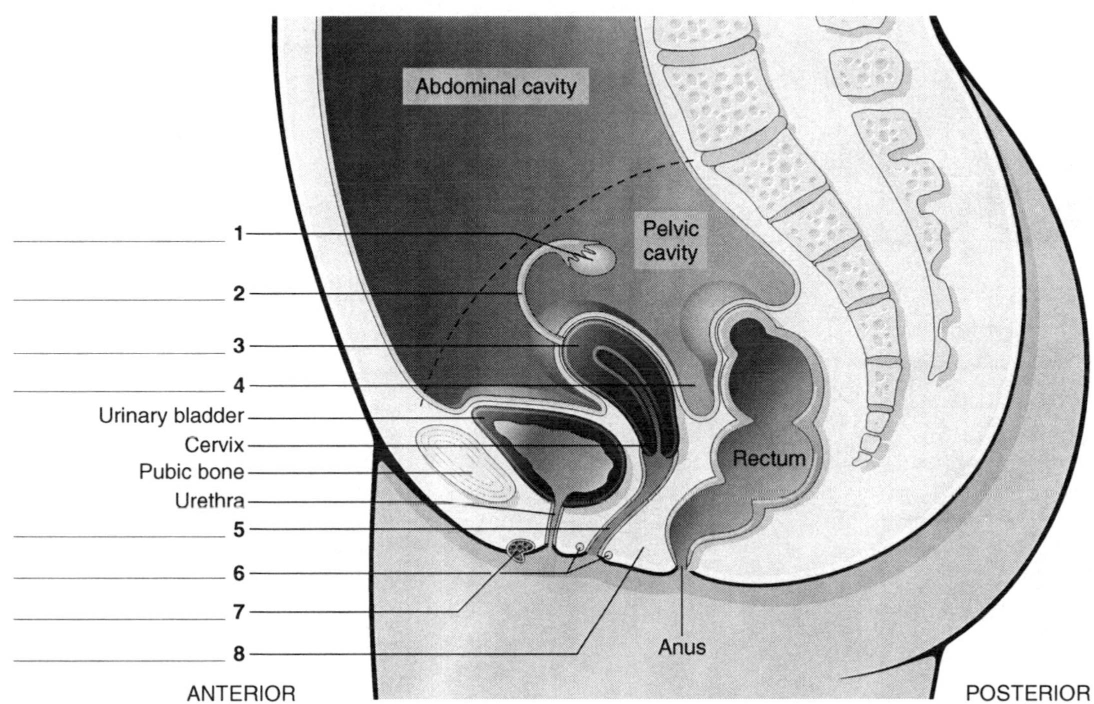

Chapter Eight
DIAGRAM QUIZ 2

Name: ______________________________

Label the diagram below using the terms listed below:

Cervix
Corpus luteum
Endometrium
Fallopian tube
Fimbriae
Myometrium
Ovarian follicles
Ovary
Ovum
Uterine serosa
Utero-ovarian ligament
Uterus
Vagina

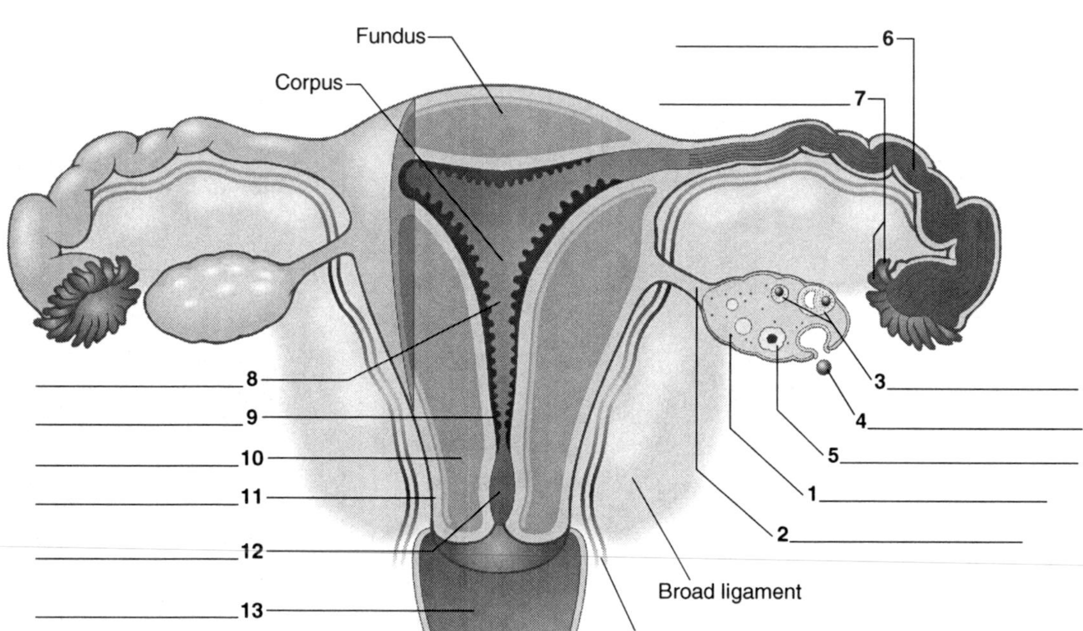

Chapter Eight

DIAGRAM QUIZ 3

Name: ______________________________

Label the diagram below using the terms listed below:

Areola
Fatty tissue
Glandular tissue
Lactiferous ducts
Mammary papilla
Sinuses

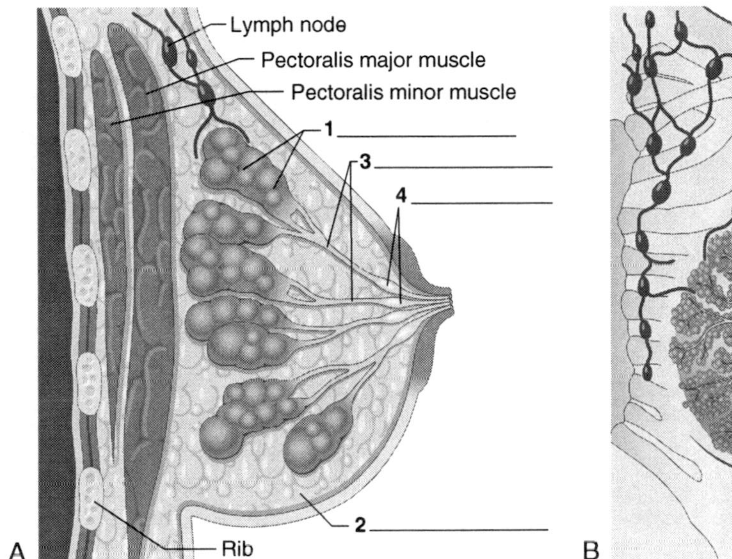

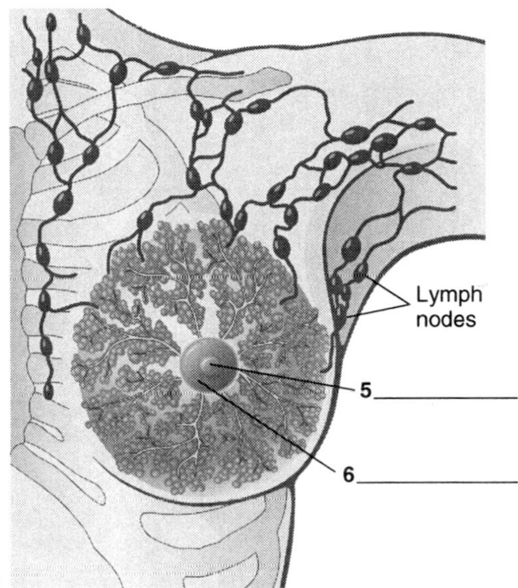

Chapter Eight
REVIEW SHEET QUIZ

Name: ______________________________

A. Give meanings for the following combining forms:

1. metr/o ____________________
2. olig/o ____________________
3. myom/o ____________________
4. galact/o ____________________
5. mast/o ____________________
6. colp/o ____________________
7. episi/o ____________________
8. oophor/o ____________________
9. hyster/o ____________________
10. perine/o ____________________
11. bartholin/o ____________________

B. Give meanings for the following suffixes:

1. -stenosis ____________________
2. -pareunia ____________________
3. -plasty ____________________
4. -ectasis ____________________
5. -cele ____________________
6. -rrhaphy ____________________
7. -stomy ____________________
8. -gravida ____________________
9. -rrhagia ____________________
10. -parous ____________________
11. -dynia ____________________

C. Give meanings for the following prefixes:

1. intra- ____________________
2. retro- ____________________
3. peri- ____________________
4. uni- ____________________
5. multi- ____________________
6. dys- ____________________
7. nulli- ____________________
8. pre- ____________________
9. pseudo- ____________________
10. endo- ____________________
11. infra- ____________________

Chapter Eight
MEDICAL SCRAMBLE

Name: ______________________________

Unscramble the letters to form medical terms from the clues. Use the letters in the squares to complete the bonus term.

1. *Clue:* Neck-like region of the womb

   ___ ___ □ ___ □ ___ R I V X E C

2. *Clue:* Lips of the vagina

   ___ □ ___ ___ ___ B A L I A

3. *Clue:* Produces eggs and hormones

   □ ___ ___ □ ___ R A O Y V

4. *Clue:* Womb

   □ □ ___ ___ ___ ___ T U S R E U

5. *Clue:* Region between the anus and the vagina

   □ ___ ___ □ □ ___ ___ ___ E N M P R E I U

6. *Clue:* Sperm cell or ovum

   ___ ___ ___ ___ □ ___ T M A G E E

BONUS TERM: *Clue:* The act of giving birth

□ □ □ □ □ □ □ □ □ □ □

Chapter Eight
CROSSWORD PUZZLE

Name: ______________________________

Fill in the crossword puzzle below using the clues listed underneath it.

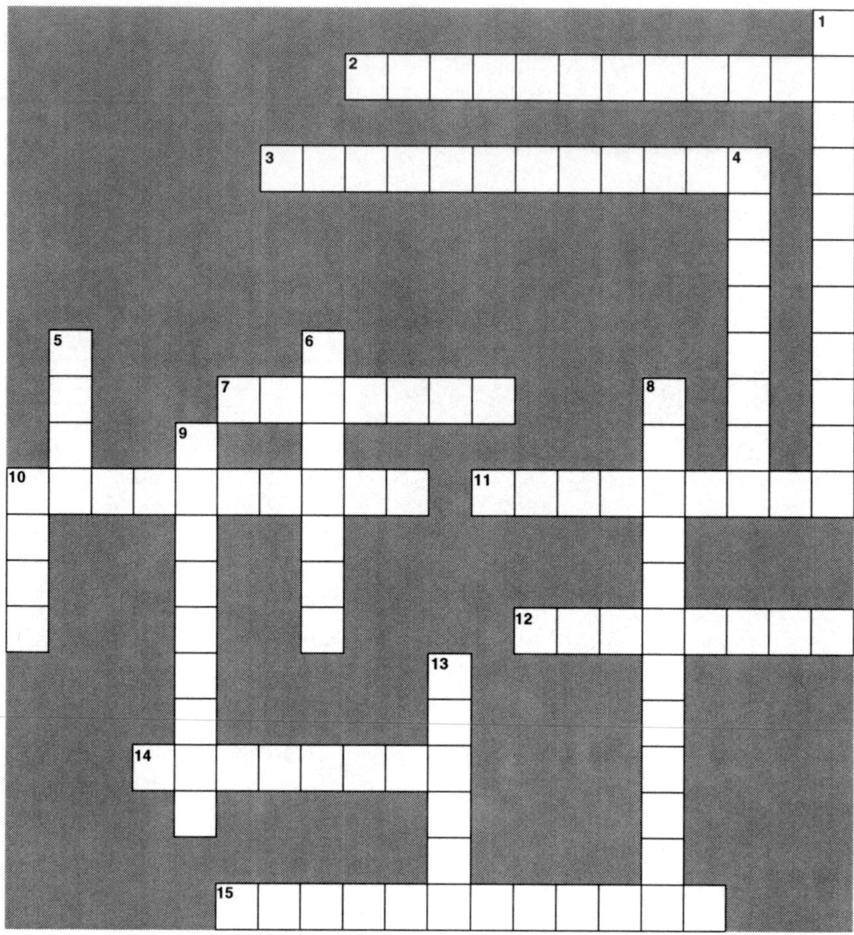

Across Clues

2. Condition of breasts (enlarged) in a male.
3. A condition during pregnancy marked by high blood pressure, proteinuria and edema.
7. Female gonads.
10. The muscle layer lining the uterus.
11. Pseudocyesis means false _____ .
12. Benign tumors in the uterus.
14. Finger-like ends of the fallopian tubes.
15. Hormone secreted by the ovaries to sustain pregnancy.

Down Clues

1. Process of taking x-rays of the breast.
4. Premature termination of pregnancy before embryo or fetus is able to exist on its own.
5. Multi- means _____.
6. A small nipple-shaped projection or elevation; the mammary_____.
8. The monthly shedding of the uterine lining
9. Reproductive organs.
10. Galact/o means _____.
13. Womb.

Chapter Eight

PRACTICAL APPLICATIONS

Name: ______________________________

Operative Report

Preoperative diagnosis:	Menorrhagia, leiomyomata
Anesthetic:	General
Material forwarded to laboratory for examination:	A. Endocervical curettings B. Endometrial curettings

Operation Performed: Dilation and Curettage of the Uterus

With the patient in the dorsal lithotomy position (legs are flexed on the thighs, thighs flexed on the abdomen and abducted) and sterilely prepped and draped, manual examination of the uterus revealed it to be 6- to 8-week size, retroflexed; no adnexal masses noted. The anterior lip of the cervix was then grasped with a tenaculum (hook-like surgical instrument for grasping and holding parts). The cervix was dilated up to a #20 Hank dilator. The uterus was sounded (widened) up to 4 inches. A sharp curettage of the endocervix showed only a scant amount of tissue. With a sharp curettage, the uterus was curetted in a clockwise fashion with an irregularity noted in the posterior floor. A large amount of hyperplastic endometrial tissue was removed. The patient tolerated the procedure well.

Operative diagnosis: Leiomyomata uteri

1. **The preoperative diagnosis indicated:** ☐
   A. Excessive bleeding between menstrual periods
   B. Possibility of malignancy in the uterine lining
   C. Fibroids and excessive bleeding during menstruation
   D. Pelvic inflammatory disease

2. **The operation described is:** ☐
   A. Scraping and burning the lining of the uterus
   B. Surgical removal of a malignant tumor
   C. Freezing and aspirating tissue from the cervix and uterus
   D. Widening the cervix and scraping the lining of the uterus

3. **What materials were sent to the laboratory for analysis?** ☐
   A. Tissue samples from vaginal and perineal region
   B. Cervical and uterine tissue samples
   C. Ovarian and abdominal tissue
   D. Uterine and ovarian tissue

4. **What were characteristics of the uterus upon examination by hand?** ☐
   A. Bent forward and prepregnancy size
   B. Bent backward and early pregnancy size
   C. Narrowed and bent forward
   D. Filled with hyperplastic tissue

5. **An adnexal mass would be located in the:** ☐
   A. Uterus
   B. Vagina
   C. Cervix
   D. Ovaries and/or fallopian tubes

6. **The diagnosis following the operative procedure indicated:** ☐
   A. Endometriosis
   B. Endocervicitis and endometritis
   C. Benign growths in the uterus
   D. Malignant fibroid tumors

FYI: When your Pap smear is positive

The Pap smear is a test for cervical cancer, but the causes of an abnormal Pap smear are more likely to be a yeast infection or STD with human papillomavirus (HPV). The following are five categories of Pap smear abnormalities:

1. ASCUS (atypical squamous cells of undetermined significance) means that the Pap smear wasn't completely normal, but did not meet diagnostic criteria for a lesion. A gynecologist may recommend repeating the Pap smear in 3 to 6 months, test for HPV, or perform colposcopy in high-risk women.
2. LSIL (low-grade squamous intraepithelial lesion) is a precancerous lesion caused by HPV. Physicians perform colposcopy for exact diagnosis (often mild dysplasia or CIN-1), and most of these lesions disappear on their own within 2 years.
3. HSIL (high-grade squamous intraepithelial lesion) is a serious precancerous lesion caused by HPV. Colposcopy is recommended, and abnormal tissue (moderate dysplasia or cervical intraepithelial neoplasia [CIN]–11) is destroyed. Conization for biopsy will rule out cervical cancer.
4. ASCUS (atypical glandular cells of undetermined significance) indicates precancerous or cancerous condition of the cervix or uterus. Colposcopy and conization are performed for biopsy and treatment to remove abnormal tissue.
5. Adenocarcinoma is cancerous glandular tissue of the cervix or uterus. Treatment is removal of the cervix and uterus and additional therapy with radiation.

Chapter Eight
ANSWERS TO THE QUIZZES

Multiple Choice Quiz

1. B
2. E
3. A
4. C
5. C
6. B
7. E
8. A
9. D
10. B
11. D
12. D
13. C
14. C
15. B
16. C
17. C
18. D
19. B
20. C
21. A
22. B
23. D
24. C
25. D

Vocabulary Quiz

A

1. cervix
2. coitus
3. amnion
4. adnexa uteri
5. cul-de-sac
6. corpus luteum
7. areola
8. clitoris
9. chorion
10. Bartholin glands

B

1. fimbriae
2. estrogen
3. fertilization
4. embryo
5. genitalia
6. fetus
7. follicle-stimulating hormone
8. endometrium
9. gamete
10. fallopian tube

C

1. lactiferous ducts
2. hCG (human chorionic gonadotropin)
3. mammary papilla
4. gynecology
5. labia
6. gonad
7. menopause
8. luteinizing hormone
9. menarche
10. gestation

D

1. neonatology
2. ovum
3. perineum
4. obstetrics
5. ovulation
6. myometrium
7. orifice
8. menstruation
9. parturition
10. ovarian follicle

E

1. zygote
2. uterine serosa
3. progesterone
4. puberty
5. placenta
6. ovary
7. vagina
8. pituitary gland
9. pregnancy
10. vulva

Terminology Quiz

A

1. inframammary
2. galactorrhea
3. lactation
4. endocervicitis
5. episiotomy
6. gynecomastia
7. colposcopy
8. amniocentesis
9. culdocentesis
10. amniotic fluid

B

1. inframammary
2. hysterectomy
3. mammoplasty
4. mastitis
5. hysteroscopy
6. mastectomy
7. oligomenorrhea
8. dysmenorrhea
9. amenorrhea
10. menorrhagia
11. bartholinitis
12. vulvodynia

C

1. myometrium
2. ovum
3. neonatal
4. oocyte
5. obstetrics
6. oophorectomy
7. oogenesis
8. myomectomy
9. metrorrhagia
10. menometrorrhagia

D

1. ovarian
2. oophoritis
3. salpingectomy
4. perineorrhaphy
5. anovulatory
6. vaginitis
7. vulvovaginitis
8. pseudocyesis
9. leukorrhea
10. menarche

E

1. oxytocia
2. menorrhea
3. primigravida
4. pyosalpinx
5. uterine prolapse
6. vaginal orifice
7. dystocia
8. primiparous
9. cephalic version
10. involution of the uterus

F

1. endometritis
2. dyspareunia
3. prenatal
4. endometrial
5. multipara
6. multigravida
7. nulligravida
8. nullipara
9. primigravida
10. retroversion

Pathology Quiz

A

1. cervicitis
2. fibroids

3. carcinoma of the breast
4. carcinoma of the cervix
5. endometriosis
6. carcinoma of the endometrium
7. ovarian cysts
8. ovarian carcinoma
9. fibrocystic breast disease
10. pelvic inflammatory disease

B

1. fibrocystic breast disease
2. ovarian carcinoma
3. pelvic inflammatory disease
4. endometriosis
5. fibroids
6. carcinoma of the cervix
7. cervicitis
8. carcinoma of the endometrium
9. ovarian cysts
10. carcinoma of the breast

C

1. erythroblastosis fetalis
2. preeclampsia
3. Down syndrome
4. placenta previa
5. abruptio placentae
6. ectopic pregnancy
7. meconium aspiration syndrome
8. pyloric stenosis
9. hydrocephalus
10. multiple gestations
11. hyaline membrane disease

Abbreviations Quiz

A

1. abortion
2. cesarean section
3. carcinoma in situ
4. chorionic villus sampling
5. cervix
6. dilation and curettage
7. follicle stimulating hormone
8. gravida
9. gynecology
10. human chorionic gonadotrophin

a. FSH
b. hCG or HCG
c. Cx
d. GYN
e. AB
f. CIS
g. CVS
h. C-section
i. G
j. D & C

B

1. hemolytic disease of the newborn
2. human papillomavirus
3. hormone replacement therapy
4. hysterosalpingography
5. intrauterine device
6. in vitro fertilization
7. loop electrocautery excision procedure
8. luteinizing hormone
9. multipara
10. obstetrics

a. HSG
b. IVF
c. LEEP
d. IUD
e. OB
f. multip
g. HDN
h. HRT
i. LH
j. HPV

C

1. Papanicolaou test
2. pelvic inflammatory disease
3. premenstrual syndrome
4. primipara
5. sentinel lymph node biopsy
6. total abdominal hysterectomy with bilateral salpingo-oophorectomy
7. uterine artery embolization
8. vaginal hysterectomy

a. PID
b. PMS
c. VH
d. UAE
e. primip
f. SNB
g. Pap test
h. TAH-BSO

Exercise Quiz

A

1. endometrium
2. mammary papilla
3. amnion
4. areola
5. vulva
6. perineum
7. ovaries
8. placenta
9. fallopian tubes
10. clitoris
11. fimbriae
12. cervix

B

13. milk
14. vagina
15. ovary
16. breast
17. uterus
18. pregnancy
19. vulva
20. egg cell

C

21. yellowish white discharge from the vagina
22. excessive discharge of blood from the uterus between menstrual periods
23. no menstrual period
24. painful sexual intercourse
25. pus in a fallopian tube

D

26. neonatal
27. culdocentesis
28. cervicitis
29. menarche
30. oxytocia

E

31. choriocarcinoma
32. preeclampsia
33. endometrial carcinoma
34. cystadenocarcinoma
35. placenta previa
36. endometriosis
37. carcinoma in situ
38. abruptio placentae

F

39. colposcopy
40. aspiration
41. cryocauterization
42. conization
43. pregnancy test
44. dilation and curettage

G

45. fibroids
46. adnexa uteri
47. progesterone
48. oophorectomy
49. vulvovaginitis
50. genitalia

Dictation and Comprehension Quiz: Vocabulary and Terminology

A

1. adnexa
2. anovulatory
3. areola
4. chorion
5. clitoris
6. colposcopy
7. amniocentesis
8. dyspareunia
9. dystocia
10. endometrium
11. genitalia
12. mastectomy
13. menarche
14. metrorrhagia
15. multipara
16. obstetrics
17. orifice
18. perineum
19. progesterone
20. pyosalpinx

B

15 Woman who has had more than one live birth
8 Painful sexual intercourse
4 Outermost membrane surrounding the developing embryo
18 Tissue lying between the anus and vagina
13 First menstrual period
19 Hormone secreted by the ovary during pregnancy
1 Ovary and fallopian tubes; accessory uterine structures
17 An opening
3 Pigmented area around the nipple of the breast
10 Inner lining of the uterus
6 Visual examination of the vagina
16 Practice of caring for women during pregnancy and delivering neonates
2 Pertaining to no egg production
7 Surgical puncture to remove fluid from the membrane surrounding the embryo
14 Excessive discharge of blood from the uterus (not during menstruation)
20 Pus in the fallopian tubes
9 Difficult labor and delivery
12 Removal of a breast
11 Reproductive organs
5 Female organ of sexual stimulation; located anterior to the urethra

Dictation and Comprehension Quiz: Pathologic Conditions, Clinical Tests and Procedures

A

1. aspiration
2. carcinoma in situ
3. cauterization
4. cervical dysplasia
5. cesarean section
6. chlamydia
7. conization
8. dilation and curettage
9. ectopic pregnancy
10. endometriosis
11. hydrocephalus
12. hysterosalpingography
13. laparoscopy
14. leiomyoma
15. mammography
16. palpation
17. placenta previa
18. preeclampsia
19. pyloric stenosis
20. tubal ligation

B

10 Tissue from the inner lining of the uterus is found in abnormal locations
14 Benign tumor in the uterus; fibroid
13 Visual examination of the abdomen; minimally invasive surgery
16 Examination by touch
1 Fluid is removed by a needle
6 Type of bacteria found as a common cause of pelvic inflammatory disease
2 Malignant tumor that is localized and not invasive
15 X-ray examination of the breast
19 Narrowing of the opening of the stomach to the intestine in a newborn
18 Condition during pregnancy marked by hypertension, proteinuria, and edema
20 Tying off the fallopian tubes; sterilization procedure
11 Accumulation of fluid in the spaces of the brain and can occur in a neonate
8 Widening the cervix and scraping the lining of the uterus
3 Burning tissue with chemicals or an electrically heated instrument
4 Abnormal growth of tissue in the neck of the uterus
5 Removal of an infant through an incision of the abdominal wall
17 Abnormal location of the organ connecting the infant and the mother
12 X-ray examination of the uterus and the fallopian tubes
9 Embryo is not implanted in the uterus
7 Removal of a cone-shaped section of the cervix for biopsy

Spelling Quiz

A

1. amenorrhea—no menstrual flow
2. oophoritis—inflammation of an ovary
3. menarche—first menstrual period
4. cervicitis—inflammation of the cervix
5. areola—pigmented area around breast nipple

Pronunciation Quiz Answers

A

1. fimbriae
2. genitalia
3. primipara
4. menarche
5. gravida
6. pelvimetry
7. perineum
8. areola
9. gamete
10. endometriosis

B

1. B
2. E
3. G
4. D
5. I
6. A
7. F

8. C
9. H
10. J

C

1. pyosalpinx
2. amenorrhea
3. colposcopy
4. mammoplasty
5. nullipara
6. oophorectomy
7. hysterectomy
8. dystocia
9. pseudocyesis
10. perineorrhaphy

Diagram Quiz 1

1. ovary
2. fallopian tube
3. uterus
4. cul-de-sac
5. vagina
6. Bartholin glands
7. clitoris
8. perineum

Diagram Quiz 2

1. ovary
2. utero-ovarian ligament
3. ovarian follicles
4. ovum
5. corpus luteum
6. fallopian tube
7. fimbriae
8. uterus
9. endometrium
10. myometrium
11. uterine serosa
12. cervix
13. vagina

Diagram Quiz 3

1. glandular tissue
2. fatty tissue
3. lactiferous ducts
4. sinuses
5. mammary papilla
6. areola

Review Sheet Quiz

A

1. uterus
2. scanty
3. muscle tumor
4. milk
5. breast
6. vagina
7. vulva
8. ovary
9. uterus
10. perineum
11. Bartholin glands

B

1. narrowing, tightening
2. sexual intercourse
3. surgical repair
4. widening, dilation
5. hernia
6. suture
7. new opening
8. pregnancy
9. bursting forth of blood
10. to bear, bring forth
11. pain

C

1. within
2. backward
3. surrounding
4. one
5. many
6. painful
7. no, not, none
8. before
9. false
10. within
11. below

Medical Scramble

1. CERVIX
2. LABIA
3. OVARY
4. UTERUS
5. PERINEUM
6. GAMETE

BONUS TERM: PARTURITION

Practical Applications

1. C
2. D
3. B
4. B
5. D
6. C

Crossword Puzzle

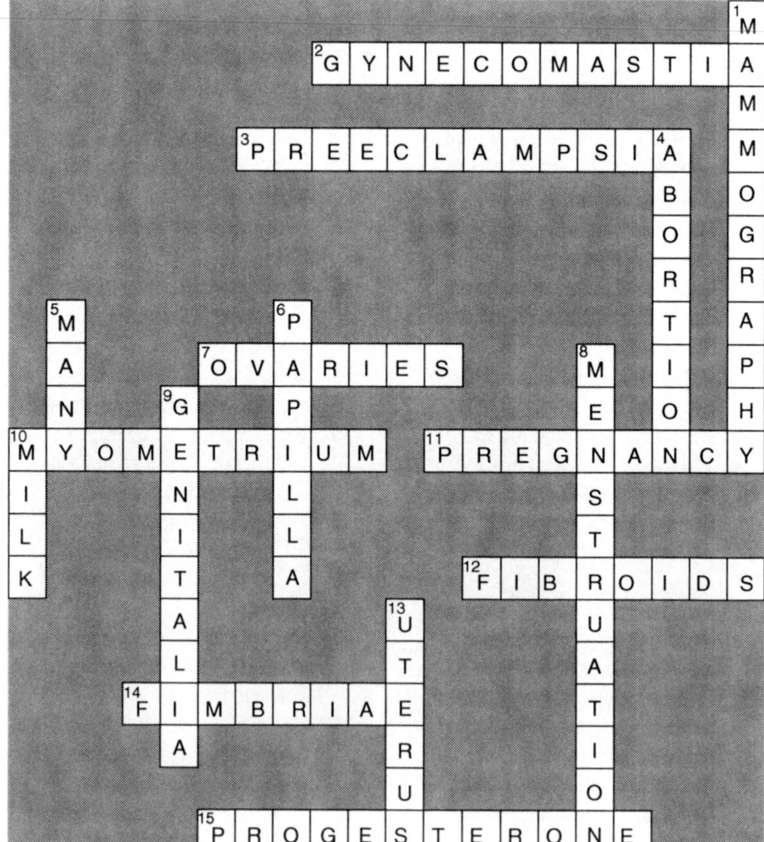

Chapter Eight
Answers to Terminology Section

(textbook pages 268–273)

Terminology	Meaning
Combining Forms	
amniocentesis	Surgical puncture to remove fluid from the amnion.
amniotic fluid	Fluid that is contained within the amnionic sac
bartholinitis	inflammation of the Bartholin glands
endocervicitis	Inflammation of the inner lining of the cervix
chorionic	Pertaining to the chorion
colposcopy	Visual examination of the vagina
culdocentesis	Surgical puncture of the cul-de-sac
episiotomy	Incision of the vulva (perineum)
galactorrhea	Discharge of milk (abnormal amount)
gynecomastia	Condition of female breasts (enlarged) in a male
hysterectomy	Removal of the uterus
hysteroscopy	Visual examination of the uterus (endoscopic)
lactation	Secretion of milk
mammary	Pertaining to the breast
mammoplasty	Surgical repair of the breast
mastitis	Inflammation of a breast
mastectomy	Removal of a breast
amenorrhea	No menstrual flow
dysmenorrhea	Pain during menstruation
oligomenorrhea	Scanty menstrual flow
menorrhagia	Excessive discharge of blood during menstruation
metrorrhagia	Excessive discharge of blood from the uterus (between menstrual periods)
menometrorrhagia	Excessive uterine bleeding at and between menstrual periods
myometrium	Muscle layer lining the uterus
myomectomy	Removal of a muscle tumor (fibroid)
neonatal	Pertaining to newborn
obstetrics	Field of medicine dealing with pregnancy and delivery of the newborn
oogenesis	Production of eggs (egg cells)
oocyte	Immature ovum
oophorectomy	Removal of an ovary
ovum	An egg cell
ovarian	Pertaining to an ovary
anovulatory	Ovulation does not occur; ovum is not released from the ovary.
perineorrhaphy	Suture of the perineum
oophoritis	Inflammation of an ovary
salpingectomy	Removal of the fallopian (uterine) tube
uterine prolapse	Sagging or falling of the uterus into the vagina
vaginal orifice	Opening of the vagina to the outside of the body
vaginitis	Inflammation of the vagina
vulvovaginitis	Inflammation of the vagina and vulva
vulvodynia	Pain of the vulvar region

Suffixes and Prefixes

menarche	Beginning of the first menstrual period.
pseudocyesis	False pregnancy
primigravida	Woman who is in her first pregnancy
primiparous	Pertaining to a woman who has delivered her first child
leukorrhea	Discharge of white vaginal secretion, which is normal or a sign of infection if becomes yellow
menorrhea	Menstrual discharge
pyosalpinx	Pus in the fallopian tube
dystocia	Difficult, painful labor and delivery
oxytocia	Rapid labor and delivery
cephalic version	Turning of the head of the fetus toward the cervix
dyspareunia	Painful sexual intercourse
endometritis	Inflammation of the inner lining of the uterus
involution of the uterus	The uterus returns to its normal nonpregnant size
intrauterine device	Object that is placed within the uterus as a contraceptive device
multipara	Woman who has had many births (deliveries)
multigravida	Woman who has had more than one pregnancy
nulligravida	Woman who has not had any pregnancies
nullipara	Woman who has not had any vaginal births
prenatal	Pertaining to before birth
primipara	Woman who has had or is giving birth to her first child
retroversion	The uterus is abnormally turned backward

Chapter 9

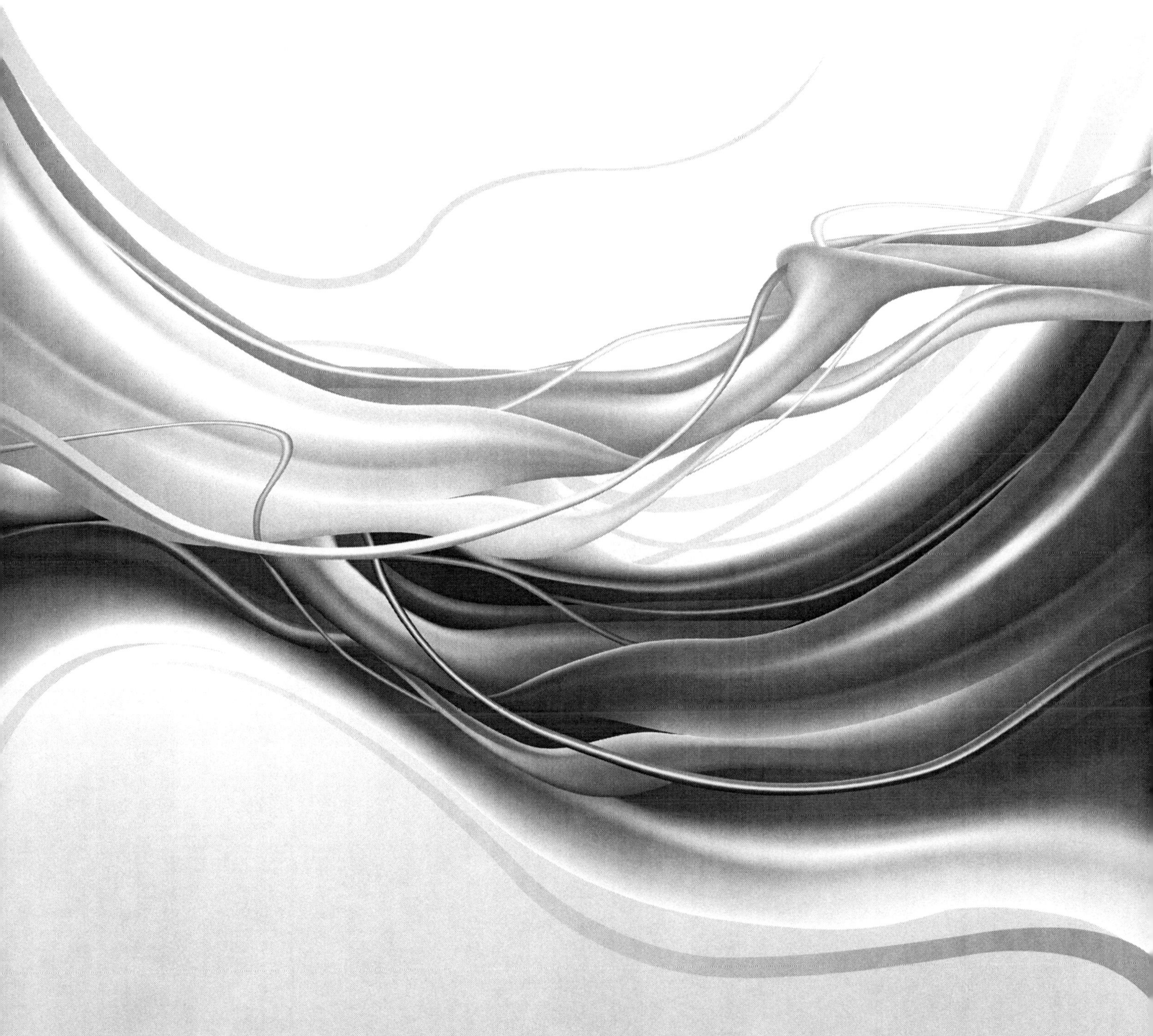

Chapter Nine
MULTIPLE CHOICE QUIZ

Name: ______________________

In the box write the letter of the choice that is the definition of the term or best answers the question. There is only one correct answer for each question.

1. The male gonad: ☐
A. Sperm cell
B. Scrotum
C. Testis
D. Penis
E. Epididymis

2. A gland below the bladder and surrounding the urethra: ☐
A. Vas deferens
B. Bulbourethral
C. Bartholin
D. Seminal vesicle
E. Prostate

3. Tissue that produces sperm cells: ☐
A. Seminiferous tubules
B. Endometrium
C. Urethra
D. Ureters
E. Scrotum

4. Hair-like tail region of the sperm is called: ☐
A. Cilia
B. Sperm head
C. Flagellum
D. Fimbriae
E. Calyx

5. Tube that leads from the epididymis to the urethra: ☐
A. Ureter
B. Seminiferous tubule
C. Cowper duct
D. Vas deferens
E. Bulbourethral duct

6. Foreskin: ☐
A. Perineum
B. Phimosis
C. Prepuce
D. Glans penis
E. Scrotum

7. Male castration would result from which of the following operations? ☐
A. Bilateral orchiectomy
B. TURP
C. Vasectomy
D. Bilateral oophorectomy
E. Unilateral orchidectomy

8. Inflammation of the glans penis: ☐
A. Orchitis
B. Hydrocele
C. Varicocele
D. Balanitis
E. Epididymitis

9. A chancre is the primary lesion in which of the following conditions? ☐
A. Pelvic inflammatory disease
B. Genital herpes
C. Nongonococcal urethritis
D. Gonorrhea
E. Syphilis

10. An androgen: ☐
A. Luteinizing hormone
B. hCG
C. Testosterone
D. Estrogen
E. Progesterone

11. Testosterone is produced by: ☐
A. Testes (interstitial tissue)
B. Prostate gland
C. Bulbourethral glands (Cowper glands)
D. Seminiferous tubules
E. Seminal vesicles

12. Undescended testicles: ☐
A. Varicocele
B. Phimosis
C. Epispadias
D. Cryptorchidism
E. Orchiotomy

13. **Benign prostatic hyperplasia is characterized by:................................** ☐
    A. Adenocarcinoma of the prostate
    B. Overgrowth of glandular tissue
    C. Hydrocele
    D. Urinary incontinence
    E. Varicocele

14. **Testicular carcinoma: ....** ☐
    A. BPH
    B. Seminoma
    C. Hypernephroma
    D. PID
    E. Chlamydia

15. **Sterilization procedure: ....** ☐
    A. Vasectomy
    B. Circumcision
    C. Orchiotomy
    D. TURP
    E. Left orchiectomy

16. **The sac containing the male gonad: ....** ☐
    A. Perineum
    B. Peritoneum
    C. Epididymis
    D. Scrotum
    E. Seminal vesicle

17. **Congenital condition of the male urethra:..** ☐
    A. Varicocele
    B. Phimosis
    C. Circumcision
    D. Hypospadias
    E. Hydrocele

18. **Parenchymal tissue in the testes:........** ☐
    A. Seminiferous tubules
    B. Bulbourethral fluid
    C. Vas deferens
    D. Connective tissue
    E. Vas deferens

19. **Scanty production of sperm:..............** ☐
    A. Azoospermia
    B. Cryptorchidism
    C. Aspermia
    D. Oligospermia
    E. Varicocele

20. **A spermolytic substance:..** ☐
    A. Produces sperm cells
    B. Destroys sperm cells
    C. Is used for benign prostatic hyperplasia
    D. Increases potency
    E. Is produced by the testes

21. **Orchiopexy:......................................** ☐
    A. Removal of a testicle
    B. Incision and removal of a piece of the vas deferens
    C. Fixation of an undescended testicle
    D. Removal of the prepuce
    E. Prolapse of a testicle

22. **Swollen, twisted veins near the testes: ....** ☐
    A. Varicocele
    B. Hydrocele
    C. Hypospadias
    D. Herpes genitalis
    E. Testicular torsion

23. **Nongonococcal urethritis is most often caused by:.................................** ☐
    A. Prostatitis
    B. Syphilis
    C. Herpes genitalis
    D. Chlamydial infection
    E. Castration

24. **Treating tissue with cold temperatures is called:..** ☐
    A. Aspiration
    B. Purulent
    C. Ejaculation
    D. Curettage
    E. Cryogenic surgery

25. **Which of the following is not an STD: ....** ☐
    A. HSV
    B. Gonorrhea
    C. BPH
    D. Syphilis
    E. Chlamydia

Chapter Nine VOCABULARY QUIZ

Name: ______________________________

A. *Match the following vocabulary terms with their meanings below:*

bulbourethral glands
ejaculation
ejaculatory duct
epididymis
erectile dysfunction
flagellum
fraternal twins
glans penis
identical twins
parenchymal tissue
perineum
prepuce

1. One of a pair of long, tightly coiled tubes on top of each testis ______________________
2. Sensitive tip of the penis ______________________
3. Two infants resulting from division of one fertilized egg into two distinct embryos ______________________
4. Pair of exocrine organs near the male urethra; secrete fluid into the urethra ______________________
5. Tube through which semen enters the male urethra ______________________
6. External region between the anus and scrotum ______________________
7. Two infants born of the same pregnancy from two separate egg cells fertilized by two different sperm cells ______________________
8. Ejection of sperm and fluid from the male urethra ______________________
9. The essential, distinctive cells of an organ ______________________
10. Hair-like projection on a sperm cell ______________________
11. Inability of an adult male to achieve an erection; impotence ______________________
12. Foreskin of the penis ______________________

B. *Match the following vocabulary terms with their meanings below:*

penis
prostate gland
scrotum
semen
seminal vesicles
seminiferous tubules
spermatozoa
sterilization
stromal tissue
testis
testosterone
vas deferens

1. Hormone secreted by the testes ______________________
2. Procedure that removes an individual's ability to produce or release reproductive cells ______________________
3. Exocrine gland at the base of the male urinary bladder ______________________
4. Male gonad that produces sperm cells and male hormone ______________________

5. Supportive, connective cells of an organ ______________________

6. Sperm cells and seminal fluid ______________________

7. Narrow, coiled tubules that produce sperm cells in the testes ______________________

8. Narrow tube that carries sperm from the epididymis
   into the body and toward the urethra ______________________

9. Sperm cells ______________________

10. External sac that contains the testes ______________________

11. Paired male exocrine glands that secrete fluid into the vas deferens ______________________

12. Male organ of reproduction ______________________

Chapter Nine
TERMINOLOGY QUIZ

Name: ______________________________

A. Match the following terms with their meanings below:

androgen
balanitis
cryogenic surgery
cryptorchidism
epididymitis
gonorrhea
hydrocele
orchiectomy
orchitis
prostatitis
prostatectomy
seminiferous tubules

1. Inflammation of a testis ______________________________
2. Undescended testicle ______________________________
3. Hernia of fluid in the scrotum ______________________________
4. Inflammation of the penis ______________________________
5. Male hormone; testosterone is an example ______________________________
6. Removal of a testis ______________________________
7. Use of cold, freezing temperatures to destroy tissue ______________________________
8. Inflammation of genital tract mucous membranes; caused by gonococcal infection ____________
9. Inflammation of the epididymis ______________________________
10. Inflammation of the gland below the urinary bladder in males ______________________________
11. Resection of a gland that produces seminal fluid ______________________________
12. Coiled tubes with the testes; form and carry sperm ______________________________

B. Give medical terms for the following definitions:

1. destruction of sperm ______________________________
2. lack of formation or ejaculation of semen ______________________________
3. scanty production of sperm ______________________________
4. hernia of swollen, twisted veins in the scrotal sac ______________________________
5. pertaining to a testis ______________________________
6. tumor resembling a "monster" (composed of many different types of tissues) ____________
7. removal of the vas deferens ______________________________
8. formation of sperm ______________________________
9. hormone produced by the testis ______________________________
10. condition of lack of sperm cells in semen ______________________________
11. fixation of the testis in place ______________________________
12. new opening between two parts of the vas deferens that were previously disconnected __________

Chapter Nine
PATHOLOGY QUIZ

Name: ______________________________

A. Match the following pathologic conditions with their descriptions below:

carcinoma of the prostate
carcinoma of the testis
cryptorchidism
hydrocele
hypospadias
phimosis
prostatic hyperplasia
testicular torsion
varicocele

1. Male urethral opening is on the undersurface of the penis ______________________
2. Twisting of the spermatic cord ______________________
3. Malignant tumor of the exocrine gland lying below the urinary bladder ______________________
4. Enlarged, dilated veins near the testis ______________________
5. Undescended testicles ______________________
6. Narrowing (stricture) of the opening of the prepuce over the glans penis ______________________
7. Malignant tumor of the male gonad ______________________
8. Benign growth of glandular tissue lying below the urinary bladder ______________________
9. Sac of clear fluid in the scrotum ______________________

B. Name the sexually transmitted disease from its description below:

1. Infection of skin and genital mucosa caused by HSV; marked by blisters ______________________
2. Infection of skin and mucous membranes in the anogenital region by HPV ______________________
3. Inflammation of the genital tract mucosa caused by gonococcal infection ______________________
4. Infection of the urethra and reproductive tract with bacteria *(Chlamydia trachomatis)* ______________________
5. Chronic infection with a spirochete bacterium ______________________

Chapter Nine

LABORATORY TESTS AND CLINICAL PROCEDURES QUIZ

Name: ______________________________

Match the following terms with their descriptions below:

circumcision
castration
digital rectal examination
photoselective vaporization of the prostate
PSA test
semen analysis
transurethral resection of the prostate
vasectomy

1. Surgical excision of testes or ovaries ______________________________
2. Finger palpation through the anal canal and rectum to examine the prostate ______________________________
3. Bilateral surgical removal of a part of the vas deferens ______________________________
4. Measurement of levels of prostate-specific antigen in the blood ______________________________
5. Removal of prostatic tissue using a green light laser ______________________________
6. Surgical procedure to remove the prepuce of the penis ______________________________
7. Excision of BPH using a resectoscope through the urethra ______________________________
8. Microscopic examination of ejaculated fluid ______________________________

Chapter Nine
ABBREVIATIONS QUIZ

Name: ______________________________

A. *On the line provided, give meanings for the following abbreviations, then write each abbreviation next to its explanation below:*

1. BPH ______________________________
2. DRE ______________________________
3. ED ______________________________
4. HPV ______________________________
5. HSV ______________________________
6. PID ______________________________
7. PSA ______________________________
8. STD ______________________________
9. TRUS ______________________________
10. TURP ______________________________

a. __________ Blood test that measures levels of a protein elevated in prostate cancer

b. __________ Inflammation of organs in the genital region associated with sexually transmitted infection

c. __________ Nonmalignant growth of tissue in the prostate gland

d. __________ Virus causing blisters on the skin and mucosa of the genital area

e. __________ Finger palpation through the anal canal to examine the prostate gland

f. __________ Virus causing genital warts

g. __________ Group of diseases transmitted by sexual intercourse

h. __________ Removal of prostatic tissue using a resectoscope through the urethra

i. __________ Impotence

j. __________ Test to assess the prostate and guide precise placement of biopsy needle

Chapter Nine
EXERCISE QUIZ

Name: ______________________

A. Build medical terms:

1. inflammation of the testes ______________________
2. resection of the prostate gland ______________________
3. condition of scanty sperm ______________________
4. process of forming (producing) sperm cells ______________________
5. fixation of an undescended testicle ______________________

B. Give meanings for the following medical terms:

6. parenchymal tissue ______________________
7. androgen ______________________
8. testicular teratoma ______________________
9. stromal tissue ______________________
10. azoospermia ______________________

C. Give medical terms for the descriptions below:

11. pair of sacs; secrete fluid into ejaculatory duct ______________________
12. coiled tube above each testis; carries and stores sperm ______________________
13. male gonad; produces hormone and sperm cells ______________________
14. foreskin ______________________

D. Match the term in Column I with its meaning in Column II:

Column I		Column II
15. castration	______	A. To tie off or bind
16. purulent	______	B. Removal of a piece of vas deferens
17. ligation	______	C. Orchiectomy
18. circumcision	______	D. Removal of the prepuce
19. ejaculation	______	E. Destruction of tissue by freezing
20. cryosurgery	______	F. Pus-filled
21. vasectomy	______	G. Test of fertility (reproductive ability)
22. semen analysis	______	H. Ejection of sperm and fluid from the urethra

E. Give medical terms for the following abnormal conditions:

23. STD; etiology is berry-shaped bacteria ______________________
24. opening of the urethra on the undersurface of the penis ______________________
25. enlarged, swollen veins near the testes ______________________
26. undescended testicles ______________________
27. STD; primary stage marked by a chancre ______________________
28. malignant tumor of the prostate gland ______________________

F. Give meanings for the following abbreviations:

29. TURP ______________________
30. PSA ______________________
31. BPH ______________________

G. Give the meaning of the following:

32. -sclerosis ______________________
33. -cele ______________________
34. -rrhagia ______________________
35. -phagia ______________________
36. -genesis ______________________
37. oophor/o ______________________
38. colp/o ______________________
39. balan/o ______________________
40. salping/o ______________________
41. -ptosis ______________________

H. Match the surgical procedures in Column I with the reasons they would be performed in Column II:

Column I		Column II
42. bilateral orchiectomy	________	A. Carcinoma of the prostate gland
43. TURP	________	B. Cryptorchidism
44. vasectomy	________	C. Sterilization (hormones remain)
45. orchiopexy	________	D. Benign prostatic hyperplasia
46. hydrocelectomy	________	E. Reversal of sterilization
47. circumcision	________	F. Removal of swollen, twisted veins near the testes
48. radical prostatectomy	________	G. Abnormal fluid collection in scrotum
49. vasovasostomy	________	H. Seminoma
50. varicocelectomy	________	I. Phimosis

Chapter Nine

DICTATION AND COMPREHENSION QUIZ

Name: ______________________________

A. Dictation of Terms

1. ______________________ 11. ______________________
2. ______________________ 12. ______________________
3. ______________________ 13. ______________________
4. ______________________ 14. ______________________
5. ______________________ 15. ______________________
6. ______________________ 16. ______________________
7. ______________________ 17. ______________________
8. ______________________ 18. ______________________
9. ______________________ 19. ______________________
10. ______________________ 20. ______________________

B. Comprehension of Terms: Match number of the above term with its meaning below.

______ Inflammation of the tube that carries sperm from the testicle to the vas deferens
______ Hard ulcer that is a sign of a sexually transmitted disease
______ Pus-filled
______ A hormone that produces male secondary sex characteristics
______ Inflammation of a testicle
______ Fluid that contains sperm cells and secretions and is produced during ejaculation
______ Hernia of fluid in the testicle
______ Malignant tumor of the testes
______ Foreskin
______ Essential cells of the testes; seminiferous tubules
______ Excision of the testicles or ovaries
______ Increase in growth of cells of a gland below the urinary bladder in males
______ Glands that secrete a fluid into the vas deferens
______ Enlarged, dilated veins near the testicle
______ Undescended testicle
______ Condition of scanty sperm cell production
______ Congenital opening of the male urethra on the under surface of the penis
______ Chronic STD caused by a type of bacteria (spirochete)
______ Inflammation of the genital tract mucosa caused by infection with berry-shaped bacteria
______ Infection of the skin and mucous membranes with HSV; small fluid-filled blisters occur

Chapter Nine
SPELLING QUIZ

Name: ______________________________

A. Circle the term that is spelled correctly, and write its meaning in the space provided.

1. chyamydia — chlamydia ______________________________
2. impotance — impotence ______________________________
3. chanker — chancre ______________________________
4. seminoma — semenoma ______________________________
5. scrotum — scrotim ______________________________
6. parynchomal — parenchymal ______________________________
7. purulent — puerluent ______________________________
8. adenocarcinoma — adenocarsinoma ______________________________
9. prostrate gland — prostate gland ______________________________
10. prepus — prepuce ______________________________

B. Circle the term that is spelled correctly. The meaning of each term is given.

11. Undescended testicle	criptororhidism	crytporchidism	cryptorchidism
12. Glands that secrete semen	bulbourethral	bulboureteral	bolboureteral
13. Tubules that produce sperm	seminiferous	semeniferious	seminefarous
14. Sexually transmitted disease	syphilis	syphillis	syfalus
15. Type of carcinoma of the testes	embrional	embryonal	enbryomal
16. Sperm cells and fluid	semin	seman	semen
17. Scanty sperm production	olagospermia	oliospermia	oligospermia
18. Pus-filled	purulent	poorulent	pureulent
19. Male sex hormone	testostarone	testosterone	testosterome
20. Male gonad	testus	testas	testis

Chapter Nine
PRONUNCIATION QUIZ

Name: ______________________________

A. Underline the accented syllable in the following terms:

1. parenchymal
2. prepuce
3. varicocele
4. scrotum
5. flagellum
6. androgen
7. seminoma
8. prostatectomy
9. testosterone
10. impotence

B. Match the term in Column I with its meaning in Column II:

Column I		Column II
1. cryptorchidism	________	A. Sac that holds the testes
2. testosterone	________	B. Hormone produced by the testes
3. spermolytic	________	C. Removal of the testes
4. circumcision	________	D. Undescended testicle
5. vasectomy	________	E. Sterilization; removal of part of the vas deferens
6. scrotum	________	F. Congenital opening of the urethra on the underside of penis
7. gonorrhea	________	G. Pus-filled
8. hypospadias	________	H. Venereal disease marked by urethral discharge
9. orchiectomy	________	I. Removal of the foreskin around the glans penis
10. purulent	________	J. Pertaining to destruction of sperm cells

C. Complete the following terms from their definitions:

1. ______________________ opexy — Fixation of a testicle in place.
2. oligo ______________________ — Condition of scanty sperm production.
3. ______________________ itis — Inflammation of the glans penis.
4. prostatic ______________________ — Excessive development; enlargement of the prostate gland.
5. hydro ______________________ — Hernia of fluid in the scrotal sac.
6. ______________________ itis — Inflammation of the epididymis.
7. vaso ______________________ — New connection between two parts of the vas deferens.
8. spermato ______________________ — Formation of sperm cells.
9. gono ______________________ — Sexually transmitted disease.
10. ______________________ osis — Narrowing of the foreskin over the glans penis.

Chapter Nine
DIAGRAM QUIZ

Name: ______________________________

Label the diagram below using the terms listed below:

Bulbourethral (Cowper) gland
Ejaculatory duct
Epididymis
Glans penis
Penis
Perineum
Prepuce (foreskin)
Prostate gland
Scrotum
Seminal vesicle
Seminiferous tubules
Testis
Urethra
Vas deferens

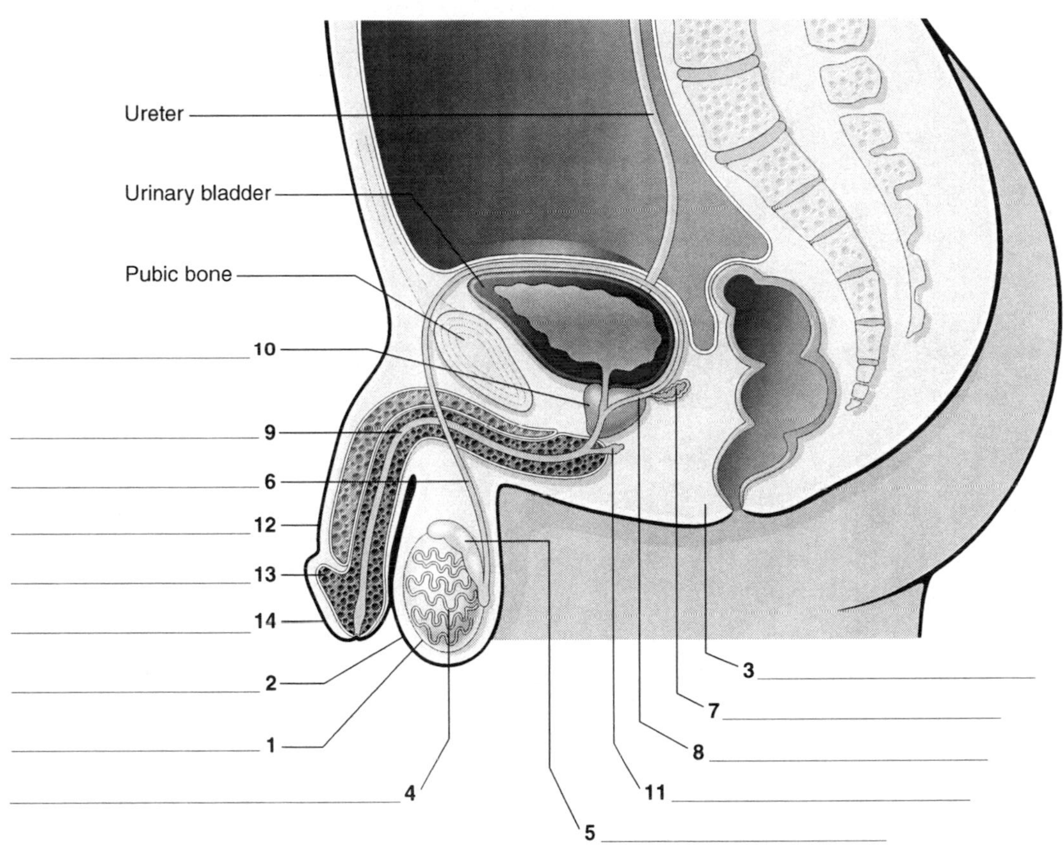

Chapter Nine
FLOW CHART QUIZ

Name: ____________________

Label the flow chart using the terms listed below:

ejaculatory duct	penis	urethra
epididymis	seminiferous tubules	vas deferens

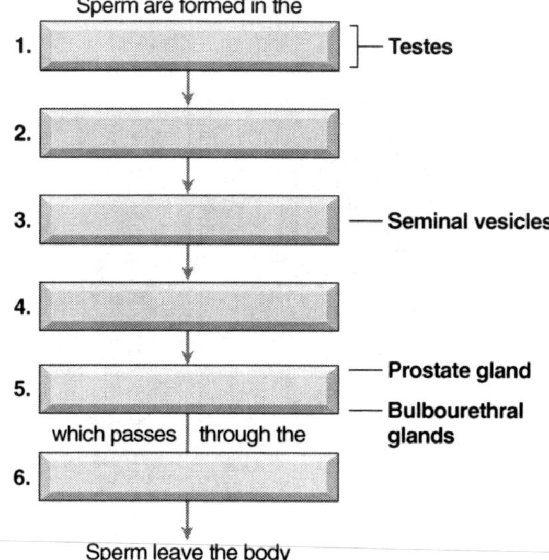

Chapter Nine
REVIEW SHEET QUIZ

Name: ______________________________

A. Give meanings for the following combining forms:

1. balan/o ____________________
2. orchi/o ____________________
3. vas/o ____________________
4. zo/o ____________________
5. andr/o ____________________
6. crypt/o ____________________
7. cry/o ____________________
8. hydr/o ____________________
9. epididym/o ____________________
10. terat/o ____________________

B. Give meanings for the following suffixes:

1. -plasia ____________________
2. -lysis ____________________
3. -cele ____________________
4. -pexy ____________________
5. -stomy ____________________
6. -tomy ____________________
7. -trophy ____________________
8. -genesis ____________________
9. -ectomy ____________________
10. -rrhea ____________________

Chapter Nine
MEDICAL SCRAMBLE

Name: ______________________

Unscramble the letters to form suffixes from the clues. Use the letters in the squares to complete the bonus term.

1. *Clue:* Ulcer associated with an STD

   ___ □ ___ ___ ___ ___ ___ RACEHCN

2. *Clue:* Collection of fluid in the scrotal sac (hernia)

   ___ □ ___ ___ ___ ___ ___ □ ___ COYLHERED

3. *Clue:* Inflammation of the testes

   ___ ___ ___ ___ □ ___ □ □ TCIOSHRI

4. *Clue:* Gland at the base of the bladder that secretes seminal fluid

   □ ___ ___ □ ___ ___ ___ ___ TOSEPART

BONUS TERM: *Clue:* A common sexually transmitted disease caused by a spirochete

□ □ □ □ □ □ □ □

Chapter Nine
CROSSWORD PUZZLE

Name: ______________________________

Fill in the crossword puzzle below using the clues listed underneath it.

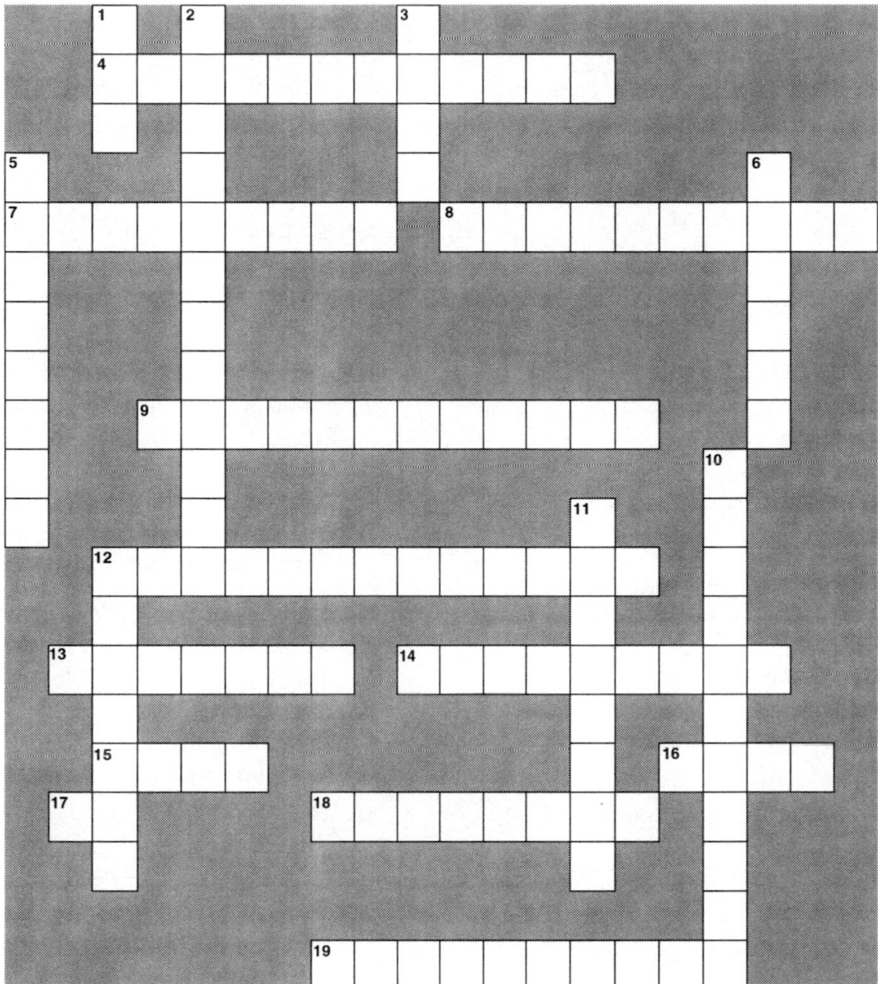

Across Clues

4. Sperm cell.
7. Sac of clear fluid in the testes.
8. Enlarged, swollen veins near the testicle.
9. Undescended testicle.
12. Procedure rendering an individual incapable of reproduction.
13. Foreskin.
14. Hair-like process on a sperm cell that makes it motile.
15. Transurethral resection of the prostate (abbrev).
16. Andr/o.
17. Genitourinary (abbrev).
18. Chronic sexually transmitted infectious disease caused by spirochete bacteria.
19. Orchiectomy.

Down Clues

1. Herpes simplex virus (abbrev).
2. Hormone secreted by the testes.
3. Cry/o.
5. Narrowing of the opening of the foreskin over the glans penis.
6. Vas/o.
10. Ejection of sperm and fluid from the male urethra.
11. Skin covering the tip of the penis.
12. External sac that contains the testes.

Chapter Nine

PRACTICAL APPLICATIONS

Name: ______________________

A. Case Report

A 22-year-old male presents with a scrotal mass that does not transilluminate. An orchiectomy reveals embryonal carcinoma with teratoma. Chest x-rays and lung tomograms are normal. Serum AFP (alpha-fetoprotein, a protein secreted by tumor cells. is elevated. Abdominal CT scan reveals minimal retroperitoneal lymphadenopathy. Retroperitoneal lymphadenectomy indicates 4 of 42 nodes positive for embryonal carcinoma.

Six months after the node dissection the patient remains asymptomatic but his chest x-ray reveals pulmonary metastases. AFP is slightly elevated. Chemotherapy (cisplatin, vinblastine, and bleomycin) is given over 12 weeks. One month after completion of chemotherapy a thoracotomy is done and residual lung lesions are removed. He remains free of disease 32 months after the start of chemotherapy.

1. **What is the diagnosis for this patient?** ☐
   A. Prostate cancer
   B. Testicular cancer
   C. Benign prostatic hyperplasia
   D. Lung cancer
2. **What was the primary method of treatment?** ☐
   A. Chemotherapy
   B. Radiation therapy
   C. Surgical removal of the prostate gland
   D. Surgical removal of a testis
3. **What other surgical procedure was done to stage the patient's condition?** ☐
   A. Removal of tumor from the lung
   B. Chest x-ray
   C. Removal of pelvic lymph nodes
   D. Removal of lymph nodes behind the membrane lining the abdominal cavity
4. **What treatment was initially given for spread of the tumor to the lungs?** ☐
   A. Drug treatment with AFP
   B. Thoracotomy
   C. Chemotherapy
   D. Retroperitoneal lymphadenectomy

B. Chart Note

History: The patient is a 55-year-old male with adenocarcinoma of the prostate. He had a TURP 1 year ago for presumed prostatic hyperplasia, but tissue fragments examined by a pathologist revealed a poorly differentiated adenocarcinoma. He received local irradiation to the prostate; however, PSA levels increased to 10 (normal is less than 4). A bone scan showed bony metastases. Bilateral orchiectomy was advised, but refused. Alternative hormonal treatment with Lupron and flutamide to decrease testosterone production will be offered.

1. **What is the patient's diagnosis?** ☐
   A. Prostate cancer
   B. Bone cancer
   C. Testicular cancer
   D. BPH
2. **What procedure revealed the diagnosis?** ☐
   A. Irradiation
   B. Removal of the testicles
   C. Bone scan
   D. Transurethral resection of the prostate
3. **Poorly differentiated means:** ☐
   A. Cells are mature
   B. Cells are very immature
   C. Cells have metastasized
   D. Cells are not malignant
4. **What type of drug treatment was offered to the patient?** ☐
   A. Standard chemotherapy with cytotoxic agents
   B. Androgens
   C. Antiandrogen drugs
   D. PSA treatment

Chapter Nine
ANSWERS TO THE QUIZZES

Multiple Choice Quiz

1. C
2. E
3. A
4. C
5. D
6. C
7. A
8. D
9. E
10. C
11. A
12. D
13. B
14. B
15. A
16. D
17. D
18. A
19. D
20. B
21. C
22. A
23. D
24. E
25. C

Vocabulary Quiz

A

1. epididymis
2. glans penis
3. identical twins
4. bulbourethral glands
5. ejaculatory duct
6. perineum
7. fraternal twins
8. ejaculation
9. parenchymal tissue
10. flagellum
11. erectile dysfunction
12. prepuce

B

1. testosterone
2. sterilization
3. prostate gland
4. testis
5. stromal tissue
6. semen
7. seminiferous tubules
8. vas deferens
9. spermatozoa
10. scrotum
11. seminal vesicles
12. penis

Terminology Quiz

A

1. orchitis
2. cryptorchidism
3. hydrocele
4. balanitis
5. androgen
6. orchiectomy
7. cryogenic surgery
8. gonorrhea
9. epididymitis
10. prostatitis
11. prostatectomy
12. seminiferous tubules

B

1. spermolytic
2. aspermia
3. oligospermia
4. varicocele
5. testicular
6. teratoma
7. vasectomy
8. spermatogenesis
9. testosterone
10. azoospermia
11. orchiopexy
12. vasovasostomy

Pathology Quiz

A

1. hypospadias
2. testicular torsion
3. carcinoma of the prostate
4. varicocele
5. cryptorchidism
6. phimosis
7. carcinoma of the testis
8. prostatic hyperplasia
9. hydrocele

B

1. herpes genitalis
2. human papilloma virus (HPV)
3. gonorrhea
4. chlamydia
5. syphilis

Laboratory Tests and Clinical Procedures Quiz

1. castration
2. digital rectal examination
3. vasectomy
4. PSA test
5. photoselective vaporization of the prostate
6. circumcision
7. transurethral resection of the prostate
8. semen analysis

Abbreviations Quiz

1. benign prostatic hyperplasia
2. digital rectal examination
3. erectile dysfunction
4. human papillomavirus
5. herpes simplex virus
6. pelvic inflammatory disease
7. prostate-specific antigen
8. sexually transmitted diseases
9. transrectal ultrasonography
10. transurethral resection of the prostate

a. PSA
b. PID
c. BPH
d. HSV
e. DRE
f. HPV
g. STD
h. TURP
i. ED
j. TRUS

Exercise Quiz

A

1. orchitis
2. prostatectomy
3. oligospermia
4. spermatogenesis
5. orchiopexy

B

6. essential cells of an organ
7. male hormone
8. tumor of the testes (malignant)
9. connective tissue in an organ
10. condition of no sperm cells in semen

C

11. seminal vesicles
12. epididymis
13. testis
14. prepuce

D

15. C
16. F
17. A
18. D
19. H
20. E
21. B
22. G

E

23. gonorrhea
24. hypospadias
25. varicocele
26. cryptorchidism
27. syphilis
28. prostatic adenocarcinoma

F

29. transurethral resection of the prostate
30. prostate specific antigen
31. benign prostatic hyperplasia

G

32. hardening
33. hernia
34. bursting forth of blood
35. eating, swallowing
36. formation
37. ovary
38. vagina
39. glans penis
40. fallopian tube
41. falling, sagging, prolapse

H

42. H
43. D
44. C
45. B
46. G
47. I
48. A
49. E
50. F

Dictation and Comprehension Quiz

A

1. androgen
2. castration
3. chancre
4. cryptorchidism
5. epididymitis
6. gonorrhea
7. herpes genitalis
8. hydrocele
9. hypospadias
10. oligospermia
11. orchitis
12. parenchymal tissue
13. prepuce
14. prostatic hyperplasia
15. purulent
16. semen
17. seminal vesicles
18. seminoma
19. syphilis
20. varicocele

B

5 Inflammation of the tube that carries sperm from the testicle to the vas deferens
3 Hard ulcer that is a sign of a sexually transmitted disease
15 Pus-filled
1 A hormone that produces male secondary sex characteristics
11 Inflammation of a testicle
16 Fluid that contains sperm cells and secretions and is produced during ejaculation
8 Hernia of fluid in the testicle
18 Malignant tumor of the testes
13 Foreskin
12 Essential cells of the testes; seminiferous tubules
2 Excision of the testicles or ovaries
14 Increase in growth of cells of a gland below the urinary bladder in males
17 Glands that secrete a fluid into the vas deferens
20 Enlarged, dilated veins near the testicle
4 Undescended testicle
10 Condition of scanty sperm cell production
9 Congenital opening of the male urethra on the undersurface of the penis
19 Chronic STI caused by a type of bacteria (spirochete)
6 Inflammation of the genital tract mucosa caused by infection with berry-shaped bacteria
7 Infection of the skin and mucous membranes with HSV; small fluid-filled blisters occur

Spelling Quiz

A

1. chlamydia—bacteria causing sexually transmitted disease
2. impotence—inability of an adult male to achieve an erection
3. chancre—ulcer associated with syphilis
4. seminoma—malignant tumor of the testes
5. scrotum—sac that holds the testes
6. parenchymal—pertaining to essential cells of an organ
7. purulent—pus-filled
8. adenocarcinoma—cancerous tumor of a gland
9. prostate gland—below the urinary bladder (males); secretes seminal fluid
10. prepuce—foreskin

B

11. cryptorchidism
12. bulbourethral
13. seminiferous
14. syphilis
15. embryonal
16. semen
17. oligospermia
18. purulent
19. testosterone
20. testis

Pronunciation Quiz

A

1. parenchymal
2. prepuce
3. varicocele
4. scrotum
5. flagellum
6. androgen
7. seminoma
8. prostatectomy
9. testosterone
10. impotence

B

1. D
2. B
3. J
4. I
5. E
6. A
7. H
8. F
9. C
10. G

C

1. orchiopexy
2. oligospermia
3. balanitis
4. prostatic hyperplasia (or hypertrophy)
5. hydrocele
6. epididymitis
7. vasovasostomy
8. spermatogenesis
9. gonorrhea
10. phimosis

Diagram Quiz

1. Testis
2. Scrotum
3. Perineum
4. Seminiferous tubules
5. Epididymis
6. Vas deferens
7. Seminal vesicle
8. Ejaculatory duct
9. Urethra
10. Prostate gland
11. Bulbourethral (Cowper) gland
12. Penis
13. Glans penis
14. Prepuce (foreskin)

Flow Chart Quiz

1. seminiferous tubules
2. epididymis
3. vas deferens
4. ejaculatory duct
5. urethra
6. penis

Review Sheet Quiz

A

1. glans penis
2. testis
3. vessel, duct; vas deferens
4. animal life
5. male
6. hidden
7. cold
8. water
9. epididymis
10. monster

B

1. formation
2. destruction; separation
3. hernia
4. fixation
5. new opening
6. incision
7. nourishment, development
8. formation
9. removal, excision, resection
10. flow, discharge

Practical Applications

A

1. B
2. D
3. D
4. C

Crossword Puzzle

Across: 4 SPERMATOZOON; 7 HYDROCELE; 8 VARICOCELE; 9 CRYPTORCHISM; 12 STERILIZATION; 13 PREPUCE; 14 FLAGELLUM; 15 TURP; 16 MALE; 17 GU; 18 SYPHILIS; 19 CASTRATION

Down: 1 HSV; 2 TESTOSTERONE; 3 COLD; 5 PHIMOSIS; 6 VESSEL; 10 EJACULATION; 11 FORESKIN; 12 SCROTUM

B

1. A
2. D
3. B
4. C

Medical Scramble

1. CHANCRE
2. HYDROCELE
3. ORCHITIS
4. PROSTATE

BONUS TERM: SYPHILIS

Chapter Nine
Answers to Terminology Section

(textbook pages 317–319)

Terminology	Meaning
androgen	Male hormone producing or stimulating male characteristics. An example is testosterone.
balanitis	Inflammation of the glans penis.
cryogenic surgery	Pertaining to destruction of tissue by producing cold temperatures.
cryptorchidism	Undescended testicles.
epididymitis	Inflammation of the epididymis.
gonorrhea	Sexually transmitted disease; disease marked by gonococci and urethral discharge.
hydrocele	Hernia (sac) of fluid in the scrotal sac.
orchiectomy	Removal of a testicle.
orchitis	Inflammation of a testicle.
penile	Pertaining to the penis.
penoscrotal	Pertaining to the penis and scrotum.
prostatitis	Inflammation of the prostate gland.
prostatectomy	Removal of the prostate gland.
seminiferous tubules	Produce sperm in the testes.
spermolytic	Pertaining to destruction of sperm.
oligospermia	Scanty production of sperm.
aspermia	Lack of formation or ejaculation of semen.
teratoma	Tumor (testicular) that is composed of many types of tissue. Terat/o means monster.
testicular	Pertaining to the testes.
varicocele	Hernia (collection) of swollen, twisted veins above the testes.
vasectomy	Removal of a portion of each vas deferens.
azoospermia	Lack of spermatozoa in semen.
spermatogenesis	Formation of sperm cells.
testosterone	Male hormone produced by the testes.
orchiopexy	Fixation of the testicle. It is put in place following a diagnosis of cryptorchidism.
vasovasostomy	New opening (anastomosis) between two parts of the vas deferens; surgery to reverse vasectomy.

Chapter 10

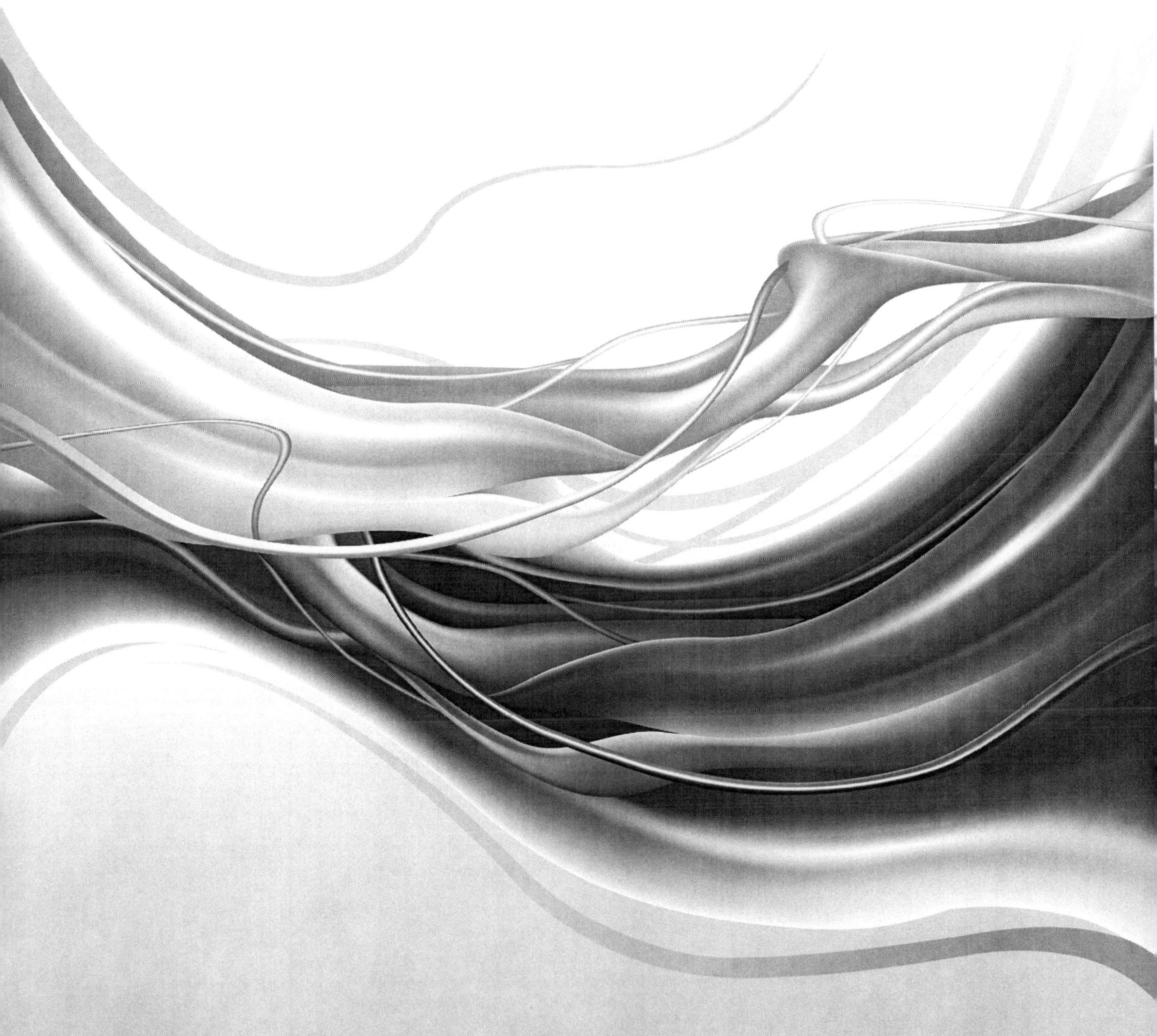

Chapter Ten
MULTIPLE CHOICE QUIZ

Name: ______________________

In the box write the letter of the choice that is the definition of the term or best answers the question. There is only one correct answer for each question.

1. **Part of the brain responsible for coordinating muscle movements and maintaining balance:..........................** ☐
   A. Pons
   B. Cerebrum
   C. Thalamus
   D. Hypothalamus
   E. Cerebellum

2. **Pertaining to muscles and nerves:.......** ☐
   A. Myoneural
   B. Neuroanastomosis
   C. Myelogram
   D. Myelomeningocele
   E. Polyneuritis

3. **Neurotransmitter:..............................** ☐
   A. Cerebrospinal fluid
   B. Myelin
   C. Acetylcholine
   D. Lymph
   E. Sulcus

4. **Part of the nerve cell that first receives the nervous impulse is the:................** ☐
   A. Axon
   B. Cell body
   C. Neurilemma
   D. Convolution
   E. Dendrite

5. **Elevated portions of the cerebral cortex are called: ....** ☐
   A. Sulci
   B. Plexuses
   C. Gyri
   D. Ventricles
   E. Glial cells

6. **Burning sensation of pain:.................** ☐
   A. Analgesia
   B. Cephalgia
   C. Anesthesia
   D. Causalgia
   E. Dysesthesia

7. **A network of interlacing nerve fibers in the peripheral nervous system: ....** ☐
   A. Microglia
   B. Astrocyte
   C. Plexus
   D. Synapse
   E. Receptor

8. **Portion of the brain that controls the pituitary gland, water balance, and body temperature: ....** ☐
   A. Medulla oblongata
   B. Cauda equina
   C. Cerebellum
   D. Thalamus
   E. Hypothalamus

9. **Glial cells: ....** ☐
   A. Neurons
   B. Astrocytes
   C. Meninges
   D. Parenchymal cells
   E. Nerve cells that conduct impulses

10. **Space between nerve cells is called the: ....** ☐
    A. Subdural space
    B. Subarachnoid space
    C. Ventricle
    D. Synapse
    E. Stimulus

11. **Part of the brain that controls breathing, heartbeat, and the size of blood vessels: ....** ☐
    A. Cerebellum
    B. Pons
    C. Cauda equina
    D. Medulla oblongata
    E. Thalamus

12. **Inability to speak: ....** ☐
    A. Apraxia
    B. Dysplasia
    C. Aphasia
    D. Aphagia
    E. Ataxia

13. **Collection of spinal nerves below the end of the spinal cord:** .... ☐
    A. Gyrus
    B. Dendrites
    C. Cauda equina
    D. Microglia
    E. Oligodendroglia

14. **Disease of the spinal cord:** .... ☐
    A. Encephalopathy
    B. Myopathy
    C. Myoparesis
    D. Meningioma
    E. Myelopathy

15. **Collection of blood within the meningeal layers:** .... ☐
    A. Leptomeningitis
    B. Cerebromalacia
    C. Subdural hematoma
    D. Hydrocephalus
    E. Hemiparesis

16. **Abnormal sensation of tingling or prickling:** .... ☐
    A. Anesthesia
    B. Paresthesia
    C. Analgesia
    D. Neurasthenia
    E. Hyperkinesis

17. **Inflammation of a spinal nerve root:** ... ☐
    A. Encephalitis
    B. Meningitis
    C. Blepharitis
    D. Radiculitis
    E. Polyneuritis

18. **A highly malignant brain tumor:** .... ☐
    A. Meningioma
    B. Epidural hematoma
    C. Glioblastoma
    D. Subdural hematoma
    E. Teratoma

19. **Paralysis of four extremities:** .... ☐
    A. Hemiparesis
    B. Hemiplegia
    C. Paraplegia
    D. Quadriplegia
    E. Apraxia

20. **Cerebral aneurysm, thrombosis, or hemorrhage can be the cause of:** .... ☐
    A. Cerebrovascular accident
    B. Concussion
    C. Multiple sclerosis
    D. Myasthenia gravis
    E. Epilepsy

21. **Fainting:** .... ☐
    A. Shingles
    B. Hypesthesia
    C. Ataxia
    D. Syncope
    E. Palsy

22. **Spina bifida is associated with:** .... ☐
    A. Poliomyelitis
    B. Myelomeningocele
    C. Multiple myeloma
    D. Hyperkinesis
    E. Narcolepsy

23. **Parkinson disease is characterized by:** .... ☐
    A. Shuffling gait
    B. Cerebellar ataxia
    C. Bell palsy
    D. Herpes zoster infection
    E. Narcolepsy

24. **Disorder of reading, writing, and learning is:** .... ☐
    A. Epilepsy
    B. Apraxia
    C. Bradykinesis
    D. Neurasthenia
    E. Dyslexia

25. **Condition of no nervous sensation:** ..... ☐
    A. Analgesia
    B. Anencephaly
    C. Anesthesia
    D. Huntington disease
    E. Alzheimer disease

Chapter Ten
VOCABULARY QUIZ

Name: ______________________________

A. Match the following vocabulary terms with their meanings below:

acetylcholine
afferent nerve
arachnoid membrane
astrocyte
autonomic nervous system
axon
blood-brain barrier
brainstem
cauda equina
cell body

1. Blood vessels (capillaries) that selectively let certain substances enter brain tissue and keep others out ______________________________
2. Type of glial (neuroglial) cell that transports water and salts from capillaries ______________
3. Collection of spinal nerves below the end of the spinal cord ______________
4. Neurotransmitter chemical released at the ends of nerve cells ______________
5. Microscopic fiber that carries the nervous impulse along a nerve cell ______________
6. Carries messages toward the brain and spinal cord from receptors ______________
7. Lower portion of the brain that connects the cerebrum with the spinal cord ______________
8. Part of a nerve cell that contains the nucleus ______________
9. Middle layer of the meninges surrounding the brain and spinal cord ______________
10. Contains nerves that control involuntary body functions or muscles, glands, and internal organs ______________________________

B. Match the following vocabulary terms with their meanings below:

central nervous system
cerebellum
cerebral cortex
cerebrospinal fluid
cerebrum
cranial nerves
dendrite
dura mater
efferent nerve
ependymal cell

1. Motor nerve that carries messages away from the brain and spinal cord ______________
2. Largest part of the brain ______________________________
3. Includes the brain and spinal cord ______________________________
4. Microscopic branching fiber of a nerve cell that is the first to receive a nervous impulse ______________________________
5. Posterior part of the brain; coordinates muscle movements and maintains balance ______________
6. Glial (neuroglial) cell that lines membranes within the brain and spinal cord; helps form cerebrospinal fluid ______________________________

7. Outer region of the cerebrum; contains sheets of nerves ______________________

8. Circulates throughout the brain and spinal cord ______________________

9. Thick, outermost layer of the meninges ______________________

10. Twelve pairs of nerves that carry messages to and from the brain ______________________

C. Match the following vocabulary terms with their meanings below:

ganglion	medulla oblongata	myelin sheath
glial cell	meninges	nerve
gyrus	motor nerve	neuron
hypothalamus		

1. Portion of the brain that controls sleep, appetite, body temperature, and secretions from the pituitary gland ______________________

2. White, fatty tissue that surrounds and insulates the axon of a nerve cell ______________________

3. Supportive and connective type of nerve cell; does not carry nervous impulses ______________________

4. Membranes surrounding the brain and spinal cord ______________________

5. Sheet of nerve cells that produces a rounded fold on the surface of the brain ______________________

6. Nerve cell that carries impulses throughout the body ______________________

7. Collection of nerve cell bodies in the PNS ______________________

8. Portion of the brain just above the spinal cord; controls breathing, heartbeat, and size of blood vessels ______________________

9. Carries messages away from the brain and spinal cord; efferent nerve ______________________

10. Macroscopic cord-like collection of fibers that carry electrical impulses ______________________

D. Match the following vocabulary terms with their meanings below:

microglial cell	parenchyma	pons
neurotransmitter	peripheral nervous system	receptor
oligodendroglial cell	pia mater	
parasympathetic nerves	plexus	

1. Part of the brain anterior to the cerebellum and between the medulla and rest of the midbrain ______________________

2. Chemical messenger, released at the end of a nerve cell ______________________

3. Essential, distinguishing tissue of an organ or system ______________________

4. Thin, delicate inner membrane of the meninges ______________________

5. Organ that receives a nervous stimulation and passes it on to afferent nerves ______________________

6. Phagocytic glial cell ______________________

7. Large, interlacing network of nerves ______________________________

8. Nerves outside the brain and spinal cord including cranial and spinal nerves ______________

9. Involuntary, autonomic nerves that regulate normal body functions such as heart rate, breathing, and gastrointestinal muscles ______________________________

10. Glial cell that forms the myelin sheath covering axons ______________________________

E. Match the following vocabulary terms with their meanings below:

sciatic nerve	sulcus	vagus nerve
sensory nerve	sympathetic nerves	ventricles of the brain
stimulus	synapse	
stroma	thalamus	

1. Depression or groove in the surface of the cerebral cortex ______________________________

2. Connective and supporting tissue of an organ; glial cells of the brain ______________________

3. Tenth cranial nerve ______________________________

4. Carries messages toward the brain and spinal cord; afferent nerve ______________________

5. Main relay center of the brain ______________________________

6. Autonomic nerves that influence bodily functions involuntarily in times of stress ____________

7. Spinal nerve extending from the base of the spine down the thigh, lower leg, and foot ______________________________

8. Agent of change (light, sound, touch) that evokes a response ______________________________

9. Space through which a nervous impulse travels between nerve cells or between nerve and muscle or glandular cells ______________________________

10. Canals in the brain that contain cerebrospinal fluid ______________________________

Chapter Ten
TERMINOLOGY QUIZ

Name: ______________________________

A. Using the following word parts, build medical terms from the definitions below:

cerebell/o	lept/o	-pathy
cerebr/o	mening/o	an-
dur/o	meningi/o	epi-
encephal/o	-al	sub-

1. inflammation of the brain: ______________________________ itis
2. collection of blood located below the dura mater: ______________________________ hematoma
3. pertaining to the cerebellum: ______________________________ ar
4. pertaining to the outer section of the cerebrum: ______________________________ cortex
5. collection of blood located above the dura mater: ______________________________ hematoma
6. disease of the brain: encephalo ______________________________
7. congenital absence of a brain: ______________________________ encephaly
8. pertaining to the pia and arachnoid membranes: ______________________________ meningeal
9. tumor of the membranes around the brain and spinal cord: ______________________________ oma

B. Using the following word parts, build medical terms from the definitions below:

gli/o	pont/o	-gram
meningi/o	radicul/o	-ine
my/o	-al	-itis
myel/o	-blast	-pathy
neur/o	-cele	poly-

1. disease of the spinal cord: ______________________________
2. disease of nerves: ______________________________
3. malignant tumor of immature glial cells: ______________________________ oma
4. pertaining to muscles and nerves: ______________________________
5. hernia of the spinal cord and meninges: ______________________________
6. inflammation of many nerves: ______________________________
7. inflammation of a nerve root: ______________________________
8. inflammation of the gray matter of the spinal cord: polio ______________________________
9. pertaining to the cerebellum and the pons: cerebello ______________________________
10. disease of a nerve root: ______________________________

C. Using the following word parts, build medical terms from the definitions below:

caus/o	vag/o	-ose
comat/o	-algia	an-
esthesi/o	-al	hyper-
thalam/o	-algesia	hypo-
thec/o	-esthesia	par-

1. intense burning pain: ____________________
2. pertaining to the tenth cranial nerve: ____________________
3. condition of lack of sensation: ____________________
4. pertaining to a state of unconsciousness: ____________________ ose
5. drugs are delivered into a space within the meninges: intra ____________________
6. pertaining to an area of the brain that is a relay station for nerve impulses: ____________________ ic
7. condition of increased sensation: ____________________ ia
8. abnormal sensation: ____________________ ia
9. condition of lack of sensitivity to pain: ____________________
10. diminished sensation to pain: ____________________

D. Using the following word parts, build medical terms from the definitions below:

narc/o	-lepsy	brady-
neur/o	-lex/o	dys-
-algia	-ia	hyper-
-kinesia	-paresis	hemi-
-kinetic	-phasia	
-kinesis	a-	

1. slow movement: ____________________ kinesia
2. abnormal movement occurring late in treatment (using antipsychotic drugs): tardive ____________________
3. nerve pain related to the fifth cranial nerve: trigeminal ____________________
4. pertaining to without movement: ____________________
5. headache: ceph ____________________
6. excessive movement: ____________________ kinesis
7. compulsion (seizure) to sleep: ____________________
8. reading, writing, and learning disorders: dys ____________________
9. weakness in the right or left side (half) of the body: ____________________
10. inability to speak: ____________________

E. Using the following word parts, build medical terms from the definitions below:

syncop/o	-praxia	hemi-
tax/o	-sthenia	quadri-
-plegia	a-	para-

1. paralysis of the lower portion of the body: ______________________
2. pertaining to fainting: ______________________ al
3. lack of coordination: ______________________ ia
4. movements and behavior are not purposeful (actions are not appropriate): ______________________
5. paralysis of one side of the body: ______________________
6. nervous exhaustion and fatigue: neur ______________________
7. paralysis of all four extremities: ______________________

Chapter Ten

PATHOLOGY QUIZ

Name: ______________________________

A. Match the following neurologic disorders with their definitions below:

Alzheimer disease	hydrocephalus	Parkinson disease
amyotrophic lateral sclerosis	multiple sclerosis	spina bifida
epilepsy	myasthenia gravis	
Huntington disease	palsy	

1. Chronic brain disorder characterized by recurrent seizure activity ________________
2. Degenerative disorder of motor neurons in the spinal cord and brainstem ________________
3. Destruction of myelin sheath on neurons in the CNS; replacement by plaques of sclerotic tissue ________________
4. Hereditary disorder marked by degenerative changes in the cerebrum leading to abrupt involuntary movements and mental deterioration ________________
5. Congenital defect in the lumbar spinal column caused by imperfect union of vertebrae; may involve myelomeningocele ________________
6. Abnormal accumulation of CSF in the ventricles of the brain ________________
7. Brain disorder marked by gradual, progressive mental deterioration; personality changes; and impairment of daily functioning ________________
8. Autoimmune neuromuscular disorder characterized by weakness of voluntary muscles ________________
9. Degeneration of neurons in the basal ganglia; occurring later in life and leading to tremors, muscle weakness, and slowness of movement ________________
10. Paralysis (partial or complete loss of motor function) ________________

B. Match the following neurologic disorders with their definitions below:

brain tumor	dementia	migraine
cerebral concussion	herpes zoster	Tourette syndrome
cerebral contusion	HIV encephalopathy	
cerebrovascular accident	meningitis	

1. Mental decline and deterioration ________________
2. Viral infection affecting peripheral nerves; marked by eruption of painful blisters ________________
3. Involuntary, spasmodic, twitching movements; uncontrollable vocal sounds ________________
4. Severe, recurrent, unilateral, vascular headache ________________

5. Disruption in the normal blood supply to the brain; stroke ______________________

6. Bruising of brain tissue as a result of direct trauma to the head ______________________

7. Abnormal growth of brain tissue (glial cells) and meninges ______________________

8. Inflammation of the membranes around the brain and spinal cord ______________________

9. Traumatic brain injury caused by a blow to the head; no evidence of structural damage to brain tissue ______________________

10. Brain disease occurring with AIDS ______________________

C. Match the following terms with their meanings below:

absence seizure	dopamine	palliative
aneurysm	embolus	thymectomy
astrocytoma	gait	tic
aura	ictal event	tonic-clonic seizure
demyelination	occlusion	

1. Peculiar sensation that occurs before the onset of an attack of migraine or an epileptic seizure ______________________

2. Manner of walking ______________________

3. Relieving symptoms, but not curing the illness ______________________

4. Major convulsive seizure marked by sudden loss of consciousness, stiffening of muscles, and twitching and jerking movements ______________________

5. Enlarged, weakened area in an artery ______________________

6. Involuntary movement of a small group of muscles, as of the face; characteristic of Tourette syndrome ______________________

7. Pertaining to a sudden, acute onset, as the convulsions of an epileptic seizure ______________________

8. Neurotransmitter that is deficient in patients with Parkinson disease ______________________

9. Clot of material that travels through the bloodstream and suddenly blocks a vessel ______________________

10. Malignant tumor of a type of neuroglial cells in the brain ______________________

11. Minor form of seizure ______________________

12. Destruction of the covering on axons of neurons in the CNS ______________________

13. Removal of a gland in the mediastinum (treatment for myasthenia gravis) ______________________

14. Blockage of a vessel ______________________

Chapter Ten

LABORATORY TESTS AND CLINICAL PROCEDURES QUIZ

Name: ______________________________

Match the following terms with their definitions below:

cerebral angiography	Doppler/ultrasound studies	myelography
CSF analysis	EEG	PET scan of the brain
CT of the brain and spinal cord	LP	
stereotactic radiosurgery	MRI of the brain and spinal cord	

1. Cerebrospinal fluid is withdrawn from between two lumbar vertebrae ____________________
2. Magnetic waves and radio wave energy create images (of the brain and spinal cord) in three planes ____________________
3. Samples of cerebrospinal fluid are examined ____________________
4. X-ray imaging of the spinal cord after injection of contrast material within the subarachnoid space ____________________
5. Radioactive glucose is injected and detected in the brain to image the metabolic activity of cells ____________________
6. X-ray imaging of arterial blood vessels in the brain after injection of contrast material ____________________
7. Sound waves detect blood flow in the carotid and intracranial arteries ____________________
8. X-ray technique that produces computerized multiple (especially cross-sectional) images of the brain and spinal cord ____________________
9. Use of a specialized instrument (Gamma knife) to locate and treat targets in the brain ____________________
10. Recording of the electrical activity of the brain ____________________

Chapter Ten

ABBREVIATIONS QUIZ

Name: ________________________________

A. On the line provided, give meanings for the following abbreviations, then write each abbreviation next to its explanation below:

1. AD ____
2. ALS ____
3. CNS ____
4. CSF ____
5. CT ____
6. CVA ____
7. EEG ____
8. ICP ____
9. LP ____
10. MG ____

a. _______ Otherwise known as Lou Gehrig disease

b. _______ Otherwise known as a stroke

c. _______ Otherwise known as a spinal tap

d. _______ X-ray imaging procedure in which multiple images and a computer produce cross-sectional pictures

e. _______ Seizure activity can be detected via this procedure that records electrical activity in the brain

f. _______ Tumor or swelling in the brain can cause an increase in this pressure

g. _______ An autoimmune disorder characterized by weakness of voluntary muscles

h. _______ This fluid circulates within the ventricles of the brain and around the spinal cord

i. _______ Consists of the brain and the spinal cord

j. _______ Brain disorder marked by gradual and progressive dementia

B. On the line provided, give meanings for the following abbreviations, then write each abbreviation next to its explanation below:

1. MRA ______________________________
2. MRI ______________________________
3. MS ______________________________
4. PET ______________________________
5. Sz ______________________________
6. TENS ______________________________
7. TIA ______________________________
8. TLE ______________________________
9. PNS ______________________________
10. PCA ______________________________

a. _______ Patient controls his/her pain medication

b. _______ Imaging techniques in which radioactive chemicals are given and traced in the body

c. _______ Temporary interference with blood supply to the brain; mini-stroke

d. _______ Seizures that originate in areas of the brain near the ear

e. _______ Technique using a battery-powered device to relieve acute and chronic pain

f. _______ Imaging of blood vessels after injection of contrast material in the arteries supplying the brain and taking pictures using magnetic waves

g. _______ Disorder marked by destruction of the myelin sheath on neurons in the CNS and replacement with hard scar tissue

h. _______ Nervous tissue outside the brain and spinal cord

i. _______ A magnetic field and pulses of radio wave energy create images of the brain and spinal cord

j. _______ A symptom of abnormal electrical activity in the brain

Chapter Ten
EXERCISE QUIZ

Name: ______________________________

A. Match the following neurologic structures with their meanings:

axon	cerebral cortex	meninges	oligodendroglia
cauda equina	dendrite	myelin sheath	plexus

1. three protective membranes surrounding the brain and spinal cord ____________________
2. microscopic fiber that carries the nervous impulse along a nerve cell ____________________
3. a large, interlacing network of nerves ____________________
4. branching fiber that is first part of a neuron to receive a nervous impulse ____________________
5. protective fatty tissue that surrounds the axon of a nerve cell ____________________
6. collection of spinal nerves below the end of the spinal cord ____________________
7. glial cell that produces myelin ____________________
8. outer region of the largest part of the brain; composed of gray matter ____________________

B. Give meanings for the following terms:

9. dura mater ____________________
10. synapse ____________________
11. medulla oblongata ____________________
12. hypothalamus ____________________

C. Match the following terms with their meanings or associated terms below:

gyri	parenchymal cell	sensory nerve
neurotransmitter	pia mater	subarachnoid space

13. carries messages toward the brain from receptors ____________________
14. essential cell of the nervous system; a neuron ____________________
15. innermost meningeal membrane ____________________
16. elevations in the cerebral cortex ____________________
17. acetylcholine is an example of this chemical released into a synapse ____________________
18. contains cerebrospinal fluid ____________________

D. Give meanings for the following terms:

19. intrathecal ______________________________
20. glioma ______________________________
21. myelopathy ______________________________
22. subdural hematoma ______________________________
23. meningioma ______________________________
24. paresthesias ______________________________

E. Match the following neurologic symptoms with their meanings below:

apraxia	bradykinesia	hemiparesis	narcolepsy
ataxia	causalgia	hyperesthesia	syncope

25. slow movement ______________________________
26. increased nervous sensation ______________________________
27. seizure of sleep ______________________________
28. movements and behavior are not purposeful ______________________________
29. fainting ______________________________
30. burning pain ______________________________
31. no coordination ______________________________
32. slight paralysis in half the body ______________________________

F. Match the following terms with their descriptions below:

Alzheimer disease	epilepsy	myasthenia gravis
Bell palsy	multiple sclerosis	Parkinson disease

33. destruction of myelin sheath; replacement by plaques of hard scar tissue ______________
34. sudden, transient disturbances of brain function marked by seizures ______________
35. loss of muscle strength; breakdown of acetylcholine, a neurotransmitter ______________
36. degeneration of nerves in the brain leading to tremors, shuffling gait, and muscle stiffness (mask-like facial expression); dopamine is deficient in the brain ______________________________
37. deterioration of mental capacity (dementia) beginning in middle age; cerebral cortex atrophy, microscopic neurofibrillary tangles ______________________________
38. unilateral facial paralysis ______________________________

G. Give meanings for the following abnormal conditions:

39. pyogenic meningitis ______________________________

40. Tourette syndrome ______________________________

41. shingles ______________________________

42. cerebral embolus ______________________________

H. Match the term in Column I with its meaning in Column II:

Column I		Column II
43. aura	_______	A. Relieving but not curing
44. palliative	_______	B. Major convulsive epileptic seizure
45. transient ischemic attack	_______	C. Peculiar symptoms appearing before more definite symptoms
46. occlusion	_______	D. Malignant brain tumor of immature glial cells
47. dopamine	_______	E. Interruption of blood supply to the cerebrum
48. glioblastoma multiforme	_______	F. Minor form of epileptic seizure
49. absence seizure	_______	G. Blockage
50. tonic-clonic seizure	_______	H. Neurotransmitter

Chapter Ten

DICTATION AND COMPREHENSION QUIZ: VOCABULARY AND TERMINOLOGY

Name: ____________________

A. Dictation of Terms

1.	______________________	11.	______________________
2.	______________________	12.	______________________
3.	______________________	13.	______________________
4.	______________________	14.	______________________
5.	______________________	15.	______________________
6.	______________________	16.	______________________
7.	______________________	17.	______________________
8.	______________________	18.	______________________
9.	______________________	19.	______________________
10.	______________________	20.	______________________

B. Comprehension of Terms: Match number of the above term with its meaning below.

______ The connective and framework tissue of any organ
______ Fatty tissue that surrounds and protects the axon of a nerve cell
______ Largest part of the brain
______ Posterior part of the brain; responsible for maintaining balance
______ A type of glial cell
______ Neurotransmitter chemical released at the ends of nerve cells
______ The space through which a nerve impulse passes from one nerve cell to another
______ Inflammation of membranes around the brain and spinal cord
______ Malignant brain tumor
______ Slow movement
______ Lack of muscle coordination
______ Condition of absence of a brain (congenital anomaly)
______ Pertaining to fainting
______ Benign tumor of the membranes around brain
______ Part of the brain that controls the secretions of the pituitary gland
______ Nervous exhaustion; "lack of nerve strength"
______ Movements and behavior are not purposeful
______ Paralysis of the lower part of the body
______ State of unconsciousness from which a patient cannot be aroused
______ Elevations on the surface of the cerebral cortex

Chapter Ten

DICTATION AND COMPREHENSION QUIZ: PATHOLOGY

Name: ____________________

A. Dictation of Terms

1. ____________________ 11. ____________________
2. ____________________ 12. ____________________
3. ____________________ 13. ____________________
4. ____________________ 14. ____________________
5. ____________________ 15. ____________________
6. ____________________ 16. ____________________
7. ____________________ 17. ____________________
8. ____________________ 18. ____________________
9. ____________________ 19. ____________________
10. ____________________ 20. ____________________

B. Comprehension of Terms: Match number of the above term with its meaning below.

______ A floating clot; mass of material suddenly blocks a blood vessel
______ Relieving symptoms, but not curing
______ Mini-stroke
______ X-ray record of blood vessels within the brain
______ Mental decline and deterioration
______ Breakage of a blood vessel within the brain
______ Demyelination of tissue around the axons of CNS neurons
______ Paralysis and loss of muscular coordination caused by brain damage in the perinatal period
______ Congenital defect of spinal column with herniation of the spinal cord and meninges
______ Major convulsive epileptic seizure
______ Malignant brain tumor
______ Relapsing weakness of skeletal muscles ("no muscle strength"); autoimmune condition
______ Collection of fluid in the ventricles of the brain
______ Degeneration of nerves in the brain; occurring in later life and leading to tremors, bradykinesia
______ Manner of walking
______ Type of neurotransmitter
______ Peculiar sensation appearing before more definite symptoms
______ Involuntary, spasmodic twitching movements; uncontrollable utterances

Chapter Ten

SPELLING QUIZ

Name: ______________________________

A. Circle the term that is spelled correctly and write its meaning in the space provided:

1. hypothalamus hypothalmus ________________________________
2. neurorrhapy neurorrhaphy ________________________________
3. motor nerve moter nerve ________________________________
4. myelin sheath mylein sheath ________________________________
5. acetylcholene acetylcholine ________________________________
6. meningoma meningioma ________________________________
7. hyperkinesis hyperkenesis ________________________________
8. neurasthenia neurastenea ________________________________
9. pareasis paresis ________________________________
10. demyleination demyelination ________________________________

B. Circle the term that is spelled correctly. The meaning of each term is given.

11. Pertaining to fainting	sincopal	syncopal	sinkaple
12. Abnormal sensation	paresthesia	parasthesia	parasthezia
13. Relieving, but not curing	pailiative	paliative	palliative
14. Peculiar symptoms appearing before more definite symptoms	aura	aurra	hora
15. Loss of mental capacity	demenshea	dementia	dementsha
16. Within the meninges	intrathecal	interthecal	intrathekal
17. Essential cells of an organ	parenchymal	parenchymel	parencyhmal
18. Space between nerve cells	sinapse	synnapse	synapse
19. Part of the brain that controls muscular coordination	cerebellum	serabellum	serebellum
20. Manner of walking	gate	gaite	gait

Chapter Ten
PRONUNCIATION QUIZ

Name: ____________________

A. Underline the accented syllable in the following terms:

1. angiography
2. encephalopathy
3. occlusion
4. myelomeningocele
5. syncope
6. dendrite
7. myelopathy
8. glioma
9. hyperesthesia
10. narcolepsy

B. Match the term in Column I with its meaning in Column II:

Column I		Column II
1. axon	_______	A. Pertaining to supportive cells of the nervous system
2. meninges	_______	B. Substance that helps transmit a nervous impulse
3. embolism	_______	C. Part of a nerve cell
4. cauda equina	_______	D. Obstruction of a blood vessel by a clot or foreign substance
5. glial	_______	E. Network of nerve fibers.
6. thalamus	_______	F. Tail end of the spinal cord
7. synapse	_______	G. Three membranes surrounding the brain and spinal cord
8. plexus	_______	H. Space between nerve cells
9. acetylcholine	_______	I. A part of the brain that serves as a relay station for impulses
10. neurasthenia	_______	J. Lack of strength in nerves; sense of weakness and exhaustion

C. Complete the following terms from their definitions:

1. dys____________________	Difficult speech
2. an____________________	A condition of insensitivity to pain
3. hemi ____________________	Slight paralysis of right or left side of the body
4. ____________________ itis	Inflammation of a spinal nerve root
5. neuro____________________	Disease of a nerve
6. vago____________________	Incision of the vagus nerve
7. a ____________________	Lack of coordination
8. dys ____________________	Condition of painful nervous sensations
9. glio ____________________	Tumor of immature brain cells (glia)
10. electro ____________________	Electrical record of the brain

Chapter Ten
DIAGRAM QUIZ

Name: ______________________________

Label the diagram using the terms listed below:

Axon
Cell body
Cell nucleus
Dendrites
Myelin sheath
Synapse
Terminal end fibers

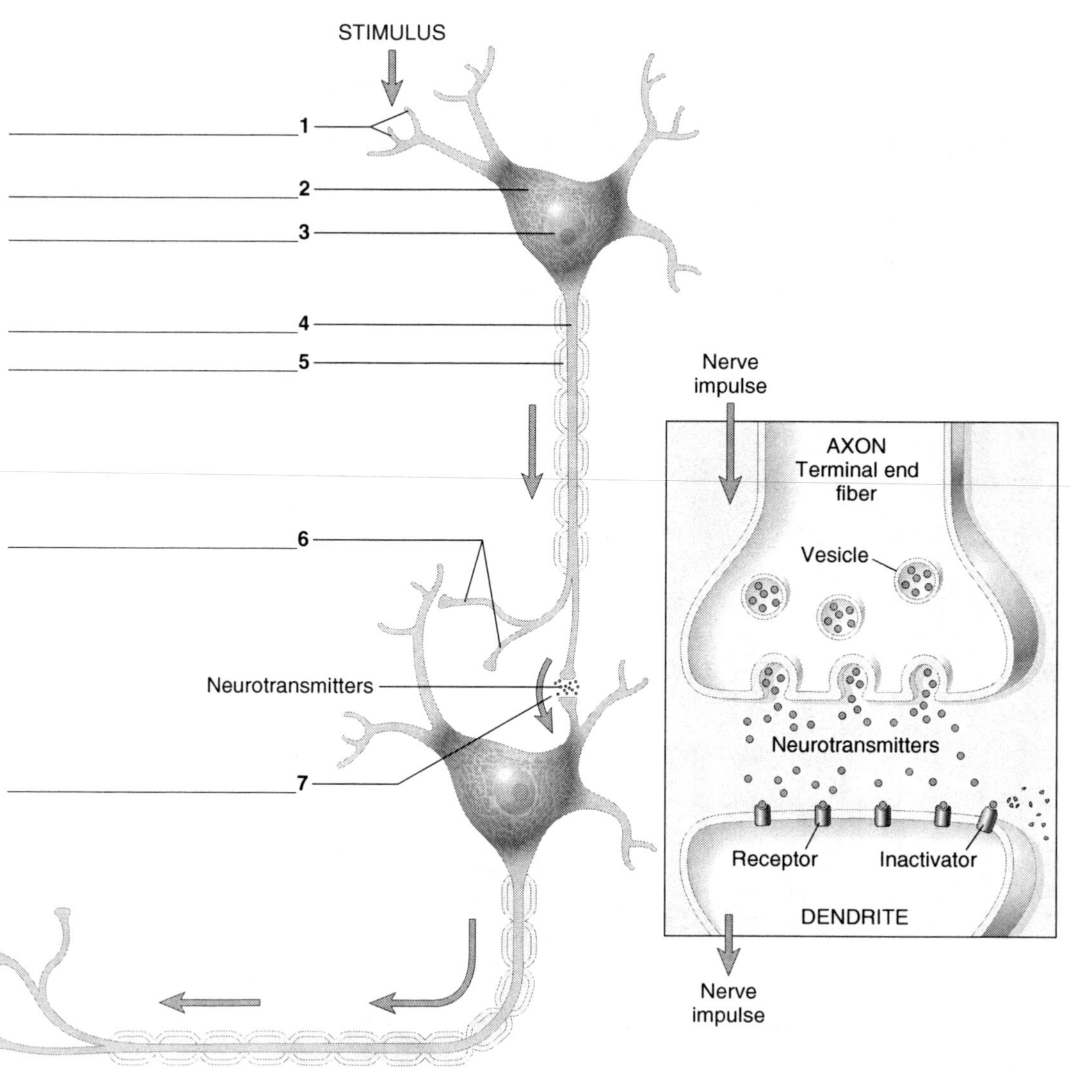

Chapter Ten
REVIEW SHEET QUIZ

Name: ______________________________

A. Give meanings for the following combining forms:

1. encephal/o ______________________________
2. kines/o ______________________________
3. mening/o ______________________________
4. neur/o ______________________________
5. my/o ______________________________
6. vag/o- ______________________________
7. radicul/o ______________________________
8. tax/o ______________________________
9. myel/o ______________________________
10. esthesi/o ______________________________

B. Give meanings for the following prefixes:

1. quadri- ______________________________
2. hypo- ______________________________
3. hemi-______________________________
4. poly- ______________________________
5. sub- ______________________________
6. micro- ______________________________
7. hyper- ______________________________
8. dys- ______________________________
9. epi- ______________________________
10. para- ______________________________

C. Give meanings for the following suffixes:

1. -algesia ______________________________
2. -paresis ______________________________
3. -phasia ______________________________
4. -ptosis ______________________________
5. -sclerosis ______________________________
6. -plegia ______________________________
7. -sthenia ______________________________
8. -praxia ______________________________
9. -blast ______________________________
10. -cele ______________________________

Chapter Ten
MEDICAL SCRAMBLE

Name: ____________________

Unscramble the letters to form suffixes related to nervous system conditions from the clues. Use the letters in the squares to complete the bonus term.

1. *Clue:* Abnormal electrical activity in the brain

   ___ ___ ___ ___ ___ ___ ☐ ☐ EYPIPESL

2. *Clue:* Inflammation of membranes surrounding the brain and spinal cord

   ___ ☐ ___ ___ ___ ___ ___ ___ ___ ___ SIETMINGNI

3. *Clue:* Paralysis

   ☐ ___ ___ ☐ ___ SAYLP

4. *Clue:* Mental decline and deterioration

   ___ ___ ___ ___ ☐ ___ ___ ☐ ENETIDAM

BONUS TERM: *Clue:* Space between nerve cells

☐ ☐ ☐ ☐ ☐ ☐ ☐

Chapter Ten
CROSSWORD PUZZLE

Name: ______________________

Fill in the crossword puzzle below using the clues listed underneath it.

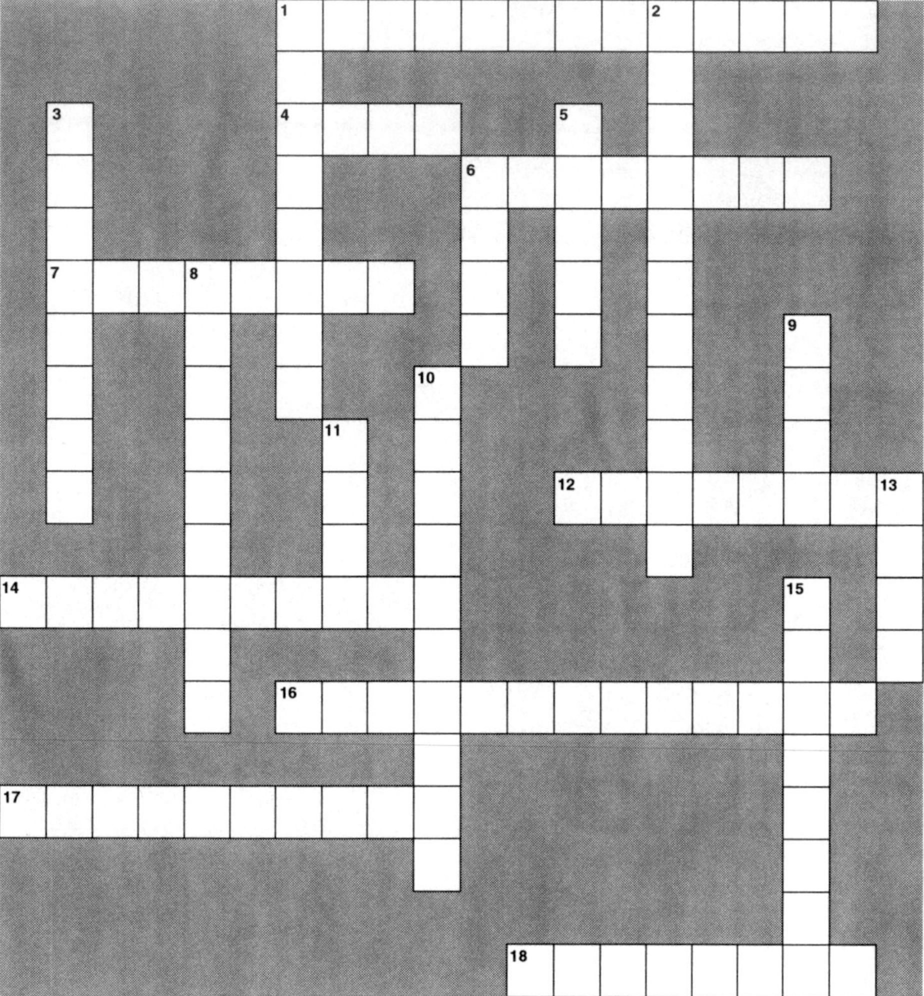

Across Clues

1. Destruction of myelin on the axons of nerves.
4. Part of the brain; means "bridge".
6. Abnormal widening of a blood vessel.
7. Mass of material travels through the bloodstream and suddenly blocks a vessel.
12. Mental decline and deterioration.
14. Relieving symptoms, but not curing.
16. Neurotransmitter released at the ends of some nerve cells.
17. Posterior part of the brain.
18. Three protective membranes that surround the brain and spinal cord.

Down Clues

1. Neurotransmitter that is deficient in Parkinson disease.
2. Malignant tumor of glial cells (astrocytes) in the brain.
3. Largest part of the brain.
5. Macroscopic structure consisting of axons and dendrites in bundle-like strands.
6. Peculiar sensation appearing before more definite symptoms.
8. Blockage.
9. Manner of walking.
10. Removal of the thymus gland; treatment for myasthenia gravis.
11. Sheets of nerve cells that produce elevation in the cerebral cortex, convolution.
13. Microscopic fiber that carries the nervous impulse along a nerve cell.
15. Microscopic branching fiber of a nerve cell that is the first part to receive the nervous impulse.

Chapter Ten

PRACTICAL APPLICATIONS

Name: ______________________________

MRI Report

MRI was performed through the brain, cervical spine, and upper thoracic region. Scans were generated in the transaxial, sagittal, and coronal (frontal) planes.

Evaluation of the brain parenchyma demonstrates the presence of multiple areas of abnormal increased signal intensity scattered through the white matter of both cerebral hemispheres. These areas are periventricular in location. The pattern is most compatible with a demyelinative process. Scans through the cervical spine and spinal cord demonstrate no definite areas of abnormal increased or decreased signal within the cord. The disks are intact. Evaluation of the upper thoracic region demonstrates an appearance similar to that of the cervical region.

1. What is MRI? .... ☐

A. Ultrasound images that show the structure of organs and tissues
B. X-rays on a transverse plane
C. Magnetic and radio waves are used to create images
D. Radioactive materials are injected and images are recorded of their uptake in tissues

2. What combining forms indicate the regions of the body imaged? .... ☐

A. Myel/o and my/o
B. Encephal/o and myel/o
C. My/o and encephal/o
D. Encephal/o

3. What is the brain parenchyma? .... ☐

A. Neuronal tissue of the brain
B. Glial tissue of the brain
C. Ventricles of the brain
D. Connective tissue of the brain

4. From the report, what is a likely diagnosis? .... ☐

A. Alzheimer disease
B. Parkinson disease
C. Amyotrophic lateral sclerosis
D. Multiple sclerosis

Chapter Ten

ANSWERS TO THE QUIZZES

Multiple Choice Quiz

1. E
2. A
3. C
4. E
5. C
6. D
7. C
8. E
9. B
10. D
11. D
12. C
13. C
14. E
15. C
16. B
17. D
18. C
19. D
20. A
21. D
22. B
23. A
24. E
25. C

Vocabulary Quiz

A

1. blood-brain barrier
2. astrocyte
3. cauda equina
4. acetylcholine
5. brainstem
6. axon
7. afferent nerve
8. cell body
9. arachnoid membrane
10. autonomic nervous system

B

1. efferent nerve
2. cerebrum
3. central nervous system
4. dendrite
5. cerebellum
6. ependymal cell
7. cerebral cortex
8. cerebrospinal fluid
9. dura mater
10. cranial nerves

C

1. hypothalamus
2. myelin sheath
3. glial cell
4. meninges
5. gyrus
6. neuron
7. ganglion
8. medulla oblongata
9. motor nerve
10. nerve

D

1. pons
2. neurotransmitter
3. parenchyma
4. pia mater
5. receptor
6. microglial cell
7. plexus
8. peripheral nervous system
9. parasympathetic nerves
10. oligodendroglial cell

E

1. sulcus
2. stroma
3. vagus nerve
4. sensory nerve
5. thalamus
6. sympathetic nerves
7. sciatic nerve
8. stimulus
9. synapse
10. ventricles of the brain

Terminology Quiz

A

1. encephalitis
2. subdural hematoma
3. cerebellar
4. cerebral cortex
5. epidural hematoma
6. encephalopathy
7. anencephaly
8. leptomeningeal
9. meningioma

B

1. myelopathy
2. neuropathy
3. glioblastoma
4. myoneural
5. myelomeningocele
6. polyneuritis
7. radiculitis
8. poliomyelitis
9. cerebellopontine
10. radiculopathy

C

1. causalgia
2. vagal
3. anesthesia
4. comatose
5. intrathecal
6. thalamic
7. hyperesthesia
8. paresthesia
9. anesthesia
10. hypalgesia

D

1. bradykinesia
2. tardive dyskinesia
3. trigeminal neuralgia
4. akinetic
5. cephalgia
6. hyperkinesis
7. narcolepsy
8. dyslexia
9. hemiparesis
10. aphasia

E

1. paraplegia
2. syncopal
3. ataxia
4. apraxia
5. hemiplegia
6. neurasthenia
7. quadriplegia

Pathology Quiz

A

1. epilepsy
2. amyotrophic lateral sclerosis
3. multiple sclerosis
4. Huntington disease
5. spina bifida
6. hydrocephalus
7. Alzheimer disease
8. myasthenia gravis
9. Parkinson disease
10. palsy

B

1. dementia
2. herpes zoster
3. Tourette syndrome

4. migraine
5. cerebrovascular accident
6. cerebral contusion
7. brain tumor
8. meningitis
9. cerebral concussion
10. HIV encephalopathy

C

1. aura
2. gait
3. palliative
4. tonic-clonic seizure
5. aneurysm
6. tic
7. ictal event
8. dopamine
9. embolus
10. astrocytoma
11. absence seizure
12. demyelination
13. thymectomy
14. occlusion

Laboratory Tests and Clinical Procedures Quiz

1. LP
2. MRI of the brain and spinal cord
3. CSF analysis
4. myelography
5. PET scan of the brain
6. cerebral angiography
7. Doppler/ultrasound studies
8. CT of the brain and spinal cord
9. stereotactic radiosurgery
10. EEG

Abbreviations Quiz

A

1. Alzheimer disease
2. amyotrophic lateral sclerosis
3. central nervous system
4. cerebrospinal fluid
5. computed tomography
6. cerebrovascular accident
7. electroencephalography
8. intracranial pressure
9. lumbar puncture
10. myasthenia gravis

a. ALS
b. CVA
c. LP
d. CT
e. EEG
f. ICP
g. MG
h. CSF
i. CNS
j. AD

B

1. magnetic resonance angiography
2. magnetic resonance imaging
3. multiple sclerosis
4. positron emission tomography
5. seizure
6. transcutaneous electrical nerve stimulation
7. transient ischemic attack
8. temporal lobe epilepsy
9. peripheral nervous system
10. patient controlled anesthesia

a. PCA
b. PET
c. TIA
d. TLE
e. TENS
f. MRA
g. MS
h. PNS
i. MRI
j. Sz

Exercise Quiz

A

1. meninges
2. axon
3. plexus
4. dendrite
5. myelin sheath
6. cauda equina
7. oligodendroglia
8. cerebral cortex

B

9. outermost layer of the meninges
10. space between nerve cells
11. lower portion of the brain; controls blood pressure, heartbeat, and respiration
12. portion of the brain under thalamus; controls sleep, appetite, pituitary gland

C

13. sensory nerve
14. parenchymal cell
15. pia mater
16. gyri
17. neurotransmitter
18. subarachnoid space

D

19. within the membranes around the brain and spinal cord
20. tumor of neuroglial cells in the brain
21. disease of the spinal cord
22. mass of blood under the dura mater
23. tumor of the meninges
24. abnormal sensations

E

25. bradykinesia
26. hyperesthesia
27. narcolepsy
28. apraxia
29. syncope
30. causalgia
31. ataxia
32. hemiparesis

F

33. multiple sclerosis
34. epilepsy
35. myasthenia gravis
36. Parkinson disease
37. Alzheimer disease
38. Bell palsy

G

39. inflammation of meninges with pus formation
40. involuntary spasmodic twitching movements
41. herpes zoster infection with blisters in a band-like pattern on the body
42. blood clot that suddenly enters a blood vessel in the brain

H

43. C
44. A
45. E
46. G
47. H
48. D
49. F
50. B

Dictation and Comprehension Quiz: Vocabulary and Terminology

A

1. acetylcholine
2. anencephaly
3. apraxia

4. astrocyte
5. ataxia
6. bradykinesia
7. cerebellum
8. cerebrum
9. comatose
10. glioma
11. gyri
12. hypothalamus
13. leptomeningitis
14. meningioma
15. myelin sheath
16. neurasthenia
17. paraplegia
18. stroma
19. synapse
20. syncopal

B

18 The connective and framework tissue of any organ
15 Fatty tissue that surrounds and protects the axon of a nerve cell
8 Largest part of the brain
7 Posterior part of the brain; responsible for maintaining balance
4 A type of neuroglial cell
1 Neurotransmitter chemical released at the ends of nerve cells
19 The space through which a nerve impulse passes from one nerve cell to another
13 Inflammation of membranes around the brain and spinal cord
10 Malignant brain tumor
6 Slow movement
5 Lack of muscle coordination
2 Condition of absence of a brain (congenital anomaly)
20 Pertaining to fainting
14 Benign tumor of the membranes around brain
12 Part of the brain that controls the secretions of the pituitary gland
16 Nervous exhaustion; "lack of nerve strength"
3 Movements and behavior are not purposeful
17 Paralysis of the lower part of the body
9 State of unconsciousness from which a patient cannot be aroused
11 Elevations on the surface of the cerebral cortex

Dictation and Comprehension Quiz: Pathology

A

1. aura
2. cerebral angiography
3. cerebral hemorrhage
4. cerebral palsy
5. dementia
6. dopamine
7. embolus
8. gait
9. glioblastoma multiforme
10. hydrocephalus
11. multiple sclerosis
12. myasthenia gravis
13. palliative
14. Parkinson disease
15. spina bifida
16. tonic-clonic
17. Tourette syndrome
18. transient ischemic attack

B

7 A floating clot; mass of material suddenly blocks a blood vessel
13 Relieving symptoms, but not curing
18 Mini-stroke
2 X-ray record of blood vessels within the brain
5 Mental decline and deterioration
3 Breakage of a blood vessel within the brain
11 Demyelination of tissue around the axons of CNS neurons
4 Paralysis and loss of muscular coordination caused by brain damage in the perinatal period
15 Congenital defect of spinal column with herniation of the spinal cord and meninges
16 Major convulsive epileptic seizure
9 Malignant brain tumor
12 Relapsing weakness of skeletal muscles ("no muscle strength"); autoimmune condition
10 Collection of fluid in the ventricles of the brain
14 Degeneration of nerves in the brain; occurring in later life and leading to tremors, bradykinesia
8 Manner of walking
6 Type of neurotransmitter
1 Peculiar sensation appearing before more definite symptoms
17 Involuntary, spasmodic twitching movements; uncontrollable utterances

Spelling Quiz

A

1. hypothalamus—region of the brain below the thalamus
2. neurorrhaphy—suture of a nerve
3. motor nerve—takes messages to muscles from brain
4. myelin sheath—covering on nerve cell axon
5. acetylcholine—neurotransmitter
6. meningioma—tumor of the meninges
7. hyperkinesis—excessive movement
8. neurasthenia—lack of strength in nerves; irritability
9. paresis—slight paralysis
10. demyelination—lack of myelin

B

11. syncopal
12. paresthesia
13. palliative
14. aura
15. dementia
16. intrathecal
17. parenchymal
18. synapse
19. cerebellum
20. gait

Pronunciation Quiz

A

1. angiography
2. encephalopathy
3. occlusion
4. myelomeningocele
5. syncope
6. dendrite
7. myelopathy
8. glioma
9. hyperesthesia
10. narcolepsy

B

1. C
2. G
3. D

4. F
5. A
6. I
7. H
8. E
9. B
10. J

C

1. dysphasia
2. analgesia
3. hemiparesis
4. radiculitis
5. neuropathy
6. vagotomy
7. ataxia
8. dysesthesia
9. glioblastoma
10. electroencephalogram

Diagram Quiz

1. Dendrites
2. Cell body
3. Cell nucleus
4. Axon
5. Myelin sheath
6. Terminal end fibers
7. Synapse

Review Sheet Quiz

A

1. brain
2. movement
3. meninges
4. nerve
5. muscle
6. vagus nerve
7. nerve root
8. order, coordination
9. spinal cord
10. feeling, nervous sensation

B

1. four
2. deficient, below
3. half
4. much, many
5. under, below
6. small
7. excessive, above
8. painful, abnormal, difficult
9. above
10. abnormal

C

1. excessive sensitivity to pain
2. weakness
3. speech
4. prolapse
5. hardening
6. paralysis
7. strength
8. action
9. immature, embryonic
10. hernia

Medical Scramble

1. EPILEPSY
2. MENINGITIS
3. PALSY
4. DEMENTIA

BONUS TERM: SYNAPSE

Practical Applications

1. C
2. B
3. A
4. D

Crossword Puzzle

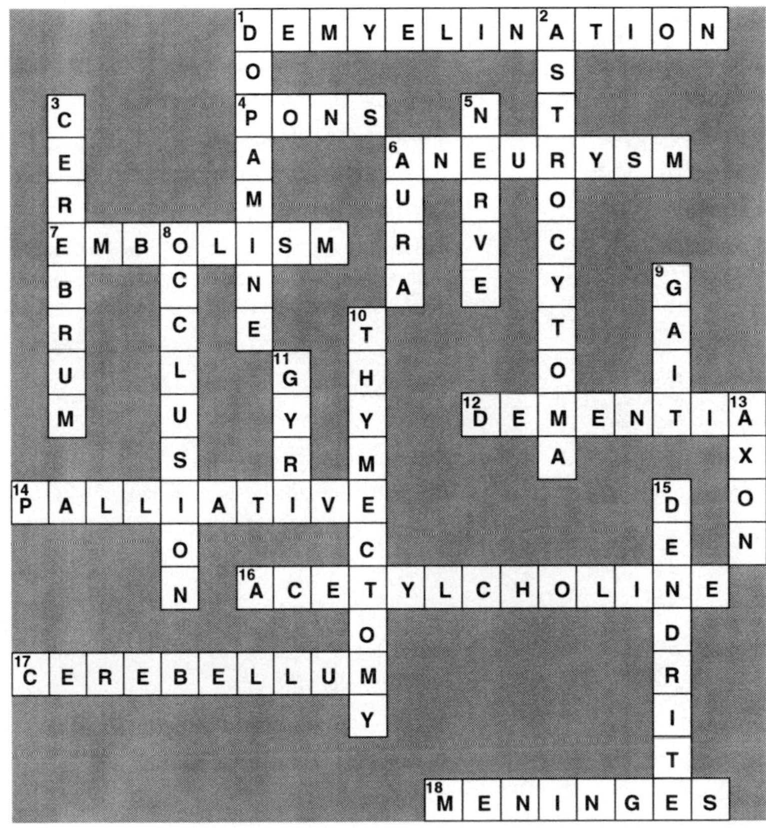

Chapter Ten

Answers to Terminology Section

(textbook pages 357-362)

Terminology	Meaning

Organ and Structures

Terminology	Meaning
cerebellar	Pertaining to the cerebellum.
cerebrospinal fluid	Fluid that surrounds the brain and spinal cord and is located within the ventricles of the brain.
cerebral cortex	The outer region (gray matter) of the cerebrum.
subdural hematoma	Collection of blood under the dura mater (outermost layer of the meninges).
epidural hematoma	Collection of blood above the dura mater.
encephalitis	Inflammation of the brain.
encephalopathy	Any disease of the brain.
anencephaly	Condition of no brain (congenital anomaly).
glioblastoma	Tumor (malignant) of glial (neuroglial or supportive) cells in the brain.
leptomeningeal	Pertaining to the pia mater and arachnoid membranes of the meninges.
meningeal	Pertaining to the meninges.
meningioma	Tumor of the meninges.
myelomeningocele	Hernia of the spinal cord and meninges; associated with spina bifida.
myoneural	Pertaining to muscle and nerve.
myelopathy	Disease of the spinal cord.
poliomyelitis	Inflammation of the gray matter of the spinal cord.
neuropathy	Disease of nerves.
polyneuritis	Inflammation of many (spinal) nerves, causing paralysis, pain, and wasting of muscles. *Guillain-Barré* syndrome (sequela of certain viral infections with paresthesias and muscular weakness) is an example.
cerebellopontine	Pertaining to the cerebellum and the pons.
radiculopathy	Disease of the spinal nerve roots.
radiculitis	Inflammation of nerve roots.
thalamic	Pertaining to the thalamus.
intrathecal injection	Placement of substances (medications) into the subarachnoid space.
vagal	Pertaining to the vagus (10th cranial) nerve.

Symptoms

Terminology	Meaning
analgesia	Condition of no sensation of pain (usually accompanied by sedation without loss of consciousness).
anesthetics	Agents that reduce or eliminate sensation.
hypalgesia	Diminished sensation to pain.
neuralgia	Nerve pain.
cephalgia	Headache (head pain).
causalgia	Burning sensation of pain (in the skin); usually following injury to sensory fibers of a peripheral nerve.
comatose	In a state of coma (profound unconsciousness from which one cannot be roused; may be due to trauma, disease, or action of ingested toxic substance).
anesthesia	Condition of no nervous sensation.
hyperesthesia	Excessive sensitivity to touch, pain, or other sensory stimuli.

paresthesia	An abnormal sensation such as numbness, tingling, or pricking.
bradykinesia	Slowness of movement.
hyperkinesis	Condition of excessive movement (muscular activity).
dyskinesia	Involuntary, spasmodic movements.
akinetic	Pertaining to without movement.
epilepsy	Chronic disorder marked by attacks of brain dysfunction due to excessive firing of nervous impulses.
narcolepsy	Sudden, uncontrollable episodes of sleep (seizures of sleep).
dyslexia	Disorder of reading, writing, or learning (despite the ability to see and recognize letters).
hemiparesis	Slight paralysis in either the right or left half of the body.
aphasia	Condition of inability to speak.
hemiplegia	Paralysis in half of the body.
paraplegia	Paralysis in the lower portion of the body.
quadriplegia	Paralysis of all four limbs of the body.
apraxia	Inability to carry out familiar purposeful movements (in the absence of paralysis or sensory or motor impairment).
neurasthenia	Condition of lack of nerve strength; nervous exhaustion and weakness.
syncopal	Pertaining to syncope (fainting).
ataxia	No muscular coordination (often caused by cerebellar dysfunction).

Chapter 11

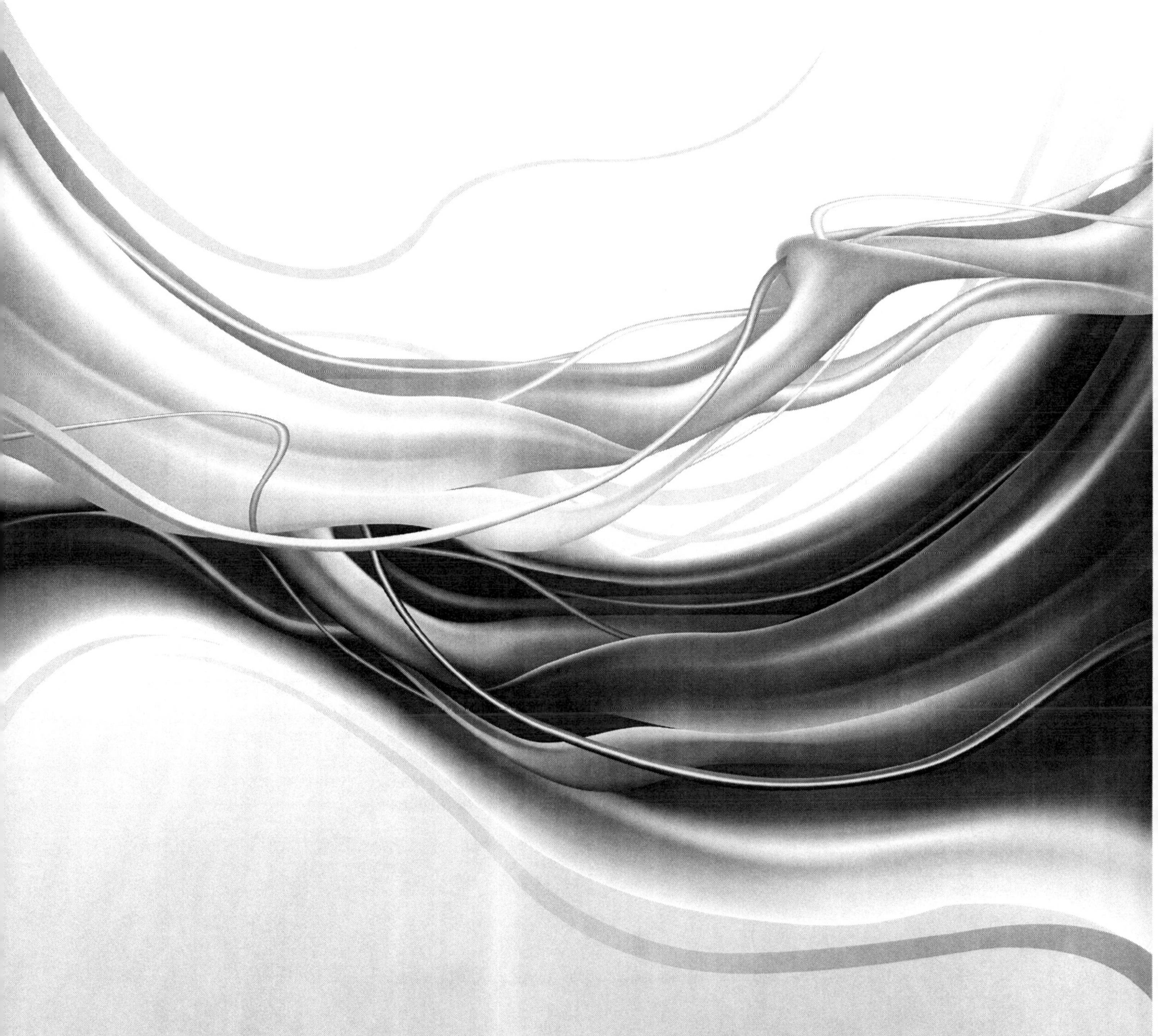

Chapter Eleven

MULTIPLE CHOICE QUIZ

Name: ______________________

In the box write the letter of the choice that is the definition of the term or best answers the question. There is only one correct answer for each question.

1. A blood vessel that carries oxygen-poor blood from heart to lungs: ☐
- A. Pulmonary vein
- B. Pulmonary artery
- C. Aorta
- D. Superior vena cava
- E. Inferior vena cava

2. Contraction phase of the heartbeat: ☐
- A. Septum
- B. Diastole
- C. Tachycardia
- D. Systole
- E. Pacemaker

3. Located between the left upper and lower chambers of the heart: ☐
- A. Mitral valve
- B. Tricuspid valve
- C. Aortic valve
- D. Pulmonary valve
- E. Superior vena cava

4. Saclike membrane surrounding the heart: ☐
- A. Endocardium
- B. Bundle of His
- C. Interatrial septum
- D. Ventricle
- E. Pericardium

5. Sensitive tissue in the right atrium wall that begins the heartbeat: ☐
- A. Tricuspid valve
- B. Atrioventricular node
- C. Bundle of His
- D. Epicardium
- E. Sinoatrial node

6. Blood vessels branching from the aorta to carry oxygen-rich blood to the heart muscle: ☐
- A. Capillaries
- B. Venae cavae
- C. Coronary arteries
- D. Carotid arteries
- E. Renal arteries

7. Disease of heart muscle: ☐
- A. Cardiomegaly
- B. Endocarditis
- C. Arteriolitis
- D. Cardiomyopathy
- E. Aortic stenosis

8. Phlebitis: ☐
- A. Narrowing of a valve with inflammation
- B. Inflammation of a capillary
- C. Blockage of a heart valve
- D. Inflammation of a vein
- E. Narrowing of an artery

9. Instrument to measure blood pressure: ☐
- A. Sphygmomanometer
- B. Electrocardiogram
- C. Stress test
- D. Stethoscope
- E. Cardiac catheterization

10. A local widening of an artery: ☐
- A. Thrombosis
- B. Infarction
- C. Arterial anastomosis
- D. Aortic stenosis
- E. Aneurysm

11. Cyanosis: ☐
- A. Bluish coloration of the skin
- B. Yellow coloration of the skin
- C. Associated with a hemangioma
- D. A form of atherosclerosis
- E. Associated with increased oxygen in the blood

12. Ischemia: ☐
- A. Can lead to myocardial infarction
- B. Blood is held back from an area
- C. Can be caused by thrombotic occlusion of a blood vessel
- D. May be a result of coronary artery disease
- E. All of the above

13. **Angina is:**..
   A. Chest pain relieved with nitroglycerin
   B. An extra heart sound
   C. An abnormal heart rhythm
   D. Caused by rheumatic fever
   E. Associated with Raynaud phenomenon

14. **Cardiac arrhythmia:**..........................
   A. Calcium channel blocker
   B. Beta-blocker
   C. Fibrillation
   D. Hypoxia
   E. Atheroma

15. **Petechiae:**..
   A. Small, pinpoint hemorrhages
   B. Vegetations
   C. Dilation of large vessels
   D. Defects, or holes in heart septa
   E. Hemorrhoids

16. **Blood clot forms in a large lower limb vessel:**..
   A. Aortic stenosis
   B. Mitral valve prolapse
   C. Deep vein thrombosis
   D. Hypercholesterolemia
   E. Acute coronary syndrome

17. **Four separate congenital heart defects:** ....
   A. Coarctation of the aorta
   B. Patent ductus arteriosus
   C. Raynaud disease
   D. Tetralogy of Fallot
   E. Peripheral vascular disease

18. **Patent means:** ....
   A. Deoxygenated
   B. Oxygenated
   C. Open
   D. Closed
   E. Half-closed

19. **The cause of essential hypertension is:** ....
   A. Due to some secondary factor
   B. Pyelonephritis
   C. Glomerulonephritis
   D. Adrenal cortex adenoma
   E. Idiopathic

20. **Digoxin:**..
   A. Drug used to strengthen the heartbeat
   B. A calcium blocker
   C. Used to dissolve emboli
   D. Used to treat varicose veins
   E. A strong antibiotic

21. **CK, LD, and AST are:** ....
   A. Lipids
   B. Lipoproteins
   C. Serum enzymes
   D. Fatty acids
   E. Nitrate-like drugs

22. **ECHO:**..
   A. Dye is injected into the blood and x-rays are taken of the heart
   B. Catheter is positioned in a vein and guided into the heart
   C. A stress test of cardiac function is performed
   D. High-frequency sound waves are transmitted into the chest
   E. Electricity is measured as it flows through the heart

23. **Incision of a vein:**..............................
   A. Phebotomy
   B. Phlebitis
   C. Phlebotomy
   D. Vasoconstriction
   E. Ventriculotomy

24. **Removal of plaque from the inner lining of an artery:**............................
   A. Endarterectomy
   B. Arteriography
   C. Aneurysmectomy
   D. Ventriculotomy
   E. Valvuloplasty

25. **A Holter monitor is:** ....
   A. An EEG test
   B. A stress test
   C. Part of a chest CT scan
   D. An ECG taken during daily activity
   E. Part of a cardiac catheterization

Chapter Eleven

VOCABULARY QUIZ

Name: ______________________________

A. Match the following terms with their meanings below:

aorta
apex
arteriole
atrioventricular bundle
atrium
capillary
carbon dioxide
diastole
endocardium
oxygen
systole

1. Gas that enters the blood through the lungs ______________________________
2. Smallest blood vessel ______________________________
3. Relaxation phase of the heartbeat ______________________________
4. Upper chamber of the heart ______________________________
5. Gas released by body cells; travels via blood to the lungs where it is exhaled. ______________
6. Small artery ______________________________
7. Inner lining of the heart ______________________________
8. Specialized muscle fibers connecting the upper and lower heart chambers; bundle of His ______________________________
9. Contraction phase of the heartbeat ______________________________
10. Largest artery in the body ______________________________
11. Lower tip of the heart ______________________________

B. Match the following terms with their meanings below:

coronary arteries
deoxygenated blood
electrocardiogram
endothelium
mitral valve
murmur
myocardium
normal sinus rhythm
pacemaker
pericardium

1. Double-layered membrane surrounding the heart ______________________________
2. Muscular, middle layer of the heart ______________________________
3. Positioned between the left upper and lower heart chambers ______________________________
4. Innermost lining of blood vessels ______________________________
5. Resting rate of 60 to 100 beats per minute ______________________________
6. Blood lacking in oxygen ______________________________
7. Blood vessels that carry oxygen-rich blood to the heart muscle ______________________________
8. Abnormal heart sound ______________________________

9. Specialized nervous tissue in the right atrium that begins the heartbeat; sinoatrial node ____________________

10. Record of the electricity flowing through the heart ____________________

C. Match the following terms with their meaning below:

pulmonary artery	septum	vena cava
pulmonary valve	sphygmomanometer	ventricle
pulmonary vein	tricuspid valve	venule
pulse		

1. Small vein ____________________
2. Beat of the heart as felt through the wall of the arteries ____________________
3. Located between the upper and lower right heart chambers ____________________
4. Instrument to measure blood pressure ____________________
5. Partition or wall dividing the chambers of the heart ____________________
6. Located between the lower right chamber and the vessel carrying blood to the lungs ____________________
7. Lower chamber of the heart ____________________
8. One of two pairs of vessels carrying oxygenated blood from the lungs to the heart ____________________
9. Vessel that carries oxygen-poor blood from the heart to the lungs ____________________
10. Largest vein in the body ____________________

Chapter Eleven

TERMINOLOGY QUIZ

Name: ______________________________

A. *Using the following word parts, build medical terms from the definitions below:*

angi/o	atri/o	-ic
aort/o	-al	-oma
arter/o	-ectomy	-plasty
arteri/o	-gram	-sclerosis
ather/o	-graphy	end-

1. Process of recording (x-ray) arteries: ______________________________
2. Surgical repair of blood vessels: ______________________________
3. Collection of yellowish plaque: ______________________________
4. Pertaining to the upper chamber of the heart: ______________________________
5. New opening between two arteries: ______________________________ anastomosis
6. Narrowing of the aorta: ______________________________ stenosis
7. Hardening of arteries (yellowish plaque collects): athero ______________________________
8. Removal of the inner lining of an artery: ______________________________
9. Record (x-ray) of blood vessels: ______________________________
10. Removal of yellowish plaque (from arteries): ______________________________

B. *Using the following word parts, build or complete medical terms to match the definitions below:*

atri/o	ventricul/o	-genic
brachi/o	brady-	-megaly
cardi/o	hyper-	-osis
cholesterol/o	tachy-	-pathy
cyan/o	-al	
my/o	-ar	
myx/o	-emia	

1. Slow heartbeat: ______________________________ cardia
2. High levels of cholesterol in the blood: ______________________________
3. Circulatory failure produced by the heart: ______________________________ shock
4. Pertaining to the upper and lower chambers of the heart: ______________________________
5. Rapid heartbeat: ______________________________
6. Disease of heart muscle: ______________________________
7. Artery in the upper arm: ______________________________ artery

8. Condition of bluish discoloration of the skin: ____________________

9. Enlargement of the heart: ____________________

10. Benign tumor (cells embedded in mucoid tissue) of the heart: ____________________ oma

C. *Using the following word parts create terms or complete terms based on the following definitions.*

coron/o	thromb/o	-itis
ox/o	valvul/o, valv/o	-lysis
pericardi/o	vas/o	-plasty
phleb/o	-ary	-tomy
sphygm/o	-centesis	
steth/o	-ia	

1. Surgical puncture to remove fluid from the space surrounding the heart: ____________________

2. Incision of a vein: ____________________

3. Arteries that surround the outside of the heart: ____________________ arteries

4. Condition of deficient oxygen in tissues: hyp ____________________

5. Inflammation of a vein with clot formation: ____________________

6. Destruction of a clot: ____________________

7. Narrowing of a blood vessel: ____________________ constriction

8. Surgical repair of a valve: ____________________

9. Instrument to measure blood pressure: ____________________ manometer

10. Instrument to listen to the chest: ____________________ scope

D. *Using the following word parts, create terms or complete terms based on the following definitions.*

rrhythm/o	ven/o	-ia
valvul/o	ven/i	-itis
vas/o	ventricul/o	a-
vascul/o	-ar	inter-

1. Pertaining to vessels: ____________________

2. Puncture of a vein: ____________________ puncture

3. Widening of a vessel: ____________________ dilation

4. Pertaining to a vein: ____________________ ous

5. Inflammation of the valve on the left side of the heart: mitral ____________________

6. Pertaining to the wall between the lower chambers of the heart: ____________________ septum

7. Abnormal heart rhythm: ____________________

Chapter Eleven
PATHOLOGY QUIZ

Name: ______________________________

A. Select from the following pathologic conditions to match the definitions below:

coarctation of the aorta
congestive heart disease
coronary artery disease
endocarditis
fibrillation
flutter
heart block
patent ductus arteriosus
septal defects
tetralogy of Fallot

1. Disease originating in the arteries surrounding the heart: ______________________________
2. Passageway between the aorta and the pulmonary artery remains open after birth: ____________
3. Rapid, but regular contractions of the heart (usually the atria): ______________________________
4. Narrowing of the aorta (congenital anomaly): ______________________________
5. Very rapid, random, inefficient, and irregular contractions of the heart: ______________________
6. Congenital malformation involving four distinct heart defects: ______________________________
7. Failure of proper conduction of impulses from the SA node through the rest of the heart: ______________________________
8. Small holes in the wall between the atria or the wall between the ventricles: ________________
9. Heart is unable to pump its required amount of blood: ______________________________
10. Inflammation of the inner lining of the heart: ______________________________

B. Select from the following pathologic conditions to match the definitions below:

aneurysm
deep vein thrombosis
hypertension
hypertensive heart disease
mitral valve prolapse
murmur
pericarditis
peripheral vascular disease
Raynaud disease
rheumatic heart disease
varicose veins

1. High blood pressure (essential and secondary) are types: ______________________________
2. Inflammation of the membrane surrounding the heart: ______________________________
3. Local widening of an arterial wall: ______________________________
4. Heart disease caused by rheumatic fever: ______________________________
5. Blood clot forms in a large vein (usually lower limb): ______________________________
6. Extra heart sound heard between normal beats: ______________________________
7. High blood pressure that affects the heart: ______________________________
8. Improper closure of the bicuspid valve: ______________________________
9. Abnormally swollen or twisted veins; usually occurring in the legs: ________________________

10. Recurrent episodes of pallor and cyanosis primarily in fingers and toes: ____________________
11. Blockage of blood vessels carrying blood to the legs, arms, kidneys, and other organs: ____________________

C. Select from the following pathologic terminology to match its description below:

acute coronary syndromes
angina
angiotensin-converting enzyme inhibitor
auscultation
beta-blocker
biventricular pacemaker
bruit
calcium channel blocker
cardiac arrest
cardiac tamponade
claudication

1. Unstable angina and heart attack; consequences are plaque rupture in coronary arteries: ____________________
2. Listening for sounds using a stethoscope: ____________________
3. Drug used to treat angina and hypertension; dilates blood vessels stopping the influx of calcium into muscle cells lining vessels ____________________
4. Abnormal blowing or swishing sound heard during auscultation of an artery: ____________________
5. Antihypertensive drug that blocks the conversion of angiotensin I to angiotensin II and dilates blood vessels ____________________
6. Sudden, unexpected stoppage of heart action: ____________________
7. Chest pain resulting from blood flow being held back from heart muscle: ____________________
8. Drug used to treat angina, hypertension, and arrhythmias by blocking the action of epinephrine at receptor sites on cells: ____________________
9. Pain, tension, and weakness in a leg after walking has begun: ____________________
10. Device that enables ventricles to beat together so that more blood is pumped out of the heart: ____________________
11. Pressure on the heart caused by fluid in the pericardial space: ____________________

D. Select from the following pathologic terminology to match its description below:

digoxin	occlusion	petechiae
embolus	palpitations	statins
infarction	patent	thrill
nitrates	pericardial friction rub	vegetations

1. Clot or other material that travels to a distant location: ____________________
2. Drugs that lower cholesterol in the blood: ____________________
3. Open: ____________________
4. Area of dead tissue: ____________________
5. Small, pinpoint hemorrhages: ____________________
6. Clumps of platelets and other material on diseased heart valves: ____________________
7. Uncomfortable sensations in the chest related to cardiac arrhythmias: ____________________
8. Drugs used in the treatment of angina by dilating blood vessels: ____________________
9. Vibration felt over an area of turmoil in blood flow: ____________________
10. Scraping or grating noise heard on auscultation of the heart: ____________________
11. Closure of a blood vessel due to a blockage: ____________________
12. Drug that treats arrhythmias and strengthens the heartbeat: ____________________

Chapter Eleven
LABORATORY TESTS AND CLINICAL PROCEDURES QUIZ

Name: ______________________________

A. *Match the following terms with their descriptions below:*

angiography
BNP test
computerized tomography angiography
digital subtraction angiography
Doppler ultrasound studies
echocardiography
electron beam computed tomography
lipid tests
lipoprotein electrophoresis
serum enzyme tests
transcatheter aortic valve replacement

1. This test can identify calcium deposits in and around coronary arteries to diagnose early coronary artery disease ______________________________
2. X-ray imaging of blood vessels after injection of contrast material ______________________________
3. Video equipment and a computer produce x-ray images of blood vessels (computer compares two images with and without contrast and subtracts one from the other) ______________________________
4. Measurement of cholesterol and triglycerides in a blood sample ______________________________
5. Chemicals (creatine kinase, troponins) are measured in the blood as evidence of a heart attack ______________________________
6. Measurement of brain natriuretic peptide in blood identifies patients with heart failure ______________________________
7. Three-dimensional x-ray images of the heart and coronary arteries are produced using a 64-slice CT scanner ______________________________
8. Placement of a balloon-expandable structure into the heart via a tube ______________________________
9. Sound waves are used to measure blood flow in blood vessels ______________________________
10. LDL and HDL are physically separated and measured in the blood sample ______________________________
11. High-frequency sound waves produce images of the structure and movement of the heart ______________________________

B. Match the following terms with their descriptions below:

cardiac catheterization
cardiac MRI
cardioversion
electrocardiography
Holter monitoring
PET scan
stress test
thallium 201 scan

1. An ECG device is worn during a 24-hour period to detect cardiac arrhythmias ______________
2. Brief discharges of electricity are applied across the chest to stop arrhythmias (defibrillation) ______________
3. Images of the heart are produced with magnetic waves ______________
4. Thin, flexible tube is guided into the heart through a vein or an artery ______________
5. Images show blood flow and myocardial function after uptake of radioactive glucose ______________
6. Recording of electricity flowing through the heart ______________
7. An exercise tolerance test determines the heart's response to physical exertion ______________
8. Concentration of a radioactive element is measured to give information about blood supply to heart muscle ______________

C. Match the following terms with their descriptions below:

catheter ablation
coronary artery bypass grafting
endarterectomy
extracorporeal circulation
heart transplantation
percutaneous coronary intervention
technetium Tc99m sestamibi scan
thrombolytic therapy

1. Balloon-tipped catheter is inserted into a coronary artery to open the artery (stents are used) ______________
2. Drugs to dissolve clots are injected into the bloodstream of patients with coronary thrombosis ______________
3. Arteries and veins are anastomosed to coronary arteries to detour around blockages ______________
4. A donor heart is transferred to a recipient ______________
5. Radioactive tracer substance is injected intravenously and taken up by cardiac tissue, where it is detected by scanning ______________
6. Brief delivery of radiofrequency or cryoenergy to destroy areas of heart tissue that may be causing arrhythmias ______________
7. Heart-lung machine diverts blood from the heart and lungs while the heart is repaired ______________
8. Surgical removal of plaque from the inner layer of an artery ______________

Chapter Eleven

ABBREVIATIONS QUIZ

Name: ______________________________

A. On the line provided, give meanings for the following abbreviations, then write each abbreviation next to its explanation below:

1. AAA ______________________________
2. ACE inhibitor ______________________________
3. ACLS ______________________________
4. ACS ______________________________
5. AED ______________________________
6. AF ______________________________
7. AICD ______________________________
8. AMI ______________________________
9. AS ______________________________
10. ASD ______________________________

a. __________ Includes unstable angina and myocardial infarction

b. __________ Arrhythmia originating in the upper chambers of the heart

c. __________ Heart attack; death of myocardial tissue

d. __________ Abnormal widening of the largest artery in the body

e. __________ Narrowing of the aorta

f. __________ Drug that is used to treat hypertension

g. __________ Device that is implanted in the chest to treat arrhythmias

h. __________ Congenital heart defect; hole in the wall between the atria or ventricles

i. __________ Portable electronic device that diagnoses and treats arrhythmias

j. __________ Skills used in the treatment of cardiac failure and arrhythmias (CPR, drugs, and defibrillation)

B. On the line provided, give meanings for the following abbreviations, then write each abbreviation next to its explanation below:

1. AV ______________________________
2. BNP ______________________________
3. ECMO ______________________________
4. ECG ______________________________
5. ECHO ______________________________

6. EF ____________________
7. ETT ____________________
8. ETT-MIBI ____________________
9. HDL ____________________
10. LAD ____________________

a. __________ Recording of the electrical activity of the heart

b. __________ Coronary artery

c. __________ This substance is elevated in congestive heart failure

d. __________ Type of lipoprotein in the blood

e. __________ Pertaining to the upper and lower heart chambers

f. __________ Method used by the heart-lung machine

g. __________ Assessment of the heart's ability to cope with increased physical activity

h. __________ Recording of sound waves as they bounce off structures within the heart

i. __________ Measure of the amount of blood that pumps out of the heart with each beat

j. __________ Treadmill and radioactive tracer test physical activity effect on heart function

C. *On the line provided, give meanings for the following abbreviations, then write each abbreviation next to its explanation below:*

1. HTN ____________________
2. BP ____________________
3. CABG ____________________
4. CCU ____________________
5. Cath ____________________
6. CHF ____________________
7. CK ____________________
8. CoA ____________________
9. CPR ____________________
10. CRT ____________________

a. __________ Area where specialized care is given for patients with heart conditions or after heart surgery

b. __________ Substance released into the bloodstream after injury to heart or muscles

c. __________ Procedure in which a tube is placed in a blood vessel

d. __________ Heart can't pump the required amount of blood

e. __________ Biventricular heart pacing

f. __________ High blood pressure

g. __________ Narrowing of the largest artery in the body

h. __________ Technique used to resume working of the heart and lungs

i. __________ Vessels are anastomosed around occlusions to restore blood flow in coronary arteries

j. __________ Normal is 120/80

D. *On the line provided, give meanings for the following abbreviations, then write each abbreviation next to its explanation below:*

1. CTNI (cTnI) ______________________________
2. DSA ______________________________
3. DVT ______________________________
4. EVAR ______________________________
5. LDL ______________________________
6. LVAD ______________________________
7. MI ______________________________
8. MUGA ______________________________
9. MVP ______________________________
10. NSR ______________________________

a. __________ The regular, normal heartbeat

b. __________ Protein released into the bloodstream after myocardial injury

c. __________ Radioactive test of heart function

d. __________ Combination of fat and protein

e. __________ Left-sided valve does not close properly

f. __________ Heart attack

g. __________ Repair of an abdominal aortic aneurysm

h. __________ Bridge to transplant

i. __________ X-ray recording of the blood vessels surrounding the heart

j. __________ Clot that originates in a deep vein

E. *On the line provided, give meanings for the following abbreviations, then write each abbreviation next to its explanation below:*

1. NSTEMI ______________________________
2. PAC ______________________________
3. PDA ______________________________
4. PCI ______________________________
5. PE ______________________________
6. SVT ______________________________
7. SA node ______________________________
8. TAVR ______________________________
9. TEE ______________________________
10. TEVAR ______________________________
11. VF ______________________________
12. UA ______________________________

a. __________ Catheter with a transducer is placed in the esophagus to obtain ultrasound images of the heart

b. __________ Congenital heart condition in which a connection between the pulmonary artery and aorta remains open after birth (does not close)

c. __________ Blood clot that lodges in the lung

d. __________ Rapid heartbeats arising from the atria and causing palpitations, shortness of breath and dizziness

e. __________ Type of heart attack

f. __________ Upper chamber of the heart is beating out of rhythm

g. __________ Angioplasty procedures are an example

h. __________ Pacemaker of the heart

i. __________ Serious arrhythmia of the lower chamber of the heart

j. __________ Chest pain associated with partial blockage of a coronary artery

k. __________ Treatment for an aneurysm of the thoracic aorta

l. __________ Treatment for aortic valve stenosis

Chapter Eleven

EXERCISE QUIZ

Name: ______________________________

A. Match the following terms with their meanings below:

aorta	mitral valve	superior vena cava
arteriole	pulmonary artery	tricuspid valve
atrium	pulmonary vein	ventricle
capillary		

1. Smallest blood vessel ______________________________
2. Largest artery in the body ______________________________
3. Lower chamber of the heart ______________________________
4. Valve between the right atrium and ventricle ______________________________
5. Carries blood from the lungs to the heart ______________________________
6. Brings blood to heart from upper parts of the body ______________________________
7. Upper chamber of the heart ______________________________
8. Valve between the left atrium and ventricle ______________________________
9. Carries blood to the lungs from the heart ______________________________
10. Small artery ______________________________

B. Complete the following sentences:

11. The pacemaker of the heart is the ______________________________
12. The sac-like membrane surrounding the heart is the ______________________________
13. The contractive phase of the heartbeat is called ______________________________
14. The relaxation phase of the heartbeat is called ______________________________
15. Abnormal heart sound caused by improper closure of heart valves is ______________________________

C. Complete the following terms from their definitions:

16. hardening of arteries: arterio ______________________________
17. enlargement of the heart: cardio ______________________________
18. inflammation of a vein with a clot: ______________________________ itis
19. disease condition of heart muscle: cardio ______________________________
20. condition of rapid heartbeat: ______________________________ cardia

D. Give meanings for the following terms:

21. cyanosis ____________________
22. Raynaud disease ____________________
23. heart block ____________________
24. ischemia ____________________
25. atheroma ____________________
26. vasoconstriction ____________________
27. myocardial infarction ____________________
28. angina ____________________
29. thrombotic occlusion ____________________

E. Match the following pathologic conditions with their meanings below:

coarctation of the aorta
congestive heart failure
coronary artery disease
fibrillation
flutter
hypertensive heart disease
mitral valve prolapse
tetralogy of Fallot

30. rapid but regular atrial or ventricular contractions ____________________
31. improper closure of the valve between the left atrium and ventricle during systole ____________________
32. blockage of the arteries surrounding the heart leading to ischemia ____________________
33. high blood pressure affecting the heart ____________________
34. congenital narrowing of the large artery leading from the heart ____________________
35. rapid, random, ineffectual, and irregular contractions of the heart ____________________
36. inability of the heart to pump its required amount of blood ____________________
37. congenital malformation involving four separate heart defects ____________________

F. Match the following terms with their descriptions:

aneurysm
auscultation
claudication
emboli
essential hypertension
petechiae
secondary hypertension
vegetations

38. listening with a stethoscope ____________________
39. lesions that form on heart valves after damage by infection ____________________
40. small pinpoint hemorrhages ____________________
41. high blood pressure due to kidney disease ____________________

42. high blood pressure with idiopathic etiology ______________________

43. local widening of an artery ______________________

44. pain, tension, and weakness in a limb after walking has begun ______________________

45. clots that travel to and suddenly block a blood vessel ______________________

G. *Give meanings for the following:*

46. HDL ______________________

47. thrombolytic therapy ______________________

48. cardiac catheterization ______________________

49. SA node ______________________

50. ECG ______________________

Chapter Eleven

DICTATION AND COMPREHENSION QUIZ: VOCABULARY AND TERMINOLOGY

Name: ________________

A. Dictation of Terms

1. ____________________ 11. ____________________
2. ____________________ 12. ____________________
3. ____________________ 13. ____________________
4. ____________________ 14. ____________________
5. ____________________ 15. ____________________
6. ____________________ 16. ____________________
7. ____________________ 17. ____________________
8. ____________________ 18. ____________________
9. ____________________ 19. ____________________
10. ____________________ 20. ____________________

B. Comprehension of Terms: Match number of the above term with its meaning below.

_______ Smallest blood vessel
_______ Instrument to measure blood pressure
_______ Incision of a vein
_______ Condition of deficient oxygen
_______ Largest vein in the body
_______ Pacemaker of the heart
_______ Largest artery in the body
_______ High levels of a fatty substance in the blood
_______ Wall between the upper chambers of the heart
_______ Widening of a blood vessel
_______ Vessel carrying blood to the arm
_______ Removal of fatty plaque (from a blood vessel)
_______ New connection between two arteries
_______ Inflammation of valve on the left side of the heart
_______ Breakdown (destruction) of a blood clot
_______ Vessel carrying blood to the lungs
_______ Surgical repair of a valve
_______ Hardening of arteries
_______ Enlargement of the heart
_______ Surgical puncture to remove fluid between the membranes surrounding the heart

Chapter Eleven

DICTATION AND COMPREHENSION QUIZ: PATHOLOGY

Name: ______________________________

A. Dictation of Terms

1.	____________________	10.	____________________
2.	____________________	11.	____________________
3.	____________________	12.	____________________
4.	____________________	13.	____________________
5.	____________________	14.	____________________
6.	____________________	15.	____________________
7.	____________________	16.	____________________
8.	____________________	17.	____________________
9.	____________________	18.	____________________

B. Comprehension of Terms: Match number of the above term with its meaning below.

______ High blood pressure of idiopathic etiology
______ Varicose veins near the anus
______ Closure (blockage) of a blood vessel
______ Collections of material (clots) that travel to and suddenly block a vessel
______ Chest pain resulting from temporary difference between supply and demand of oxygen to the heart muscle
______ Short episodes of pallor and numbness in fingers and toes due to temporary constriction of arterioles
______ Examples are flutter, fibrillation, and heart block
______ A small duct between the aorta and pulmonary artery, which normally closes soon after birth, remains open
______ The heart is unable to pump its required amount of blood; pulmonary edema may result
______ Congenital malformation of the heart involving four distinct defects
______ An extra heart sound heard between normal beats
______ Inflammation of the inner lining of the heart
______ Local widening of an artery caused by weakness in the arterial wall
______ Improper closure of a heart valve when the heart is pumping blood
______ Drugs used to treat abnormal heart rhythms and high blood pressure
______ Blockage of arteries in the lower extremities due to atherosclerosis
______ Bluish discoloration of the skin
______ Uncomfortable sensations in the chest

Chapter Eleven
SPELLING QUIZ

Name: ______________________________

A. Circle the term that is spelled correctly, and write its meaning in the space provided.

1. capillary — capilliary ______________________________
2. ventricle — ventracle ______________________________
3. carbon dyoxide — carbon dioxide ______________________________
4. vien — vein ______________________________
5. myocardium — myocardiam ______________________________
6. arterosclerosis — arteriosclerosis ______________________________
7. pulmunary — pulmonary ______________________________
8. tricuspid valve — trikuspid valve ______________________________
9. arterioles — arteroiles ______________________________
10. aortia — aorta ______________________________

B. Circle the term that is spelled correctly. The meaning of each term is given.

11.	Pertaining to the heart	coronery	coronary	corenary
12.	Relaxation phase of the heartbeat	diastole	diostole	dieastole
13.	Pain	angina	anjena	anjina
14.	Abnormal rapid heart rhythm	fibrilation	filbrilation	fibrillation
15.	Swollen blood vessels in the rectal region	hemmorhoids	hemmorrhoids	hemorrhoids
16.	Incision of a vein	phlebotomy	phebotomy	phliebotomy
17.	Widening of a vessel	vasodialation	vassodialation	vasodilation
18.	Bluish coloration of the skin	cianosis	cyanosis	cyianosis
19.	Traveling clot that suddenly blocks a blood vessel	embulus	embulos	embolus
20.	Contraction phase of the heartbeat	systole	sistolle	sistole

Chapter Eleven
PRONUNCIATION QUIZ

Name: ______________________________

A. Underline the accented syllable in the following terms:

1. diastole
2. arteriolitis
3. sphygmomanometer
4. pericarditis
5. coronary
6. capillary
7. anastomosis
8. phlebotomy
9. idiopathic
10. coarctation

B. Match the term in Column I with its meaning in Column II:

Column I		Column II
1. ventricle	_______	A. Contraction phase of the heartbeat
2. petechiae	_______	B. Small, pinpoint hemorrhages
3. hemangioma	_______	C. Largest artery in the body
4. embolus	_______	D. Tumor of blood vessels
5. systole	_______	E. Widening or dilation of a blood vessel
6. septum	_______	F. Lower chamber of the heart
7. aorta	_______	G. Swollen, twisted veins in the rectal region
8. aneurysm	_______	H. Wall or partition within the heart
9. digoxin	_______	I. Floating blood clot or other material
10. hemorrhoids	_______	J. Drug used to reduce abnormal heart rhythms

C. Complete the following terms from their definitions:

1. ______________________ itis	Inflammation of a vein
2. ______________________ cardia	Fast heartbeat
3. ______________________ ectomy	Removal of the inner lining of an artery
4. ______________________ ia	Condition of abnormal heart rhythm
5. ______________________ osis	Abnormal condition of blue coloration of the skin
6. ______________________ emia	High levels of cholesterol in the bloodstream
7. ______________________ ium	Muscle layer of the heart
8. vaso ______________________	Widening of a blood vessel
9. thrombo ______________________	Destruction of clots
10. hyp______________________	Decreased oxygen condition

Chapter Eleven
DIAGRAM QUIZ

Name: ______________________________

Label the diagram below using the following terms:

Aorta
Aortic valve
Inferior vena cava
Left atrium
Left ventricle
Mitral valve
Pulmonary artery
Pulmonary valve
Pulmonary vein
Right atrium
Right ventricle
Superior vena cava
Tricuspid valve

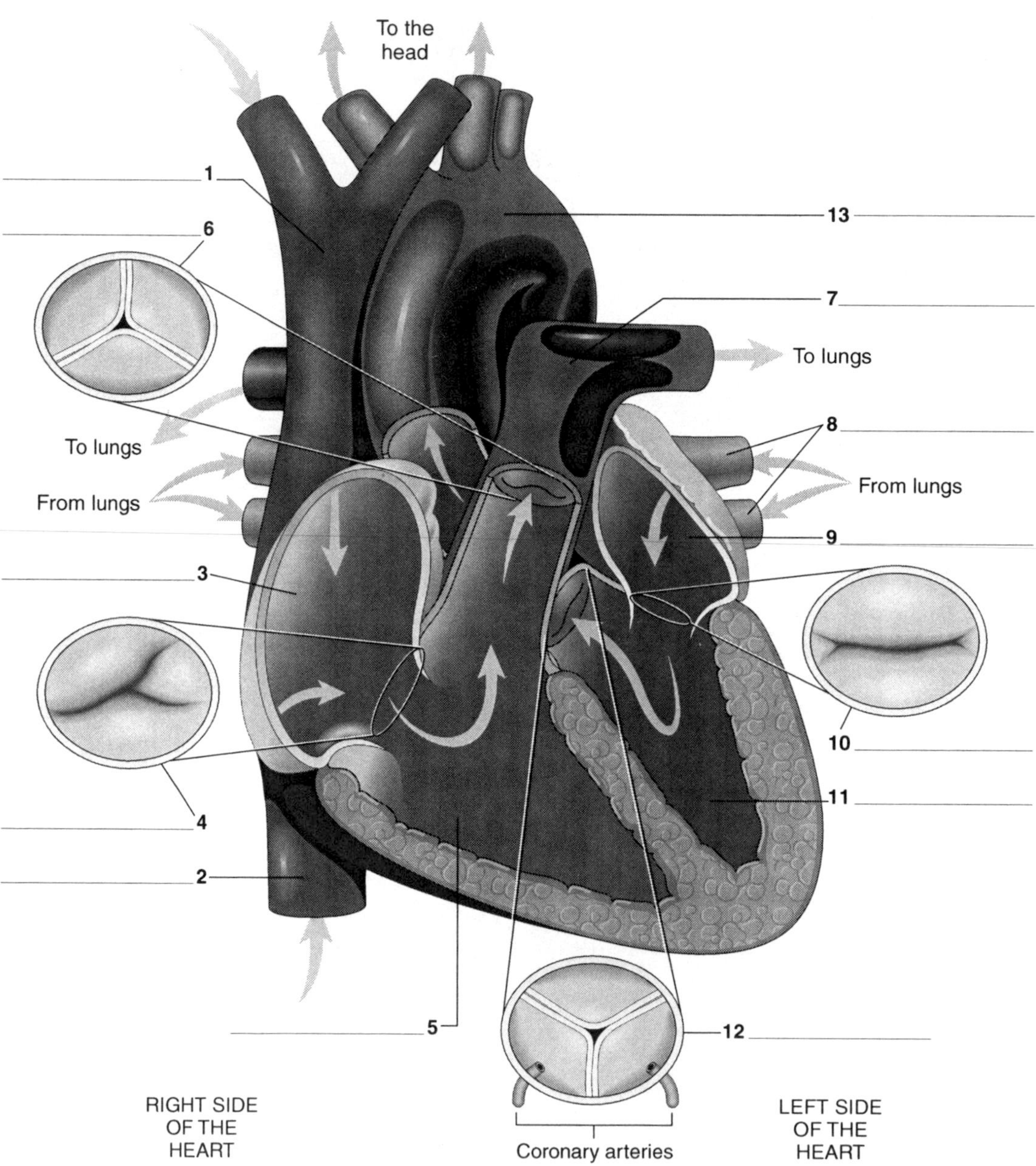

Chapter Eleven
FLOW CHART QUIZ

Name: ____________________

Label the flow chart using the following terms:

Aorta	Lung capillaries	Right atrium
Inferior vena cava	Mitral valve	Right ventricle
Left atrium	Pulmonary artery	Superior vena cava
Left ventricle	Pulmonary vein	Tricuspid valve

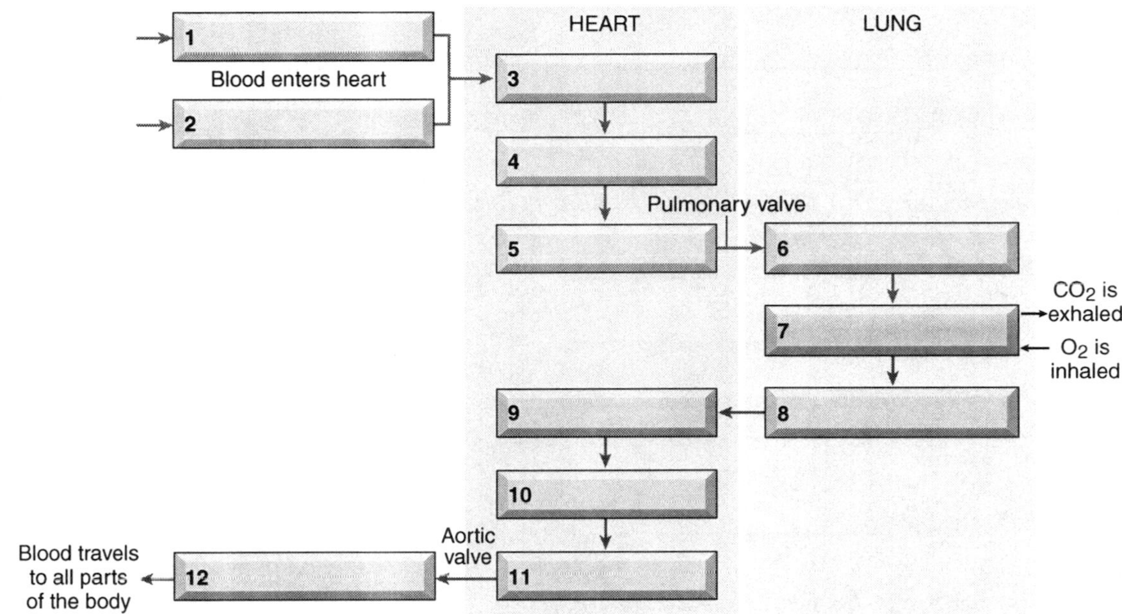

Chapter Eleven

REVIEW SHEET QUIZ

Name: ______________________

A. Give meanings for the following combining forms:

1. angi/o ______________
2. ather/o ______________
3. brachi/o ______________
4. my/o ______________
5. phleb/o ______________
6. aort/o ______________
7. axill/o ______________
8. coron/o ______________
9. pulmon/o ______________
10. ox/o ______________

B. Give meanings for the following combining forms:

1. cyan/o ______________
2. thromb/o ______________
3. atri/o ______________
4. valvul/o ______________
5. sphygm/o ______________
6. vas/o ______________
7. myx/o ______________
8. ventricul/o ______________
9. ven/o ______________
10. vascul/o ______________

C. Give meanings for the following suffixes:

1. -constriction ______________
2. -dilation ______________
3. -graphy ______________
4. -megaly ______________
5. -plasty ______________
6. -sclerosis ______________
7. -stenosis ______________
8. -tomy ______________
9. -lysis ______________
10. -emia ______________

D. Give meanings for the following prefixes:

1. brady- ______________
2. hyper- ______________
3. hypo- ______________
4. endo- ______________
5. dys- ______________
6. inter- ______________
7. tri- ______________
8. tachy- ______________
9. peri- ______________
10. a-, an- ______________

Chapter Eleven
MEDICAL SCRAMBLE

Name: ______________________

Unscramble the letters to form cardiovascular terms from the clues. Use the letters in the squares to complete the bonus term.

1. *Clue:* Localized widening of an arterial wall
   ☐ ___ ___ ___ ☐ ☐ ___ ___ R M E Y U A S N

2. *Clue:* Contraction phase of the heartbeat
   ___ ___ ___ ☐ ___ ___ ___ E O S L S T Y

3. *Clue:* Swollen, dilated veins in the rectal region
   ☐ ___ ☐ ___ ☐ ___ ☐ ___ ☐ ___ ___ R I H E O D R S H M O

4. *Clue:* Blue discoloration of skin due to hypoxia
   ___ ___ ☐ ___ ___ ___ ___ ___ O C N S Y S A I

BONUS TERM: *Clue:* Flutter and fibrillation are examples

☐ ☐ ☐ ☐ ☐ ☐ ☐ ☐ ☐ ☐

Chapter Eleven
CROSSWORD PUZZLE

Name: ______________________

Fill in the crossword puzzle below using the clues listed underneath it.

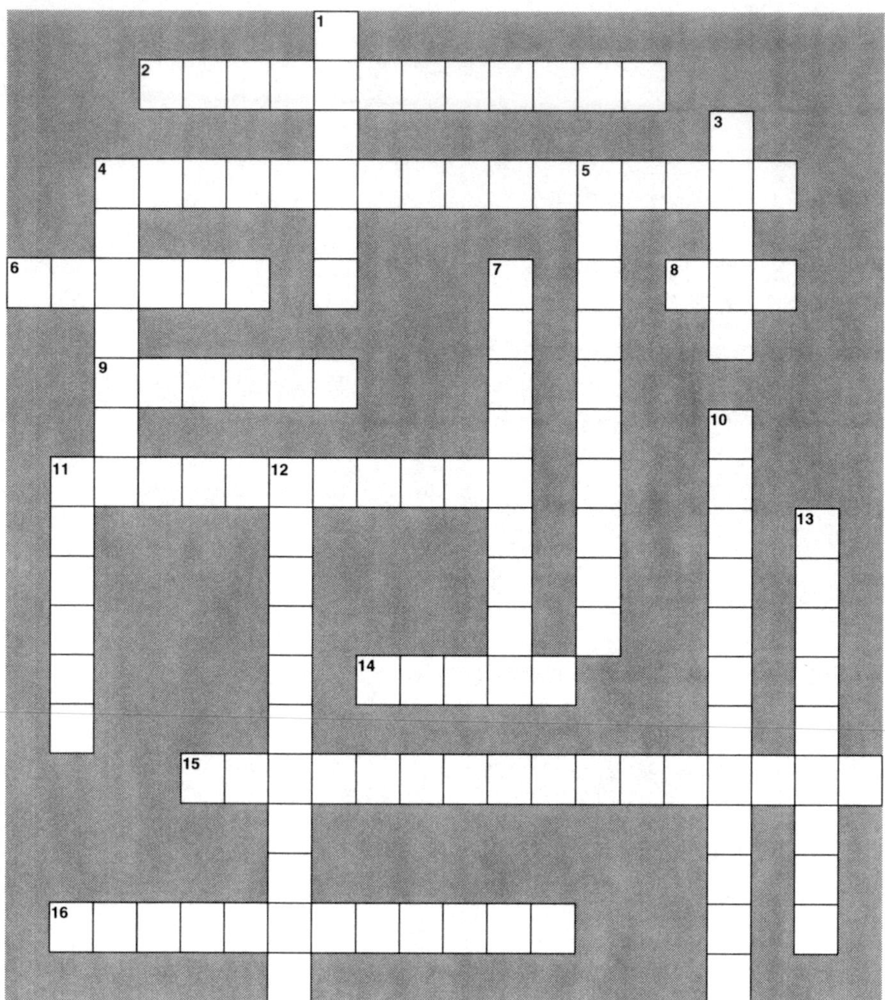

Across Clues

2. Listening with a stethoscope.
4. Instrument to measure blood pressure.
6. Angi/o means ________.
8. Brachi/o means ________.
9. Gas that enters the blood through the lungs.
11. Saclike membrane surrounding the heart.
14. Coron/o.
15. Process of using ultrasound to record images of the heart.
16. Inflammation of the inner lining of the heart; etiology is bacterial.

Down Clues

1. An abnormal heart sound.
3. Cardi/o means ________.
4. Contraction phase of the heartbeat.
5. Muscle layer of the heart.
7. Sensitive tissue in the right atrium. that begins the heartbeat; sinoatrial node.
10. Pain, tension, and weakness in a leg after. walking has begun, but absence of pain at rest.
11. Open; as in _____ ductus arteriosus.
12. Abnormal heart rhythms.
13. Small, pinpoint hemorrhages.

Chapter Eleven

PRACTICAL APPLICATIONS

Name: ______________________

A. Emergency Room—Patient Report

Mr. Smith was seen by the emergency medical technicians (EMTs) and found to have tachycardia. Lidocaine (a cardiac antiarrhythmic) was started and by the time he reached the ER his heart rate was between 75 and 80 with a sinus rhythm. He had excellent ST segments and T waves. Blood pressure was 156/88. He had a good carotid pulse bilaterally. No cardiomegaly and no murmurs.

He was started on a cardiac monitor and observed for any ECG change. He had no episode of hypotension and no further arrhythmia. There was no evidence to do cardiac enzyme studies, and the patient was discharged to be followed by his regular physician.

1. **What type of problem did the patient have before coming to the ER? ....** ☐
   - A. Chest pain
   - B. Low blood pressure
   - C. High blood pressure
   - D. Rapid heartbeat

2. **What did the EMTs do for the patient?** ☐
   - A. They administered an electrocardiogram and put him on a heart monitor
   - B. They administered a drug to reverse his arrhythmia
   - C. They checked his cardiac enzymes and got him to the hospital
   - D. They shocked his heart into a normal rhythm

3. **What is a sinus rhythm? ....** ☐
   - A. A normal heart rhythm
   - B. A rapid heartbeat
   - C. A very slow heartbeat
   - D. An abnormal heartbeat caused by respiratory problems

4. **ST and T waves are elements of: ....** ☐
   - A. An EEG
   - B. An ECG
   - C. A cardiac scan
   - D. Echocardiography

B. Patient Assessment

The patient is a 58-year-old male who has had angina for 3 years. His symptom of substernal (stern/o means breastbone) tightness occurs with exertion and is relieved promptly by rest (typical of angina). A treadmill stress test showed definite ST segment abnormalities consistent with myocardial ischemia at stage 3 of the test. In addition, the patient has multiple risk factors including hypertension, hypercholesterolemia, and history of smoking.

I have started the patient on Cardizem (a calcium channel blocker) as antianginal medication. If the patient has evidence of significant stenosis in the future, he should undergo coronary angiography and possibly PCI.

1. **What is the patient's major symptom?** ☐
   - A. Pain in his left arm
   - B. High blood pressure
   - C. High blood levels of cholesterol
   - D. Chest pain

2. **What did the treadmill test show? ....** ☐
   - A. Hypertension
   - B. Decrease in blood flow to heart muscle
   - C. Fracture of the breastbone
   - D. History of smoking

3. **What is the effect of Cardizem? ....** ☐
   - A. Increases blood pressure
   - B. Lowers blood cholesterol
   - C. Decreases myocardial ischemia
   - D. Promotes aortic stenosis

4. **What procedures are recommended? ...** ☐
   - A. X-ray of heart blood vessels and balloon angioplasty with stent placement
   - B. Coronary artery bypass surgery
   - C. Thrombolytic therapy
   - D. Exercise tolerance test and radioactive scan

C. General Hospital Nuclear Cardiology Center Stress Test Imaging Report

Patient Name:	SALLY SMITH	Procedure Date:	14-APR-1998
Procedure:	MYOCARDIAL IMAGING, SPECT	Date of Birth:	21-OCT-1956
Ref Physician:	TOM JONES, MD		

CLINICAL HISTORY:
Family history of CAD. Ex-smoker, palpitations. Sudden onset of SSCP and shortness of breath with radiation to back and down both arms at rest.

INDICATION(S):
Diagnosis of ischemia.

MEDICATIONS:
ASA, Premarin.

PROCEDURE:
The patient underwent a ^{99m}Tc sestamibi exercise treadmill stress test using standard Bruce protocol [patient must get to 85% of maximum heart rate for age]. Sestamibi at 8 AM.

302MBq [radioactive dose] ^{99m}Tc sestamibi was injected intravenously at peak exercise and tomographic imaging data acquired. Additional data were acquired following intravenous injection of another 893MBq ^{99m}Tc sestamibi at rest on the same day.

ENDPOINT(S):
Exercise was limited by fatigue. Chest pain did not occur.

REST ECG:
The baseline cardiac rhythm was normal sinus rhythm. The rest electrocardiogram revealed nonspecific ST segment and T-wave abnormalities.

STRESS ECG:
No ST segment changes were observed during this test.
Arrhythmias: None.

STRESS TEST COMMENTS
Negative for ischemia.

CONCLUSIONS:
The patient has excellent exercise capacity. The ECG response to stress was negative for ischemia. The perfusion images show equivocal mild anterior ischemia.

1. **What type of test is the patient receiving?..** ☐
   A. Cardiac MRI and stress test
   B. Radioactive scan to image blood flow to heart muscle with an exercise stress test
   C. Image of cardiac structures with ultrasound and exercise stress test
   D. Computed tomography after exercise stress test
   E. Holter monitor with stress test

2. **Why was the procedure indicated?.......** ☐
   A. History of previous MI
   B. Symptoms of intermittent claudication
   C. Congestive heart failure
   D. Substernal chest pain and SOB
   E. Family history of essential hypertension

3. **What are the results of the test? ....** ☐
   A. Patient experienced angina
   B. Patient experienced palpitations and tiredness
   C. Heart function is good and ischemia is not clearly evident
   D. Abnormal heart rhythms were evident with ST and T-wave abnormalities
   E. Heart block and ischemia occurred

Chapter Eleven
ANSWERS TO THE QUIZZES

Multiple Choice Quiz

1. B
2. D
3. A
4. E
5. E
6. C
7. D
8. D
9. A
10. E
11. A
12. E
13. A
14. C
15. A
16. C
17. D
18. C
19. E
20. A
21. C
22. D
23. C
24. A
25. D

Vocabulary Quiz

A

1. oxygen
2. capillary
3. diastole
4. atrium
5. carbon dioxide
6. arteriole
7. endocardium
8. atrioventricular bundle
9. systole
10. aorta

B

1. pericardium
2. myocardium
3. mitral valve
4. endothelium
5. normal sinus rhythm
6. deoxygenated blood
7. coronary arteries
8. murmur
9. pacemaker
10. electrocardiogram

C

1. venule
2. pulse
3. tricuspid valve
4. sphygmomanometer
5. septum
6. pulmonary valve
7. ventricle
8. pulmonary vein
9. pulmonary artery
10. vena cava

Terminology Quiz

A

1. arteriography
2. angioplasty
3. atheroma
4. atrial
5. arterial anastomosis
6. aortic stenosis
7. atherosclerosis
8. endarterectomy
9. angiography
10. atherectomy
11. apex

B

1. bradycardia
2. hypercholesterolemia
3. cardiogenic shock
4. atrioventricular
5. tachycardia
6. cardiomyopathy
7. brachial artery
8. cyanosis
9. cardiomegaly
10. myxoma

C

1. pericardiocentesis
2. phlebotomy
3. coronary arteries
4. hypoxia
5. thrombophlebitis
6. thrombolysis
7. vasoconstriction
8. valvuloplasty
9. sphygmomanometer
10. stethoscope

D.

1. vascular
2. venipuncture
3. vasodilation
4. venous
5. mitral valvulitis
6. interventricular septum
7. arrhythmia

Pathology Quiz

A

1. coronary artery disease
2. patent ductus arteriosus
3. flutter
4. coarctation of the aorta
5. fibrillation
6. tetralogy of Fallot
7. heart block
8. septal defects
9. congestive heart disease
10. endocarditis

B

1. hypertension
2. pericarditis
3. aneurysm
4. rheumatic heart disease
5. deep vein thrombosis
6. murmur
7. hypertensive heart disease
8. mitral valve prolapse
9. varicose veins
10. Raynaud disease
11. peripheral vascular disease

C

1. acute coronary syndromes
2. auscultation
3. calcium channel blocker
4. bruit
5. angiotensin-converting enzyme inhibitor
6. cardiac arrest
7. angina
8. beta-blocker
9. claudication
10. biventricular pacemaker
11. cardiac tamponade

D

1. embolus
2. statins
3. patent
4. infarction
5. petechiae
6. vegetations
7. palpitations
8. nitrates
9. thrill
10. pericardial friction rub
11. occlusion
12. digoxin

Laboratory Tests and Clinical Procedures Quiz

A

1. electron beam computed tomography
2. angiography
3. digital subtraction angiography
4. lipid tests
5. serum enzyme tests
6. BNP test
7. computerized tomography
8. transcatheter aortic valve replacement
9. Doppler ultrasound studies
10. lipoprotein electrophoresis
11. echocardiography

B

1. Holter monitoring
2. cardioversion
3. cardiac MRI
4. cardiac catheterization
5. PET scan
6. electrocardiography
7. stress test
8. thallium 201 scan

C

1. percutaneous coronary intervention
2. thrombolytic therapy
3. coronary artery bypass grafting
4. heart transplantation
5. technetium Tc99m sestamibi scan
6. catheter ablation
7. extracorporeal circulation
8. endarterectomy

Abbreviations Quiz

A

1. abnormal aortic aneurysm
2. angiotensin-converting enzyme inhibitor
3. advanced cardiac life support
4. acute coronary syndromes
5. automatic external defibrillator
6. atrial fibrillation
7. automatic implantable cardioverter-defibrillator
8. acute myocardial infarction
9. aortic stenosis
10. atrial septal defect

a. ACS
b. AF
c. AMI
d. AAA
e. AS
f. ACE inhibitor
g. AICD
h. ASD
i. AED
j. ACLS

B

1. atrioventricular
2. brain natriuretic peptide
3. extracorporeal membrane oxygenation
4. electrocardiography
5. echocardiography
6. ejection fraction
7. exercise tolerance test
8. exercise tolerance test combined with a radioactive tracer (sestamibi) scan
9. high-density lipoprotein
10. left anterior descending

a. ECG
b. LAD
c. BMP
d. HDL
e. AV
f. ECMO
g. ETT
h. ECHO
i. EF
j. ETT-MIBI

C

1. hypertension (high blood pressure)
2. blood pressure
3. coronary artery bypass grafting
4. coronary care unit
5. catheterization
6. congestive heart failure
7. creatine kinase
8. coarctation of the aorta
9. cardiopulmonary resuscitation
10. cardiac resynchronization therapy

a. CCU
b. CK
c. Cath
d. CHF
e. CRT
f. HTN
g. CoA
h. CPR
i. CABG
j. BP

D

1. cardiac troponin I
2. digital subtraction angiography
3. deep vein thrombosis
4. endovascular aneurysm repair
5. low-density lipoprotein
6. left ventricular assist device
7. myocardial infarction
8. multiple-gated acquisition scan
9. mitral valve prolapse
10. normal sinus rhythm

a. NSR
b. CTNI (cTnI)
c. MUGA
d. LDL
e. MVP
f. MI
g. EVAR
h. LVAD
i. DSA
j. DVT

E

1. non-ST elevation myocardial infarction
2. premature atrial contraction
3. patent ductus arteriosus
4. percutaneous coronary intervention
5. pulmonary embolus
6. supraventricular tachycardia
7. sinoatrial node
8. transcatheter aortic valve replacement
9. transesophageal echocardiography
10. thoracic endovascular aneurysm repair
11. ventricular fibrillation
12. unstable angina

a. TEE
b. PDA
c. PE
d. SVT
e. NSTEMI
f. PAC
g. PCI
h. SA node
i. VF
j. UA
k. TEVAR
l. TAVR

Exercise Quiz

A

1. capillary
2. aorta
3. ventricle
4. tricuspid valve
5. pulmonary vein
6. superior vena cava
7. atrium
8. mitral valve
9. pulmonary artery
10. arteriole

B

11. sinoatrial node
12. pericardium
13. systole
14. diastole
15. murmur

C

16. arteriosclerosis
17. cardiomegaly
18. thrombophlebitis
19. cardiomyopathy
20. tachycardia

D

21. bluish coloration of the skin
22. recurrent episodes of cyanosis and pallor in fingers and toes
23. failure of conduction of impulses from the AV node to bundle of His
24. blood is held back from tissues
25. mass of plaque (cholesterol)
26. narrowing of a vessel
27. dead tissue in heart muscle
28. chest pain
29. blockage of a vessel due to a clot

E

30. flutter
31. mitral valve prolapse
32. coronary artery disease
33. hypertensive heart disease
34. coarctation of the aorta
35. fibrillation
36. congestive heart failure
37. tetralogy of Fallot

F

38. auscultation
39. vegetations
40. petechiae
41. secondary hypertension
42. essential hypertension
43. aneurysm
44. claudication
45. emboli

G

46. high-density lipoproteins
47. treatment to dissolve clots in blood vessels
48. tube is introduced into a vessel and guided into the heart to detect pressures and blood flow
49. sinoatrial node (pacemaker)
50. electrocardiogram

Dictation and Comprehension Quiz: Vocabulary and Terminology

A

1. aorta
2. arterial anastomosis
3. arteriosclerosis
4. atherectomy
5. brachial artery
6. capillary
7. cardiomegaly
8. hypercholesterolemia
9. hypoxia
10. interatrial septum
11. mitral valvulitis
12. pericardiocentesis
13. phlebotomy
14. pulmonary artery
15. sinoatrial node
16. sphygmomanometer
17. thrombolysis
18. valvuloplasty
19. vasodilation
20. vena cava

B

6 Smallest blood vessel
16 Instrument to measure blood pressure
13 Incision of a vein
9 Condition of deficient oxygen
20 Largest vein in the body
15 Pacemaker of the heart
1 Largest artery in the body
8 High levels of a fatty substance in the blood
10 Wall between the upper chambers of the heart
19 Widening of a blood vessel
5 Vessel carrying blood to the arm
4 Removal of fatty plaque (from a blood vessel)
2 New connection between two arteries
11 Inflammation of a valve on the left side of the heart
17 Breakdown (destruction) of a blood clot
14 Vessel carrying blood to the lungs
18 Surgical repair of a valve
3 Hardening of arteries
7 Enlargement of the heart
12 Surgical puncture to remove fluid between the membranes surrounding the heart

Dictation and Comprehension Quiz: Pathology

A

1. aneurysm
2. angina
3. arrhythmias
4. beta blockers
5. claudication
6. congestive heart failure
7. cyanosis
8. emboli
9. endocarditis
10. essential hypertension
11. hemorrhoids
12. mitral valve prolapse
13. murmur
14. occlusion
15. palpitations
16. patent ductus arteriosus
17. Raynaud disease
18. tetralogy of Fallot

B

10 High blood pressure of idiopathic etiology
11 Varicose veins near the anus
14 Closure (blockage) of a blood vessel
8 Collections of material (clots) that travel to and suddenly block a vessel
2 Chest pain resulting from temporary difference between supply and demand of oxygen to the heart muscle
17 Short episodes of pallor and numbness in fingers and toes due to temporary constriction of arterioles
3 Examples are flutter, fibrillation, and heart block
16 A small duct between the aorta and pulmonary artery, which normally closes soon after birth, remains open
6 The heart is unable to pump its required amount of blood; pulmonary edema may result

18 Congenital malformation of the heart involving four distinct defects
13 An extra heart sound heard between normal beats
9 Inflammation of the inner lining of the heart
1 Local widening of an artery caused by weakness in the arterial wall
12 Improper closure of a heart valve when the heart is pumping blood
4 Drugs used to treat abnormal heart rhythms and high blood pressure
5 Blockage of arteries in the lower extremities due to atherosclerosis
7 Bluish discoloration of the skin
15 Uncomfortable sensations in the chest

Spelling Quiz

A

1. capillary—smallest blood vessel
2. ventricle—lower heart chamber
3. carbon dioxide—gas released from lungs
4. vein—vessel carrying blood to the heart from tissues
5. myocardium—heart muscle
6. arteriosclerosis—hardening of arteries
7. pulmonary—pertaining to the lung
8. tricuspid valve—between the upper and lower right chambers of the heart
9. arterioles—small arteries
10. aorta—largest artery

B

11. coronary
12. diastole
13. angina
14. fibrillation
15. hemorrhoids
16. phlebotomy
17. vasodilation
18. cyanosis
19. embolus
20. systole

Pronunciation Quiz

A

1. diastole
2. arteriolitis
3. sphygmomanometer
4. pericarditis
5. coronary
6. capillary
7. anastomosis
8. phlebotomy
9. idiopathic
10. coarctation

B

1. F
2. B
3. D
4. I
5. A
6. H
7. C
8. E
9. J
10. G

C

1. phlebitis
2. tachycardia
3. endarterectomy
4. arrhythmia
5. cyanosis
6. hypercholesterolemia
7. myocardium
8. vasodilation
9. thrombolysis
10. hypoxia

Diagram Quiz

1. Superior vena cava
2. Inferior vena cava
3. Right atrium
4. Tricuspid valve
5. Right ventricle
6. Pulmonary valve
7. Pulmonary artery
8. Pulmonary vein
9. Left atrium
10. Mitral valve
11. Left ventricle
12. Aortic valve
13. Aorta

Flow Chart Quiz

1. Superior vena cava
2. Inferior vena cava
3. Right atrium
4. Tricuspid valve
5. Right ventricle
6. Pulmonary artery
7. Lung capillaries
8. Pulmonary vein
9. Left atrium
10. Mitral valve
11. Left ventricle
12. Aorta

Review Sheet Quiz

A

1. vessel
2. yellowish plaque; fatty substance
3. arm
4. muscle
5. vein
6. aorta
7. armpit
8. heart
9. lung
10. oxygen

B

1. blue
2. clot
3. atrium; upper chamber of the heart
4. valve
5. pulse
6. vessel
7. mucus
8. ventricle; lower chamber of the heart
9. vein
10. vessel

C

1. to tighten or narrow
2. to widen or enlarge
3. process of recording
4. enlargement
5. surgical repair
6. hardening
7. narrowing
8. incision
9. separation; breakdown
10. blood condition

D

1. slow
2. too much; above
3. too little; below
4. within
5. painful, difficult, abnormal
6. between
7. three
8. fast
9. surrounding
10. no, not, without

Medical Scramble

1. ANEURYSM
2. SYSTOLE
3. HEMORRHOIDS
4. CYANOSIS

BONUS TERM: ARRHYTHMIA

Practical Applications

A

1. D
2. B
3. A
4. B

B

1. D
2. B
3. C
4. A

C

1. B
2. D
3. C

Crossword Puzzle

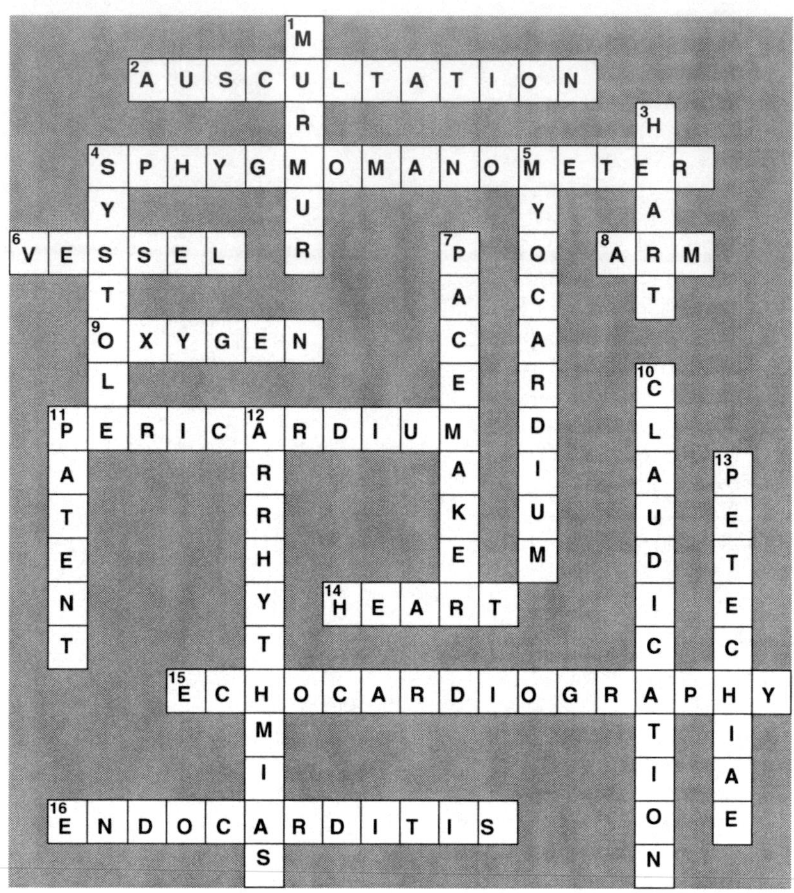

Chapter Eleven
Answers to Terminology Section

(textbook pages 409–412)

Terminology	Meaning
angiogram	Record (x-ray) of a blood vessel.
angioplasty	Surgical repair of a blood vessel.
aortic stenosis	Narrowing of the aorta.
arteriosclerosis	Hardening of arteries.
arterial anastomosis	Surgical connection between arteries.
arteriography	Process of recording (x-ray) arteries after injecting contrast material.
endarterectomy	Removal of the inner lining of the artery (when it is filled with plaque).
atheroma	Collection of fatty material in an artery.
atherosclerosis	Hardening of arteries with deposit of fatty substance.
atherectomy	Removal of a fatty mass in a vessel.
atrial	Pertaining to an upper chamber of the heart.
atrioventricular	Pertaining to an atrium and ventricle (upper and lower chambers of the heart).
brachial artery	Artery that branches from the aorta to bring blood to the arm.
cardiomegaly	Enlargement of the heart.
cardiomyopathy	Disease of heart muscle.
bradycardia	Condition of slow heartbeat.
tachycardia	Condition of fast heartbeat.
hypercholesterolemia	Condition of excessive cholesterol in the blood.
coronary arteries	Arteries branch from the aorta to bring oxygen-rich blood to the heart muscle.
cyanosis	Abnormal condition of bluish discoloration due to poor oxygenation of blood.
myxoma	Benign tumor of the heart (myx/o = mucus). The tumor is embedded in soft mucoid stromal tissue.
hypoxia	Condition of decreased oxygen in inspired air; as occurs in high altitudes.
pericardiocentesis	Surgical puncture of the membrane surrounding the heart (to remove fluid).
phlebotomy	Incision of a vein.
thrombophlebitis	Inflammation of a vein with clots.
arrhythmia	Arrhythmia and dysrhythmia are used to describe abnormal heart rhythm.
sphygmomanometer	Instrument to measure blood pressure.
stethoscope	Instrument to examine the chest.
thrombolysis	Destruction of clots.
valvuloplasty	Surgical repair of a valve (within the heart).
mitral valvulitis	Inflammation of the mitral valve.
valvotomy	Incision of a valve.
vasoconstriction	Narrowing of vessels.
vasodilation	Widening of vessels.
vascular	Pertaining to blood vessels.
venous	Pertaining to veins.
venipuncture	Incision of a vein for phlebotomy or to start an intravenous infusion.
interventricular septum	The wall separating the ventricles of the heart (lower chambers).

Chapter 12

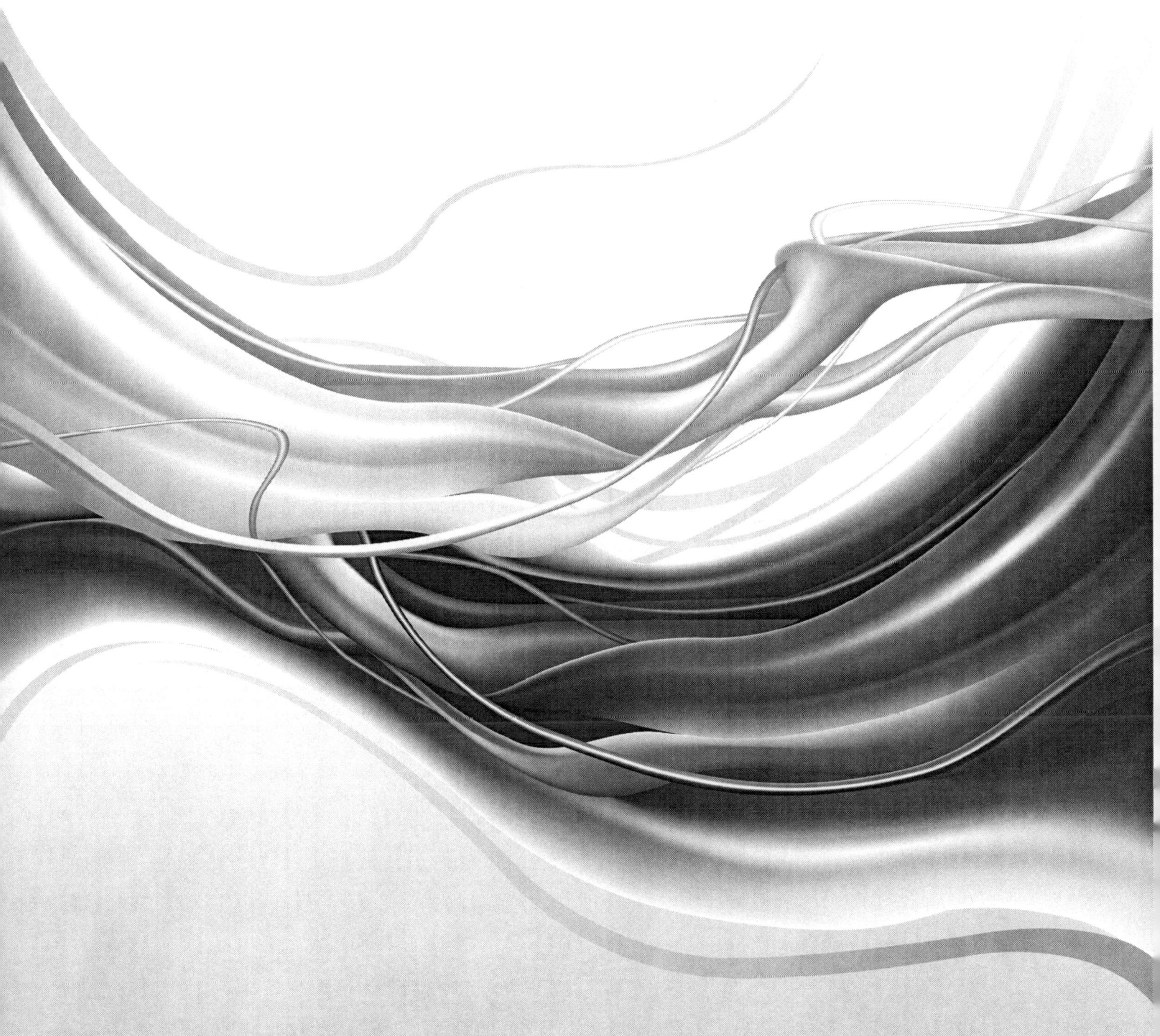

Chapter Twelve
MULTIPLE CHOICE QUIZ

Name: ______________________________

In the box write the letter of the choice that is the definition of the term or best answers the question. There is only one correct answer for each question.

1. **Tubes that bifurcate from the windpipe:..** ☐
   A. Alveoli
   B. Bronchioles
   C. Sinuses
   D. Adenoids
   E. Bronchi

2. **Uppermost portion of the lung:..........** ☐
   A. Hilum
   B. Apex
   C. Base
   D. Lobe
   E. Diaphragm

3. **Space between the lungs in the chest:..** ☐
   A. Pleura
   B. Peritoneum
   C. Mediastinum
   D. Trachea
   E. Bronchial tubes

4. **Nasopharyngeal lymphatic tissue: ....** ☐
   A. Mucosa
   B. Adenoids
   C. Visceral pleura
   D. Paranasal sinuses
   E. Epiglottis

5. **Pulmonary parenchyma: ....** ☐
   A. Trachea
   B. Pharynx
   C. Alveoli and bronchioles
   D. Red blood cells
   E. Cilia

6. **Removal of the voice box: ....** ☐
   A. Larnygectomy
   B. Pharnygectomy
   C. Laryngectomy
   D. Esophagectomy
   E. Pharyngectomy

7. **Phren/o means: ....** ☐
   A. Lung
   B. Chest
   C. Membrane around the lung
   D. Air sac
   E. Diaphragm

8. **Medical term for a condition of decreased oxygen in the blood:...........** ☐
   A. Hematemesis
   B. Paroxysmal
   C. Hypoxemia
   D. Hemorrhage
   E. Hemoptysis

9. **Type of pneumoconiosis: ....** ☐
   A. Asbestosis
   B. Pyothorax
   C. Atelectasis
   D. Pneumonia
   E. Epiglottis

10. **Breathing is easier in an upright position:...** ☐
    A. Dysphonia
    B. Hemothorax
    C. Dyspnea
    D. Orthopnea
    E. Anosmia

11. **Collection of pus in the pleural cavity: ....** ☐
    A. Cyanosis
    B. Pleuritis
    C. Hemoptysis
    D. Pyothorax
    E. Pneumothorax

12. **Sharp, short blows to the surface of the chest: ....** ☐
    A. Auscultation
    B. Percussion
    C. Stridor
    D. Rales
    E. Expectoration

13. **The "P" in DPT stands for: ....** ☐
    A. Pneumonia
    B. Pertussis
    C. Pleurisy
    D. Pneumothorax
    E. Pulmonary

14. Stridor occurs in which upper respiratory disorder?
A. Croup
B. Diphtheria
C. Asthma
D. Epistaxis
E. Pneumonia

15. Difficult breathing:
A. Anosmia
B. Dyspnea
C. Dysphonia
D. Tachypnea
E. Hypoxia

16. Bronchial airway obstruction marked by paroxysmal dyspnea, wheezing, and cough:
A. Pleurisy
B. Epistaxis
C. Cor pulmonale
D. Diphtheria
E. Asthma

17. Collapsed lung:
A. Pneumonitis
B. Endotracheal
C. Thoracotomy
D. Atelectasis
E. Tracheoesophageal fistula

18. Material is expelled from the lungs:
A. Rhinorrhea
B. Bronchiolitis
C. Sinusitis
D. Expiration
E. Expectoration

19. Localized area of pus formation in the lungs:
A. Pulmonary edema
B. Pulmonary embolism
C. Pleural effusion
D. Pulmonary abscess
E. Pleurisy

20. Spitting up blood from the lungs:
A. Pleurodynia
B. Hematemesis
C. Hemothorax
D. Hydrothorax
E. Hemoptysis

21. Tube is placed through the mouth to the trachea to establish an airway:
A. Endotracheal intubation
B. Tracheostomy
C. Tracheotomy
D. Thoracentesis
E. Laryngoscopy

22. PPD:
A. Pulmonary function test
B. Type of lung x-ray
C. Drug used to treat pneumonia
D. Tuberculin test
E. None of the above

23. Airway obstruction associated with emphysema and chronic bronchitis
A. RDS
B. COPD
C. CPR
D. SOB
E. IPPB

24. Which of the following is an endoscopic examination?
A. Tracheostomy
B. Lung scan
C. Thoracentesis
D. Bronchoscopy
E. Auscultation

25. Hypercapnia:
A. Increased oxygen to the tissues
B. High blood pressure
C. High carbon dioxide levels in the blood
D. Decreased carbon dioxide in the blood
E. Decreased oxygen in the blood

Chapter Twelve
VOCABULARY QUIZ

Name: ______________________________

A. Match the following terms with their meanings below:

adenoids	bronchi
alveolus	cilia
apex of the lung	diaphragm
base of the lung	epiglottis
bronchioles	expiration

1. Thin hairs attached to the mucous membrane epithelium lining the respiratory tract ______________________________
2. Lower portion of the lung ______________________________
3. Branches of the trachea leading into the lungs ______________________________
4. Lymphatic tissue in the nasopharynx ______________________________
5. Tip or uppermost portion of the lung ______________________________
6. Breathing out (exhalation) ______________________________
7. Small branches of the tubes leading into the lungs ______________________________
8. Muscle separating the chest and abdomen ______________________________
9. Air sac in the lung ______________________________
10. Lid-like piece of cartilage covering the larynx ______________________________

B. Match the following terms with their meanings below:

glottis	mediastinum
hilum of the lung	nares
inspiration	palatine tonsil
larynx	paranasal sinus
lobe of the lung	pharynx

1. Voice box ______________________________
2. One of a pair of masses of lymphatic tissue in the oropharynx ______________________________
3. Openings through the nose carrying air into the air passageways ______________________________
4. Breathing in ______________________________
5. Slit-like opening to the voice box ______________________________
6. Region between the lungs in the thoracic cavity ______________________________
7. Throat ______________________________

8. One of the air cavities in the bones near the nose ____________________

9. Division of the lung ____________________

10. Midline region where the bronchi, blood vessels, and nerves enter and exit the lungs ____________________

C. Match the following terms with their meanings below:

carbon dioxide
oxygen
parietal pleura
pleural cavity
pulmonary parenchyma
respiration
trachea
visceral pleura

1. Gas that passes into the bloodstream at the lungs and travels to all body cells ____________________

2. Space between the double-folded membrane surrounding each lung ____________________

3. Inner fold of membrane surrounding each lung and closest to the lung tissue ____________________

4. Windpipe ____________________

5. Essential parts of the lung responsible for respiration; bronchioles and alveoli ____________________

6. Gas that is exhaled through the lungs ____________________

7. Process of moving air into and out of the lungs; breathing ____________________

8. Outer fold of membrane surround each lung and lying closest to the ribs ____________________

Chapter Twelve
TERMINOLOGY QUIZ

Name: ______________________________

A. Using the following word parts, build or complete medical terms from the definitions below:

adenoid/o	capn/o	-al	-itis
alveol/o	coni/o	-ar	-osis
bronch/o	epiglott/o	-ectasis	-spasm
bronchi/o	pleur/o	-ectomy	-trophy
bronchiol/o	pneum/o	-ia	hyper-

1. Pertaining to an air sac: ______________________________
2. Dilation of a bronchial tube: ______________________________
3. Increased development of adenoids: adenoid hyper ______________________________
4. Inflammation of small bronchi: ______________________________
5. Tightening (involuntary contraction of muscles) of a bronchus: ______________________________
6. Abnormal condition of dust in the lungs: ______________________________
7. Removal of the adenoids: ______________________________
8. An abnormal connection between a bronchial tube and the pleural cavity: ______________ fistula
9. High levels of carbon dioxide in the blood: ______________________________
10. Inflammation of the piece of cartilage over the trachea: ______________________________

B. Using the following word parts, build or complete medical terms from the definitions below:

cyan/o	ox/o	-itis
laryng/o	pector/o	-pnea
lob/o	-al	-scopy
mediastin/o	-ectomy	-spasm
nas/o	-eal	ex-
orth/o	-ia	para-

1. Inflammation of the voice box: ______________________________
2. Visual examination of the central area of the chest: ______________________________
3. Involuntary contraction of muscles in the voice box: ______________________________
4. Bluish discoloration of the skin: ______________________________ osis
5. Cavities within the skull near the nose: ______________________________ sinuses
6. Removal of a lobe of the lung: ______________________________
7. Pertaining to the voice box: ______________________________

8. Breathing is easier in an upright position: ____________________
9. Process of expelling sputum from the chest: ____________________ tion
10. Condition of decreased oxygen: hyp ____________________

C. Using the following word parts, build or complete medical terms from the definitions below:

pharyng/o	pneum/o	-al	-ectomy
phon/o	pneumon/o	-ary	-ia
phren/o	pulmon/o	-dynia	-rrhea
pleur/o	rhin/o	-eal	-plasty

1. Pain associated with the chest muscles: pleuro ____________________
2. Hoarseness (abnormal sound) of the voice: dys ____________________
3. Pertaining to the throat: ____________________
4. Discharge from the nose: ____________________
5. Nerve that sends messages to the diaphragm: ____________________ ic nerve
6. Removal of a lung: ____________________
7. Accumulation of air in the chest: ____________________ thorax
8. Collection of fluid in the space surrounding the lungs: ____________________ effusion
9. Pertaining to the lungs: ____________________
10. Surgical repair of the nose: ____________________

D. Using the following word parts, build or complete medical terms from the definitions below:

py/o	tel/o	-ectasis	-itis
sinus/o	thorac/o	-ectomy	-meter
spir/o	tonsill/o	-ema	-tomy
sten/o	trache/o	-ic	re-

1. Condition of collapsed lung: a ____________________
2. Incision of the chest: ____________________
3. Inflammation of cavities in the skull: ____________________
4. Rhythmic changes in breathing: Cheyne-Stokes ____________________ ion
5. Removal of the tonsils: ____________________
6. Instrument to measure breathing: ____________________
7. Incision of the windpipe: ____________________
8. Pertaining to the chest: ____________________
9. Narrowing of the windpipe: ____________________ eal ____________________ osis
10. Collection of pus in the pleural cavity: em ____________________

E. Using the following word parts, build or complete medical terms from the definitions below:

hem/o	hyper-	tachy-
py/o	-ptysis	a-
-osmia	-sphyxia	an-
-pnea	-thorax	dys-

1. Increase in depth of breathing: ____________________
2. Excessive or rapid breathing: ____________________
3. Blood in the chest (pleural space): hemo ____________________
4. Not breathing: ____________________
5. Pus in the chest (pleural space): ____________________
6. Spitting up blood: ____________________
7. Abnormal breathing (shortness of breath): ____________________
8. No sense of smell: ____________________
9. Lack of pulse: ____________________

Chapter Twelve
PATHOLOGY QUIZ

Name: ______________________________

A. Match the following diagnostic terms with their meanings below:

auscultation	rhonchi
percussion	sputum
pleural rub	stridor
rales	wheezes

1. Material expelled from the lungs or upper respiratory tract by spitting ____________________
2. Continuous high-pitched whistling sounds produced during breathing ____________________
3. Tapping on a surface to determine the difference in density of the underlying structure ____________________
4. Loud, rumbling sound heard on auscultation over bronchi obstructed by sputum ____________________
5. Fine crackling sound heard on auscultation during inhalation ____________________
6. Scratchy sound produced by pleural surfaces roughened by inflammation rubbing against each other ____________________
7. Listening to sounds within the body ____________________
8. Strained, high-pitched sound made on inspiration; caused by obstruction in the pharynx or larynx ____________________

B. Match the following respiratory disorders with their explanations below.

asthma	cystic fibrosis
atelectasis	diphtheria
bronchiectasis	emphysema
chronic bronchitis	epistaxis
croup	pertussis

1. Nosebleed ____________________
2. Acute viral infection of infants and children with laryngeal obstruction and stridor ____________________
3. Chronic dilation of a bronchus secondary to infection in the bronchial tree ____________________
4. Inherited disorder of exocrine glands resulting in thick, mucous secretions in the respiratory tract that do not drain normally ____________________
5. Chronic inflammatory disorder of bronchi with airway obstruction, bronchial edema, constriction, and increased mucus production ____________________

6. Collapsed lung ____________________
7. Inflammation of bronchi persisting over a long period of time; type of COPD ____________________
8. Acute infection (membrane forms) of the throat and upper respiratory tract caused by *Corynebacterium* ____________________
9. Whooping cough: highly infectious bacterial infection of the pharynx, larynx, and trachea marked by spasms of coughing ____________________
10. Hyperinflation of air sacs with destruction of alveolar walls ____________________

C. *Match the following respiratory pathologic terminology with the descriptions below:*

lung cancer	sarcoidosis
mesothelioma	pneumonia
pleural effusion	pulmonary abscess
pleurisy	pulmonary edema
pneumoconiosis	pulmonary embolism
pulmonary fibrosis	tuberculosis

1. Inflammation of pleura ____________________
2. Chronic inflammatory disease in which small nodules (granulomas) develop in lungs, lymph nodes and other organs ____________________
3. Clot or other material lodges in vessels of the lung ____________________
4. Infectious disease of the lungs caused by bacilli (mycobacteria) ____________________
5. Acute inflammation and infection of alveoli, which fill with pus or inflammatory products ____________________
6. Malignant tumor arising from the lungs and bronchi; non–small cell and small cell are types ____________________
7. Collection of fluid in air sacs and bronchioles ____________________
8. Dust in the lungs; chronic inflammation, infection, and bronchitis ____________________
9. Large collection of pus (bacterial infection) in the lungs ____________________
10. Formation of scar tissue in the connective tissue of the lungs ____________________
11. Abnormal accumulation of fluid the pleural space ____________________
12. Rare malignant tumor arising in the pleura ____________________

D. Match the following pathologic terms with their meanings below:

anthracosis
asbestosis
bacilli
chronic obstructive pulmonary disease
palliative
paroxysmal
pneumothorax
cor pulmonale
exudate
hydrothorax
infiltrate
pulmonary infarction
purulent
silicosis

1. Failure of the right side of the heart to pump sufficient amount of blood to the lungs ____________________
2. Containing pus ____________________
3. Collection of air in the pleural space ____________________
4. Pertaining to a sudden occurrence ____________________
5. Rod-shaped bacteria ____________________
6. Glass dust in the lungs ____________________
7. Collection of fluid or other material within the lung, as seen on x-ray or other radiologic evaluation ____________________
8. Chronic bronchitis and emphysema are examples ____________________
9. Coal dust accumulation in the lungs ____________________
10. Collection of fluid in the pleural space ____________________
11. Asbestos particles accumulate in the lungs ____________________
12. Relieving, but not curing symptoms ____________________
13. Necrotic dead tissue in the lung ____________________
14. Fluid and other substances that filter from cells or capillaries oozes into lesions or areas of inflammation ____________________

Chapter Twelve

CLINICAL PROCEDURES QUIZ

Name: ______________________________

A. Match the following tests and procedures with their descriptions below:

bronchoscopy	laryngoscopy
chest x-ray	lung biopsy
CT angiography	MRI of the chest
CT scan	PET scan of the lung
endotracheal intubation	V/Q scan

1. Visual examination of the voice box ______________________________
2. Detection device records radioactivity in the lung after injection of a radioisotope or inhalation of radioactive gas ______________________________
3. Magnetic waves create detailed images of the chest in different planes of the body ______________________________
4. Computer-generated series of x-ray images show thoracic structures in cross-section and other planes ______________________________
5. Fiberoptic endoscopic examination of the bronchial tubes ______________________________
6. Radioactive glucose is injected and images show metabolic activity in the lungs ______________________________
7. Removal of lung tissue followed by microscopic examination ______________________________
8. Placement of a tube through the mouth, pharynx, larynx, and trachea to establish an airway ______________________________
9. PA and lateral films show radiographic images of the thoracic cavity ______________________________
10. Combination of computed tomography and images of blood vessels (with injected contrast) ______________________________

B. Match the following tests and procedures with their descriptions below:

mediastinoscopy	tube thoracostomy
pulmonary function tests	thoracoscopy
thoracentesis	tracheostomy
thoracotomy	tuberculin tests

1. Endoscopic visual examination of the area between the lungs ______________________________
2. Heaf, tine and Mantoux tests (based on positive skin reactions) are examples ______________________________
3. Large surgical incision of the chest ______________________________

4. Chest tube is passed through an opening in the chest to continuously drain a pleural effusion ____________________
5. Surgical puncture to remove fluid from the pleural space ____________________
6. Tests that measure the ventilation mechanics of the lungs ____________________
7. Visual examination of the chest via small incisions and use of an endoscope ____________________
8. Surgical creation of an opening into the trachea through the neck ____________________

Chapter Twelve

ABBREVIATIONS QUIZ

Name: ______________________

A. On the line provided, give meanings for the following abbreviations, then write each abbreviation next to its explanation below:

1. ABGs ______________________
2. ARDS ______________________
3. BAL ______________________
4. Bronch ______________________
5. CF ______________________
6. CO_2 ______________________
7. COPD ______________________
8. CPAP ______________________
9. CPR ______________________
10. C&S ______________________

a. __________ Fluid is injected and withdrawn from the bronchial tubes

b. __________ Growing and testing contents of sputum for bacterial analysis

c. __________ Hereditary disease that causes accumulation of mucus in the respiratory tract

d. __________ Gases are measured in the blood

e. __________ Airway is opened; breathing is restored; circulation restored by external cardiac compression

f. __________ Chronic bronchitis and emphysema are examples

g. __________ Visual examination of the bronchi

h. __________ Group of signs and symptoms of respiratory failure

i. __________ Gas that is expelled in expiration

j. __________ Mask and machine help to avoid obstructive sleep apnea

B. On the line provided, give meanings for the following abbreviations, then write each abbreviation next to its explanation below:

1. CXR ______________________
2. CTPA ______________________
3. DOE ______________________
4. DPT ______________________
5. FVC ______________________
6. ICU ______________________

7. MDI ______________________________

8. NSCLC ______________________________

9. O_2 ______________________________

10. OSA ______________________________

a. __________ Device used to deliver aerosolized medication to patients

b. __________ Toxoids for vaccination of infants

c. __________ Inability to breathe during sleep because of blockage in the airway

d. __________ Gas that is inhaled and absorbed through alveoli into the bloodstream

e. __________ PA and lateral views are taken in this procedure

f. __________ Amount of gas that can be rapidly exhaled after a full inspiration

g. __________ Major type of malignancy originating in the lung

h. __________ Seriously ill patients are treated in this area of the hospital

i. __________ Multiple computerized x-ray views of pulmonary blood vessels are taken

j. __________ Difficult breathing with strong physical activity

C. *On the line provided, give meanings for the following abbreviations, then write each abbreviation next ot its explanation below:*

1. PE ______________________________

2. PEEP ______________________________

3. PFTs ______________________________

4. PND ______________________________

5. PPD ______________________________

6. SCLC ______________________________

7. SOB ______________________________

8. TB ______________________________

9. URI ______________________________

10. VATS ______________________________

a. __________ Mechanical ventilator setting

b. __________ Infectious lung disease caused by bacilli

c __________ Clot or other material lodges in vessels of the lung

d. __________ Respiratory disease that originates in the throat, larynx, or trachea

e. __________ Sudden attack of difficult breathing at night

f. __________ Visual examination of the chest using special video assistance

g. __________ Spirometer is used for these tests

h. __________ Type of lung cancer; "oat cell" cancer

i. __________ Difficulty in breathing

j. __________ Substance used in test for tuberculosis

Chapter Twelve
EXERCISE QUIZ

Name: ______________________

A. Select from the following anatomical structures to complete the sentences below:

alveoli	larynx
bronchi	mediastinum
cilia	palatine tonsils
epiglottis	paranasal sinuses
hilum	parietal pleura

1. Branches of the windpipe that lead into the lungs are the ______________________
2. The region between the lungs in the chest cavity is the ______________________
3. Collections of lymph tissue in the oropharynx are the ______________________
4. Air sacs of the lung are called ______________________
5. The outer fold of pleura lying closest to the ribs is called ______________________
6. Thin hairs attached to the mucous membrane lining the respiratory tract are ______________________
7. The voice box is called the ______________________
8. Middle region where bronchi, blood vessels, and nerves enter and exit lungs is the ______________________
9. Air-containing cavities in the bones around the nose are the ______________________
10. The lid-like piece of cartilage that covers the voice box is the ______________________

B. Complete the following sentences:

11. The gas produced by cells and exhaled through the lungs is called ______________________
12. Divisions of the lungs are called ______________________
13. The essential cells of the lung that perform its main function are the pulmonary ______________________
14. Breathing in air is called ______________________

C. Give meanings for the following medical terms:

15. bronchiectasis ______________________
16. anosmia ______________________
17. phrenic ______________________
18. pneumothorax ______________________

D. Complete the medical terms for the following respiratory symptoms:

19. excessive carbon dioxide in the blood: hyper ______________________________
20. spitting up blood: hemo ______________________________
21. hoarseness; voice impairment: dys ______________________________
22. breathing is possible only in an upright position: ______________________________ pnea
23. nosebleed: epi ______________________________

E. Give meanings for the following medical terms:

24. purulent ______________________________
25. rales ______________________________
26. auscultation ______________________________
27. pulmonary infarction ______________________________

F. Match the following terms with their descriptions:

asbestosis	chronic bronchitis
asthma	cystic fibrosis
atelectasis	emphysema
bronchogenic carcinoma	pertussis

28. Hyperinflation of air sacs with destruction of alveolar walls ______________________________
29. Inflammation of tubes leading from the trachea (over a long period of time) ______________________________
30. Spasm and narrowing of bronchi leading to airway obstruction ______________________________
31. Lung or portion of a lung is collapsed ______________________________
32. Malignant neoplasm originating in a bronchus ______________________________
33. Whooping cough; bacterial infection of the pharynx ______________________________
34. Inherited disease of exocrine glands leading to airway obstruction ______________________________
35. Type of pneumoconiosis; dust particles are inhaled ______________________________

G. Give meanings for the following medical terms:

36. adenoid hypertrophy ______________________________
37. tachypnea ______________________________
38. pleurodynia ______________________________
39. pulmonary embolism ______________________________
40. pulmonary edema ______________________________
41. pulmonary abscess ______________________________

H. Match the clinical procedure or abbreviation with its description:

bronchioalveolar lavage	lung scan (V/Q)
CT pulmonary angiography	thoracentesis
endotracheal intubation	tracheostomy

42. Tube is placed through the mouth into the trachea to establish an airway ____________________
43. Radioactive material is injected or inhaled and images are recorded ____________________
44. After contrast is injected into blood vessels of the lungs, computerized tomographic x-rays are taken____________________
45. Opening into the trachea through the neck to establish an airway____________________
46. Chest wall is punctured with a needle to obtain fluid from the pleural space____________________
47. Fluid is injected into the bronchi and then removed for examination ____________________

I. Give meanings for the following abbreviations:

48. COPD____________________
49. PFT ____________________
50. URI ____________________

Chapter Twelve

DICTATION AND COMPREHENSION QUIZ: VOCABULARY AND TERMINOLOGY

Name: ____________________

A. Dictation of Terms

1. ____________________ 11. ____________________
2. ____________________ 12. ____________________
3. ____________________ 13. ____________________
4. ____________________ 14. ____________________
5. ____________________ 15. ____________________
6. ____________________ 16. ____________________
7. ____________________ 17. ____________________
8. ____________________ 18. ____________________
9. ____________________ 19. ____________________
10. ____________________ 20. ____________________

B. Comprehension of Terms: Match number of the above term with its meaning below.

_______ Condition of increased carbon dioxide in the blood
_______ Space in the chest between the lungs
_______ Essential tissue of the lung
_______ Surgical repair of the nose
_______ Drug that opens up (widens) the bronchial tubes
_______ Spitting up blood
_______ Instrument to measure breathing
_______ Incision of the chest
_______ Inflammation of the flap of cartilage over the windpipe
_______ Pertaining to the throat
_______ Resection of a lung
_______ Inflammation of the small bronchial tubes
_______ Pertaining to the voice box
_______ Inflammation of the membrane lining the lungs
_______ Widening of bronchial tubes
_______ Difficult, painful breathing
_______ Absence of a sense of smell
_______ Pus in the chest (between the membranes around the lung)
_______ Incision of the windpipe
_______ Muscle that aids in breathing and is located between the chest and the abdomen

Chapter Twelve

DICTATION AND COMPREHENSION QUIZ: PATHOLOGY

Name: ______________________________

A. Dictation of Terms

1.	______________________	11.	______________________
2.	______________________	12.	______________________
3.	______________________	13.	______________________
4.	______________________	14.	______________________
5.	______________________	15.	______________________
6.	______________________	16.	______________________
7.	______________________	17.	______________________
8.	______________________	18.	______________________
9.	______________________	19.	______________________
10.	______________________	20.	______________________

B. Comprehension of Terms: Match the number of the above term with its meaning below.

_____ Pertaining to containing pus
_____ Escape of fluid into the pleural cavity
_____ Visual examination of the voice box
_____ Adenocarcinoma and small cell carcinoma are examples
_____ Musical sounds heard during expiration
_____ Whooping cough
_____ Swelling and fluid in alveoli and bronchioles
_____ Spasm and narrowing of bronchi leading to airway obstruction
_____ Creation of an opening into the windpipe
_____ Coal dust accumulation in the lungs
_____ Malignant tumor arising in the pleura
_____ Collapsed lung
_____ Infectious disease of the lungs; caused by bacilli
_____ Nosebleed
_____ Strained, high-pitched noisy breathing
_____ Listening to sounds within the body
_____ Surgical puncture to remove fluid from the chest (pleural cavity)
_____ Hyperinflation of alveoli with damage to alveolar walls; type of COPD
_____ Pertaining to a sudden occurrence
_____ Injecting and retrieving fluid from the bronchial tubes

Chapter Twelve
SPELLING QUIZ

Name: ______________________________

A. Circle the term that is spelled correctly and write its meaning in the space provided.

1. epiglottis epiglottus ______________________________
2. diaphrame diaphragm ______________________________
3. ascultation auscultation ______________________________
4. astmah asthma ______________________________
5. emphysema emphyzema ______________________________
6. cilia cili ______________________________
7. traychea trachea ______________________________
8. plural pleural ______________________________
9. pnuemonia pneumonia ______________________________
10. alveoli alveroli ______________________________

B. Circle the term that is spelled correctly. The meaning of each term is given.

11. Incision of the chest .... thorocotomy thorecotomy thoracotomy
12. Collapsed lung .... atelactasis atelectasis atelelectisis
13. Rod-shaped bacteria .... bacilli basilli basceilli
14. Collection of pus....................................... absess absecess abscess
15. Surgical repair of the nose .... rhinoplasty rrhinoplasty rinoplasty
16. Removal of the tonsils .... tonsilectomy tonselectomy tonsillectomy
17. Whooping cough .... pertusis pertussis partussus
18. Visual examination of the voice box.......... larnygoscopy larnygoscipe laryngoscopy
19. Pain of the pleura (chest wall) .... phrenodynia frenodynia phrenodinia
20. Incision of the windpipe........................... trachiotomy tracheotomy traycheotomy

Chapter Twelve
PRONUNCIATION QUIZ

Name: ______________________________

A. Underline the accented syllable in the following terms:

1. dyspnea
2. bacilli
3. larynx
4. rhinoplasty
5. pleural effusion
6. adenoids
7. bronchoscopy
8. expectoration
9. hypoxia
10. tonsillectomy

B. Match the term in Column I with its meaning in Column II:

Column I		Column II
1. mediastinum	_______	A. Throat
2. empyema	_______	B. Collection of fluid in tissues
3. auscultation	_______	C. Membranes surrounding the lungs
4. edema	_______	D. Central cavity between the lungs in the chest
5. atelectasis	_______	E. The windpipe
6. pleura	_______	F. Condition of imperfect lung expansion; collapsed lung
7. pharynx	_______	G. Thin hairs attached to the lining of the respiratory tract
8. trachea	_______	H. Pus in the pleural cavity
9. cilia	_______	I. Listening to the sounds in the chest
10. diphtheria	_______	J. Infectious disease of the throat and upper respiratory tract; caused by bacteria

C. Complete the following terms using the definitions given:

1. dys______________________________	Difficult breathing
2. hemo______________________________	Spitting up blood
3. ______________________________itis	Inflammation of a small bronchial tube
4. ______________________________ osis	Abnormal condition of dust in the lung
5. ______________________________ otomy	Incision of the windpipe
6. par______________________________	Essential cells of an organ
7. pleuro ______________________________	Pain of the pleura (chest wall)
8. ______________________________itis	Inflammation of the nose and throat
9. em ______________________________	Lung disease marked by distention or swelling of the alveoli
10. ______________________________ pnea	Breathing is easier in an upright position

Chapter Twelve
DIAGRAM QUIZ

Name: ______________________________

Label the diagram below using the following terms:

Adenoids	Erythrocytes	Nasal cavity	Parietal pleura
Alveoli	Esophagus	Nasopharynx	Terminal bronchiole
Bronchi	Laryngopharynx	Nose	Trachea
Capillary	Larynx	Oropharynx	Visceral pleura
Diaphragm	Lung	Palatine tonsils	
Epiglottis	Mediastinum	Paranasal sinuses	

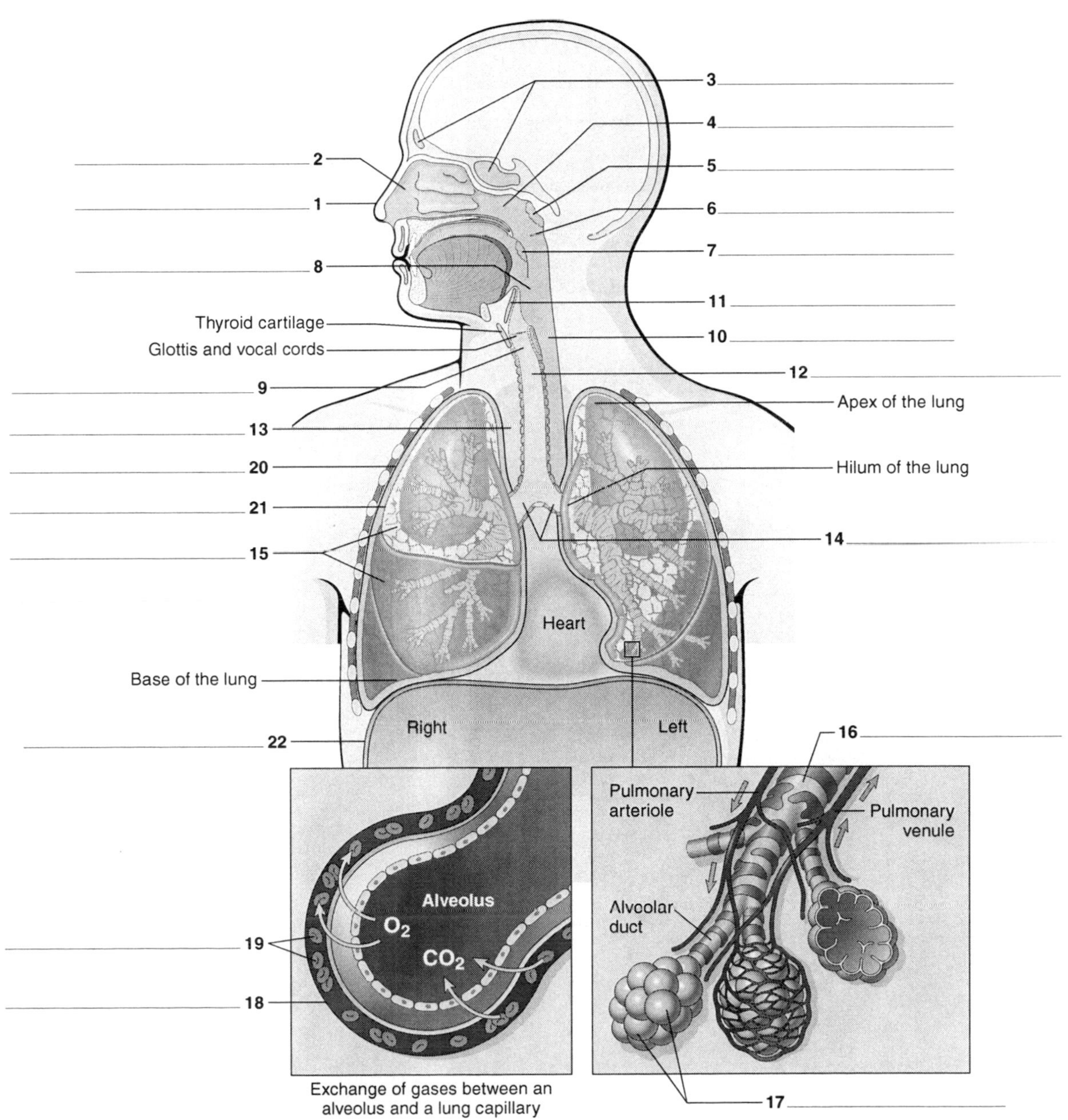

Exchange of gases between an alveolus and a lung capillary

Chapter Twelve
FLOW CHART QUIZ

Name: ______________________________

Alveoli
Bronchi
Bronchioles
Larynx
Lung capillaries (bloodstream)
Nasal cavities and paranasal sinuses
Nose
Pharynx
Trachea

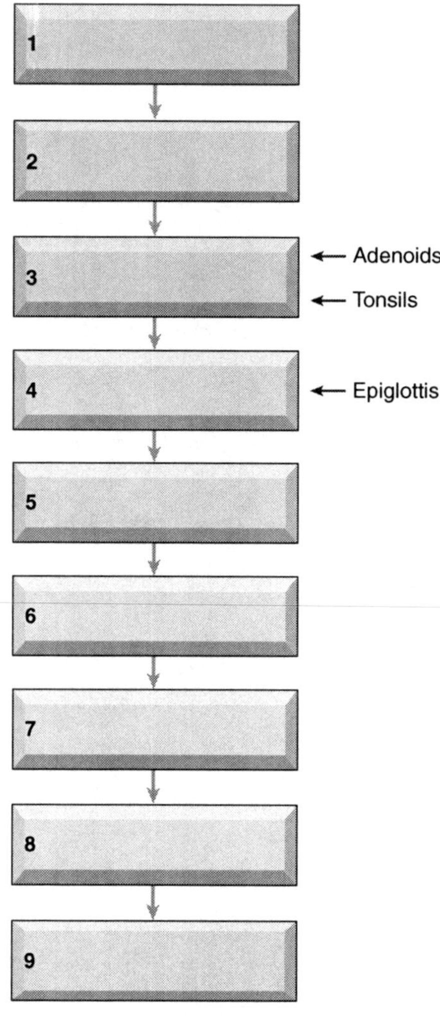

Chapter Twelve
REVIEW SHEET QUIZ

Name: ______________________

A. Give meanings for the following combining forms:

1. adenoid/o ____________
2. alveol/o ____________
3. bronch/o ____________
4. bronchiol/o ____________
5. pulmon/o ____________
6. nas/o ____________
7. or/o ____________
8. ox/o ____________
9. pector/o ____________
10. orth/o ____________

B. Give combining forms for the following meanings:

1. voice box ____________
2. throat ____________
3. blue ____________
4. voice ____________
5. diaphragm ____________
6. dust ____________
7. pus ____________
8. complete ____________
9. windpipe ____________
10. tonsils ____________

C. Give meanings for the following suffixes and prefixes:

1. -centesis ______________________
2. -osmia ______________________
3. -pnea ______________________
4. -stenosis ______________________
5. -ectasis ______________________
6. -ptysis ______________________
7. brady- ______________________
8. per- ______________________
9. hypo- ______________________
10. para- ______________________

Chapter Twelve

MEDICAL SCRAMBLE

Name: ______________________

Unscramble the letters to form respiratory system–related terms from the clues. Use the letters in the squares to complete the bonus term.

1. *Clue:* Flap of cartilage above the trachea

   ☐ ___ ___ ___ ___ ___ ☐ ___ ___ ☐ I O P T L G E T S I

2. *Clue:* Bacteria causing tuberculosis

   ___ ___ ☐ ☐ ___ ☐ ___ L A L C B I I

3. *Clue:* Small airway leading to air sacs

   ___ ___ ___ ___ ___ ___ ___ ___ ___ ☐ O N E B H L R I C O

4. *Clue:* Chronic allergic condition marked by airway obstruction

   ☐ ☐ ☐ ___ ___ ☐ S M T A H A

BONUS TERM: *Clue:* Collapsed lung

☐ ☐ ☐ ☐ ☐ ☐ ☐ ☐ ☐ ☐ ☐

Chapter Twelve

CROSSWORD PUZZLE

Name: ______________________________

Fill in the crossword puzzle below using the clues listed underneath it.

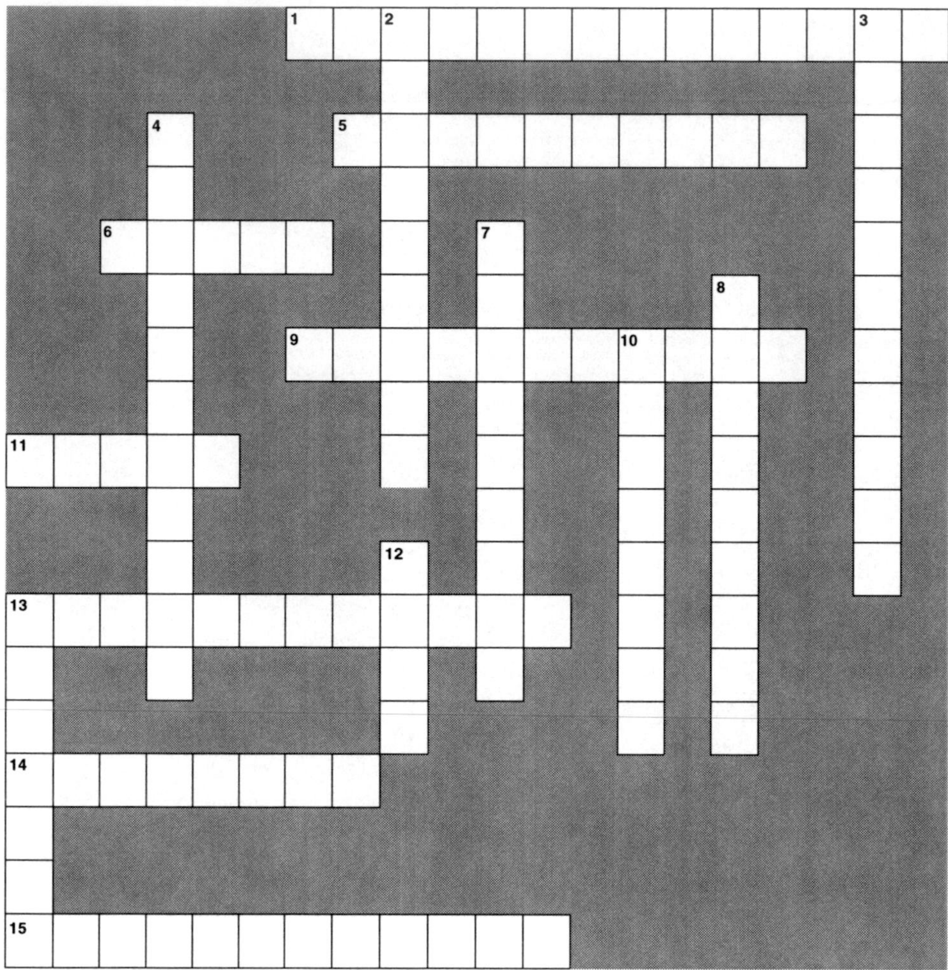

Across Clues

1. Abnormal condition caused by dust in the lungs.
5. Lid-like piece of cartilage that covers the larynx.
6. Phon/o means sound or _____.
9. Collapsed lung; or incomplete expansion of lung.
11. Thin hairs attached to the mucous membranes.
13. An infectious disease caused by bacilli and treated with INH (isoniazid).
14. Tel/o means _____, as in atelectasis.
15. Listening to sounds within the body.

Down Clues

2. Air is trapped in lungs, and bronchioles are plugged with mucus; a type of COPD.
3. Breathing in.
4. Smallest branches of the bronchi.
7. Acute inflammation and infection of the lung caused by bacteria (pneumococci), viruses, or fungi.
8. Muscle separating the chest and abdomen.
10. Collection of lymph tissue in the nasopharynx.
12. Rhin/o means ________.
13. Windpipe.

Chapter Twelve
PRACTICAL APPLICATIONS

Name: ______________________________

A. Questions for the Case Report on page 482 of the text

1. **What did the initial chest x-ray show?** ☐
   A. Collapsed lung
   B. Shallow respirations
   C. Pleurodynia
   D. Collection of fluid between the pleura

2. **What term indicates that the condition was caused by fractured ribs?** ☐
   A. Secondary
   B. Comatose
   C. Heroin
   D. Effusion

3. **What procedure was used to relieve the condition?** ☐
   A. Chest x-ray
   B. Thoracotomy and tube insertion
   C. Paracentesis
   D. Pericardiocentesis

4. **What is the lesson from this case report?** ☐
   A. Get a chest x-ray immediately upon entering the ER
   B. Removal of fluid from the pleural space showed no blood was present
   C. Be sure that a chest x-ray is read correctly
   D. Be careful when injecting heroin

B. Two Chart Notes

Bill Smith: The patient is being treated palliatively with irradiation to the left ilium for metastatic lung cancer.

1. **Where is the treatment being given?** ☐
   A. To the lungs
   B. To the whole chest
   C. To the hip
   D. To the abdomen (small intestine)

2. **What does palliative mean?** ☐
   A. Strong treatment is given
   B. Treatment will relieve, but not cure
   C. Treatment is given often
   D. Treatment is weak so that the patient does not suffer

3. **What type of physician gives this treatment?** ☐
   A. Radiologist
   B. Medical oncologist
   C. Radiation oncologist
   D. Pulmonologist

Mary Jones: Recurrent episodes of dyspnea, coughing, and wheezing. She has never been hospitalized but she requires daily therapy with a bronchodilator.

4. **What do you think the patient's condition might be?** ☐
   A. Small cell lung cancer
   B. Epistaxis
   C. Sinusitis
   D. Asthma

PATHOLOGY REPORT

Date:	November 16, 2003	Pathology No. 450231
Patient:	Carolyn Jones	Room No. 422
Physician:	Howard T. Waxman, MD	Hospital No. 550330
Specimen:	Biopsy of left bronchus	

GROSS DESCRIPTION: The specimen consisted of a very tiny, wispy portion of soft whitish pink tissue measuring 3 × 2 × 1 mm in toto. The entire specimen is submitted.

MICROSCOPIC DESCRIPTION: The sections of the bronchial biopsy show approximately half of the mucosa to be composed of pseudostratified, ciliated, respiratory-type epithelium, and the second half to be composed of respiratory epithelium that has undergone squamous metaplasia. There is one small area of cells that has become detached from the mucosa, which is composed of rather pleomorphic and hyperchromatic cells with loss of polarity. This small area of tissue would be classified as the squamous carcinoma. However, I see no evidence of (the) infiltration through the basement membrane in this section. Additional tissue may show more extensive involvement with the carcinoma.

DIAGNOSIS: Small fragment of squamous carcinoma without evidence of infiltration into the underlying submucosa, left bronchus, biopsy (see description).

Pathologist ______________________

Mark M. Mosley, MD

New Terms:

hyperchromatic — Pertaining to cells that stain intensely (chrom/o = color)

loss of polarity — Cells lose normal sense of organization (characteristic of malignancy)

pleomorphic — Pertaining to cells with many (ple/o = more) different shapes and form characteristic of malignancy

pseudostratified — Type of layered epithelium in which nuclei of adjacent cells are at different levels.

squamous metaplasia — Reversible conversion of normal cells into another, less specialized cell type. Often, these cells can transform into cancerous cells.

Chapter Twelve
ANSWERS TO THE QUIZZES

Multiple Choice Quiz

1. E
2. B
3. C
4. B
5. C
6. C
7. E
8. C
9. A
10. D
11. D
12. B
13. B
14. A
15. B
16. E
17. D
18. E
19. D
20. E
21. A
22. D
23. B
24. D
25. C

Vocabulary Quiz

A

1. cilia
2. base of the lung
3. bronchi
4. adenoids
5. apex of the lung
6. expiration
7. bronchioles
8. diaphragm
9. alveolus
10. epiglottis

B

1. larynx
2. palatine tonsil
3. nares
4. inspiration
5. glottis
6. mediastinum
7. pharynx
8. paranasal sinus
9. lobe of the lung
10. hilum of the lung

C

1. oxygen
2. pleural cavity
3. visceral pleura
4. trachea
5. pulmonary parenchyma
6. carbon dioxide
7. respiration
8. parietal pleura

Terminology Quiz

A

1. alveolar
2. bronchiectasis
3. adenoid hypertrophy
4. bronchiolitis
5. bronchospasm
6. pneumoconiosis
7. adenoidectomy
8. bronchopleural fistula
9. hypercapnia
10. epiglottitis

B

1. laryngitis
2. mediastinoscopy
3. laryngospasm
4. cyanosis
5. paranasal sinuses
6. lobectomy
7. laryngeal
8. orthopnea
9. expectoration
10. hypoxia

C

1. pleurodynia
2. dysphonia
3. pharyngeal
4. rhinorrhea
5. phrenic nerve
6. pneumonectomy
7. pneumothorax
8. pleural effusion
9. pulmonary
10. rhinoplasty

D

1. atelectasis
2. thoracotomy
3. sinusitis
4. Cheyne-Stokes respiration
5. tonsillectomy
6. spirometer
7. tracheotomy
8. thoracic
9. tracheal stenosis
10. empyema

E

1. hyperpnea
2. tachypnea
3. hemothorax
4. apnea
5. pyothorax
6. hemoptysis
7. dyspnea
8. anosmia
9. asphyxia

Pathology Quiz

A

1. sputum
2. wheezes
3. percussion
4. rhonchi
5. rales
6. pleural rub
7. auscultation
8. stridor

B

1. epistaxis
2. croup
3. bronchiectasis
4. cystic fibrosis
5. asthma
6. atelectasis
7. chronic bronchitis
8. diphtheria
9. pertussis
10. emphysema

C

1. pleurisy
2. sarcoidosis
3. pulmonary embolism
4. tuberculosis
5. pneumonia
6. lung cancer
7. pulmonary edema
8. pneumoconiosis
9. pulmonary abscess
10. pulmonary fibrosis
11. pleural effusion
12. mesothelioma

D

1. cor pulmonale
2. purulent
3. pneumothorax
4. paroxysmal
5. bacilli
6. silicosis
7. infiltrate
8. chronic obstructive pulmonary disease
9. anthracosis

10. hydrothorax
11. asbestosis
12. palliative
13. pulmonary infarction
14. exudate

Clinical Procedures Quiz

A

1. laryngoscopy
2. V/Q scan
3. MRI of the chest
4. CT scan
5. bronchoscopy
6. PET scan of the lung
7. lung biopsy
8. endotracheal intubation
9. chest x-ray
10. CT angiography

B

1. mediastinoscopy
2. tuberculin tests
3. thoracotomy
4. tube thoracostomy
5. thoracentesis
6. pulmonary function tests
7. thoracoscopy
8. tracheostomy

Abbreviations Quiz

A

1. arterial blood gases
2. acute respiratory distress syndrome
3. bronchioalveolar lavage
4. bronchoscopy
5. cystic fibrosis
6. carbon dioxide
7. chronic obstructive pulmonary disease
8. continuous positive airway pressure
9. cardiopulmonary resuscitation
10. culture and sensitivity testing

a. BAL
b. CNS
c. CF
d. ABGs
e. CPR
f. COPD
g. Bronch
h. ARDS
i. CO2
j. CPAP

B

1. chest x-ray
2. computed tomography pulmonary angiography
3. dyspnea on exertion
4. diphtheria, pertussis, tetanus
5. forced expiratory volume
6. intensive care unit
7. metered-done inhaler
8. non-small cell lung cancer
9. oxygen
10. obstructive sleep apnea

a. MDI
b. DPT
c. OSA
d. O_2
e. CXR
f. FVC
g. NSCLC
h. ICU
i. CTPA
j. DO

C

1. pulmonary embolism
2. positive end-expiratory pressure
3. pulmonary function tests
4. paroxysmal nocturnal dyspnea
5. purified protein derivative
6. small cell lung cancer
7. shortness of breath
8. tuberculosis
9. upper respiratory infection
10. video-assisted thoracic surgery

a. PEEP
b. TB
c. PE
d. URI
e. PND
f. VATS
g. PFTs
h. SCLC
i. SOB
j. PPD

Exercise Quiz

A

1. bronchi
2. mediastinum
3. palatine tonsils
4. alveoli
5. parietal pleura
6. cilia
7. larynx
8. hilum
9. paranasal sinuses
10. epiglottis

B

11. carbon dioxide
12. lobes
13. parenchyma
14. inspiration

C

15. dilation of bronchi
16. lack of sense of smell
17. pertaining to the diaphragm
18. collection of air in the pleural space (chest)

D

19. hypercapnia
20. hemoptysis
21. dysphonia
22. orthopnea
23. epistaxis

E

24. pus-filled
25. abnormal crackling sounds during inspiration
26. listening with a stethoscope
27. dead tissue in the lung

F

28. emphysema
29. chronic bronchitis
30. asthma
31. atelectasis
32. bronchogenic carcinoma
33. pertussis
34. cystic fibrosis
35. asbestosis

G

36. enlargement of adenoids
37. rapid breathing
38. pain in the chest wall (pleura)
39. blood clot suddenly blocks a vessel in the lungs
40. swelling, collection of fluid in the lungs
41. collection of pus (infection in the lungs)

H

42. endotracheal intubation
43. lung scan (V/Q)
44. CT pulmonary angiography
45. tracheostomy
46. thoracentesis
47. bronchioalveolar lavage

I

48. chronic obstructive pulmonary disease
49. pulmonary function test
50. upper respiratory infection

Dictation and Comprehension Quiz: Vocabulary

A

1. anosmia
2. bronchiectasis
3. bronchiolitis
4. bronchodilator
5. diaphragm
6. dyspnea
7. epiglottitis
8. hemoptysis
9. hypercapnia
10. laryngeal
11. mediastinum
12. pharyngeal
13. pleuritis
14. pneumonectomy
15. pulmonary parenchyma
16. pyothorax
17. rhinoplasty
18. spirometer
19. thoracotomy
20. tracheotomy

B

9 Condition of increased carbon dioxide in the blood
11 Space in the chest between the lungs
15 Essential tissue of the lung
17 Surgical repair of the nose
4 Drug that opens up (widens) the bronchial tubes
8 Spitting up blood
18 Instrument to measure breathing
19 Incision of the chest
7 Inflammation of the flap of cartilage over the windpipe
12 Pertaining to the throat
14 Resection of a lung
3 Inflammation of the small bronchial tubes
10 Pertaining to the voice box
13 Inflammation of the membrane lining the lungs
2 Widening of bronchial tubes
6 Difficult, painful breathing
1 Absence of a sense of smell
16 Pus in the chest (between the membranes around the lung)
20 Incision of the windpipe
5 Muscle that aids in breathing and is located between the chest and the abdomen

Dictation and Comprehension Quiz: Pathology

A

1. anthracosis
2. asthma
3. atelectasis
4. auscultation
5. bronchioalveolar lavage
6. bronchogenic carcinoma
7. emphysema
8. epistaxis
9. laryngoscopy
10. mesothelioma
11. paroxysmal
12. pertussis
13. pleural effusion
14. pulmonary edema
15. purulent
16. stridor
17. thoracentesis
18. tracheostomy
19. tuberculosis
20. wheezes

B

15 Pertaining to containing pus
13 Escape of fluid into the pleural cavity
9 Visual examination of the voice box
6 Adenocarcinoma and small cell carcinoma are examples
20 Continuous high-pitched whistling sounds
12 Whooping cough
14 Swelling and fluid in alveoli and bronchioles
2 Spasm and narrowing of bronchi leading to airway obstruction
18 Creation of an opening into the windpipe
1 Coal dust accumulation in the lungs
10 Malignant tumor arising in the pleura
3 Collapsed lung
19 Infectious disease of the lungs; caused by bacilli
8 Nosebleed
16 Strained, high-pitched noisy breathing
4 Listening to sounds within the body
17 Surgical puncture to remove fluid from the chest (pleural cavity)
7 Hyperinflation of alveoli with damage to alveolar walls; type of COPD
11 Pertaining to a sudden occurrence
5 Injecting and retrieving fluid from the bronchial tubes

Spelling Quiz

A

1. epiglottis—flap of cartilage over the windpipe
2. diaphragm—muscle between the chest and abdomen
3. auscultation—listening with a stethoscope
4. asthma—spasm and narrowing of bronchi
5. emphysema—hyperinflation of air sacs; destruction of alveoli
6. cilia—tiny hairs in the respiratory tract
7. trachea—windpipe
8. pleural—pertaining to the membrane around the lungs
9. pneumonia—acute inflammation and infection of air sacs
10. alveoli—air sacs

B

11. thoracotomy
12. atelectasis
13. bacilli
14. abscess
15. rhinoplasty
16. tonsillectomy
17. pertussis
18. laryngoscopy
19. phrenodynia
20. tracheotomy

Pronunciation Quiz

A

1. dyspnea
2. bacilli
3. larynx
4. rhinoplasty
5. pleural effusion
6. adenoids
7. bronchoscopy
8. expectoration
9. hypoxia
10. tonsillectomy

B

1. D
2. H
3. I
4. B
5. F
6. C

7. A
8. E
9. G
10. J

C

1. dyspnea
2. hemoptysis
3. bronchiolitis
4. pneumoconiosis
5. tracheotomy
6. parenchyma
7. pleurodynia
8. nasopharyngitis
9. emphysema
10. orthopnea

Diagram Quiz

1. Nose
2. Nasal cavity
3. Paranasal sinuses
4. Nasopharynx
5. Adenoids
6. Oropharynx
7. Palatine tonsils
8. Laryngopharynx
9. Larynx
10. Esophagus
11. Epiglottis
12. Trachea
13. Mediastinum
14. Bronchi
15. Lung
16. Terminal bronchiole
17. Alveoli
18. Capillary
19. Erythrocytes
20. Parietal pleura
21. Visceral pleura
22. Diaphragm

FLOW CHART QUIZ

1. Nose (Nares)
2. Nasal cavities and paranasal sinuses
3. Pharynx
4. Larynx
5. Trachea
6. Bronchi
7. Bronchioles
8. Alveoli
9. Lung capillaries (bloodstream)

Review Sheet Quiz

A

1. adenoids
2. alveolus (air sac)
3. bronchial tube
4. bronchiole
5. lung
6. nose
7. mouth
8. oxygen
9. chest
10. straight

B

1. laryng/o
2. pharyng/o
3. cyan/o
4. phon/o
5. phren/o
6. coni/o
7. py/o
8. tel/o
9. trache/o
10. tonsill/o

C

1. surgical puncture to remove fluid
2. smell
3. breathing
4. narrowing, tightening
5. widening, expansion
6. spitting
7. slow
8. through
9. under, below; less than
10. near

Medical Scramble

1. EPIGLOTTIS
2. BACILLI
3. BRONCHIOLE
4. ASTHMA

BONUS TERM: ATELECTASIS

Practical Applications

A	*B*
1. D	1. C
2. A	2. B
3. B	3. C
4. C	4. D

Crossword Puzzle

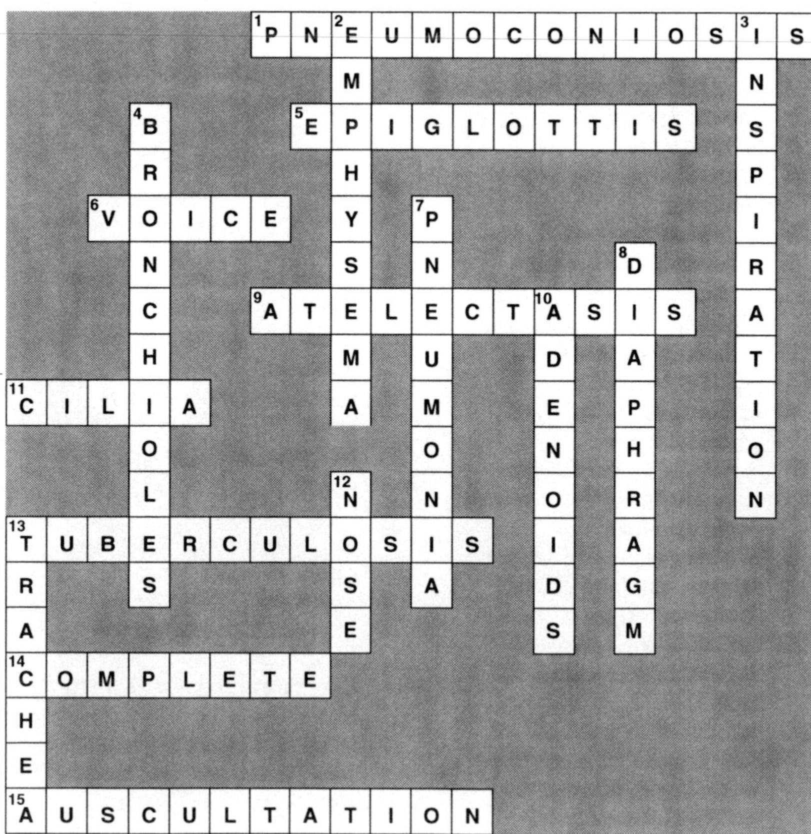

Chapter Twelve

Answers to Terminology Section

(textbook pages 463–468)

Terminology	Meaning
Combining Forms	
adenoidectomy	Removal of adenoids.
adenoid hypertrophy	Excessive development (enlargement) of adenoids.
alveolar	Pertaining to an alveolus.
bronchospasm	Involuntary contraction of muscles in the walls of bronchial tubes.
bronchiectasis	Dilation of bronchial tubes.
bronchodilator	A substance (chemical or drug) that widens bronchial tubes to make breathing easier.
bronchopleural	Pertaining to a bronchial tube and pleura or pleural cavity.
bronchiolitis	Inflammation of bronchioles.
hypercapnia	Excessive carbon dioxide in the blood.
pneumoconiosis	Abnormal condition of dust in the lungs.
cyanosis	Condition of bluish coloration of skin caused by decreased oxygen in the blood.
epiglottitis	Inflammation of the epiglottis.
laryngeal	Pertaining to the larynx.
laryngospasm	Contraction of the muscles of the larynx.
laryngitis	Inflammation of the voice box.
lobectomy	Removal of a lobe (of the lung).
mediastinoscopy	Visual examination of the mediastinum.
paranasal sinuses	Pertaining to spaces in the skull that are near, alongside, the nose and nasal cavities.
nasogastric intubation	Tube placed from the nose into the stomach.
orthopnea	Breathing discomfort in any position but erect, sitting, or standing straight.
hypoxia	Deficiency of oxygen (anoxia) due to decreased oxygen in blood.
expectoration	Expulsion of material (mucus or phlegm).
pharyngeal	Pertaining to the throat.
dysphonia	Difficult (abnormal) voice; hoarseness or any voice impairment.
phrenic nerve	Nerve carrying messages from the brain to the diaphragm.
pleurodynia	Pain associated with inflammation of irritation of pleura (or pain from intercostal muscles).
pleural effusion	Fluid collects in the pleural cavity (space).
pneumothorax	Air within the pleural cavity surrounding the lungs.
pneumonectomy	Removal of a lung.
pulmonary	Pertaining to lungs.
rhinoplasty	Surgical repair of the nose.
rhinorrhea	Discharge from the nose.
sinusitis	Inflammation of sinuses.
spirometer	Instrument to measure breathing (the air taken into and exhaled from the lungs).
expiration	The expulsion of air from the lungs.
respiration	Breathing (inspiration and expiration).
atelectasis	Incomplete expansion of a lung (collapsed lung).
thoracotomy	Incision of the chest.
thoracic	Pertaining to the chest.

tonsillectomy	Removal of tonsils.
tracheotomy	Incision of the trachea.
tracheal stenosis	Pertaining to narrowing of the trachea.

Suffixes

empyema	Pus in the pleural cavity.
anosmia	Absence of the sense of smell.
apnea	Stoppage of breathing.
dyspnea	Difficult breathing.
hyperpnea	Increase in depth of breathing.
tachypnea	Increase in rate of breathing; shallow respirations.
hemoptysis	Spitting up blood.
asphyxia	Decrease in the amount of oxygen and increase in amount of carbon dioxide in the blood leading to absence of pulse.
hemothorax	Blood in the pleural cavity; seen in pneumonia, tuberculosis, or carcinoma.
pyothorax	Pus in the pleural cavity (empyema of the chest).

Chapter 13

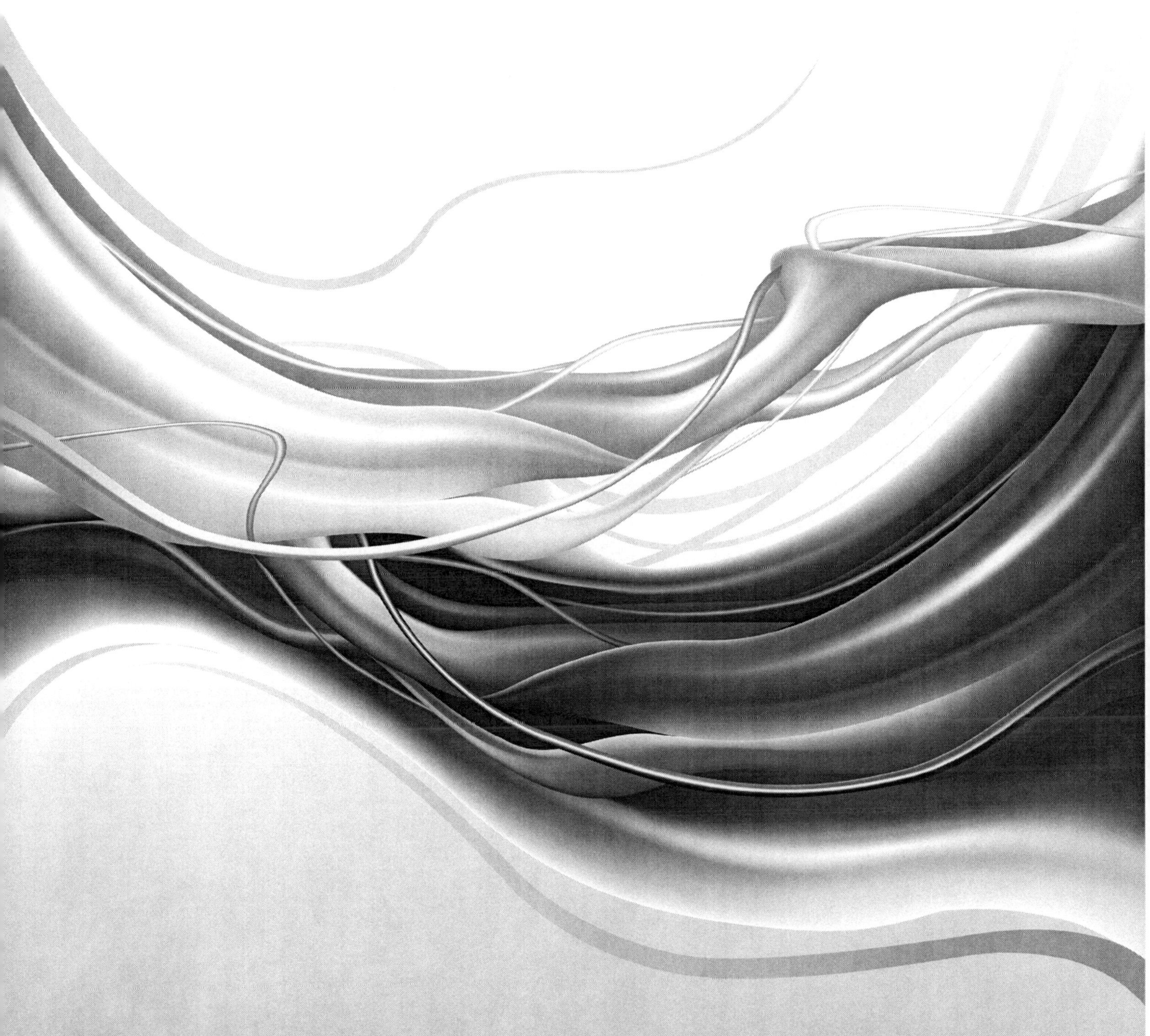

Chapter Thirteen

MULTIPLE CHOICE QUIZ

Name: ______________________

In the box write the letter of the choice that is the definition of the term or best answers the question. There is only one correct answer for each question.

1. White blood cell with reddish granules; numbers increase in allergic reactions: ☐
A. Lymphocyte
B. Eosinophil
C. Neutrophil
D. Erythrocyte
E. Basophil

2. Protein threads that form the basis of a clot: ☐
A. Fibrinogen
B. Globulin
C. Hemoglobin
D. Thrombin
E. Fibrin

3. Method of separating out plasma proteins by electrical charge: ☐
A. Plasmapheresis
B. Hemolysis
C. Electrophoresis
D. Coagulation time
E. Leukapheresis

4. Foreign material that invades the body: ☐
A. Neutrophils
B. Macrophages
C. Antibodies
D. Antigens
E. Granulocytes

5. Pigment produced from hemoglobin when red blood cells are destroyed: ☐
A. Serum
B. Albumin
C. Globulin
D. Plasma
E. Bilirubin

6. An undifferentiated blood cell is called a(an): ☐
A. Granulocyte
B. Segmented cell
C. Hematopoietic stem cell
D. Thrombocyte
E. Lymphocyte

7. Anticoagulant found in the blood: ☐
A. Heparin
B. Prothrombin
C. Thrombin
D. Gamma globulin
E. Vitamin B_{12}

8. A disorder of red blood cell morphology is: ☐
A. Multiple myeloma
B. Poikilocytosis
C. Monocytosis
D. Acute myelocytic leukemia
E. Hemochromatosis

9. Deficiency in numbers of white blood cells: ☐
A. Neutropenia
B. Hypochromia
C. Leukocytosis
D. Chronic lymphocytic leukemia
E. Spherocytosis

10. Immature red blood cell: ☐
A. Thrombocyte
B. Monoblast
C. Segmented
D. Erythroblast
E. Megakaryoblast

11. Derived from bone marrow: ☐
A. Myeloid
B. Lymphoid
C. Granulocytopenic
D. Polymorphonuclear
E. Phagocytic

12. Breakdown of recipient's red blood cells when incompatible bloods are mixed: ☐
A. Erythrocytosis
B. Hemolysis
C. Embolism
D. Anticoagulation
E. Erythropoiesis

13. **Sideropenia occurs causing deficient production of hemoglobin:..................** ☐
   A. Pernicious anemia
   B. Iron deficiency anemia
   C. Aplastic anemia
   D. Hemolytic anemia
   E. Thalassemia

14. **Reduction in red cells due to excessive cell destruction:...................** ☐
   A. Pernicious anemia
   B. Iron deficiency anemia
   C. Aplastic anemia
   D. Hemolytic anemia
   E. Thalassemia

15. **Failure of blood cell production due to absence of formation of cells in the bone marrow: ....** ☐
   A. Pernicious anemia
   B. Iron deficiency anemia
   C. Aplastic anemia
   D. Hemolytic anemia
   E. Thalassemia

16. **Inherited defect in ability to produce hemoglobin: ....** ☐
   A. Pernicious anemia
   B. Iron deficiency anemia
   C. Aplastic anemia
   D. Hemolytic anemia
   E. Thalassemia

17. **Lack of mature red cells due to inability to absorb vitamin B12 into the body:**
   A. Pernicious anemia
   B. Iron deficiency anemia
   C. Aplastic anemia
   D. Hemolytic anemia
   E. Thalassemia

18. **Excessive deposits of iron throughout the body: ....** ☐
   A. Polycythemia vera
   B. Cooley anemia
   C. Purpura
   D. Hemochromatosis
   E. Thrombocytopenia

19. **Symptoms of pallor, shortness of breath, infection, bleeding gums, predominance of immature and abnormally functioning leukocytes, and low numbers of mature neutrophils in a young child may indicate a likely diagnosis of: ....** ☐
   A. Sickle cell anemia
   B. Hemostasis
   C. Acute lymphocytic leukemia
   D. Chronic lymphocytic leukemia
   E. Hemoglobinopathy

20. **Excessive bleeding caused by congenital lack of factor VIII or IX:.....** ☐
   A. Autoimmune thrombocytopenic purpura
   B. Granulocytosis
   C. Polycythemia vera
   D. Erythremia
   E. Hemophilia

21. **Venous blood is clotted in a test tube:** ☐
   A. Hematocrit
   B. White blood cell differential
   C. Erythrocyte sedimentation rate
   D. Coagulation time
   E. Red blood cell morphology

22. **Sample of blood is spun in a test tube so that red cells fall to the bottom and percentage of RBCs is taken: ....** ☐
   A. Hematocrit
   B. White blood cell differential
   C. Erythrocyte sedimentation rate
   D. Coagulation time
   E. Red blood cell morphology

23. **Blood smear is examined to determine the shape or form of cells: ....** ☐
   A. Hematocrit
   B. White blood cell differential
   C. Erythrocyte sedimentation rate
   D. Coagulation time
   E. Red blood cell morphology

24. Leukocytes are stained and counted under a microscope to see numbers of mature and immature forms: ☐
A. Hematocrit
B. White blood cell differential
C. Erythrocyte sedimentation rate
D. Coagulation time
E. Red blood cell morphology

25. Venous blood is collected; anticoagulant added and the distance cells fall in a period of time is determined: ☐
A. Hematocrit
B. White blood cell differential
C. Erythrocyte sedimentation rate
D. Coagulation time
E. Red blood cell morphology

26. Blood protein that maintains the proper proportion and concentration of water in blood: ☐
A. Bilirubin
B. Prothrombin
C. Fibrinogen
D. Albumin
E. Globulin

27. Swelling; fluid leaks out into tissue spaces: ☐
A. Petechiae
B. Edema
C. Ecchymoses
D. Dyscrasia
E. Autologous transfusion

28. IgM, IgG, IgA, IgD, IgE: ☐
A. Megakaryocytes
B. Eosinophils
C. Neutrophils
D. Stem cells
E. Immunoglobulins

29. Symptoms of disease return: ☐
A. Palliative
B. Relapse
C. Hemoglobinopathy
D. Remission
E. Spherocytosis

30. Relieving symptoms, but not curing disease: ☐
A. Coagulopathy
B. Hemostasis
C. Hemolysis
D. Palliative
E. Myelopoiesis

Chapter Thirteen
VOCABULARY QUIZ

Name: ______________________

A. Match the following vocabulary terms with their meanings below:

albumin	bilirubin	eosinophil
antibody	coagulation	erythrocyte
antigen	differentiation	erythropoietin
basophil	electrophoresis	fibrin

1. Orange-yellow pigment in bile; formed by the breakdown of hemoglobin ______________
2. Blood protein that maintains the proper amount of water in the blood ______________
3. White blood cell containing granules that stain red; associated with allergic reactions ______________
4. Blood clotting ______________
5. Method of separating serum proteins by electrical charge ______________
6. Foreign substance that stimulates the production of an antibody ______________
7. Red blood cell ______________
8. Change in structure and function of a cell as it matures ______________
9. White blood cell containing granules that stain blue; associated with release of histamine and heparin ______________
10. Hormone secreted by the kidneys that stimulates red blood cell formation ______________
11. Immunoglobulin produced by lymphocytes to combat specific antigens ______________
12. Protein threads that form the basis of a blood clot ______________

B. Match the following terms with their definitions below:

fibrinogen	hemolysis	macrophage
globulins	heparin	plasma
granulocyte	immune reaction	
hemoglobin	lymphocyte	

1. Monocyte that migrates from the blood to tissue spaces; a phagocyte ______________
2. Response of the immune system to foreign invasion ______________
3. Mononuclear leukocyte that produces antibodies ______________
4. Anticoagulant found in blood and tissue cells ______________
5. Destruction or breakdown of blood ______________
6. Liquid portion of the blood ______________

7. Blood protein containing iron ______________________
8. Plasma protein that is converted to fibrin in the clotting process ______________________
9. White blood cell with numerous dark-staining granules; neutrophil, basophil, and eosinophil ______________________
10. Plasma proteins; alpha, beta, and gamma are examples ______________________

C. Match the following terms with their meanings below:

hematopoietic stem cell	plasmapheresis	serum
immunoglobulin	platelet (thrombocyte)	
neutrophil	reticulocyte	

1. White blood cell containing granules and formed in bone marrow ______________________
2. Small blood fragment that collects at sites of injury to begin the clotting process ______________________
3. Unspecialized cell that gives rise to mature, specialized forms; found in bone marrow ______________________
4. Removal of plasma from withdrawn blood by centrifuge ______________________
5. Plasma minus clotting proteins and cells ______________________
6. Protein with antibody activity; IgG, IgA, IgM, IgD, and IgE are examples ______________________
7. Immature erythrocyte ______________________

Chapter Thirteen

TERMINOLOGY QUIZ

Name: ______________________________

A. Match the following terms with their meanings given below:

anticoagulant	eosinophil	hemolysis
basophil	erythrocytopenia	hypochromic
coagulopathy	hematocrit	
cytology	hemoglobinopathy	

1. White blood cell with dark-staining blue granules; releases heparin and histamine ______________________________
2. Pertaining to a deficiency in color (of red blood cells) ______________________________
3. White blood cell with dark-staining red granules; elevated in allergic reactions ______________________________
4. Disorder marked by abnormality in hemoglobin ______________________________
5. Destruction or breakdown of blood (red blood cells) ______________________________
6. Study of cells ______________________________
7. Percentage of red blood cells in a volume of blood ______________________________
8. Disorder or disease of clotting ______________________________
9. Deficiency of red blood cells ______________________________
10. Substance that stops blood clotting ______________________________

B. Complete the medical terms from the definitions given:

1. Deficiency of white blood cells: leukocyto ______________________________
2. Immature bone marrow cell: myelo ______________________________
3. Study of the shape (of cells): ______________________________ ology
4. Deficiency of neutrophils: neutro ______________________________.
5. Abnormal formation of bone marrow: ______________________________ dysplasia
6. White blood cell with one large nucleus: ______________________________ cyte
7. Cell that eats or swallows bacteria and debris: ______________________________ cyte
8. Deficiency of iron: ______________________________ penia
9. Deficiency of platelets: ______________________________ penia
10. Pertaining to a white blood cell with multilobed (shaped) nucleus: ____________________ nuclear

C. Match the following terms with their meanings below:

erythroblast
hemoglobin
leukapheresis
macrocytosis
microcytosis
monoblast
plasmapheresis
plateletpheresis
poikilocytosis
spherocytosis

1. Immature white blood cell ______________________
2. Abnormal condition of small red blood cells ______________________
3. Immature red blood cell ______________________
4. Abnormal condition of red blood cells that are irregularly shaped ______________________
5. Plasma is separated from other parts of the blood ______________________
6. Abnormal condition of rounded red blood cells ______________________
7. Abnormal condition of large red blood cells ______________________
8. White blood cells are separated from other parts of the blood ______________________
9. Clotting cells are separated from other parts of the blood ______________________
10. Iron-containing protein in red blood cells ______________________

D. Complete the medical terms from the definitions given:

1. Antibody-containing protein in blood: immuno ______________________
2. Therapy used to dissolve (breakdown) clots: thrombo ______________________ therapy
3. Resembling bone marrow cells: myel ______________________
4. Deficiency of granulocytes: granulo ______________________
5. Increase in numbers of neutrophils: neutro ______________________
6. Abnormal condition of clotting: thromb ______________________
7. Formation of blood: hemato ______________________
8. Deficiency of all types of blood cells: pan ______________________
9. Formation of bone marrow cells: myelo ______________________
10. Stopping or controlling the flow of blood: hemo ______________________

Chapter Thirteen
PATHOLOGY QUIZ

Name: ______________________

A. Match the following conditions with their definitions below:

aplastic anemia
hemochromatosis
hemolytic anemia
hemophilia
mononucleosis
pernicious anemia
polycythemia vera
purpura
sickle cell anemia
thalassemia

1. Multiple pinpoint hemorrhages and accumulation of blood under the skin ______________
2. General increase in red blood cells (erythremia) ______________
3. Excess iron deposits throughout the body ______________
4. Hereditary condition characterized by abnormal crescent shape of erythrocytes and by hemolysis ______________
5. Inherited defect in the ability to produce hemoglobin, usually seen in persons of Mediterranean background ______________
6. Infectious disease marked by increased numbers of leukocytes and enlarged cervical lymph nodes ______________
7. Reduction in red cells due to excessive destruction ______________
8. Failure of blood cell production due absence of formation of bone marrow cells ______________
9. Excessive bleeding caused by hereditary lack of factor VIII or factor IX necessary for blood clotting ______________
10. Lack of mature erythrocytes caused by inability to absorb vitamin B_{12} into the body ______________

B. Name the types of leukemia from their descriptions and abbreviations below:

1. Abnormal numbers of relatively mature lymphocytes predominate in the bone marrow, lymph nodes, and spleen (CLL) ______________
2. Immature granulocytes predominate in the bone marrow (AML) ______________
3. Both mature and immature granulocytes are present in the bone marrow and bloodstream (CML) ______________
4. Immature lymphocytes predominate in the bone marrow and lymph nodes (ALL) ______________

C. Match the following terms with their meanings below:

dyscrasia	iron deficiency anemia	relapse
ecchymoses	multiple myeloma	remission
eosinophilia	palliative	
Epstein-Barr virus	petechiae	

1. Tiny purple or red flat spots on the skin as a result of hemorrhages ______________________
2. Causative agent in mononucleosis ______________________
3. Large blue or purplish patches on the skin (bruises) ______________________
4. Sideropenia is the cause of this condition ______________________
5. Any disease of the blood or bone marrow ______________________
6. Disappearance of signs and symptoms of disease ______________________
7. Relieving, but not curing disease ______________________
8. Disease symptoms and signs reappear ______________________
9. Malignant neoplasm of bone marrow ______________________
10. Increase in numbers of granulocytes associated with allergic conditions ______________________

Chapter Thirteen

LABORATORY TESTS AND CLINICAL PROCEDURES QUIZ

Name: ______________________________

A. Match the following laboratory test with its definition below:

antiglobulin test
bleeding time
coagulation time
complete blood count
erythrocyte sedimentation rate
hematocrit
hemoglobin test
platelet count
red blood cell count
red blood cell morphology

1. Microscopic examination of a stained blood smear to determine the shape of RBCs ______________________________
2. Time required for blood to stop flowing from a tiny puncture wound ______________________________
3. Determination of number of blood cells, hemoglobin and hematocrit, and other RBC values ______________________________
4. Test for the presence of antibodies that coat and damage erythrocytes ______________________________
5. Time required for venous blood to clot in a test tube ______________________________
6. Total amount of hemoglobin in a sample of peripheral blood ______________________________
7. Speed at which erythrocytes settle out of plasma ______________________________
8. Number of erythrocytes per cubic millimeter or microliter of blood ______________________________
9. Number of thrombocytes per cubic millimeter or microliter of blood ______________________________
10. Percentage of erythrocytes in a volume of blood ______________________________

B. Select from the following laboratory tests and clinical procedures to match the definitions below:

1. apheresis
2. blood transfusion
3. bone marrow biopsy
4. hematopoietic stem cell transplantation
5. prothrombin time
6. white blood cell count
7. white blood cell differential

A. __________ Microscopic examination of a core of bone marrow removed with a needle

B. __________ Separation of blood into component parts and removal of a select portion from the blood

C. __________ Percentages of the different types of leukocytes in the blood

D. __________ Whole blood or cells are taken from a donor and infused into a patient

E. __________ Test of the ability of blood to clot

F. __________ Peripheral stem cells from a donor are administered into a recipient

G. __________ Number of leukocytes per cubic millimeter of blood

Chapter Thirteen
ABBREVIATIONS QUIZ

Name: ______________________________

A. On the line provided, give meanings for the following abbreviations, then write each abbreviation next to its explanation below:

1. ALL ______________________________
2. AML ______________________________
3. ASCT ______________________________
4. baso ______________________________
5. BMT ______________________________
6. CBC ______________________________
7. CLL ______________________________
8. CML ______________________________
9. diff. ______________________________
10. EBV ______________________________

a. __________ Granulocytic white blood cells

b. __________ Abnormal numbers of relatively mature lymphocytes predominate

c. __________ A patient is his or her own donor for stem cell transplant

d. __________ Abnormal numbers of immature granulocytes predominate

e. __________ Recipient receives donation of bone marrow

f. __________ Percentages of different types of WBCs are given

g. __________ Cause of mononucleosis

h. __________ Mature and immature granulocytes are present in the marrow and bloodstream

i. __________ Calculation of numbers of blood cells, hemoglobin, hematocrit and red cell values

j. __________ Immature lymphocytes (lymphoblasts) predominate

B. *On the line provided, give meanings for the following abbreviations, then write each abbreviation next to its explanation below:*

1. eos ______________________________
2. EPO ______________________________
3. ESR ______________________________
4. Fe ______________________________
5. GVHD ______________________________
6. Hct ______________________________
7. Hgb ______________________________
8. IgA, IgD, IgE ______________________________
9. lymph cells ______________________________
10. mono ______________________________

a. __________ Percentage of red cells in a volume of blood

b. __________ Stimulates red blood cell formation

c. __________ Element that makes up hemoglobin

d. __________ Mononuclear white blood cell; phagocyte

e. __________ Granulocytic white blood cell elevated in allergic reactions

f. __________ Speed at which erythrocytes settle out of plasma

g. __________ White blood cells that make antibodies; mononuclear agranulocyte

h. __________ Protein found in red blood cells; carries oxygen

i. __________ Immune reaction of donor's cells to recipient's tissues

j. __________ Proteins that have antibody activity

C. On the line provided, give meanings for the following abbreviations, then write each abbreviation next to its explanation below:

1. H and H ______________________________
2. MDS ______________________________
3. polys ______________________________
4. PT ______________________________
5. RBC ______________________________
6. sed rate ______________________________
7. WBC ______________________________

a. __________ Carries oxygen in the bloodstream

b. __________ Time it takes for red cells to settle out of plasma

c. __________ Neutrophils; segmented leukocytes

d. __________ Time it takes for blood to clot

e. __________ Determination of numbers of leukocytes

f. __________ Levels of a blood protein and percentage of red blood cells are determined

g. __________ Preleukemic condition

Chapter Thirteen
EXERCISE QUIZ

Name: ______________________________

A. *Match the following cells with their meanings below:*

basophil
eosinophil
erythrocyte
hematopoietic stem cell
lymphocyte
monocyte
neutrophil
platelet

1. red blood cell ______________________________
2. white blood cell; phagocyte and precursor of a macrophage ______________________________
3. thrombocyte ______________________________
4. bone marrow cell; gives rise to many types of blood cells ______________________________
5. leukocyte formed in lymph tissue; produces antibodies ______________________________
6. leukocyte with dense reddish granules; associated with allergic reactions ______________________________
7. leukocyte (poly) formed in bone marrow and having neutral-staining granules ______________________________
8. leukocyte whose granules have an affinity for basic stain; releases histamine and heparin ______________________________

B. *Give medical terms for the following descriptions:*

9. liquid portion of blood ______________________________
10. hormone secreted by the kidney to stimulate erythrocyte production in bone marrow ______________________________
11. proteins in plasma; can be separated into alpha, beta, and gamma types ______________________________
12. plasma protein that maintains the proper amount of water in blood ______________________________
13. proteins made by lymphocytes in response to antigens in the blood ______________________________

C. *Divide the following terms into component parts, and give the meaning of the term:*

14. leukocytopenia ______________________________
15. myelopoiesis ______________________________
16. anticoagulant ______________________________
17. thrombolytic ______________________________

D. Match the following terms concerning red blood cells with their meanings:

erythroblast	hypochromia	poikilocytosis
erythropoiesis	macrocytosis	polycythemia vera
hemolysis	microcytosis	

18. irregularity in shape ______________________
19. immature red cells ______________________
20. reduction of hemoglobin ("color") ______________________
21. increase in numbers of small cells ______________________
22. erythremia ______________________
23. increase in numbers of large cells ______________________
24. formation of red cells ______________________
25. destruction of red cells ______________________

E. Describe the problem in the following forms of anemia:

26. sickle cell anemia ______________________
27. aplastic anemia ______________________
28. thalassemia ______________________

F. Give the meanings for the following abbreviations and blood dyscrasias:

29. CLL ______________________
30. AML ______________________
31. autoimmune thrombocytopenic purpura ______________________
32. hemophilia ______________________

G. Match the term in Column I with its meaning in Column II:

Column I	Column II
33. relapse ____________	A. Relieving, but not curing
34. remission ____________	B. Deficiency of all blood cells
35. purpura ____________	C. Increase in numbers of granulocytes; seen in allergic conditions
36. pancytopenia ____________	D. Symptoms of disease return
37. palliative ____________	E. Multiple pinpoint hemorrhages; blood accumulates under the skin.
38. eosinophilia ____________	F. Separation of blood into its components
39. apheresis ____________	G. Symptoms of disease disappear

H. Match the following laboratory test or clinical procedure with its description:

autologous transfusion	Coombs test	platelet count
bleeding time	erythrocyte sedimentation rate	red blood cell morphology
bone marrow biopsy	hematocrit	WBC differential
coagulation time	hematopoietic stem cell transplantation	

40. A stained blood smear is examined to determine the shape of individual red blood cells ______
41. Measures the percentage of red blood cells in a volume of blood ______
42. Determines the number of clotting cells per cubic millimeter ______
43. Ability of venous blood to clot in a test tube ______
44. Measures the speed at which erythrocytes settle out of plasma ______
45. Determines the numbers of different types of WBCs ______
46. Determines the presence of antibodies in infants of Rh-negative women or patients with autoimmune hemolytic anemia ______
47. Undifferentiated blood cells from a donor are infused into a patient being treated for leukemia or aplastic anemia ______
48. Time it takes for a small puncture wound to stop bleeding ______
49. Needle is introduced into the bone marrow cavity, and a small amount of marrow is aspirated and then examined under the microscope ______
50. Blood is collected from and later reinfused into the same patient ______

Chapter Thirteen

DICTATION AND COMPREHENSION QUIZ: VOCABULARY

Name: ______________________________

A. Dictation of Terms

1.	______________________	11.	______________________
2.	______________________	12.	______________________
3.	______________________	13.	______________________
4.	______________________	14.	______________________
5.	______________________	15.	______________________
6.	______________________	16.	______________________
7.	______________________	17.	______________________
8.	______________________	18.	______________________
9.	______________________	19.	______________________
10.	______________________	20.	______________________

B. Comprehension of Terms: Match number of the above term with its meaning below.

______ Abnormal condition of blood clotting
______ Change in structure and function of a cell as it matures; specialization
______ Platelet precursor found in bone marrow
______ Protein found in blood; maintains the proper amount of water in blood
______ Deficiency of iron
______ Immature bone marrow cell that develops into a white blood cell
______ Deficiency of a type of white blood cell
______ Protein threads that form the basis of a blood clot
______ White blood cell with dense, reddish granules (associated with allergic reactions)
______ A large cell that engulfs and destroys foreign material
______ Separation of white blood cells from the rest of the blood (using a centrifuge)
______ Plasma protein that contains antibodies
______ Blood protein found in red blood cells
______ Plasma minus clotting proteins and cells
______ Condition of irregularly shaped cells (red blood cells)
______ Condition of cells of unequal size (red blood cells)
______ A substance that prevents clotting of blood
______ Breakdown of recipient's red blood cells when incompatible bloods are mixed
______ Separation of clotting cells from the rest of the blood (using a centrifuge)
______ Formation of red blood cells

Chapter Thirteen

DICTATION AND COMPREHENSION QUIZ: PATHOLOGY AND TESTS

Name: ______________________________

A. Dictation of Terms

1.	______________________	11.	______________________
2.	______________________	12.	______________________
3.	______________________	13.	______________________
4.	______________________	14.	______________________
5.	______________________	15.	______________________
6.	______________________	16.	______________________
7.	______________________	17.	______________________
8.	______________________	18.	______________________
9.	______________________	19.	______________________
10.	______________________	20.	______________________

B. Comprehension of Terms: Match number of the above term with its meaning below.

______ Determines the numbers of different types of leukocytes
______ Determines the shape or form of erythrocytes
______ Percentage of erythrocytes in a volume of blood
______ Any abnormal or pathologic condition of the blood
______ Inherited defect in the ability to produce hemoglobin
______ Multiple pinpoint hemorrhages; thrombocytopenia
______ Erythremia
______ Excessive bleeding caused by lack of factor VIII or IX
______ Lymphoblasts predominate in the blood; most often seen in children
______ Malignant tumor of bone marrow
______ Separation of blood into its parts
______ Time required for venous blood to clot in a test tube
______ Small amount of bone marrow is aspirated and examined under a microscope
______ Relieving pain, but not curing an illness
______ Lack of mature erythrocytes owing to inability to absorb vitamin B_{12}
______ Both mature and immature granulocytes are present in bone marrow and blood
______ Total amount of a blood protein is measured in a sample of blood
______ Symptoms of disease return
______ Symptoms of disease disappear
______ Speed at which red cells settle out of plasma

Chapter Thirteen
SPELLING QUIZ

Name: ______________________________

A. Circle the term that is spelled correctly, and write its meaning in the space provided:

1. myeloma   myleoma ______________________________
2. erythropoeisis   erythropoiesis ______________________________
3. billirubin   bilirubin ______________________________
4. fibrinogen   fibrinogin ______________________________
5. platlet   platelet ______________________________
6. poykilocytosis   poikilocytosis ______________________________
7. leukopheresis   leukapheresis ______________________________
8. heparin   heparine ______________________________
9. electropheresis   electrophoresis ______________________________
10. thallassemia   thalassemia ______________________________

B. Circle the term that is spelled correctly. The meaning of each term is given.

11. Deficiency of clotting cells................thrombocitopenia   thrombositopenea   thrombocytopenia
12. Process of clotting.............................coagulation   coagglulation   coaglulation
13. Large cell that engulfs foreign material and worn-out red cells........macrophage   macropage   makrophage
14. White blood cell that destroys foreign material by phagocytosis......neutrophil   neutrophill   nuetrophil
15. Blood protein....................................allbumen   albumen   albumin
16. Lack of mature red cells owing to inability to absorb vitamin B_{12}..........pernicious anemia   perniscious anemia   panescius anemia
17. Relieving symptoms but not curing...palliative   pallitive   paliative
18. Improper formation of bone marrow cells.....................................myeleodysplasia   myleodisplasia   myelodysplasia
19. A protein with antibody activity........immunoglobulen   immunoglobulin   inmunoglobulen
20. Increase in red blood cells................polycythemia vera   polycytemia vera   polysithemia vera

Chapter Thirteen
PRONUNCIATION QUIZ

Name: ______________________________

A. Underline the accented syllable in the following terms:

1. hemolysis
2. anisocytosis
3. erythropoietin
4. purpura
5. anticoagulant
6. eosinophil
7. albumin
8. differentiation
9. myelodysplasia
10. leukocytopenia

B. Match the term in Column I with its meaning in Column II:

Column I		Column II
1. megakaryocyte	_______	A. Orange-yellow pigment formed from destruction of hemoglobin
2. reticulocyte	_______	B. Separation of clotting cells from rest of the blood
3. myeloid	_______	C. Plasma minus clotting proteins and cells
4. fibrin	_______	D. Derived from bone marrow
5. electrophoresis	_______	E. An anticoagulant substance
6. plateletpheresis	_______	F. An immature red blood cell
7. bilirubin	_______	G. Percentage of red blood cells in a volume of blood
8. heparin	_______	H. Separation of plasma proteins using electricity
9. hematocrit	_______	I. An immature clotting cell
10. serum	_______	J. Protein threads that form the essence of a blood clot

C. Complete the following terms using the definitions given:

1. hemo ______________________________	Stoppage or control of blood flow
2. dys ______________________________	Any blood disorder
3. re ______________________________	Symptoms of disease return
4. ______________________________ ology	Study of the shape of cells
5. anti ______________________________	A foreign substance that stimulates the formation of antibodies
6. anti ______________________________	Protein substances formed in the blood to destroy foreign substances
7. ______________________________ cyte	A cell that engulfs another cell
8. ______________________________ emia	A type of inherited anemia marked by defective type of hemoglobin in people of Mediterranean background

Chapter Thirteen
DIAGRAM QUIZ

Name: ______________________________

Label the diagram below using the terms listed below:

Band cell	Hematopoietic stem cell	Monocyte	Platelets
Erythroblast	Lymphocyte	Myeloblast	
Erythrocytes	Megakaryocyte	Neutrophil	

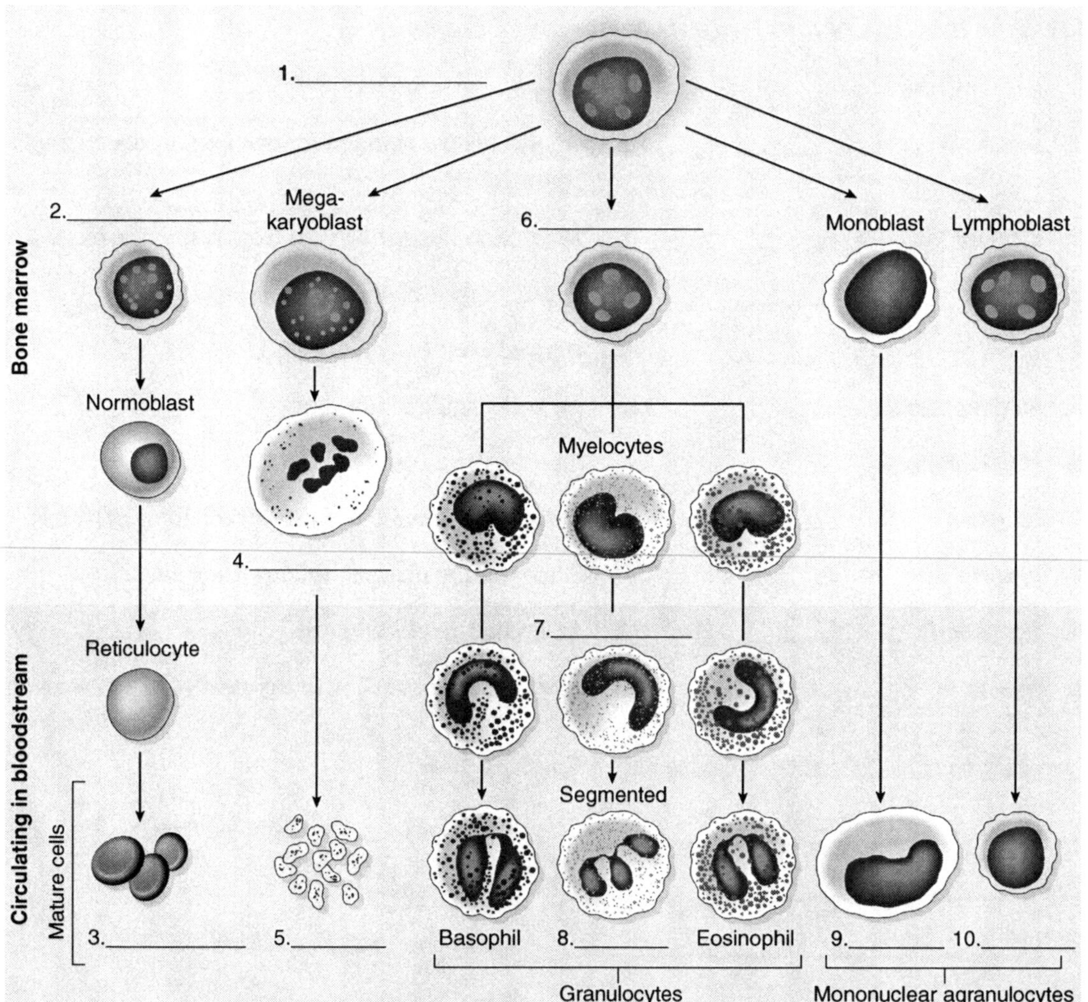

Chapter Thirteen

REVIEW SHEET QUIZ

Name: ______________________________

A. Give meanings for the following combining forms:

1. coagul/o ____________________
2. cyt/o ____________________
3. erythr/o ____________________
4. hem/o ____________________
5. kary/o ____________________
6. leuk/o ____________________
7. myel/o ____________________
8. morph/o ____________________
9. neutr/o ____________________
10. sider/o ____________________
11. phag/o ____________________
12. thromb/o ____________________

B. Give meanings for the following suffixes:

1. -apheresis ____________________
2. -blast ____________________
3. -cytosis ____________________
4. -emia ____________________
5. -globin ____________________
6. -lytic ____________________
7. -penia ____________________
8. -phage ____________________
9. -phoresis ____________________
10. -poiesis ____________________
11. -stasis ____________________
12. -oid ____________________

C. Give meanings for the following prefixes:

1. anti- ______________________________
2. hypo- ______________________________
3. macro- ______________________________
4. mega- ______________________________
5. micro- ______________________________
6. mono- ______________________________
7. pan- ______________________________
8. poly- ______________________________

Chapter Thirteen
MEDICAL SCRAMBLE

Name: ______________________________

Unscramble the letters to form blood system terms from the clues. Use the letters in the squares to complete the bonus term.

1. *Clue:* Blood protein

☐ ☐ ___ ☐ ___ ___ ___ M L U I N A B

2. *Clue:* Percentage of red blood cells in a volume of blood

___ ___ ___ ☐ ___ ☐ ☐ ___ ___ ☐ C A H O T R E T M I

3. *Clue:* Blood protein in erythrocytes

___ ___ ___ ☐ ☐ ___ ___ ___ ___ ☐ G I M O H O N E B L

4. *Clue:* Threads of a clot

___ ___ ___ ___ ☐ ___ B I F N I R

BONUS TERM: *Clue:* Process of blood clotting

☐ ☐ ☐ ☐ ☐ ☐ ☐ ☐ ☐ ☐ ☐

Chapter Thirteen
CROSSWORD PUZZLE

Name: ______________________________

Fill in the crossword puzzle below using the clues listed underneath it.

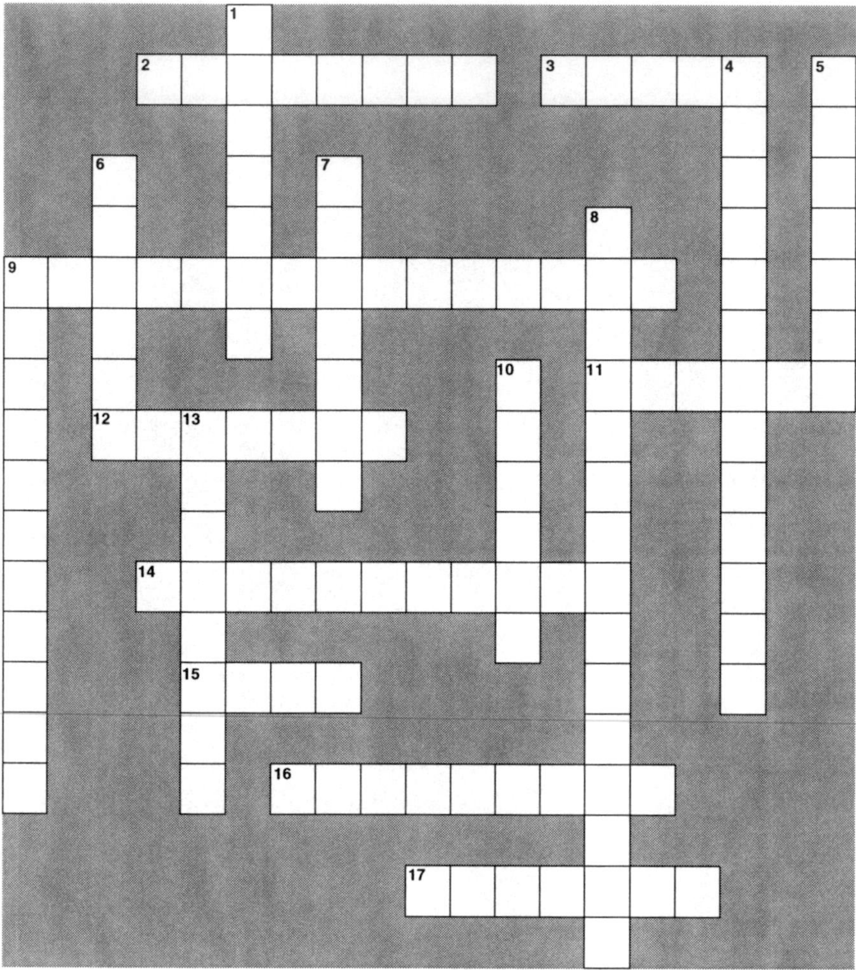

Across Clues

2. Excessive increase in white blood cells with immature forms.
3. Plasma minus clotting proteins and blood cells.
9. Method of separating plasma proteins by electrical charge.
11. Protein threads that form the base of a clot.
12. Protein found in blood.
14. Process of blood clotting.
15. Iron-containing nonprotein portion of the hemoglobin molecule.
16. White blood cell.
17. Derived from bone marrow.

Down Clues

1. Multiple pinpoint hemorrhages and accumulation of blood under the skin.
4. Platelet precursor formed in the bone marrow.
5. -globulin means______.
6. Deficiency in erythrocytes or hemoglobin.
7. An anticoagulant produced by liver cells and found in blood and tissues.
8. Change in structure and function of a cell as it matures
9. Red blood cell.
10. The protein part of hemoglobin.
13. White blood cell with large dark-staining granules.

Chapter Thirteen

PRACTICAL APPLICATIONS

Name: ______________________

A. Research Report

Colony-stimulating factors are hormones that regulate hematopoiesis. Erythropoietin (Epogen), secreted by the kidney, increases bone marrow erythropoiesis. Granulocyte colony-stimulating factor (G-CSF) stimulates bone marrow leukopoiesis. The most recent colony-stimulating factor is thrombopoietin (TPO), which acts on bone marrow to promote the growth of platelets. These hormones are now produced biosynthetically by recombinant DNA techniques and have shown some impact in the prevention of chemotherapy-induced neutropenia, treatment of cytopenias associated with myelodysplasias, and aplastic anemia.

1. **What is erythropoietin?......................** ☐
   A. A drug that causes bone marrow suppression
   B. A chemical that promotes white cell production
   C. A recombinant product that stimulates platelet growth
   D. A renal hormone that stimulates growth of RBCs

2. **G-CSF is helpful in:...........................** ☐
   A. Preventing decrease in WBCs during drug treatment for cancer
   B. Replacing red cells after hemorrhage
   C. Stimulating formation of thrombocytes
   D. Stimulating lymphocytes

3. **Myelodysplasia means:........................** ☐
   A. The spleen is not functioning
   B. Liver formation is impaired
   C. Blood cells are not made
   D. The bone marrow is not forming blood cells properly

4. **TPO is: ....** ☐
   A. A neutrophil growth factor
   B. An erythrocyte growth factor
   C. A clotting cell growth factor useful in the treatment of thrombocytopenia
   D. Useful in the treatment of hemophilia

B. Case Report

A 17-year-old white female was admitted to the ER for melena. A CBC showed the hemoglobin to be 9.0%, hematocrit 27%, WBC 32,000/mm^3 with 21% polys, 7% bands, 70% lymphocytes, and 2% monocytes. Platelet count was 20,000/ mm^3. Bone marrow aspiration and smear shows evidence of lymphoblasts.

1. **What was the patient's admitting symptom?** ☐
   A. Diarrhea
   B. Blood in her stool
   C. Vomiting blood
   D. Spitting up blood

2. **What do the lab data tell about RBCs?** ☐
   A. None of the tests reflect information about RBCs
   B. RBCs are normal
   C. RBCs are elevated
   D. RBCs are decreased as evidenced by low hematocrit and hemoglobin

3. **What is a likely diagnosis for the patient?** ☐
   A. Sickle cell anemia
   B. Hemophilia
   C. Acute lymphoblastic leukemia
   D. Chronic myelocytic leukemia

4. **The bone marrow was filled with:** ☐
   A. Immature white blood cells
   B. Mature neutrophils
   C. Platelets
   D. Immature red blood cells

Chapter Thirteen
ANSWERS TO THE QUIZZES

Multiple Choice Quiz

1. B
2. E
3. C
4. D
5. E
6. C
7. A
8. B
9. A
10. D
11. A
12. B
13. B
14. D
15. C
16. E
17. A
18. D
19. C
20. E
21. D
22. A
23. E
24. B
25. C
26. D
27. B
28. E
29. B
30. D

Vocabulary Quiz

A

1. bilirubin
2. albumin
3. eosinophil
4. coagulation
5. electrophoresis
6. antigen
7. erythrocyte
8. differentiation
9. basophil
10. erythropoietin
11. antibody
12. fibrin

B

1. macrophage
2. immune reaction
3. lymphocyte
4. heparin
5. hemolysis
6. plasma
7. hemoglobin
8. fibrinogen
9. granulocyte
10. globulins

C

1. neutrophil
2. platelet (thrombocyte)
3. hematopoietic stem cell
4. plasmapheresis
5. serum
6. immunoglobulin
7. reticulocyte

Terminology Quiz

A

1. basophil
2. hypochromic
3. eosinophil
4. hemoglobinopathy
5. hemolysis
6. cytology
7. hematocrit
8. coagulopathy
9. erythrocytopenia
10. anticoagulant

B

1. leukocytopenia
2. myeloblast
3. morphology
4. neutropenia
5. myelodysplasia
6. monocyte
7. phagocyte
8. sideropenia
9. thrombocytopenia
10. polymorphonuclear

C

1. monoblast
2. microcytosis
3. erythroblast
4. poikilocytosis
5. plasmapheresis
6. spherocytosis
7. macrocytosis
8. leukapheresis
9. plateletpheresis
10. hemoglobin

D

1. immunoglobulin
2. thrombolytic therapy
3. myeloid
4. granulocytopenia
5. neutrophilia
6. thrombosis
7. hematopoiesis
8. pancytopenia
9. myelopoiesis
10. hemostasis

Pathology Quiz

A

1. purpura
2. polycythemia vera
3. hemochromatosis
4. sickle cell anemia
5. thalassemia
6. mononucleosis
7. hemolytic anemia
8. aplastic anemia
9. hemophilia
10. pernicious anemia

B

1. chronic lymphocytic leukemia
2. acute myelogenous leukemia
3. chronic myelogenous leukemia
4. acute lymphocytic leukemia

C

1. petechiae
2. Epstein-Barr virus
3. ecchymoses
4. iron deficiency anemia
5. dyscrasia
6. remission
7. palliative
8. relapse
9. multiple myeloma
10. eosinophilia

Laboratory Tests and Clinical Procedures Quiz

A

1. red blood cell morphology
2. bleeding time
3. complete blood count
4. antiglobulin test
5. coagulation time
6. hemoglobin test
7. erythrocyte sedimentation rate
8. red blood cell count
9. platelet count
10. hematocrit

B

A. 3
B. 1
C. 7
D. 2
E. 5
F. 4
G. 6

Abbreviations Quiz

A

1. acute lymphocytic leukemia
2. acute myelogenous leukemia
3. autologous stem cell transplantation
4. basophils
5. bone marrow transplantation
6. complete blood count
7. chronic lymphocytic leukemia
8. chronic myelogenous leukemia
9. differential count
10. Epstein-Barr virus

a. baso
b. CLL
c. ASCT
d. AML
e. BMT
f. diff.
g. EBV
h. CML
i. CBC
j. ALL

B

1. eosinophils
2. erythropoietin
3. erythrocyte sedimentation rate
4. iron
5. graft versus host disease
6. hematocrit
7. hemoglobin
8. immunoglobulins
9. lymphocytes
10. monocyte

a. Hct
b. EPO
c. Fe
d. mono
e. eos
f. ESR
g. lymph cells
h. Hgb
i. GVHD
j. IgA, IgD, IgE

C

1. hemoglobin and hematocrit
2. myelodysplastic syndrome
3. polymorphonuclear leukocytes
4. prothrombin time
5. red blood cell
6. erythrocyte sedimentation rate
7. white blood cell

a. RBC
b. sed rate
c. polys
d. PT
e. WBC
f. H and H
g. MDS

Exercise Quiz

A

1. erythrocyte
2. monocyte
3. platelet
4. hematopoietic stem cell
5. lymphocyte
6. eosinophil
7. neutrophil
8. basophil

B

9. plasma
10. erythropoietin
11. globulin
12. albumin
13. immunoglobulins (antibodies)

C

14. deficiency of white blood cells
15. formation of bone marrow
16. substance that stops clotting
17. pertaining to destruction of clots

D

18. poikilocytosis
19. erythroblast
20. hypochromia
21. microcytosis
22. polycythemia vera
23. macrocytosis
24. erythropoiesis
25. hemolysis

E

26. abnormally shaped red blood cells cause hemolysis (hereditary condition)
27. blood cells are not formed or produced in the bone marrow
28. inherited defect in ability to produce hemoglobin

F

29. chronic lymphocytic leukemia
30. acute myelogenous leukemia
31. deficiency of platelets with hemorrhages into the skin; no known cause
32. Excessive bleeding caused by hereditary lack of clotting factor VIII or IX

G

33. D
34. G
35. E
36. B
37. A
38. C
39. F

H

40. red blood cell morphology
41. hematocrit
42. platelet count
43. coagulation time
44. erythrocyte sedimentation rate
45. WBC differential
46. Coombs test
47. hematopoietic stem cell transplantation
48. bleeding time
49. bone marrow biopsy
50. autologous transfusion

Dictation and Comprehension Quiz: Vocabulary

A

1. hemolysis
2. albumin
3. anisocytosis
4. anticoagulant
5. differentiation
6. eosinophil
7. erythropoiesis
8. fibrin
9. gamma globulins
10. hemoglobin
11. leukapheresis
12. macrophage
13. megakaryocyte
14. myeloblast
15. neutropenia
16. plateletpheresis
17. poikilocytosis
18. serum
19. sideropenia
20. thrombosis

B

20 Abnormal condition of blood clotting
5 Change in structure and function of a cell as it matures; specialization
13 Platelet precursor found in bone marrow
2 Protein found in blood; maintains the proper amount of water in blood

19 Deficiency of iron
14 Immature bone marrow cell that develops into a white blood cell
15 Deficiency of a type of white blood cell
8 Protein threads that form the basis of a blood clot
6 White blood cell with dense, reddish granules (associated with allergic reactions)
12 A large cell that engulfs and destroys foreign material
11 Separation of white blood cells from the rest of the blood (using a centrifuge)
9 Plasma proteins that contain antibodies
10 Blood protein found in red blood cells
18 Plasma minus clotting proteins and cells
17 Condition of irregularly shaped cells (red blood cells)
3 Condition of cells of unequal size (red blood cells)
4 A substance that prevents clotting of blood
1 Breakdown of recipient's red blood cells when incompatible bloods are mixed
16 Separation of clotting cells from the rest of the blood (using a centrifuge)
7 Formation of red blood cells

Dictation and Comprehension Quiz: Pathology and Tests

A

1. acute lymphocytic leukemia
2. apheresis
3. bone marrow biopsy
4. chronic myelogenous leukemia
5. coagulation time
6. dyscrasia
7. erythrocyte sedimentation rate
8. hematocrit
9. hemoglobin test
10. hemophilia
11. multiple myeloma
12. palliative
13. pernicious anemia
14. polycythemia vera
15. purpura
16. red blood cell morphology
17. relapse
18. remission
19. thalassemia
20. white blood cell differential

B

20 Determines the numbers of different types of leukocytes
16 Determines the shape or form of erythrocytes
8 Percentage of erythrocytes in a volume of blood
6 Any abnormal or pathologic condition of the blood
19 Inherited defect in the ability to produce hemoglobin
15 Multiple pinpoint hemorrhages; thrombocytopenia
14 Erythremia
10 Excessive bleeding caused by lack of factor VIII or IX
1 Lymphoblasts predominate in the blood; most often seen in children
11 Malignant tumor of bone marrow
2 Separation of blood into its parts
5 Time required for venous blood to clot in a test tube
3 Small amount of bone marrow is aspirated and examined under a microscope
12 Relieving pain, but not curing an illness
13 Lack of mature erythrocytes owing to inability to absorb vitamin B_{12}
4 Both mature and immature granulocytes are present in bone marrow and blood
9 Total amount of a blood protein is measured in a sample of blood
17 Symptoms of disease return
18 Symptoms of disease disappear
7 Speed at which red cells settle out of plasma

Spelling Quiz

A

1. myeloma—tumor of bone marrow
2. erythropoiesis—formation of red blood cells
3. bilirubin—pigment released with RBC destruction
4. fibrinogen—clotting protein in blood
5. platelet—clotting cell
6. poikilocytosis—abnormal shape of RBCs
7. leukapheresis—separation of WBCs
8. heparin—anticoagulant found in tissues
9. electrophoresis—separation of proteins by electrical charge
10. thalassemia—deficiency of hemoglobin (hereditary)

B

11. thrombocytopenia
12. coagulation
13. macrophage
14. neutrophil
15. albumin
16. pernicious anemia
17. palliative
18. myelodysplasia
19. immunoglobulin
20. polycythemia vera

Pronunciation Quiz

A

1. hemolysis
2. anisocytosis
3. erythropoietin
4. purpura
5. anticoagulant
6. eosinophil
7. albumin
8. differentiation
9. myelodysplasia
10. leukocytopenia

B

1. I
2. F
3. D
4. J
5. H
6. B
7. A
8. E
9. G
10. C

C

1. hemostasis
2. dyscrasia
3. relapse
4. morphology
5. antigen
6. antibodies
7. phagocyte
8. thalassemia

Diagram Quiz

1. Hematopoietic stem cell
2. Erythroblast
3. Erythrocytes

4. Megakaryocyte
5. Platelets
6. Myeloblast
7. Band cell
8. Neutrophil
9. Monocyte
10. Lymphocyte

Review Sheet Quiz

A

1. clotting
2. cell
3. red
4. blood
5. nucleus
6. white
7. bone marrow
8. shape, form
9. neutral (neutrophils.
10. iron
11. eat, swallow
12. clot

B

1. removal, carry away
2. immature cell, embryonic
3. abnormal condition of cells
4. blood condition
5. protein
6. pertaining to destruction
7. deficiency
8. eat, swallow
9. carrying, transmission
10. formation
11. stop, control
12. derived from

C

1. against
2. under, deficiency
3. large
4. large
5. small
6. one
7. all
8. many, much

Medical Scramble

1. ALBUMIN
2. HEMATOCRIT
3. HEMOGLOBIN
4. FIBRIN

BONUS TERM: COAGULATION

Practical Applications

A	B
1. D	1. B
2. A	2. D
3. D	3. C
4. C	4. A

Crossword Puzzle

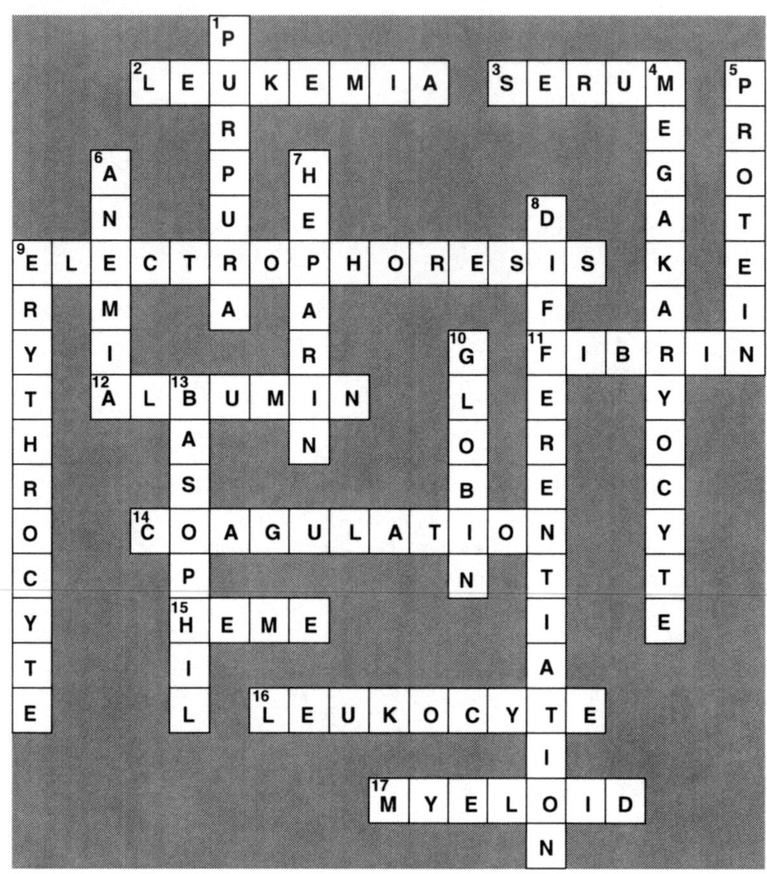

Chapter Thirteen
Answers to Terminology Section

(textbook pages 512–514)

Terminology	Meaning
basophil	White blood cell with dark-staining granules that have an affinity for basic dyes.
hypochromic	Pertaining to deficiency of color (reduction of hemoglobin in red blood cells).
anticoagulant	A substance that works against coagulation (blood clotting).
coagulopathy	Disease of the clotting process.
cytology	Study of cells.
eosinophil	White blood cell with dark-staining granules that have an affinity for acid dyes; granules turn red (eosin. in the presence of dye).
erythroblast	Immature red blood cell.
granulocyte	White blood cell with large, dark-staining granules in its cytoplasm.
hemolysis	Destruction of blood cells.
hematocrit	Separation of blood; percentage of red blood cells in a given volume of blood.
hemoglobinopathy	Disease of abnormal hemoglobins (sickle cell anemia, thalassemia).
anisocytosis	Abnormal condition of unequal size of cells (erythrocytes).
megakaryocyte	Cell with multiple large nuclei; immature platelet.
leukocytopenia	Deficiency of white blood cells.
monocyte	White blood cell with one large nucleus; an agranulocyte and phagocyte.
morphology	Study of shape or form (of blood cells).
myeloblast	Bone marrow cell that develops into a myelocyte and then a leukocyte.
myelodysplasia	Abnormal development of bone marrow cells; preleukemic condition.
neutropenia	Deficiency in neutrophils.
polymorphonuclear	Pertaining to a white blood cell with a multilobed nucleus (neutrophil).
phagocyte	Cell that ingests other cells or microorganisms.
poikilocytosis	Irregularity in the shape of red blood cells.
sideropenia	Deficiency in iron in serum.
spherocytosis	Condition (abnormal) in which erythrocytes assume a spheroidal (rounded) shape.
thrombocytopenia	Deficiency of clotting cells.

Suffixes

plasmapheresis	Removal of plasma from the rest of the blood by mechanical means (centrifuge).
leukapheresis	Removal of white blood cells from the rest of the blood by centrifugation.
plateletpheresis	Removal of platelets from the rest of the blood by centrifugation.
monoblast	Immature white blood cell (monocyte).
macrocytosis	Abnormal condition (slight increase in numbers) of macrocytes (red blood cells that are larger than normal).
microcytosis cells	Abnormal condition (slight increase in numbers) of microcytes (red blood cells that are smaller than normal).
leukemia	Abnormal condition of white blood cells (increase in numbers of malignant cells).
hemoglobin	Blood protein in erythrocytes; enables the cell to carry oxygen.
immunoglobulin	Protein (antibody produced by plasma cells) that acts to protect the body by destroying antigens.
thrombolytic therapy	Treatment that destroys blood clots.
myeloid	Derived from bone marrow.

thrombosis	Abnormal condition of clotting.
granulocytopenia	Deficiency of granulocytes (white blood cells).
pancytopenia	Deficiency of all (blood) cells.
macrophage	Large cell (in blood and tissues) that eats (engulfs) other cells; derived from a monocyte.
eosinophilia	Increase in numbers of eosinophils.
neutrophilia	Increase in numbers of neutrophils.
electrophoresis	Separation of proteins in a solution by using an electric current (used to separate protein fractions of serum, urine, or cerebrospinal fluid).
hematopoiesis	Formation of blood cells.
erythropoiesis	Formation of erythrocytes.
myelopoiesis	Formation of bone marrow.
hemostasis	Stoppage of the flow of blood.

Chapter 14

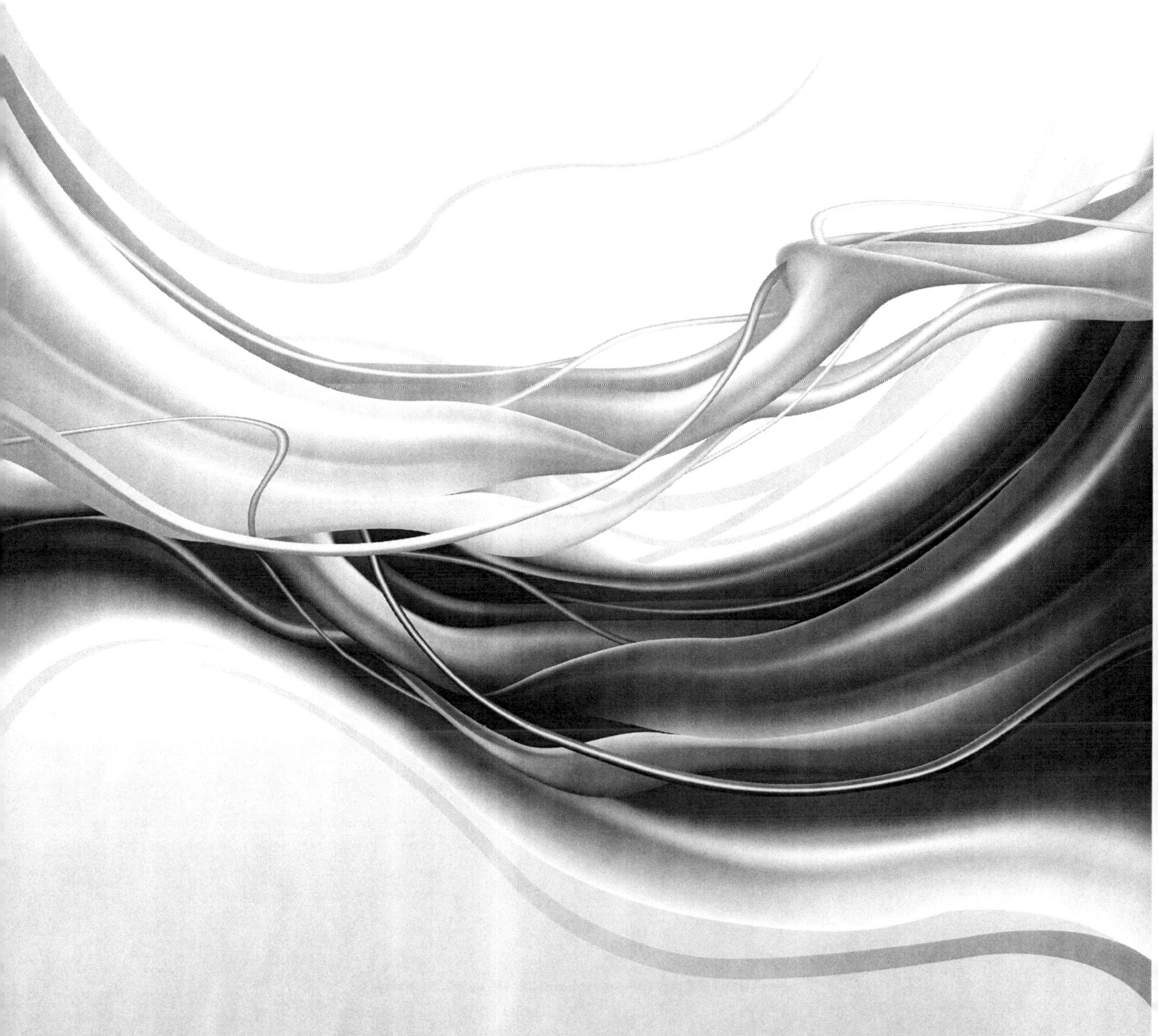

Chapter Fourteen

MULTIPLE CHOICE QUIZ

Name: ______________________________

In the box write the letter of the choice that is the definition of the term or best answers the question. There is only one correct answer for each question.

1. **Formation of lymph:** .... ☐
   A. Lymphocytopenia
   B. Lymphadenitis
   C. Lymphedema
   D. Lymphopoiesis
   E. Lymphoid

2. **Interstitial fluid contains or is:** .... ☐
   A. Antibodies produced by white blood cells
   B. Red and white blood cells
   C. Found in the spaces between cells and becomes lymph when it enters lymph capillaries
   D. Connective tissue
   E. Blood clotting factors

3. **All of the following are part of the immune system EXCEPT:** .... ☐
   A. Lymphocytes
   B. Platelets
   C. Monocytes
   D. Phagocytes
   E. Antibodies

4. **All of the following describe areas of lymph node concentration EXCEPT:** ... ☐
   A. Inguinal
   B. Axillary
   C. Bone marrow
   D. Mediastinal
   E. Cervical

5. **Atopy is:** .... ☐
   A. An early stage of AIDS
   B. A hypersensitivity or allergic state
   C. A type of lymphoma
   D. A disease found in tropical areas
   E. Acute infectious disease caused by Epstein-Barr virus

6. **Helper or suppressor cells are types of:** .... ☐
   A. B cells
   B. T cells
   C. Platelets
   D. Antigens
   E. Antibiotics

7. **Examples of immunoglobulins:** .... ☐
   A. IgA, IgG, IgE
   B. Monocytes
   C. Lymphocytes
   D. Hepatocytes
   E. Clotting factors

8. **Oropharyngeal lymph tissue:** .... ☐
   A. Spleen
   B. Thymus
   C. Bone marrow
   D. Tonsils
   E. Adenoids

9. **Mediastinal T-cell producer:** .... ☐
   A. Spleen
   B. Thymus
   C. Bone marrow
   D. Tonsils
   E. Adenoids

10. **Nasopharyngeal lymph tissue:** .... ☐
    A. Spleen
    B. Thymus
    C. Bone marrow
    D. Tonsils
    E. Adenoids

11. **Abdominal organ that filters erythrocytes and activates lymphocytes:** .... ☐
    A. Spleen
    B. Thymus
    C. Bone marrow
    D. Tonsils
    E. Adenoids

12. **Produces lymphocytes and monocytes and all other blood cells:** .... ☐
    A. Spleen
    B. Thymus
    C. Bone marrow
    D. Tonsils
    E. Adenoids

13. Cytotoxic cells are: ....
A. B cell lymphocytes
B. T-cell lymphocytes
C. Platelets
D. Thrombocytes
E. Eosinophils

14. Interferons and interleukins are: ....
A. Gamma globulins
B. Interstitial fluid
C. Antiviral proteins produced by T-cell lymphocytes
D. Produced by B-cell lymphocytes
E. Helper cells

15. Slight increase in numbers of lymphocytes: ....
A. Lymphocytopenia
B. Lymphopoiesis
C. Lymphoid
D. Lymphocytosis
E. Lymphedema

16. Pertaining to poison: ....
A. Necrotic
B. Hypoxic
C. Cyanotic
D. Toxic
E. Stenotic

17. Computerized x-ray imaging in the transverse plane: ....
A. CT scan
B. Lymphangiogram
C. Ultrasonography
D. MRI
E. Lymphadenectomy

18. HIV is: ....
A. A malignancy associated with AIDS
B. A drug used to treat AIDS
C. The virus that causes AIDS
D. The test used to detect AIDS
E. A type of lymphoma

19. Malignant tumor of lymph nodes: ....
A. Sarcoidosis
B. Lymphedema
C. Hodgkin disease
D. Hypersplenism
E. Lymphocytopenia

20. Viral infection causing blisters on skin of lips, nose, or genitals: ....
A. Kaposi sarcoma
B. Herpes simplex
C. Cryptococcus
D. Toxoplasmosis
E. *Pneumocystis jiroveci* pneumonia

21. Cancer arising from the lining cells of capillaries, producing bluish red skin nodules: ....
A. Kaposi sarcoma
B. Herpes simplex
C. Cryptococcus
D. Toxoplasmosis
E. *Pneumocystis jiroveci* pneumonia

22. Major lung infection with fever, cough, chest pain, and sputum. Treatment is with Bactrim ....
A. Kaposi sarcoma
B. Herpes simplex
C. Cryptococcus
D. Toxoplasmosis
E. *Pneumocystis jiroveci* pneumonia

23. Protozoal (parasitic) infection associated with AIDS. Produces pneumonitis, hepatitis, and encephalitis: ....
A. Kaposi sarcoma
B. Herpes simplex
C. Cryptococcosis
D. Toxoplasmosis
E. *Pneumocystis jiroveci* pneumonia

24. Fungal infection associated with AIDS. Involves brain and meninges, lungs, and skin: ....
A. Kaposi sarcoma
B. Herpes simplex
C. Cryptococcosis
D. Toxoplasmosis
E. *Pneumocystis jiroveci* pneumonia

Chapter Fourteen
VOCABULARY QUIZ

Name: ______________________________

A. Match the following vocabulary terms with their meanings below:

acquired immunity	B cell	dendritic cell
adenoids	cervical nodes	helper T cell
antigen	cytokines	
axillary nodes	cytotoxic T cell	

1. Lymph nodes in the neck region ______________________________
2. Substance that the body recognizes as foreign and evokes an immune response ______________________________
3. Production of antibodies and lymphocytes in response to exposure to an antigen ______________________________
4. Lymphocyte that aids B cells in recognizing antigens and stimulating antibody production (CD4+ cell) ______________________________
5. Mass of lymphatic tissue in the nasopharynx ______________________________
6. Cell (specialized macrophage) that digests foreign cells and helps B and T cells recognize and mark antigens for destruction ______________________________
7. T lymphocyte that directly kills antigens (CD8+ cell) ______________________________
8. Lymph nodes in the armpit ______________________________
9. Proteins that aid and regulate the immune response ______________________________
10. Lymphocyte that originates in the bone marrow and transforms into a plasma cell to secrete antibodies ______________________________

B. Match the following vocabulary terms with their meanings below:

immunity	inguinal nodes	lymph capillaries
immunoglobulins	interferons and interleukins	lymph node
immunotherapy	interstitial fluid	mesenteric nodes
lymphoid organs	lymph	paraaortic nodes

1. Thin, watery fluid found within lymphatic vessels ____________________
2. Tiniest lymphatic vessels ____________________
3. Proteins (cytokines) secreted by T cells to aid and regulate the immune response ____________________
4. Antibodies that are secreted by plasma cells in response to the presence of an antigen ____________________
5. Body's ability to resist foreign organisms and toxins (immune response) ____________________
6. Lymph nodes in the groin ____________________
7. Stationary, solid lymphatic tissue along lymph vessels ____________________
8. Fluid in the spaces between cells ____________________
9. Lymph nodes, spleen, and thymus gland; tissue through which lymph travels ____________________
10. Use of immune cells and antibodies or vaccines to treat and prevent disease ____________________
11. Lymph nodes associated with a major artery ____________________
12. Lymph nodes in the intestinal region ____________________

C. Match the following vocabulary terms with their meanings below:

lymph vessel	natural immunity	suppressor T cell
macrophage	plasma cell	tolerance
mediastinal nodes	right lymphatic duct	
monoclonal antibody	spleen	

1. Lymphocyte that produces and secretes antibodies ______________________
2. Carrier of lymph throughout the body ______________________
3. Lymph nodes in the area between the lungs in the thoracic cavity ______________________
4. The ability of T lymphocytes to recognize and accept the body's own antigens as "self" ______________________
5. Large phagocyte found in lymph nodes and other tissues of the body ______________________
6. Antibody produced in a laboratory to attack antigens and destroy cells ______________________
7. Organ near the stomach that produces, stores, and eliminates blood cells ______________________
8. Protection that an individual is born with to fight infection ______________________
9. Lymphocyte that inhibits the activity of B and T lymphocytes (Treg) ______________________
10. Large lymphatic vessel in the chest that receives lymph from the upper right portion of the body ______________________

D. Match the following vocabulary terms with their meanings below:

cell-mediated immunity	thymus gland	vaccination
humoral immunity	tonsils	vaccine
thoracic duct	toxin	

1. Mass of lymphatic tissue in the back of the oropharynx ____________________
2. Organ in the mediastinum that conditions T lymphocytes to react to foreign cells ____________________
3. A poison ____________________
4. Weakened or killed microorganisms, toxins, or other proteins (antigens) given to provoke an immune response ____________________
5. Large lymphatic vessel in the chest that receives lymph from below the diaphragm and from the left side of the body above the diaphragm ____________________
6. Exposure of an individual to a foreign protein (antigen) that provokes an immune response ____________________
7. Involves B cells that produce antibodies ____________________
8. Involves T cells that respond to antigens and destroy them ____________________

Chapter Fourteen

TERMINOLOGY QUIZ

Name: ______________________________

A. *Complete the following terms to match the definitions below; select from the following medical word parts:*

-cyt/o	-globulin	-pathy
-cytosis	-itis	-penia
-ectomy	-megaly	-poiesis
-edema	-oid	

1. Deficiency of lymphocytes: lympho ______________________________
2. Antibody (protein) secreted by plasma cells: immuno ______________________________
3. Formation of lymph: lympho ______________________________
4. Increase in numbers of lymphoctyes: lympho ______________________________
5. Swelling within tissue spaces (collection of interstitial fluid): lymph ______________________________
6. Organs that are part of the lymph system: lymph ______________________________ organs
7. Disease of lymph nodes: lymphadeno ______________________________
8. Enlargement of the spleen: spleno ______________________________
9. Inflammation of lymph nodes: lymphaden ______________________________
10. Excision of the spleen: splen ______________________________

B. *Select from the following terms to match the definitions below:*

anaphylaxis	hypersplenism	thymectomy
asplenia	immunosuppression	toxic
autoimmune disease	interstitial fluid	

1. Removal of the thymus gland ______________________________
2. Exaggerated or unusual hypersensitivity to previously encountered proteins or antigens ______________________________
3. Pertaining to a poison ______________________________
4. Syndrome marked by enlarged spleen, anemia, blood cell destruction ______________________________
5. Liquid that bathes and surrounds cells ______________________________
6. Abnormal production of antibodies against normal body tissues ______________________________
7. Normal reaction of the immune system to foreign agents is impaired ______________________________
8. Condition of absence of the spleen ______________________________

Chapter Fourteen

PATHOLOGY QUIZ

Name: ______________________________

A. Match the following pathologic conditions and associated terms with their meanings below:

acquired immunodeficiency syndrome	Kaposi sarcoma	reverse transcriptase inhibitor
CD4+ cells	opportunistic infections	wasting syndrome
human immunodeficiency virus	protease inhibitor	

1. Infections diseases associated with AIDS ______________________________
2. Drug that treats AIDS by blocking the production of a proteolytic enzyme that creates new viral pieces for HIV ______________________________
3. Malignant condition associated with AIDS; colored skin nodules appear ______________________________
4. Infectious agent that causes AIDS ______________________________
5. Weight loss, decrease in muscular strength, appetite and mental activity ______________________________
6. Drug that treats AIDS by blocking an enzyme needed to make copies of HIV ______________________________
7. Group of symptoms associated with suppression of the immune system; infections, new growths, and neurologic problems ______________________________
8. Helper T cells that are destroyed by the AIDS virus ______________________________

B. Match the following pathologic terms with their definitions below:

allergen	Hodgkin disease	severe combined immunodeficiency disease
allergy	multiple myeloma	thymoma
atopic dermatitis	non-Hodgkin lymphoma	

1. Malignant tumor of a lymphoid organ in the mediastinum ______________________________
2. Malignant tumor of bone marrow cells (plasma cells) ______________________________
3. Substance capable of causing a specific hypersensitivity reaction in the body ______________________________
4. Group of malignant tumors involving lymphoid tissue; follicular and large cell are types ______________________________
5. Malignant tumor of lymph tissue in the spleen and lymph nodes; Reed-Sternberg cell is often found on microscopic analysis ______________________________
6. Hypersensitivity or allergic state involving an inherited predisposition; inflammation of the skin ______________________________
7. Infants are born with deficiency of B and T cells ______________________________
8. Abnormal hypersensitivity acquired by exposure to an antigen ______________________________

Chapter Fourteen

LABORATORY TESTS, CLINICAL PROCEDURES, AND ABBREVIATIONS QUIZ

Name: ______________________________

A. Match the following with their definitions below:

CD4+ cell count	immunoelectrophoresis	T4 cell
computed tomography	MoAb	Treg
ELISA	T8 cell	viral load test

1. Measures the amount of AIDS virus in the bloodstream ______________________
2. Measures the number of helper T lymphocytes in the bloodstream of patients with AIDS ______________________
3. X-ray imaging produces cross-sectional and other views of anatomic structures ______________________
4. Test that separates immunoglobulins and detects abnormalities in antibody levels ______________________
5. Helper T lymphocyte ______________________
6. Antibody produced in a laboratory to attack antigens and destroy cells ______________________
7. Cytotoxic T lymphocyte ______________________
8. Suppressor T cell that inhibits the activity of B and T cells ______________________
9. Screening test to detect anti-HIV antibodies in the bloodstream ______________________

B. On the line provided, give meanings for the following abbreviations, then write each abbreviation next to its explanation below:

1. AIDS ____________________
2. NHL ____________________
3. HAART ____________________
4. HD ____________________
5. HIV ____________________
6. IgA ____________________
7. KS ____________________
8. SCID ____________________

a. __________ Use of combinations of drugs that are effective against AIDS

b. __________ Malignant tumor of lymph tissue in spleen and lymph nodes; Reed-Sternberg cell is often found on microscopic analysis

c. __________ Malignant condition associated with AIDS; dark-colored skin nodules appear

d. __________ Group of malignant tumors involving lymphoid tissue; follicular and large cell are types

e. __________ Infants are born with a deficiency of B and T cells

f. __________ Infectious agent that causes AIDS

g. __________ Group of symptoms associated with suppression of the immune system

h. __________ Antibody in the blood

Chapter Fourteen
EXERCISE QUIZ

Name: ______________________________

The questions on this quiz have all been taken from the exercises at the end of this chapter.

A. Give the name of the structure or fluid from its meaning below:

1. Stationary lymph tissue along the path of lymph vessels ____________________
2. Large thoracic lymph vessel draining lymph from lower and left side of the body ____________________
3. Organ near the stomach that produces, stores, and eliminates blood cells ____________________
4. Mass of lymph tissue in the nasopharynx ____________________
5. Organ in the mediastinum that produces T-cell lymphocytes ____________________
6. Tiniest of lymph vessels ____________________
7. Large lymph vessel in the chest that drains lymph from right upper part of the body ____________________
8. Fluid that lies between cells and becomes lymph as it enters lymph capillaries ____________________

B. Give the locations of the following lymph nodes:

9. inguinal nodes ____________________
10. axillary nodes ____________________
11. cervical nodes ____________________
12. mediastinal nodes ____________________

C. Match the term in Column I with its description in Column II

	Column I			Column II
13.	immunoglobulins	________	A.	T-cell lymphocytes that inhibit the activity of B-cell lymphocytes
14.	toxins	________	B.	Antibodies—IgG, IgE, IgM, IgD
15.	helper T cells	________	C.	T-cell lymphocytes; aids B cells and antibody production; T4 cells
16.	cytotoxic cells	________	D.	Poisons (antigens)
17.	interferons	________	E.	T-cell lymphocytes that directly kill foreign cells; T8 cells
18.	plasma cells	________	F.	Antiviral proteins secreted by T cells
19.	suppressor T cells	________	G.	Transformed B cells that secrete antibodies

D. Build medical terms:

20. removal of the spleen ____________________
21. inflammation of lymph glands (nodes) ____________________
22. tumor of the thymus gland ____________________
23. disease of lymph glands (nodes) ____________________
24. formation of lymph ____________________
25. deficiency of lymph cells ____________________
26. pertaining to poison ____________________
27. enlargement of the spleen ____________________

E. Match the following terms with their meanings below:

AIDS	Hodgkin disease	lymphoid organs
allergen	hypersplenism	thymectomy
anaphylaxis	lymphedema	

28. Syndrome marked by enlargement of the spleen and associated with anemia, leukopenia, and thrombocytopenia ____________________
29. An extraordinary hypersensitivity to a foreign protein; marked by hypotension, shock, respiratory distress ____________________
30. An antigen capable of causing allergy (hypersensitivity) ____________________
31. Disorder in which the immune system is suppressed by exposure to HIV ____________________
32. Removal of a mediastinal organ ____________________
33. Malignant tumor of lymph nodes and spleen marked by Reed-Sternberg cell identified in lymph nodes ____________________
34. Tissues that produce lymphocytes—spleen, thymus, tonsils, and adenoids ____________________
35. Swelling of tissues due to interstitial fluid accumulation ____________________

F. Give meanings for the following terms or abbreviations:

36. HIV ____________________
37. Histo ____________________
38. KS ____________________
39. PCP ____________________
40. CT scan ____________________
41. Toxo ____________________

G. Match the following terms with their meanings below:

ELISA
immunoelectrophoresis
helper T cells
opportunistic infections
zidovudine

42. White blood cells that are destroyed by HIV ____________________
43. Test to separate immunoglobulins ____________________
44. Drug used to treat AIDS by blocking the growth of AIDS virus ____________________
45. Test used to detect anti-HIV antibodies ____________________
46. Group of infectious diseases associated with AIDS ____________________

Chapter Fourteen

DICTATION AND COMPREHENSION QUIZ

Name: ______________________________

A. Dictation of Terms

1.	____________________	11.	____________________
2.	____________________	12.	____________________
3.	____________________	13.	____________________
4.	____________________	14.	____________________
5.	____________________	15.	____________________
6.	____________________	16.	____________________
7.	____________________	17.	____________________
8.	____________________	18.	____________________
9.	____________________	19.	____________________
10.	____________________	20.	____________________

B. Comprehension of Terms: Match the number of the above term with its meaning below.

______ Malignant tumor associated with AIDS; appears as bluish red skin nodules
______ Hypersensitive or allergic state involving hereditary predisposition
______ Disease condition of lymph nodes
______ Enlargement of the spleen
______ Collection of lymph tissue in the groin
______ Substance capable of causing a specific hypersensitivity reaction in the body
______ A drug that is used to treat AIDS by blocking the production of an enzyme
______ An exaggerated or unusual hypersensitivity to a foreign protein
______ Lymphocyte that aids B cells and cytotoxic T cells in recognizing antigens and stimulating antibody production: also called T4 cell or CD4+ cell
______ Antiviral proteins secreted by T cells
______ Malignant tumor of a gland in the chest
______ Found within lymphatic vessels and surrounding tissues throughout the body
______ Lymphatic tissue in the oropharynx
______ Collection of lymph tissue under the arm (armpit)
______ Proteins that aid and regulate the immune response
______ Malignant tumor of lymph nodes and tissue
______ Antibodies such as IgG, IgA, IgD that are secreted by plasma cells
______ Introduction of altered antigens to produce an immune response
______ Repression of the immune response
______ Fluid collects within the spaces between cells secondary to lymph vessel obstruction

Chapter Fourteen
SPELLING QUIZ

Name: ______________________________

A. Circle the term that is spelled correctly, and write its meaning:

1. mackrophage — macrophage ____________________
2. lypmh — lymph ____________________
3. immunoglobulins — immunoglobins ____________________
4. alergy — allergy ____________________
5. inguinal nodes — ingiunal nodes ____________________
6. anaphylaxis — anaphilaxis ____________________
7. Hogdkin disease — Hodgkin disease ____________________
8. axilliary nodes — axillary nodes ____________________
9. lymphocytopenis — lymphocytopenia ____________________
10. splenectomy — spleenectomy ____________________

B. Circle the term that is spelled correctly. The meaning of each term is given.

11. Organ in the chest that produces T cells.......... thymus gland — thymis gland — thimus gland
12. Fluid in the spaces between cells.......... intrastitial fluid — interstitial fluid — interstitiel fluid
13. Collection of fluid in tissues.......... lymphaedmea — lypmhfedema — lymphedema
14. Proteins that stimulate the growth of T cells.......... interleukins — interleukens — interluekins
15. Masses of lymph tissue in the nasopharynx.......... adneoidz — adeniods — adenoids
16. Introduction of altered antigens to produce an immune response.......... vaccination — vacination — vakcination
17. Inflammation of tonsils.......... tonsilitis — toncilitis — tonsillitis
18. Formation of lymph.......... lymphopoesis — lymphopoiesis — lymphopeosis

Chapter Fourteen
PRONUNCIATION QUIZ

Name: ______________________________

A. Underline the accented syllables in the following terms:

1. immunology
2. hypersensitivity
3. inguinal nodes
4. lymphedema
5. interstitial fluid
6. Kaposi sarcoma
7. macrophage
8. anaphylaxis
9. thoracic duct
10. lymphadenopathy

B. Match the term in Column I with its meaning in Column II:

Column I		Column II
1. anaphylaxis	_______	A. Mass of lymph tissue in the nasopharynx
2. AIDS	_______	B. Syndrome marked by enlargement of the spleen
3. cervical nodes	_______	C. Suppression or deficiency of the immune response caused by exposure to HIV
4. adenoids	_______	D. A hypersensitivity or allergic state involving an inherited predisposition
5. interferons	_______	E. Exaggerated hypersensitivity reaction
6. macrophage	_______	F. Antibodies secreted by plasma cells
7. Hodgkin disease	_______	G. Antiviral proteins secreted by T cells
8. hypersplenism	_______	H. Lymph nodes in the neck
9. atopy	_______	I. Malignancy of lymph nodes
10. immunoglobulins	_______	J. Large phagocyte found in lymph nodes

C. Complete the following terms using the definitions given:

1. ______________________ ectomy — Removal of the spleen
2. ________________________oma — Tumor of the thymus gland
3. _______________________ gram — Record (x-ray) of lymph vessels
4. ___________________ infections — Infectious diseases associated with AIDS
5. lympho ______________________ — Formation of lymph
6. __________________________ ic — Pertaining to poison

Chapter Fourteen
DIAGRAM QUIZ

Name: ______________________________

Label the diagram below using the terms listed below:

Axillary region
Cervical region
Inguinal region
Large veins in the neck
Lymph capillaries
Lymph nodes
Lymph vessels
Mediastinal region
Right lymphatic duct
Thoracic duct

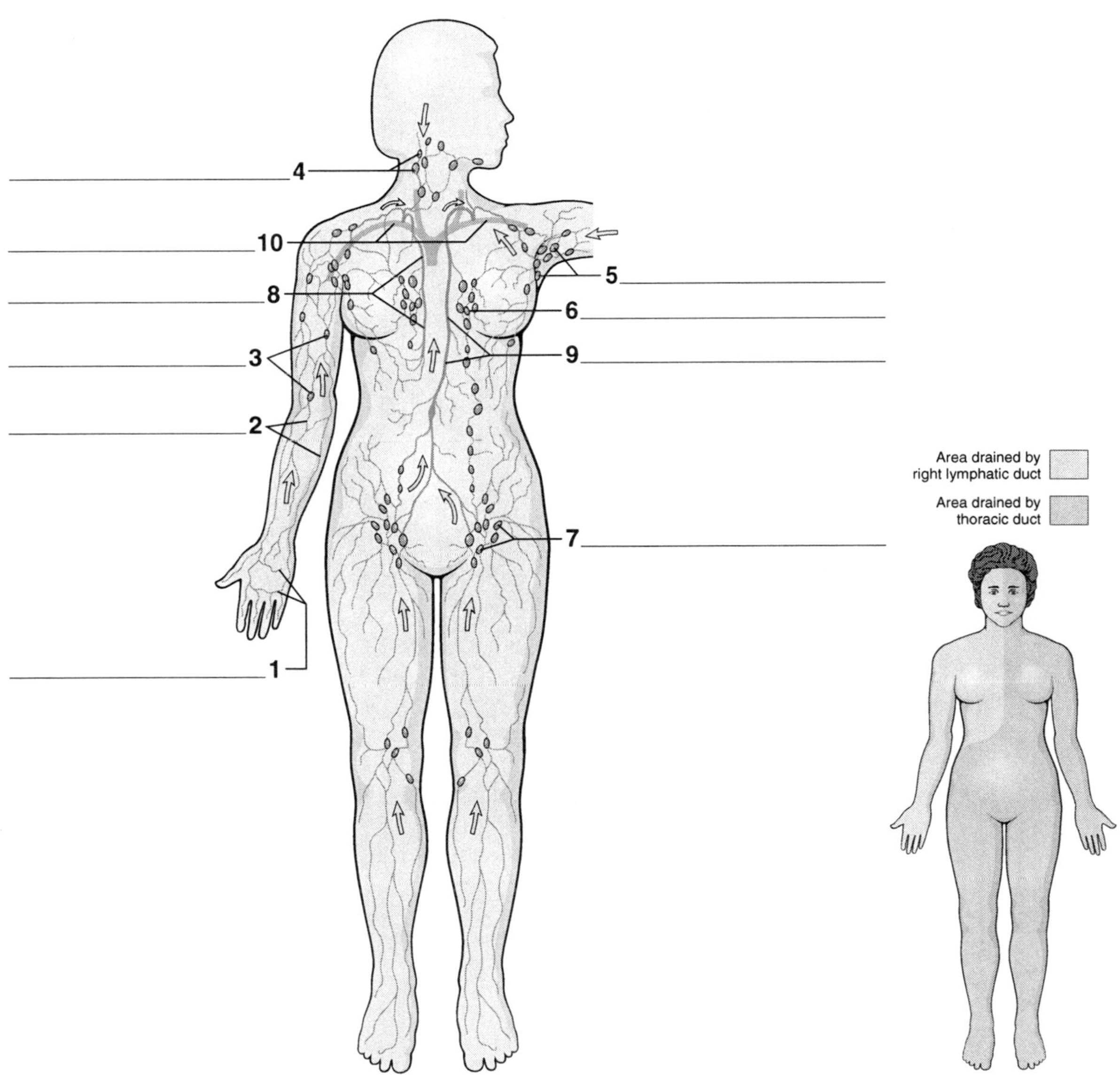

Chapter Fourteen
FLOW CHART QUIZ

Name: ______________________________

Label the flow chart using the terms listed below:

B cells
Complement system
Dendritic cells
T cells

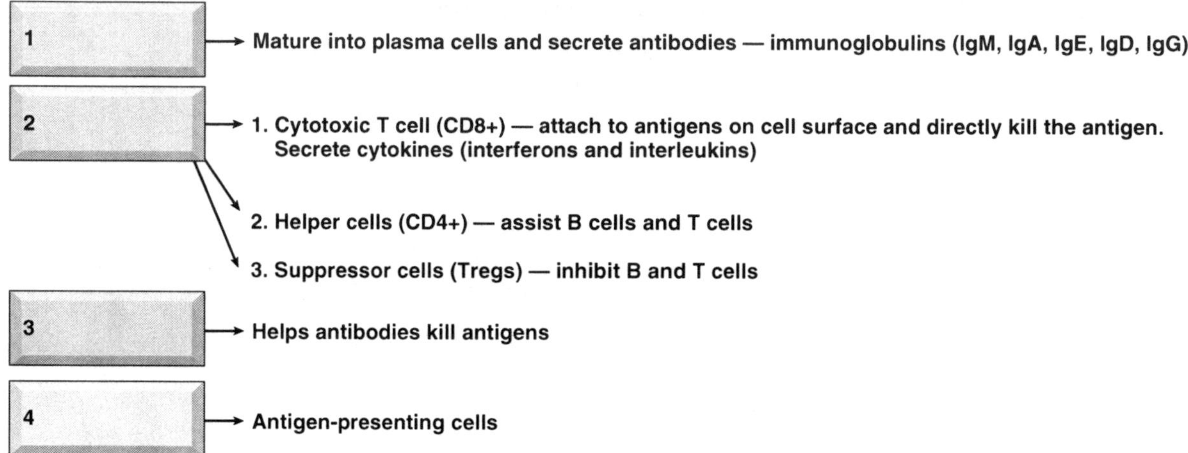

1
Mature into plasma cells and secrete antibodies — immunoglobulins (IgM, IgA, IgE, IgD, IgG)
2
1. Cytotoxic T cell (CD8+) — attach to antigens on cell surface and directly kill the antigen. Secrete cytokines (interferons and interleukins)
2. Helper cells (CD4+) — assist B cells and T cells
3. Suppressor cells (Tregs) — inhibit B and T cells
3
Helps antibodies kill antigens
4
Antigen-presenting cells

Chapter Fourteen
REVIEW SHEET QUIZ

Name: ______________________________

A. Give meanings for the following combining forms:

1. inguin/o ______________________
2. thym/o ______________________
3. axill/o ______________________
4. cervic/o ______________________
5. tox/o ______________________
6. immun/o ______________________
7. splen/o ______________________
8. lymphaden/o ______________________

B. Give meanings for the following suffixes and prefixes:

1. -edema ______________________
2. -megaly ______________________
3. -poiesis ______________________
4. -penia ______________________
5. -phylaxis ______________________
6. -oid ______________________
7. -pathy ______________________
8. inter- ______________________
9. hyper- ______________________
10. retro- ______________________

Chapter Fourteen
OPPORTUNISTIC INFECTIONS QUIZ

Name: ______________________

Match the following opportunistic infections associated with AIDS with their descriptions below:

candidiasis	histoplasmosis
Cryptococcus	*Mycobacterium avium-intracellulare*
cryptosporidiosis	*Pneumocystis carinii* pneumonia
cytomegalovirus	toxoplasmosis
herpes simplex	tuberculosis

1. Viral infection (HSV) causing small blisters on the lips, nose, or genitals: ______________________
2. Yeast-like fungal infection overgrows in the mouth (thrush), respiratory tract, and skin: ______________________
3. Bacterial disease (TB) predominant in the lungs. Symptoms include fever, weight loss, anorexia, and low energy: ______________________
4. Yeast-like fungal infection (crypto) causes lung, brain, and blood infections; found in pigeon droppings, air, water, soil: ______________________
5. Fungal infection caused by inhalation of dust contaminated with *Histoplasma capsulatum;* symptoms include fever, chills and lung infection (Histo): ______________________
6. One-celled organism causes lung infection (PCP) with fever, cough, and chest pain: ______________________
7. Parasitic infection involving the CNS and causing fever, chills, confusion, hemiparesis and seizures; parasite is found in uncooked pork, raw eggs, and vegetables (Toxo): ______________________
8. One-celled parasitic infection of the gastrointestinal tract, brain, and spinal cord: ______________________
9. Bacterial disease (MAI) with fever, malaise, night sweats, diarrhea, and lung and blood infections: ______________________
10. Virus (CMV) causes enteritis and retinitis; found in semen, saliva, urine, feces, blood, and breast milk: ______________________

Chapter Fourteen
MEDICAL SCRAMBLE

Name: ______________________

Unscramble the letters to form lymphatic/immune system–related terms from the clues. Use the letters in the squares to complete the bonus term.

1. *Clue:* Swelling due to fluid collection in spaces between tissue

   ☐ ___ ___ ___ ☐ ___ ___ ___ ___ ☐ P E L A M H Y E M D

2. *Clue:* Enlargement of a lymphoid organ in the LUQ

   ☐ ☐ ___ ___ ☐ ___ ___ ___ ___ ___ ___ ☐ N A S L O P Y E L G E M

3. *Clue:* Large phagocyte that engulfs other cells; found in lymph nodes and tissues

   ___ ☐ ___ ___ ___ ___ ___ ☐ ___ ___ G A R P A M O H E C

4. *Clue:* A poison

   ___ ___ ☐ ☐ ___ N O X I T

BONUS TERM: *Clue:* Hypersensitivity reaction

☐ ☐ ☐ ☐ ☐ ☐ ☐ ☐ ☐ ☐ ☐

Chapter Fourteen
CROSSWORD PUZZLE

Name: ______________________________

Fill in the crossword puzzle below using the clues listed underneath it.

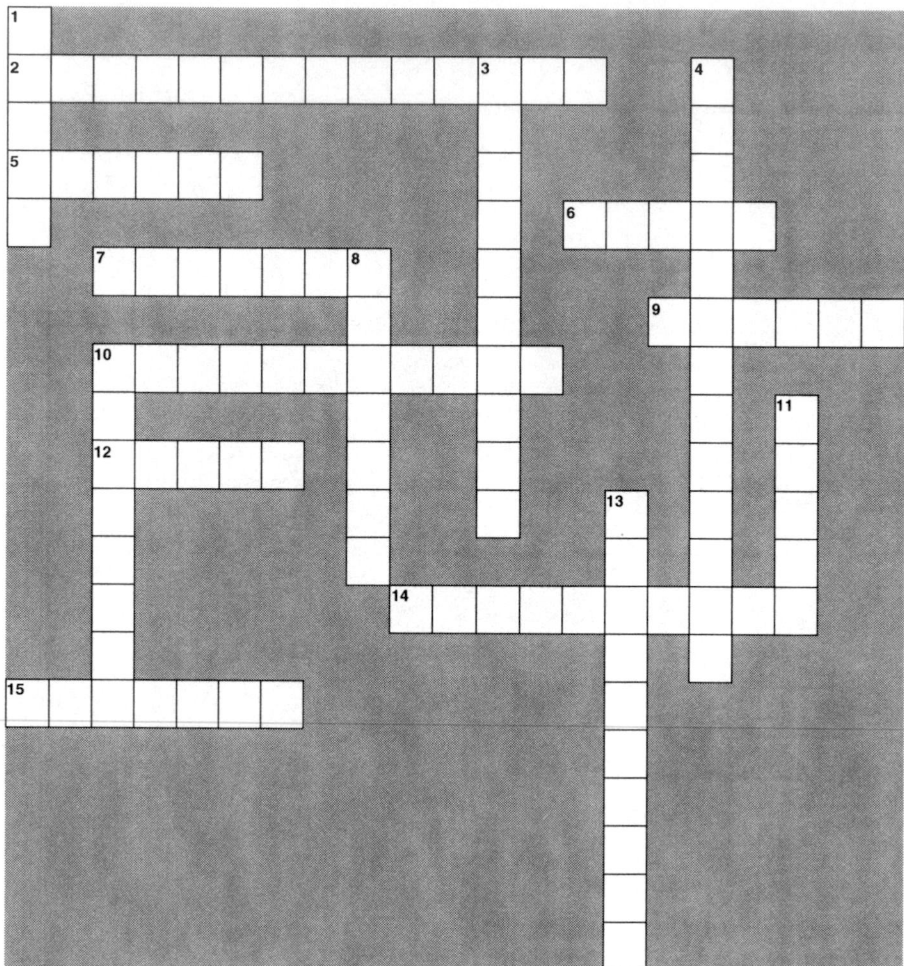

Across Clues

2. Record of lymph vessels after contrast is injected in the foot, and x-rays are taken to show the lymph.
5. Organ near the stomach that produces, stores, and eliminates blood cells.
6. Hypersensitivity or allergic state with an inherited predisposition. From a Greek word meaning "strangeness".
7. Malignant tumor of the thymus gland.
9. Tox/o means ______.
10. An exaggerated or unusual hypersensitivity to foreign protein or other substance.
12. Fluid found within lymphatic vessels.
14. Immun/o means ______.
15. Masses of lymph tissue in the oropharynx.

Down Clues

1. Enzyme-linked immunosorbent assay (abbrev).
3. An RNA virus that makes copies of itself by using the path of host cell's DNA.
4. Formation of lymph.
8. A state of abnormal hypersensitivity acquired through exposure to particular allergen.
10. Substance capable of causing specific hypersensitivity in the body; pollen, dust.
11. A poison; a protein produced by certain bacteria, animals, and plants.
13. A large phagocyte found in lymph nodes and other tissues of the body.

Chapter Fourteen

PRACTICAL APPLICATIONS

Name: ______________________

A. Case Report

This 48-year-old woman had an unexplained anemia with low-grade fever 4 years before her death. Six months before, bronchopneumonia developed, followed by return of severe anemia and continued pyrexia (fever). She was febrile (feverish), appeared pale, and had slight hepatomegaly and splenomegaly. Lymph nodes were palpated in the axillary and inguinal areas, and ascites developed. The chronic anemia did not respond to iron therapy. There was no evidence of blood loss or hemolysis. Diagnosis of lymphoma was confirmed by autopsy.

1. **What two organs were enlarged in the patient?** .... ☐
   A. Liver and lungs
   B. Lungs and spleen
   C. Liver and spleen
   D. Spleen and bone marrow

2. **Where were lymph nodes felt?** .... ☐
   A. Groin and armpit
   B. Armpit and chest
   C. Groin and abdomen
   D. Abdomen and armpit

3. **What is ascites?** .... ☐
   A. Blockage of the intestine
   B. Edema in the extremities
   C. Collection of fluid in the chest
   D. Collection of fluid in the abdomen

4. **What was the probable cause of the patient's anemia?** .... ☐
   A. Chronic blood loss
   B. Destruction of blood
   C. Malignant tumor of lymph nodes
   D. Iron deficiency

B. Symptoms of Hodgkin Disease

The most common initial feature of Hodgkin disease is painless, asymmetrical enlargement of cervical lymph nodes. Symptoms may also originate from compression of neighboring structures by growing tumor masses. For example, cough, dyspnea, dysphagia, and upper extremity edema may result from a mediastinal mass impinging on the tracheobronchial tree, esophagus, or superior vena cava. Edema of lower extremities and urinary or gastrointestinal disturbances may result from retroperitoneal lymphatic involvement. Splenomegaly is present in about half the cases.

1. **How do most patients present with Hodgkin disease?** .... ☐
   A. Lymph nodes enlarged under the arm
   B. Enlargement of the spleen
   C. Compression of the trachea
   D. Lymphadenopathy in the neck

2. **How could upper extremity edema occur?** .... ☐
   A. Tumor pressing on the esophagus
   B. Tumor blocking the main vein bringing blood to the heart
   C. Because of dysphagia
   D. Because of dyspnea

3. **What could cause bladder problems?** .... ☐
   A. Tumor behind the abdomen
   B. Tumor pressing on the bronchial tubes
   C. Enlargement of the spleen
   D. Upper extremity edema

Chapter Fourteen
ANSWERS TO THE QUIZZES

Multiple Choice Quiz

1. D	4. C	7. A	10. E	13. B	16. D	19. C	22. E
2. C	5. B	8. D	11. A	14. C	17. A	20. B	23. D
3. B	6. B	9. B	12. C	15. D	18. C	21. A	24. C

Vocabulary Quiz

A

1. cervical nodes
2. antigen
3. adaptive immunity
4. helper T cell
5. adenoids
6. dendritic cell
7. cytotoxic T cell
8. axillary nodes
9. cytokines
10. B cell

B

1. lymph
2. lymph capillaries
3. interferons and interleukins
4. immunoglobulins
5. immunity
6. inguinal nodes
7. lymph node
8. interstitial fluid
9. lymphoid organs
10. immunotherapy
11. paraaortic nodes
12. mesenteric nodes

C

1. plasma cell
2. lymph vessel
3. mediastinal nodes
4. tolerance
5. macrophage
6. monoclonal antibody
7. spleen
8. natural immunity
9. suppressor T cell
10. right lymphatic duct

D

1. tonsils
2. thymus gland
3. toxin
4. vaccine
5. thoracic duct
6. vaccination
7. humoral immunity
8. cell-mediated immunity

Terminology Quiz

A

1. lymphocytopenia
2. immunoglobulin
3. lymphopoiesis
4. lymphocytosis
5. lymphedema
6. lymphoid organs
7. lymphadenopathy
8. splenomegaly
9. lymphadenitis
10. splenectomy

B

1. thymectomy
2. anaphylaxis
3. toxic
4. hypersplenism
5. interstitial fluid
6. autoimmune disease
7. immunosuppression
8. asplenia

Pathology Quiz

A

1. opportunistic infections
2. protease inhibitor
3. human immunodeficiency virus
4. Kaposi sarcoma
5. wasting syndrome
6. reverse transcriptase inhibitor
7. acquired immunodeficiency syndrome
8. CD4+ cells

B

1. thymoma
2. multiple myeloma
3. allergen
4. non-Hodgkin lymphoma
5. Hodgkin disease
6. atopic dermatitis
7. severe combined immunodeficiency disease
8. allergy

Laboratory Tests and Clinical Procedures Quiz

A

1. viral load test
2. CD4+ cell count
3. computed tomography
4. immunoelectrophoresis
5. T4 cell
6. MoAb
7. T8 cell
8. Treg
9. ELISA

B

1. acquired immunodeficiency syndrome
2. non-Hodgkin lymphoma
3. highly active antiretroviral therapy
4. Hodgkin disease
5. human immunodeficiency virus
6. immunoglobulins
7. Kaposi sarcoma
8. severe combined immunodeficiency disease

a. HAART
b. HD
c. KS
d. NHL
e. SCID
f. HIV
g. AIDS
h. IgA

Exercise Quiz

A

1. lymph nodes
2. thoracic duct
3. spleen
4. adenoids
5. thymus
6. lymph capillaries
7. right lymphatic duct
8. interstitial fluid

B

9. groin
10. armpit
11. neck
12. chest

C

13. B
14. D
15. C
16. E
17. F
18. G
19. A

D

20. splenectomy
21. lymphadenitis
22. thymoma
23. lymphadenopathy
24. lymphopoiesis
25. lymphocytopenia
26. toxic
27. splenomegaly

E

28. hypersplenism
29. anaphylaxis
30. allergen
31. AIDS
32. thymectomy
33. Hodgkin disease
34. lymphoid organs
35. lymphedema

F

36. human immunodeficiency virus
37. histoplasmosis
38. Kaposi sarcoma
39. *Pneumocystis jiroveci* pneumonia
40. computed tomography
41. toxoplasmosis

G

42. helper T cells
43. immunoelectrophoresis
44. zidovudine
45. ELISA
46. opportunistic infections

Dictation and Comprehension Quiz

A

1. allergen
2. anaphylaxis
3. atopy
4. axillary nodes
5. cytokines
6. helper T cell
7. immunoglobulins
8. immunosuppression
9. inguinal nodes
10. interferons
11. interstitial fluid
12. Kaposi sarcoma
13. lymphadenopathy
14. lymphedema
15. lymphoma
16. protease inhibitor
17. splenomegaly
18. thymoma
19. tonsils
20. vaccination

B

12 Malignant tumor associated with AIDS; appears as bluish red skin nodules
3 Hypersensitive or allergic state involving hereditary predisposition
13 Disease condition of lymph nodes
17 Enlargement of the spleen
9 Collection of lymph tissue in the groin
1 Substance capable of causing a specific hypersensitivity reaction in the body
16 A drug that is used to treat AIDS by blocking the production of an enzyme
2 An exaggerated or unusual hypersensitivity to a foreign protein
6 Lymphocyte that aids B cells and cytotoxic T cells in recognizing antigens and stimulating antibody production: also called T4 cell or CD4+ cell
10 Antiviral proteins secreted by T cells
18 Malignant tumor of a gland in the chest
11 Found within lymphatic vessels and surrounding tissues throughout the body
19 Lymphatic tissue in the oropharynx
4 Collection of lymph tissue under the arm (armpit)
5 Proteins that aid and regulate the immune response
15 Malignant tumor of lymph nodes and tissue
7 Antibodies such as IgG, IgA, IgD that are secreted by plasma cells
20 Introduction of altered antigens to produce an immune response
8 Repression of the immune response
14 Fluid collects within the spaces between cells secondary to lymph vessel obstruction

Spelling Quiz

A

1. macrophage—large phagocyte found in lymph nodes and other tissue
2. lymph—fluid found in lymph vessels
3. immunoglobulin—antibody secreted by plasma cells
4. allergy—hypersensitivity reaction
5. inguinal nodes—lymph nodes in the groin
6. anaphylaxis—extraordinary hypersensitivity reaction
7. Hodgkin disease—malignant tumor of lymph nodes
8. axillary nodes—lymph nodes in the armpit
9. lymphocytopenia—decrease in lymphocytes
10. splenectomy—removal of the spleen

B

11. thymus gland
12. interstitial fluid
13. lymphedema
14. interleukin
15. adenoids
16. vaccination
17. tonsillitis
18. lymphopoiesis

Pronunciation Quiz

A

1. immunology
2. hypersensitivity
3. inguinal nodes
4. lymphedema
5. interstitial fluid
6. Kaposi sarcoma
7. macrophage
8. anaphylaxis
9. thoracic duct
10. lymphadenopathy

B

1. E
2. C
3. H
4. A
5. G
6. J
7. I
8. B
9. D
10. F

C

1. splenectomy
2. thymoma
3. lymphangiogram
4. opportunistic
5. lymphopoiesis
6. toxic

Diagram Quiz

1. Lymph capillaries
2. Lymph vessels
3. Lymph nodes
4. Cervical region
5. Axillary region
6. Mediastinal region
7. Inguinal region
8. Right lymphatic duct
9. Thoracic duct
10. Large veins in the neck

Flow Chart Quiz

1. B cells
2. T cells
3. Complement system
4. Dendritic cells

Review Sheet Quiz

A

1. groin
2. thymus gland
3. armpit
4. neck
5. poison
6. protection
7. spleen
8. lymph node (gland)

B

1. swelling
2. enlargement
3. formation
4. deficiency
5. protection
6. resembling, derived from
7. disease
8. between
9. excessive
10. backward

Opportunistic Infections Quiz

A

1. herpes simplex
2. candidiasis
3. tuberculosis
4. Cryptococcus
5. histoplasmosis
6. *Pneumocystis jiroveci* pneumonia
7. toxoplasmosis
8. cryptosporidiosis
9. *Mycobacterium avium-intracellulare*
10. cytomegalovirus

Crossword Puzzle

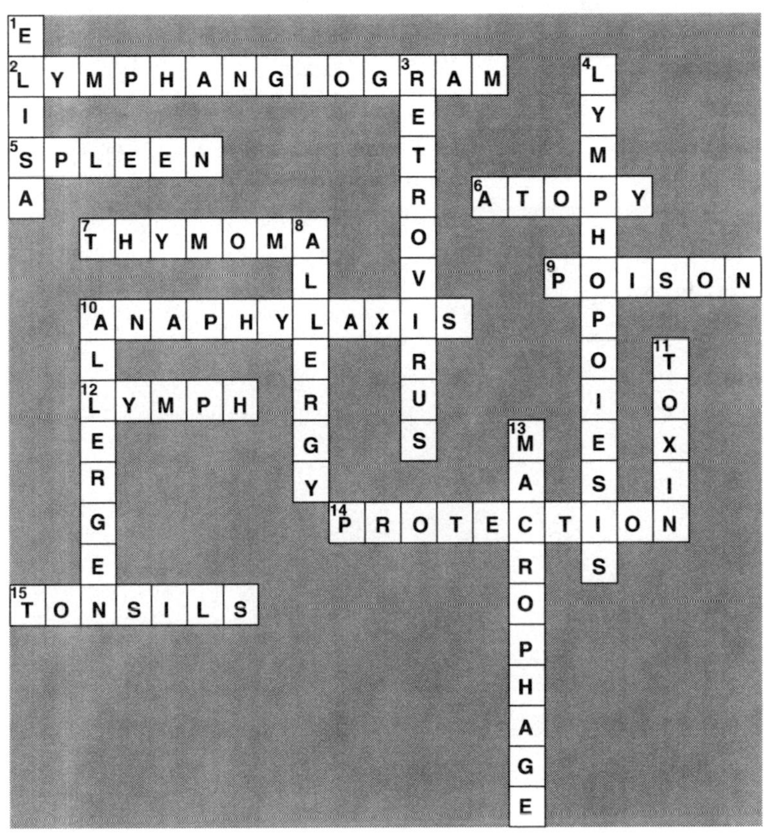

Practical Applications

A

1. C
2. A
3. D
4. C

B

1. D
2. B
3. A

Medical Scramble

1. LYMPHEDEMA
2. SPLENOMEGALY
3. MACROPHAGE
4. TOXIN

BONUS TERM: ANAPHYLAXIS

Chapter Fourteen

Answers to Terminology Section

(textbook pages 556–557)

Terminology	Meaning
autoimmune disease	Chronic, disabling disease in which the body produces antibodies against its own tissues. Examples are rheumatoid arthritis and lupus erythematosus.
immunoglobulin	Protein (antibody produced by plasma cells) that acts to protect the body by destroying antigens.
immunosuppression	Suppression (stopping) of the immune response.
lymphopoiesis	Formation of lymph.
lymphedema	Swelling of tissue due to accumulation of lymph fluid in intercellular spaces.
lymphocytopenia	Deficiency of lymphocytes in the blood.
lymphocytosis	Abnormal condition of increase in lymphocytes.
lymphoid	Derived from lymph tissue.
lymphadenopathy	Disease of lymph glands (nodes).
lymphadenitis	Inflammation of lymph glands (nodes).
splenomegaly	Enlargement of the spleen.
splenectomy	Removal of the spleen.
asplenia	Absence of the spleen. This condition may be congenital or result from surgical removal.
hypersplenism	A syndrome marked by splenomegaly (associated with anemia, leukopenia and thrombocytopenia).
thymectomy	Removal of the thymus gland.
toxic	Pertaining to poison.

Prefix

anaphylaxis	An exaggerated hypersensitivity reaction to foreign proteins.
interstitial fluid	Pertaining to fluid that lies between body cells and eventually becomes lymph fluid.

Chapter 15

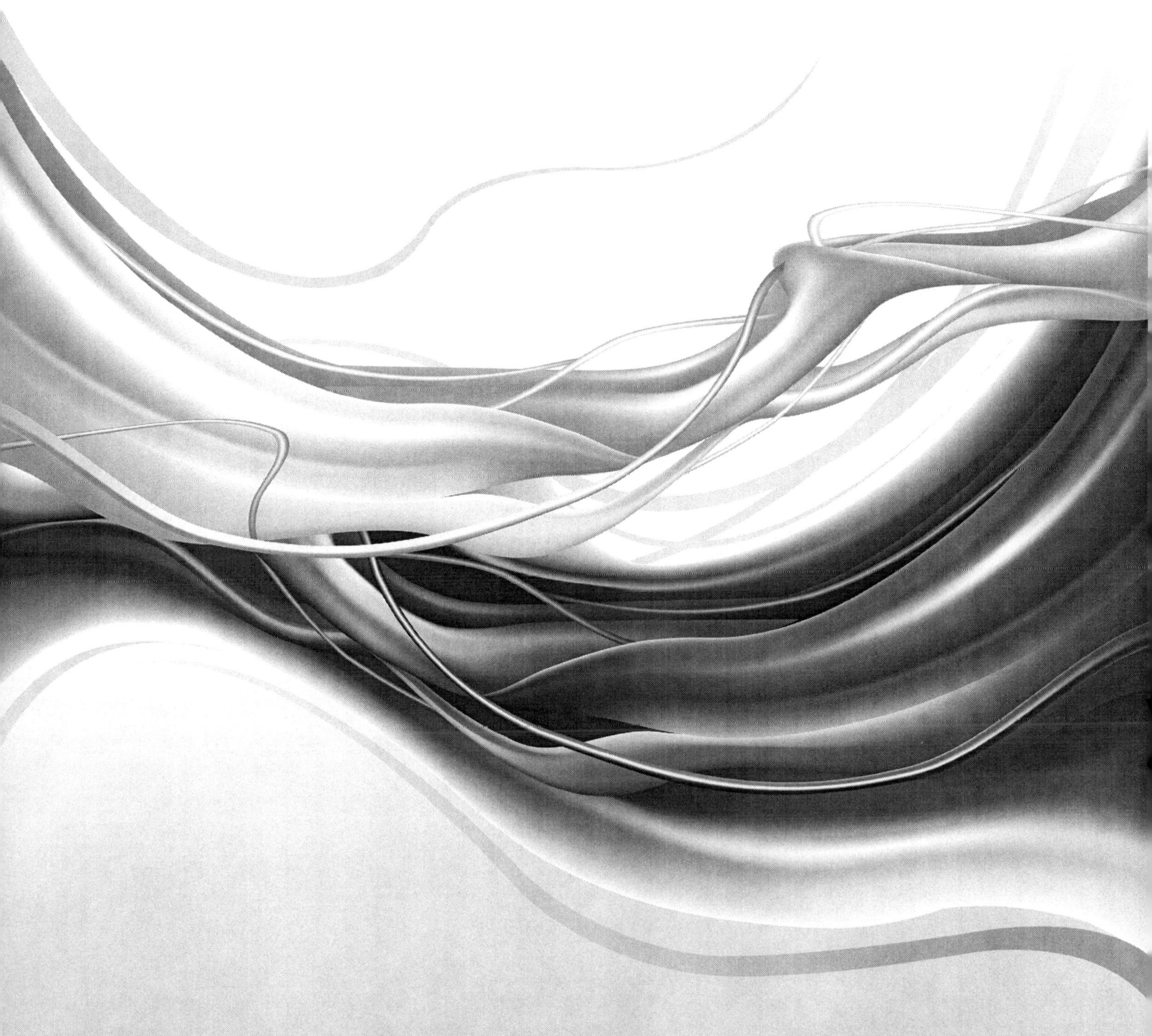

Chapter Fifteen

MULTIPLE CHOICE QUIZ

Name: ____________________

In the box write the letter of the choice that is the definition of the term or best answers the question. There is only one correct answer for each question.

1. Spongy, porous bone tissue is also called: ☐
A. Yellow bone marrow
B. Bone fissure
C. Compact bone
D. Bone sinus
E. Cancellous bone

2. Outward extension of the shoulder bone is the: ☐
A. Xiphoid process
B. Acetabulum
C. Acromion
D. Vertebral arch
E. Patella

3. An opening or passage in bones where blood vessels and nerves enter and leave is a: ☐
A. Fissure
B. Sulcus
C. Tuberosity
D. Foramen
E. Fossa

4. The projection of the temporal bone is the: ☐
A. Malleolus
B. Epiphysis
C. Xiphoid process
D. Mastoid process
E. Tubercle

5. Knuckle-like process at the end of a bone is called a: ☐
A. Fontanelle
B. Tuberosity
C. Trochanter
D. Xiphoid process
E. Condyle

6. Mandible, vomer, maxilla, and zygomatic are all bones of the: ☐
A. Face
B. Cranium
C. Spine
D. Pelvis
E. Thorax

7. Occipital, sphenoid, frontal, temporal, and ethmoid are bones of the: ☐
A. Face
B. Cranium
C. Spine
D. Pelvis
E. Thorax

8. The shaft of a long bone is called a(an): ☐
A. Olecranon
B. Periosteum
C. Osteoclast
D. Epiphysis
E. Diaphysis

9. Poor formation of bone: ☐
A. Osteolysis
B. Osteodystrophy
C. Decalcification
D. Myelopoiesis
E. Osteoclasis

10. Slipping or subluxation of a vertebra: ☐
A. Spondylitis
B. Rachitis
C. Kyphosis
D. Spondylolisthesis
E. Lordosis

11. Operation performed to relieve the symptoms of a slipped disk: ☐
A. Patellapexy
B. Arthroscopy
C. Osteoclasis
D. Laminectomy
E. Metacarpectomy

12. Lateral curvature of the spinal column: ☐
A. Lordosis
B. Scoliosis
C. Kyphosis
D. Spina bifida
E. Pubic symphysis

13. Vitamin D deficiency leads to softening of bone, which is known as: ....
A. Osteomalacia
B. Lumbago
C. Osteogenesis imperfecta
D. Osteoporosis
E. Hypercalcemia

14. Pertaining to the upper arm bone: ....
A. Humeral
B. Tibial
C. Radial
D. Ulnar
E. Carpal

15. The shoulder bone is the: ....
A. Patella
B. Sternum
C. Scapula
D. Clavicle
E. Vertebra

16. The smaller of the two lower leg bones is the: ....
A. Calcaneus
B. Tibia
C. Fibula
D. Tarsal bone
E. Malleolus

17. Inflammation of bone and bone marrow: ....
A. Osteitis fibrosa cystica
B. Multiple myeloma
C. Osteomyelitis
D. Osteoporosis
E. Osteochondroma

18. Clubfoot: ....
A. Exostosis
B. Osteogenic sarcoma
C. Bunion
D. Talipes
E. Bursitis

19. A splintered or crushed bone: ....
A. Comminuted fracture
B. Greenstick fracture
C. Crepitation
D. Compression fracture
E. Impacted fracture

20. Surgical repair of a joint: ....
A. Arthroplasty
B. Fasciectomy
C. Achondroplasia
D. Tenorrhaphy
E. Arthrosis

21. Condition of stiffening and immobility of a joint: ....
A. Hemarthrosis
B. Fibrositis
C. Bursitis
D. Kyphosis
E. Ankylosis

22. Chronic inflammation of bones and joints due to degenerative changes in cartilage: ....
A. Ankylosing spondylitis
B. Rheumatoid arthritis
C. Chondromalacia
D. Osteoarthritis
E. Systemic lupus erythematosus

23. Inflammation of joints caused by excessive uric acid accumulation: ....
A. Bunion
B. Bursitis
C. Gouty arthritis
D. Sciatica
E. Myositis

24. Malignant tumor of smooth muscle: ....
A. Rhabdomyosarcoma
B. Leiomyosarcoma
C. Rhabdomyoma
D. Leiomyoma
E. Myorrhaphy

25. Wasting away (no development) of muscle: ....
A. Myasthenia
B. Myalgia
C. Hypertrophy
D. Atrophy
E. Myositis

Chapter Fifteen

VOCABULARY QUIZ: BONES

Name: ______________________________

A. Match the following terms with their meanings below:

acetabulum
acromion
cartilage articular
calcium
cancellous bone
cartilage
collagen
compact bone
condyle
cranial bones

1. Flexible connective tissue found in the immature skeleton, epiphyseal plate, and on joint surfaces ______________________________
2. Skull bones; ethmoid, frontal, occipital, parietal, sphenoid, and temporal ______________________________
3. Mineral constituent of bone ______________________________
4. Outward extension of the shoulder bone ______________________________
5. Spongy, porous bone tissue in the inner part of bone ______________________________
6. Rounded depression or socket in the pelvis; forms the hip joint ______________________________
7. Dense connective tissue protein strands found in bone ______________________________
8. Knuckle-like process at the end of a bone near a joint ______________________________
9. Thin layer of cartilage surrounding the bones in a joint space ______________________________
10. Hard, dense bone tissue usually found around the outer portion of a bone ______________________________

B. Match the following terms with their meanings below:

diaphysis
disk (disc)
epiphysis
facial bones
fissure
fontanelle
foramen
fossa
haversian canals
ligament
malleolus

1. Shallow cavity in a bone ______________________________
2. Shaft, or midportion of a long bone ______________________________
3. Flat, round plate-like structure between two vertebrae ______________________________
4. Soft spot between the skull bones of an infant ______________________________
5. Narrow slit-like opening in or between bones ______________________________
6. Bones of the face; lacrimal, mandibular, maxillary, nasal, vomer, and zygomatic bones ______________________________
7. Minute spaces filled with blood vessels; found in compact bone ______________________________

8. Each end of a long bone ____________________
9. Opening or passage in bones where blood vessels and nerves enter and leave ____________________
10. Rounded process on both sides of the ankle joint ____________________
11. Fibrous tissue connecting bones to other bones ____________________

C. Match the following terms with their meanings below:

manubrium	olecranon	osteoblast
mastoid process	orthopedist	osteoclast
medullary cavity	osseous tissue	periosteum
metaphysis	ossification	physiatrist

1. Process of bone formation ____________________
2. Bone cell that absorbs and removes unwanted bone tissue ____________________
3. Round projection on the temporal bone behind the ear ____________________
4. Central hollowed-out area in the shaft of a long bone ____________________
5. Upper portion of the sternum ____________________
6. Bone cell that helps form bone tissue ____________________
7. Membrane surrounding bones ____________________
8. Bone tissue ____________________
9. Flared portion of a long bone between the diaphysis and the epiphyseal plate ____________________
10. Large process on the proximal end of the ulna; part of the elbow joint ____________________
11. Medical doctor specializing in bone, joint, and muscle rehabilitation ____________________
12. Surgical specialist treating bone, joint, and muscle conditions ____________________

D. Match the following terms with their meanings below:

phosphorus	sinus	temporomandibular joint
pubic symphysis	styloid process	trabeculae
red bone marrow	tendons	trochanter
sella turcica	tubercle	

1. Soft bone tissue found in cancellous bone; contains hematopoietic stem cells and blood cells ____________________
2. Supporting bundles of bony fibers in cancellous bone ____________________
3. Depression in the sphenoid bone; location of the pituitary gland ____________________

4. Rounded, small process on a bone; attachment site for muscles and tendons ______________________
5. Pole-like process extending downward from the temporal bone on each side of the skull ______________________
6. Area where the two pubic bones come together in the pelvis ______________________
7. Connection on either side of the head between the temporal bone of the skull and the mandibular bone of the jaw ______________________
8. Large process at the neck of the femur ______________________
9. Mineral substance found in bones in combination with calcium ______________________
10. Hollow air cavity with a bone ______________________
11. Fibrous connective tissue connecting muscles and bones ______________________

E. Match the following terms with their meanings below:

epiphyseal plate	tuberosity	xiphoid process
ribs	vertebra	yellow bone marrow

1. ______________________ Lower, narrow portion of the sternum
2. ______________________ Rounded process on bone; attachment for muscles and tendons
3. ______________________ Twelve pairs of elongated, curved bones that form the chest wall
4. ______________________ Fatty tissue found in the medullary cavity of most adult long bones
5. ______________________ Individual backbone
6. ______________________ Cartilaginous area at the ends of long bones

Chapter Fifteen

TERMINOLOGY QUIZ: BONES

Name: ______________________________

A. Complete the following terms to match the definitions below; select from the following word parts:

calc/o	lumb/o	spondyl/o
kyph/o	myel/o	-emia
lamin/o	oste/o	de-
lord/o	scoli/o	

1. Removal of a portion of a vertebra to relieve compression on nerves: ______________ ectomy
2. Abnormal condition of exaggerated anterior curvature of the spine: ______________ osis
3. Condition of high blood calcium: hyper ______________
4. Abnormal condition of posterior curvature of the spine: ______________ osis
5. Pertaining to the lower back: ______________ar
6. Formation of bone marrow: ______________ poiesis
7. Inflammation of bone: ______________ itis
8. Formation of bone: ______________ genesis
9. Abnormal condition of lateral curvature of the spine: ______________ osis
10. Abnormal condition of vertebrae: ______________ osis

B. Complete the following terms to match the definitions below; select from the following word parts:

vertebr/o	-malacia	-trophy
-blast	-physis	dys-
-clast	-porosis	epi-
-listhesis	-tome	sym-

1. Pertaining to a backbone: ______________al
2. Abnormal development of bone: osteo ______________
3. Immature bone cell: osteo ______________
4. Softening of bone: osteo ______________
5. Instrument to cut bone: osteo ______________
6. Forward slipping of a vertebra over a lower one: spondylo ______________
7. Bone cell that breaks down bone to remove bone tissue: osteo ______________
8. Abnormal condition of loss of bone tissue and decrease in bone mass: osteo ______________
9. Cartilaginous joint connecting two sections of the pubic bone: pubic ______________
10. Each end of a long bone: ______________ physis

Chapter Fifteen

PATHOLOGY QUIZ: BONES

Name: ______________________________

Match the following vocabulary terms with their meanings below:

Colles fracture	exostosis	osteomyelitis
comminuted fracture	greenstick fracture	osteopenia
compression fracture	impacted fracture	osteoporosis
crepitus	osteogenic sarcoma	pathologic fracture
Ewing sarcoma	osteomalacia	talipes

1. Bony benign growth arising from the surface of bone ______________________________
2. Rare, malignant tumor arising in bone; occurring in children ______________________________
3. Partially broken bone ______________________________
4. Break in a bone caused by disease ______________________________
5. Broken bone near the wrist joint at the distal end of the radius ______________________________
6. Bone is splintered or crushed into several pieces ______________________________
7. Common malignant tumor arising from osteoblasts ______________________________
8. Broken bone in which one fragment is driven firmly into the other ______________________________
9. Crackling sound produced when ends of bones rub against each other ______________________________
10. Bone collapses with trauma or as a result of osteoporosis ______________________________
11. Inflammation of bone and bone marrow secondary to infection ______________________________
12. Congenital abnormality of the hindfoot (involving the talus) ______________________________
13. Decrease in bone density with thinning and weakening of bone ______________________________
14. Softening of bone with inadequate amounts of calcium in bone ______________________________
15. Deficiency of bone; a precursor to osteoporosis ______________________________

Chapter Fifteen

VOCABULARY QUIZ: JOINTS

Name: ______________________________

Match the following vocabulary terms with their meanings below:

articulation	meniscus	synovial joint
articular cartilage	suture joint	synovial membrane
bursa	synovial cavity	tendon
ligament	synovial fluid	

1. Immovable joint between the bones of the skull ______________________________
2. Smooth, glistening, white tissue that covers the surface of a joint ______________________________
3. Connective tissue binding bones to other bones ______________________________
4. Tissue lining the synovial cavity; it produces synovial fluid ______________________________
5. Connective tissue that binds muscles to bones ______________________________
6. Sac of fluid near a joint ______________________________
7. A freely movable joint ______________________________
8. Any type of joint ______________________________
9. Viscous fluid within the synovial space ______________________________
10. Space between bones at a synovial joint ______________________________
11. Crescent-shaped fibrocartilaginous structure in the knee ______________________________

Chapter Fifteen
TERMINOLOGY QUIZ: JOINTS

Name: ______________________________

Complete the following terms to match the definitions below; select from the following word parts:

ankyl/o	ten/o	-plasia
arthr/o	tendin/o	-plasty
burs/o	-desis	-rrhaphy
chondr/o	-malacia	-stenosis
ligament/o	-oma	
rheumat/o	-osis	

1. Abnormal condition of blood in a joint: hem ______________________________
2. Narrowing of the spinal canal: spinal ______________________________
3. Surgical repair of a joint: arthro ______________________________.
4. Fusion, by surgery, of bones across a joint space: arthro ______________________________
5. Inflammation of a sac of fluid near the joint: ______________________________itis
6. Specialist in diagnosis and treatment of arthritis: ______________________________ologist
7. Inflammation of connective tissue binding muscles to bones: ______________________________itis
8. Type of dwarfism: achondro______________________________.
9. Softening of cartilage: chondro ______________________________
10. Stiffness of a joint: ______________________________ osis
11. Suture of a tendon: teno ______________________________
12. Pertaining to the connective tissue that binds bones to bones: ______________________________ ous

Chapter Fifteen
PATHOLOGY QUIZ: JOINTS

Name: ______________________________

A. *Match the following vocabulary terms with their meanings below:*

ankylosing spondylitis
bunion
carpal tunnel syndrome
dislocation
ganglion
gouty arthritis
herniation of an intervertebral disk
Lyme disease
osteoarthritis
rheumatoid arthritis
sprain
systemic lupus erythematosus

1. Progressive, degenerative joint disease with loss of articular cartilage and hypertrophy of bone ______________________________
2. Chronic, progressive arthritis with stiffening of joints, primarily of the spine ______________________________
3. Trauma to joint ligaments without rupture ______________________________
4. Disorder marked by arthritis, myalgia, malaise; cause is a bacterium carried by a tick ______________________________
5. Chronic, inflammatory autoimmune disease involving joints, skin, kidneys, nervous system, heart and lungs; butterfly rash on the face is typical ______________________________
6. Fluid-filled cyst arising from the joint capsules or tendons in the hand ______________________________
7. Inflammatory, painful swelling of joints caused by excessive uric acid in the body ______________________________
8. Chronic joint condition with inflammation and pain; caused by an autoimmune reaction against joint tissue, particularly the synovial membrane ______________________________
9. Enlargement of bone or tissue around the joint at the base of the big toe ______________________________
10. Displacement of a bone from its joint ______________________________
11. Compression of the median nerve as it passes between the ligament and the bones and tendons of the wrist ______________________________
12. Abnormal protrusion of cartilaginous tissue into the spinal canal or spinal nerves ______________________________

B. Match the following vocabulary terms with their meanings below:

hyperuricemia
laminectomy
podagra
pyrexia
sciatica
subluxation

1. High levels of uric acid in the blood ______________________________
2. Removal of a portion of a vertebra to relieve pain from a herniated disk ______________________________
3. Pain in the big toe caused by collection of uric acid crystals ______________________________
4. Pain radiating down the leg due to herniated disk ______________________________
5. Partial or incomplete dislocation of a joint ______________________________
6. Fever ______________________________

Chapter Fifteen

VOCABULARY QUIZ: MUSCLES

Name: ______________________________

Match the following vocabulary terms with their meanings below:

abduction	flexion	rotation
adduction	insertion of a muscle	skeletal muscle
dorsiflexion	origin of a muscle	supination
extension	plantar flexion	visceral muscle
fascia	pronation	

1. Bending a muscle, a limb ______________________________
2. Movement away from the midline of the body ______________________________
3. Bending the foot upward (backward) ______________________________
4. Connection of a muscle to a stationary bone ______________________________
5. Circular movement around a central point (axis) ______________________________
6. Muscle connected to bones; striated or voluntary muscle ______________________________
7. Turning the palm of the hand downward ______________________________
8. Movement toward the midline of the body ______________________________
9. Bending the sole of the foot downward toward the ground ______________________________
10. Turning the palm of the hand upward ______________________________
11. Straightening of a flexed limb ______________________________
12. Connection of a muscle to a bone that moves ______________________________
13. Muscle connected to internal organs; involuntary or smooth muscle ______________________________
14. Fibrous membrane separating and enveloping muscles ______________________________

Chapter Fifteen

TERMINOLOGY AND PATHOLOGY QUIZ: MUSCLES

Name: ______________________________

Complete the following terms to match the definitions below; select from the following word parts:

fasci/o	rhabdomy/o	a-
fibr/o	sarc/o	ab-
leiomy/o	-asthenia	ad-
my/o	-itis	dorsi-
myocardi/o	-oma	dys-
-myos/o	-penia	hyper-
plant/o	-trophy	poly-

1. Inflammation of muscle: ______________________________ itis
2. Incision into the sheath enveloping muscles: ______________________________ tomy
3. Malignant tumor of skeletal muscle: ______________________________ oma
4. Pain of muscle and fibrous tissue: ______________________________ algia
5. Benign tumor of visceral muscle: ______________________________ oma
6. Lack of development (in muscles): a ______________________________
7. Condition of lack of muscle strength: ______________________________ gravis
8. Carrying or leading away from the body: ______________________________ duction
9. Excessive development (in muscles): ______________________________ trophy
10. Pertaining to bending the sole of the foot downward: ______________________________ ar flexion
11. Bending the foot backward: ______________________________ flexion
12. Pertaining to heart muscle: ______________________________ al
13. Group of inherited diseases characterized by progressive weakness and degeneration of muscle fibers without involvement of the nervous system: muscular ______________________________
14. Chronic inflammatory myopathy (many muscles): ______________________________ itis
15. Deficiency of muscle (flesh): sarco ______________________________

Chapter Fifteen

LABORATORY TESTS AND CLINICAL PROCEDURES QUIZ

Name: ______________________________

A. *Match the following tests with the definitions below:*

antinuclear antibody test	serum calcium
erythrocyte sedimentation rate	serum creatine kinase
rheumatoid factor test	uric acid test

1. Measurement in blood of a mineral constituent of bone ______________________________
2. Measurement in blood of a substance associated with gouty arthritis ____________________
3. Time it takes for red blood cells to settle to the bottom of a test tube ____________________
4. Measurement of an enzyme in serum as an indicator of muscle disease or injury ______________________________
5. Detects antibody present in serum of patients with SLE ______________________________
6. Detects antibody found in patients with rheumatoid arthritis ______________________________

B. *Match the following procedures with the explanations below:*

arthrocentesis	arthroscopy	CT	MRI
arthrography	bone density test	diskography	muscle biopsy
arthroplasty	bone scan	electromyography	

1. Visual examination of a joint with an endoscope and camera ______________________________
2. Surgical puncture to remove fluid from a joint ______________________________
3. X-ray beam and computer provides cross-sectional and other images of soft tissue and bone ______________________________
4. Use of a magnetic field to create images of soft tissue in the body ____________________
5. X-ray images are taken after injection of contrast material into the joint ____________________
6. X-ray examination of an intervertebral disk after injection of contrast into the nucleus pulposus ______________________________
7. Removal of muscle tissue for microscopic examination ______________________________
8. Uptake of radioactive substance is measured in bone ______________________________
9. Recording the strength of muscle contraction as a result of electrical stimulation ______________________________
10. Low-energy x-ray absorption in bones is used to measure bone mass ____________________
11. Surgical repair or replacement of a joint ______________________________

Chapter Fifteen

ABBREVIATIONS QUIZ

Name: ______________________________

A. On the line provided, give meanings for the following abbreviations, then write each abbreviation next to its explanation below:

1. AC ______________________________
2. ACL ______________________________
3. ANA ______________________________
4. C1-C7 ______________________________
5. Ca ______________________________
6. CK ______________________________
7. CMC ______________________________
8. CTS ______________________________
9. DEXA ______________________________
10. DMARD ______________________________

a. __________ Mineral constituent of bone

b. __________ Connective tissue in the knee

c. __________ Compression of the median nerve in the wrist

d. __________ Medications used to treat a type of arthritis

e. __________ Shoulder joint

f. __________ Enzyme elevated in muscle disease

g. __________ Indicator of SLE

h. __________ Backbones in the neck

i. __________ Provides evidence for osteopenia and osteoporosis

j. __________ Wrist joint

B. *On the line provided, give meanings for the following abbreviations, then write each abbreviation next to its explanation below:*

1. DO ____________________
2. DTRs ____________________
3. EMG ____________________
4. ESR ____________________
5. HNP ____________________
6. IM ____________________
7. L1-L5 ____________________
8. NSAID ____________________
9. OA ____________________
10. ORIF ____________________
11. Ortho ____________________

a. __________ Professional who treats medical conditions and performs surgery

b. __________ Speed at which RBCs settle out of blood

c. __________ Pertaining to within muscles

d. __________ Prescribed to treat musculoskeletal disorders

e. __________ Bulging of the inner section of an intervertebral disk

f. __________ Measurement of connective tissue (tendon) movement, as indicator of nerve and muscle strength

g. __________ Vertebrae in the lower back

h. __________ Electrical measurement of muscle functioning

i. __________ Repair of a broken bone

j. __________ Branch of medicine dealing with evaluation and treatment of musculoskeletal disorders

k. __________ Condition in which articular cartilage wears away and joint replacement may be necessary

C. On the line provided, give meanings for the following abbreviations, then write each abbreviation next to its explanation below:

1. OT ______________________
2. P ______________________
3. PT ______________________
4. RA ______________________
5. RF ______________________
6. ROM ______________________
7. SLE ______________________
8. T1-T12 ______________________
9. TKR ______________________
10. THR ______________________
11. TMJ ______________________

a. __________ Vertebrae in the area of the chest

b. __________ Helps patients regain use of muscles and joints after injury or surgery

c. __________ Replacement of the patellar joint

d. __________ Assessment of flexibility of a joint

e. __________ Mineral element in bone

f. __________ Autoimmune condition affecting skin, joints, and internal organs

g. __________ Replacement of the pelvic joint

h. __________ Antibody associated with a type of arthritis

i. __________ Joint between the skull and the lower jaw bone

j. __________ Chronic type of arthritis marked by swelling and inflammation of joints

k. __________ Treatment that helps patients perform activities of daily living and function in work-related situations

Chapter Fifteen
EXERCISE QUIZ

Name: ______________________________

PART I: BONES

A. Complete the following sentences:

1. Two mineral substances necessary for proper development of bones are ____________________ and ______________________________
2. The shaft of a long bone is called the ______________________________
3. The ends of a long bone are called the ______________________________
4. The bones of a fetus are mainly composed of ______________________________ tissue
5. During bone development, immature bone cells called ________________ produce bony tissue
6. Red bone marrow is found in spongy or ______________________________ bone
7. The strong membrane surrounding the surface of a bone is the ____________________
8. Hard, dense bone tissue lying under the periosteum is called ____________________
9. The physician who treats bones and bone diseases is a(an) ____________________
10. Series of bone canals containing blood vessels are the ____________________
11. Medical doctor who specializes in restoring patients to functional activities after injuries to bones, nerves, and muscles is ______________________________

B. Match the following cranial and facial bones with their meanings:

frontal bone	mandible	occipital bone	temporal bone
lacrimal bone	maxilla	parietal bone	zygomatic bone

12. Forms the forehead ______________________________
13. Cheek bone ______________________________
14. Upper jaw bone ______________________________
15. Forms the back and base of the skull ______________________________
16. Lower jaw bone ______________________________
17. Forms the roof and upper side of the skull ______________________________
18. Two paired bones at the corner of each eye ______________________________
19. Bone near the ear; connected to the lower jaw ______________________________

C. Give the medical names for the following bones:

20. shoulder bone ______________________
21. upper arm bone ______________________
22. breastbone______________________
23. thigh bone ______________________
24. finger bones ______________________
25. collarbone ______________________
26. wrist bones ______________________
27. kneecap ______________________
28. foot bones ______________________
29. backbone ______________________

D. Give the meanings for the following terms associated with bones:

30. calcaneus ______________________
31. acetabulum ______________________
32. acromion ______________________
33. malleolus ______________________
34. lamina ______________________
35. olecranon ______________________
36. pubic symphysis ______________________
37. osteoporosis ______________________
38. osteogenic sarcoma ______________________

E. Match the following terms with their descriptions:

exostoses
kyphosis
lordosis
myelopoiesis
scoliosis
spondylolisthesis
talipes

39. Lateral curvature of the spine ______________________
40. Formation of bone marrow ______________________
41. Abnormal anterior curvature of the spine ______________________
42. Benign tumors arising from the bone surface ______________________
43. Humpback ______________________
44. Clubfoot ______________________
45. Subluxation of a vertebra ______________________

Chapter Fifteen
EXERCISE QUIZ

Name: ______________________________

PART II: JOINTS AND MUSCLES

A. Complete the following sentences:

1. Connective tissue that binds bones to other bones is a(an) ______________________________
2. Connective tissue that binds muscles to bones is a(an) ______________________________
3. Fluid found within the joint is called ______________________________
4. A sac of fluid near a joint is a(an) ______________________________
5. Smooth cartilage that surrounds the surface of bones at joints is ______________________________
6. Surgical repair of a joint is called ______________________________

B. Complete the medical term from its meaning and word parts given:

7. inflammation of a tendon: ______________________________ itis
8. doctor specializing in joint disorders: ______________________________ logist
9. tumor (benign) of cartilage: ______________________________ oma
10. incision of a joint: arthr ______________________________
11. stiffened, immobile joint: ______________________________ osis
12. suture of a tendon: ten ______________________________
13. softening of cartilage: chondro ______________________________
14. tumor (malignant) of cartilage: ______________________________ oma
15. inflammation of a sac of fluid near a joint: ______________________________ itis

C. Give meanings for the following terms:

16. subluxation ______________________________
17. arthrodesis ______________________________
18. podagra ______________________________
19. pyrexia ______________________________
20. sciatica ______________________________

D. Select the term that best fits the definition given.

21. fibrous membrane separating muscles: (fascia, flexion)
22. movement away from the midline: (abduction, adduction)
23. pertaining to heart muscle: (myasthenia, myocardial)
24. pain of many muscles: (myositis, polymyalgia)
25. act of turning the palm forward or upward: (supination, pronation)
26. muscle connected to internal organs: (skeletal, visceral)
27. connection of muscle to the bone that moves: (origin, insertion)
28. connection of muscle to a stationary bone: (origin, insertion)

E. Select from the following terms to name the abnormal conditions described below:

achondroplasia	dislocation	osteoarthritis
ankylosing spondylitis	ganglion	rheumatoid arthritis
bunion	gouty arthritis	systemic lupus erythematosus
carpal tunnel syndrome	Lyme disease	

29. An inherited condition in which bones of the arms and legs fail to grow normally because of a defect in cartilage and bone formation ____________________
30. Cystic mass arising from a tendon in the wrist ____________________
31. Inflammation of joints caused by accumulation of uric acid ____________________
32. Degenerative joint disease; chronic inflammation of bones and joints ____________________
33. Chronic, progressive arthritis with stiffening of joints, especially of the spine ____________________
34. Compression of the median nerve in the wrist ____________________
35. Abnormal swelling of a metatarsophalangeal joint ____________________
36. Tick-borne bacterium causes this type of arthritis ____________________
37. Chronic joint disease with inflamed and painful joints; marked by swollen and thickened synovial membranes ____________________
38. Chronic inflammatory disease affecting skin (red rash on the face), kidneys, heart, and lungs as well as joints ____________________
39. Displacement of a bone from its joint ____________________

F. Give the meanings for the following abnormal conditions affecting muscles:

40. fibromyalgia ________________________________
41. leiomyosarcoma ________________________________
42. muscular dystrophy ________________________________
43. polymyositis ________________________________
44. fasciitis ________________________________

G. Match the term in Column I with its meaning in Column II.

	Column I			Column II
45.	extension	_______	A.	Bending a limb
46.	rotation	_______	B.	Movement away from the midline
47.	flexion	_______	C.	Movement toward the midline
48.	adduction	_______	D.	Circular movement around an axis
49.	pronation	_______	E.	Straightening out a limb
50.	abduction	_______	F.	Turning the palm backward

Chapter Fifteen

DICTATION AND COMPREHENSION QUIZ: BONES

Name: ______________________________

A. Dictation of Terms

1.	____________________	11.	____________________
2.	____________________	12.	____________________
3.	____________________	13.	____________________
4.	____________________	14.	____________________
5.	____________________	15.	____________________
6.	____________________	16.	____________________
7.	____________________	17.	____________________
8.	____________________	18.	____________________
9.	____________________	19.	____________________
10.	____________________	20.	____________________

B. Comprehension of Terms: Match number of the above term with its meaning below.

______ Lateral curvature of the spinal column
______ Bat-shaped cranial bone behind the eyes
______ Large process below the neck of the femur
______ End of a long bone
______ Flexible connective tissue at joints
______ Bone break at the wrist
______ Round process on both sides of ankle
______ Forms the back and base of the skull
______ Poor development of bone
______ Pertaining to the smaller lower leg bone
______ Hip socket
______ Thin, delicate cranial bone; supports the nasal cavity
______ Formation of bone marrow
______ Malignant bone tumor
______ Upper part of the hip bone
______ Forward vertebral subluxation
______ Bone is splintered or crushed
______ Heel bone
______ Elbow bone
______ Clubfoot

Chapter Fifteen

DICTATION AND COMPREHENSION QUIZ: JOINTS AND MUSCLES

Name: ______________________________

A. Dictation of Terms

1. ______________________ 11. ______________________
2. ______________________ 12. ______________________
3. ______________________ 13. ______________________
4. ______________________ 14. ______________________
5. ______________________ 15. ______________________
6. ______________________ 16. ______________________
7. ______________________ 17. ______________________
8. ______________________ 18. ______________________
9. ______________________ 19. ______________________
10. ______________________ 20. ______________________

B. Comprehension of Terms: Match number of the above term with its meaning below.

_____ Process of recording the electrical activity of muscles
_____ Chronic, progressive arthritis with stiffening of joints (primarily the spine)
_____ Bones are fused across the joint space
_____ Inflammation of the tissue connecting bones and muscles
_____ Bones of the arms and legs fail to grow to normal size (defect in cartilage formation)
_____ Bending of the foot backward (upward)
_____ Act of turning the palm forward
_____ Movement away from the midline of the body
_____ Inflammation of the membrane lining the joint
_____ Malignant tumor of smooth muscle
_____ Trauma to a muscle from violent contraction or excessive stretching
_____ Inflammation of many muscles
_____ Trauma to a joint due to injury to ligaments
_____ Fever
_____ Blood condition found in gouty arthritis
_____ Malignant tumor of skeletal muscle
_____ Chronic disease of joint inflammation (primarily the small joints of the hands and feet); an autoimmune reaction
_____ Abnormal swelling of the metatarsophalangeal joint
_____ Sac of fluid near a joint
_____ Extreme pain of the big toe associated with gouty arthritis

Chapter Fifteen
SPELLING QUIZ

Name: ______________________________

A. Circle the term that is spelled correctly, and write its meaning in the space provided:

1. arthrocentesis arthrosentesis ______________________________
2. osteoperosis osteoporosis ______________________________
3. cartiledge cartilage ______________________________
4. atropy atrophy ______________________________
5. chondrocostal chrondrocostal ______________________________
6. scoliosis scoleosis ______________________________
7. Uwing sarcoma Ewing sarcoma ______________________________
8. osteomyleitis osteomyelitis ______________________________
9. ascetabulum acetabulum ______________________________
10. osteodystrophy osteodystropy ______________________________

B. Circle the term that is spelled correctly. The meaning of each term is given.

11. Upper arm bone .... humerus humerous humorous
12. Thigh bone .... femor femur femmur
13. End of a long bone .... epiphysis epiphisis epiphifisis
14. Humpback .... kyphiosis kiphosis kyphosis
15. Heel bone .... calcaneus calcaneous calcaineus
16. Finger or toe bones .... phalanges pharynges plalanges
17. Collarbone .... clavical klavicle clavicle
18. Kneecap .... patella petella patela
19. Larger lower leg bone .... tibbia tibea tibia
20. Mineral substance in bone .... phosphorus phosphorous phospherus

Chapter Fifteen
PRONUNCIATION QUIZ

Name: ______________________________

A. Underline the accented syllables in the following terms:

1. acetabulum
2. osteodystrophy
3. epiphysis
4. scapular
5. kyphosis
6. malleolus
7. fibromyalgia
8. phalanges
9. podagra
10. rheumatologist

B. Match the term in Column I with its meaning in Column II:

Column I		Column II
1. ulna	_______	A. Collarbone
2. ilium	_______	B. Larger of the two lower leg bones
3. diaphysis	_______	C. Upper part of the hip bone
4. clavicle	_______	D. Lower arm bone
5. bursa	_______	E. Condition of anterior curvature of the spine
6. lordosis	_______	F. The elbow
7. fibula	_______	G. Sac of fluid near joints
8. tibia	_______	H. The shaft of a long bone
9. olecranon	_______	I. A foot bone
10. metatarsal	_______	J. Smaller of the two leg bones

C. Complete the following terms using the definitions given:

1. teno______________________________ Suture of a tendon
2. ______________________________pexy Fixation of the kneecap
3. ______________________________ al Pertaining to the heel bone
4. ______________________________oma Tumor (benign) of smooth, visceral muscle
5. ______________________________ emia High levels of blood calcium
6. ______________________________itis Inflammation of bone and bone marrow
7. ______________________________ osis Lateral curvature of the spine
8. osteo ______________________________ Malignant bone tumor
9. ______________________________ ing Inflammation of the backbone with stiffness in the joints (2 words)
   ______________________________ itis

Chapter Fifteen
DIAGRAM QUIZ

Name: ______________________

Label the diagram below using the terms listed below:

Articular cartilage
Cancellous bone
Compact cortical bone
Diaphysis
Epiphyseal plate (line)
Epiphysis
Haversian canals
Medullary cavity
Metaphysis
Periosteum

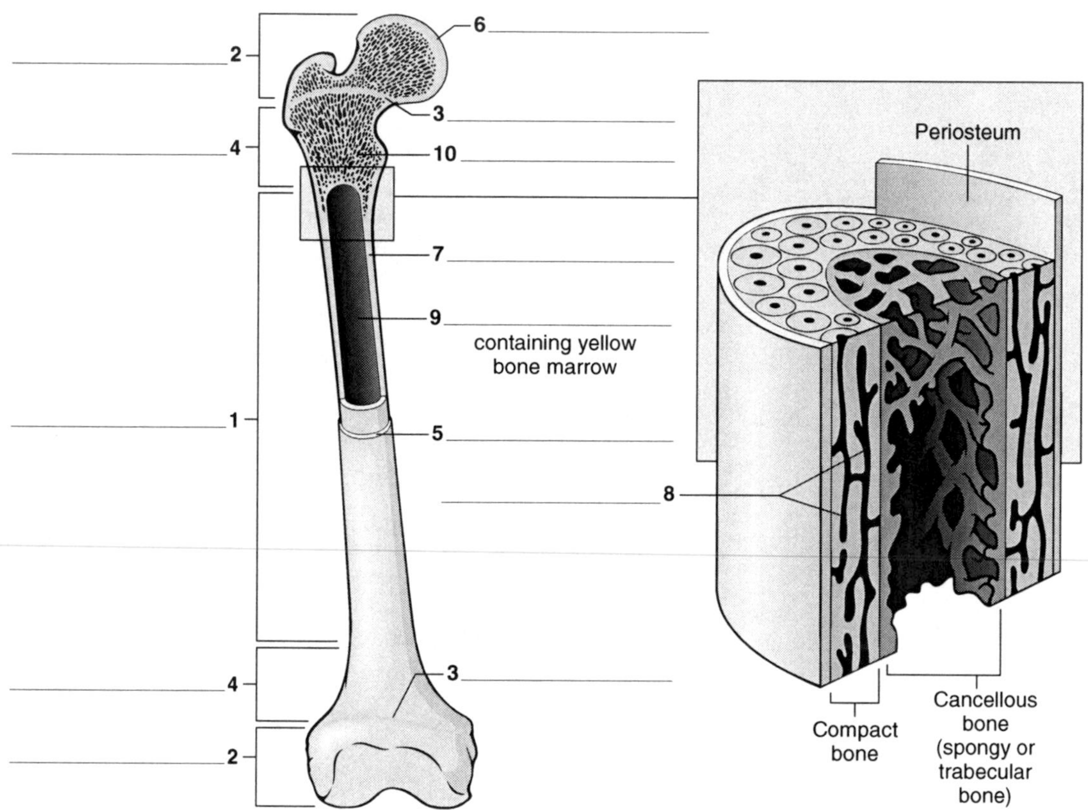

Chapter Fifteen

REVIEW SHEET QUIZ

Name: ______________________________

A. Give meanings for the following combining forms:

1. acetabul/o ____________________
2. ankyl/o ____________________
3. arthr/o ____________________
4. articul/o ____________________
5. burs/o ____________________
6. calc/o ____________________
7. calcane/o ____________________
8. carp/o ____________________
9. cervic/o ____________________
10. chondr/o ____________________

B. Give combining forms for the following meanings:

1. collarbone ____________________
2. tailbone ____________________
3. ribs ____________________
4. skull ____________________
5. fascia ____________________
6. thigh bone ____________________
7. smooth muscle ____________________
8. upper arm bone ____________________
9. ilium ____________________
10. ischium ____________________

C. Give meanings for the following combining forms:

1. kyph/o ____________________
2. lamin/o ____________________
3. lord/o ____________________
4. lumb/o ____________________
5. malleol/o ____________________
6. maxill/o ____________________
7. metacarp/o ____________________
8. metatars/o ____________________
9. my/o ____________________
10. myel/o ____________________

D. Give meanings for the following combining forms:

1. myos/o ______________
2. olecran/o ______________
3. orth/o ______________
4. oste/o ______________
5. patell/o ______________
6. perone/o ______________
7. phalang/o ______________
8. vertebr/o ______________
9. rhabdomy/o ______________
10. spondyl/o ______________

E. Give combining forms for the following meanings:

1. sacrum ______________
2. flesh ______________
3. shoulder blade ______________
4. crooked, bent (lateral curvature of spine) ______________
5. breast bone ______________
6. chest ______________
7. larger lower leg bone ______________
8. lower arm bone (little finger side) ______________
9. lower arm bone (thumb side) ______________
10. lower jaw bone ______________

F. Give meanings for the following suffixes:

1. -algia ______________________
2. -asthenia ______________________
3. -blast ______________________
4. -clast ______________________
5. -desis ______________________
6. -emia ______________________
7. -listhesis ______________________
8. -malacia ______________________
9. -penia ______________________
10. -plasty ______________________
11. -porosis ______________________
12. -stenosis ______________________
13. -tome ______________________
14. -trophy ______________________

G. Give meanings for the following prefixes:

1. a-, an- ______________________
2. ab- ______________________
3. ad- ______________________
4. dia- ______________________
5. dorsi- ______________________
6. epi- ______________________
7. exo- ______________________
8. meta- ______________________
9. peri- ______________________
10. poly- ______________________
11. sub- ______________________
12. supra- ______________________

Chapter Fifteen

MEDICAL SCRAMBLE

Name: ______________________________

Unscramble the letters to form musculoskeletal system–related terms from the clues. Use the letters in the squares to complete the bonus term.

1. *Clue:* One of the jaw bones

   ☐ ☐ ___ ___ ☐ ___ ___ ___ BALMINED

2. *Clue:* One of the bones in the arm

   ___ ___ ☐ ☐ ___ ___ ___ SUHEMUR

3. *Clue:* Group of bones at the tailbone of the spinal column

   ___ ☐ ___ ___ ☐ ___ YCOCXC

4. *Clue:* Anterior bone of the skull

   ___ ___ ☐ ___ ___ ___ ☐ TRAFOLN

BONUS TERM: *Clue:* Benign tumor of smooth muscle

☐ ☐ ☐ ☐ ☐ ☐ ☐ ☐ ☐

Chapter Fifteen

CROSSWORD PUZZLE

Name: ______________________________

Fill in the crossword puzzle below using the clues listed underneath it.

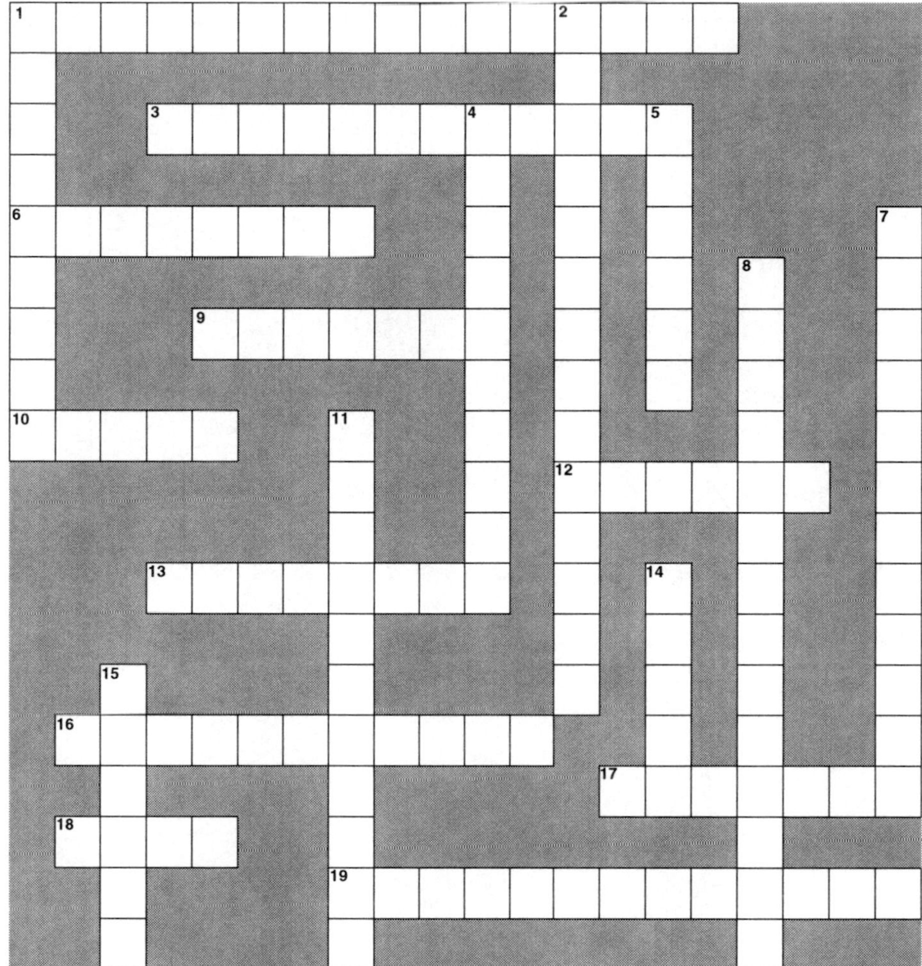

Across Clues

1. The process of recording the strength of muscle contraction.
3. Chronic inflammatory myopathy of uncertain etiology (inflammation of many muscles).
6. Rounded process on a bone; attachment for muscles and tendons.
9. Decreasing the angle between two bones; bending of the bone.
10. Cavity within a bone (cranial and facial bones).
12. Connective tissue that binds muscles to bones.
13. A cystic mass arising from a tendon in the wrist.
16. A partial or incomplete dislocation.
17. Clubfoot.
18. Flat, round, plate-like cartilaginous structure between vertebrae.
19. Inflammation of the bone and bone marrow.

Down Clues

1. Bony growth arising from the surface of bone.
2. Surgical puncture of the joint space with a needle.
4. As applied to the hand, the act of turning the palm upward.
5. Trauma to a joint with pain, swelling, and injury to ligaments.
7. Decrease in bone density; thinning and weakening a limb.
8. Progressive, degenerative joint disease characterized by loss of articular cartilage; literally, inflammation of bone and joint.
11. Displacement of a bone from its joint. For example, a shoulder ____________.
14. Shallow cavity in a bone.
15. Abnormal swelling of the joint between the big toe and the first metatarsal bone.

Chapter Fifteen

PRACTICAL APPLICATIONS

Name: ______________________

A. Chart Note

The patient is having pain around the medial aspect of his left knee. About 12 years ago he had a tear of his medial meniscus (crescent-shaped fibrocartilage), which was removed. On examination, he has a well-healed medial scar to his left knee; there was no effusion; full range of motion; and it is stable. X-rays show very slight scarring of the medial femoral condyle and a small accessory bone medially, but nothing in the interior of the joint. The great toe shows a healed fracture. There was no obvious exostosis impinging on the base of the nail.

1. **Effusion in a joint means:** .... ☐
   A. The bones at the joint are broken
   B. The meniscus is torn
   C. The patella is fractured
   D. There is fluid in the joint space

2. **Where is the femoral condyle?** .... ☐
   A. At the ankle joint
   B. At the knee joint
   C. At the distal end of the tibia
   D. At the distal end of the fibula

3. **An exostosis is:** .... ☐
   A. A bony growth
   B. A fluid-filled cyst
   C. A healed fracture
   D. Type of tendon

4. **Where is the medial meniscus?** .... ☐
   A. Near the big toe
   B. At the hip socket
   C. In the middle of the knee
   D. At the base of the nail of the big toe

B. Chart Note

Follow-up for the complications of osteoporosis as they affect the spine. Mrs. Smith had a 6-month history of progressive disabling back pain visibly associated with progressive kyphotic deformity of the thoracolumbar spine, with an attendant cervical lordosis. X-rays of the thoracic spine reveal a compression fracture of T11 and L1. I advised the patient that such fractures even without trauma may be complications of underlying osteoporosis as severe as hers.

1. **Which term best describes Mrs. Smith's condition?......................** ☐
   A. Osteoarthritis
   B. Gouty arthritis
   C. Osteomalacia
   D. Osteopenia

2. **What type of spinal deformity is present? ....** ☐
   A. Posterior curvature of the chest and anterior curvature of the neck
   B. Lateral curvature of the chest
   C. Cervical fracture
   D. Anterior curvature of the thorax

Chapter Fifteen
ANSWERS TO THE QUIZZES

Multiple Choice Quiz

1. E
2. C
3. D
4. D
5. E
6. A
7. B
8. E
9. B
10. D
11. D
12. B
13. A
14. A
15. C
16. C
17. C
18. D
19. A
20. A
21. E
22. D
23. C
24. B
25. D

Vocabulary Quiz: Bones

A

1. cartilage
2. cranial bones
3. calcium
4. acromion
5. cancellous bone
6. acetabulum
7. collagen
8. condyle
9. articular cartilage
10. compact bone

B

1. fossa
2. diaphysis
3. disk (disc)
4. fontanelle
5. fissure
6. facial bones
7. haversian canals
8. epiphysis
9. foramen
10. malleolus
11. ligaments

C

1. ossification
2. osteoclast
3. mastoid process
4. medullary cavity
5. manubrium
6. osteoblast
7. periosteum
8. osseous tissue
9. metaphysic
10. olecranon
11. physiatrist
12. orthopedist

D

1. red bone marrow
2. trabeculae
3. sella turcica
4. tubercle
5. styloid process
6. pubic symphysis
7. temporomandibular joint
8. trochanter
9. phosphorus
10. sinus
11. tendons

E

1. xiphoid process
2. tuberosity
3. ribs
4. yellow bone marrow
5. vertebra
6. epiphyseal plate

Terminology Quiz: Bones

A

1. laminectomy
2. lordosis
3. hypercalcemia
4. kyphosis
5. lumbar
6. myelopoiesis
7. osteitis
8. osteogenesis
9. scoliosis
10. spondylosis

B

1. vertebral
2. osteodystrophy
3. osteoblast
4. osteomalacia
5. osteotome
6. spondyloschisis
7. osteoclast
8. osteoporosis
9. pubic symphysis
10. epiphysis

Pathology Quiz: Bones

1. exostosis
2. Ewing sarcoma
3. greenstick fracture
4. pathologic fracture
5. Colles fracture
6. comminuted fracture
7. osteogenic sarcoma
8. impacted fracture
9. crepitus
10. compression fracture
11. osteomyelitis
12. talipes
13. osteoporosis
14. osteomalacia
15. osteopenia

Vocabulary Quiz: Joints

1. suture joint
2. articular cartilage
3. ligament
4. synovial membrane
5. tendon
6. bursa
7. synovial joint
8. articulation
9. synovial fluid
10. synovial cavity
11. meniscus

Terminology Quiz: Joints

1. hemarthrosis
2. spinal stenosis
3. arthroplasty
4. arthrodesis
5. bursitis
6. rheumatologist
7. tendinitis
8. achondroplasia
9. chondromalacia
10. ankylosis
11. tenorrhaphy
12. ligament

Pathology Quiz: Joints

A

1. osteoarthritis
2. ankylosing spondylitis

3. sprain
4. Lyme disease
5. systemic lupus erythematosus
6. ganglion
7. gouty arthritis
8. rheumatoid arthritis
9. bunion
10. dislocation
11. carpal tunnel syndrome
12. herniation of an intervertebral disk

B

1. hyperuricemia
2. laminectomy
3. podagra
4. sciatica
5. subluxation
6. pyrexia

Vocabulary Quiz: Muscles

1. flexion
2. abduction
3. dorsiflexion
4. origin of a muscle
5. rotation
6. skeletal muscle
7. pronation
8. adduction
9. plantar flexion
10. supination
11. extension
12. insertion of a muscle
13. visceral muscle
14. fascia

Terminology and Pathology Quiz: Muscles

1. myositis
2. fasciotomy
3. rhabdomyosarcoma
4. fibromyalgia
5. leiomyoma
6. atrophy
7. myasthenia gravis
8. abduction
9. hypertrophy
10. plantar flexion
11. dorsiflexion
12. myocardial
13. muscular dystrophy
14. polymyositis
15. sarcopenia

Laboratory Tests and Clinical Procedures Quiz

A

1. serum calcium
2. uric acid test
3. erythrocyte sedimentation rate
4. serum creatine kinase
5. antinuclear antibody test
6. rheumatoid factor test

B

1. arthroscopy
2. arthrocentesis
3. CT
4. MRI
5. arthrography
6. diskography
7. muscle biopsy
8. bone scan
9. electromyography
10. bone density test
11. arthroplasty

Abbreviations Quiz

A

1. acromioclavicular joint
2. anterior cruciate ligament
3. antinuclear antibody
4. cervical vertebrae
5. calcium
6. creatine kinase
7. carpometacarpal
8. carpal tunnel syndrome
9. dual-energy x-ray absorptiometry
10. disease-modifying antirheumatic drug

a. Ca
b. ACL
c. CTS
d. DMARD
e. AC
f. CK
g. ANA
h. C1-C7
i. DEXA
j. CMC

B

1. doctor of osteopathy
2. deep tendon reflexes
3. electromyography
4. erythrocyte sedimentation rate
5. herniated nucleus pulposus
6. intramuscular
7. lumbar vertebrae
8. nonsteroidal anti-inflammatory drug
9. osteoarthritis
10. open reduction/internal fixation
11. orthopedics (or orthopaedics)

a. DO
b. ESR
c. IM
d. NSAID
e. HNP
f. DTRs
g. L1-L5
h. EMG
i. ORIF
j. Ortho
k. OA

C

1. occupational therapy
2. phosphorus
3. physical therapy
4. rheumatoid arthritis
5. rheumatoid factor
6. range of motion
7. systemic lupus erythematosus
8. thoracic vertebrae
9. total knee replacement
10. total hip replacement
11. temporomandibular joint

a. T1-T12
b. PT
c. TKR
d. ROM
e. P
f. SLE
g. THR
h. RF
i. TMJ
j. RA
k. OT

Exercise Quiz

Part I:

A

1. calcium and phosphorus
2. diaphysis
3. epiphyses
4. cartilage
5. osteoblasts
6. cancellous
7. periosteum
8. compact bone
9. orthopedist
10. haversian canals
11. physiatrist

B

12. frontal bone
13. zygomatic bone
14. maxilla
15. occipital bone
16. mandible
17. parietal bone
18. lacrimal
19. temporal

C

20. scapula
21. humerus
22. sternum
23. femur
24. phalanges
25. clavicle
26. carpals
27. patella
28. metatarsals
29. vertebra

D

30. heel bone
31. socket for femur in hip
32. projection of scapula
33. rounded process at the ankle
34. part of the vertebral arch
35. elbow bone
36. anterior part of the hip bone
37. decrease in bone density; thinning and weakening of bone
38. malignant tumor of bone

E

39. scoliosis
40. myelopoiesis
41. lordosis
42. exostoses
43. kyphosis
44. talipes
45. spondylolisthesis

Part II:

A

1. ligament
2. tendon
3. synovial fluid
4. bursa
5. articular cartilage
6. arthroplasty

B

7. tendinitis
8. rheumatologist
9. chondroma
10. arthrotomy
11. ankylosis
12. tenorrhaphy
13. chondromalacia
14. chondrosarcoma
15. bursitis

C

16. partial or incomplete dislocation
17. binding of a joint
18. sharp pain of big toe; associated with gouty arthritis
19. fever
20. pain radiating down the leg

D

21. fascia
22. abduction
23. myocardial
24. polymyalgia
25. supination
26. visceral
27. insertion
28. origin

E

29. achondroplasia
30. ganglion
31. gouty arthritis
32. osteoarthritis
33. ankylosing spondylitis
34. carpal tunnel syndrome
35. bunion
36. Lyme disease
37. rheumatoid arthritis
38. systemic lupus erythematosus
39. dislocation

F

40. pain of fibrous tissue and muscle
41. tumor (malignant) of smooth muscle
42. poor development of muscle; group of inherited diseases with progressive muscle weakness and degeneration
43. chronic inflammation of many muscles
44. inflammation of fascia

G

45. E
46. D
47. A
48. C
49. F
50. B

Dictation and Comprehension: Bones

A

1. acetabulum
2. calcaneus
3. cartilage
4. Colles fracture
5. comminuted fracture
6. epiphysis
7. ethmoid bone
8. osteogenic sarcoma
9. ischium
10. malleolus
11. myelopoiesis
12. occipital bone
13. olecranon
14. osteodystrophy
15. peroneal
16. scoliosis
17. sphenoid bone
18. spondylolisthesis
19. talipes
20. trochanter

B

16 Lateral curvature of the spinal column
17 Bat-shaped cranial bone behind the eyes
20 Large process below the neck of the femur
6 End of a long bone
3 Flexible connective tissue at joints
4 Bone break at the wrist
10 Round process on both sides of ankle
12 Forms the back and base of the skull
14 Poor development of bone
15 Pertaining to the smaller lower leg bone
1 Hip socket
7 Thin, delicate cranial bone; supports the nasal cavity
11 Formation of bone marrow
8 Malignant bone tumor
9 Upper part of the hip bone
18 Forward vertebral subluxation
5 Bone is splintered or crushed
2 Heel bone
13 Elbow bone
19 Clubfoot

Dictation and Comprehension: Joints and Muscles

A

1. abduction
2. achondroplasia
3. ankylosing spondylitis
4. arthrodesis
5. bunion
6. bursa
7. dorsiflexion
8. electromyography
9. hyperuricemia
10. leiomyosarcoma
11. podagra
12. polymyositis
13. pyrexia
14. rhabdomyosarcoma
15. rheumatoid arthritis
16. sprain
17. strain
18. supination
19. synovitis
20. tendinitis

B

8 Process of recording the electrical activity of muscles
3 Chronic, progressive arthritis with stiffening of joints (primarily the spine)
4 Bones are fused across the joint space
20 Inflammation of the tissue connecting bones and muscles
2 Bones of the arms and legs fail to grow to normal size (defect in cartilage formation)
7 Bending of the foot backward (upward)
18 Act of turning the palm forward
1 Movement away from the midline of the body
19 Inflammation of the membrane lining the joint
10 Malignant tumor of smooth muscle
17 Trauma to a muscle from violent contraction or excessive stretching
12 Inflammation of many muscles
16 Trauma to a joint due to injury to ligaments
13 Fever
9 Blood condition found in gouty arthritis
14 Malignant tumor of skeletal muscle
15 Chronic disease of joint inflammation (primarily the small joints of the hands and feet); an autoimmune reaction
5 Abnormal swelling of the metatarsophalangeal joint
6 Sac of fluid near a joint
11 Extreme pain of the big toe associated with gouty arthritis

Spelling Quiz

A

1. arthrocentesis—surgical puncture to remove fluid from a joint
2. osteoporosis—decrease in bone density and weakening of bone
3. cartilage—connective tissue at joints
4. atrophy—lack of development; shrinkage of muscle
5. chondrocostal—pertaining to rib cartilage
6. scoliosis—lateral curvature of the spine
7. Ewing sarcoma—malignant bone tumor
8. osteomyelitis—inflammation of bone and bone marrow
9. acetabulum—socket in the hip bone
10. osteodystrophy—poor development of bone

B

11. humerus
12. femur
13. epiphysis
14. kyphosis
15. calcaneus
16. phalanges
17. clavicle
18. patella
19. tibia
20. phosphorus

Pronunciation Quiz

A

1. acetabulum
2. osteodystrophy
3. epiphysis
4. scapular
5. kyphosis
6. malleolus
7. fibromyalgia
8. phalanges
9. podagra
10. rheumatologist

B

1. D
2. C
3. H
4. A
5. G
6. E
7. J
8. B
9. F
10. I

C

1. tenorrhaphy
2. patellapexy
3. calcaneal
4. leiomyoma
5. hypercalcemia
6. osteomyelitis
7. scoliosis
8. osteogenic sarcoma
9. ankylosing spondylitis

Diagram Quiz

1. Diaphysis
2. Epiphysis
3. Epiphyseal plate (line)
4. Metaphysis
5. Periosteum
6. Articular cartilage
7. Compact cortical bone
8. Haversian canals
9. Medullary cavity
10. Cancellous bone

Review Sheet Quiz

A

1. acetabulum
2. stiff
3. joint
4. joint
5. bursa (sac of fluid near a joint)
6. calcium
7. calcaneus
8. wrist
9. neck
10. cartilage

B

1. clavicul/o
2. coccyg/o
3. cost/o
4. crani/o
5. fasci/o
6. femor/o
7. leiomy/o
8. humer/o
9. ili/o
10. ischi/o

C

1. humpback
2. lamina (part of the vertebral arch)
3. curve, swayback
4. loins, lower back
5. malleolus (rounded portion of ankle bone)
6. maxilla (upper jaw bone)
7. hand bones
8. foot bones
9. muscle
10. bone marrow

D

1. muscle
2. olecranon (elbow)
3. straight
4. bone
5. patella (kneecap)
6. fibula (smaller lower leg bone)
7. finger and toe bones
8. vertebra, backbone
9. skeletal, striated muscle
10. vertebra, backbone

E

1. sacr/o
2. sarc/o
3. scapul/o
4. scoli/o
5. stern/o
6. thorac/o
7. fibul/o
8. uln/o
9. radi/o
10. mandibul/o

F

1. pain
2. lack of strength
3. immature cell, embryonic
4. to break
5. to bind, tie together
6. blood condition
7. slipping
8. softening
9. deficiency
10. surgical repair
11. pore, passage
12. narrowing

13. instrument to cut
14. nourishment, development

G

1. no, not, without
2. away from
3. toward
4. complete, through
5. back
6. above, upon
7. out, outside
8. between, beyond
9. surrounding
10. many, much
11. under, below
12. above

Medical Scramble

1. MANDIBLE
2. HUMERUS
3. COCCYX
4. FRONTAL

BONUS TERM: LEIOMYOMA

Crossword Puzzle

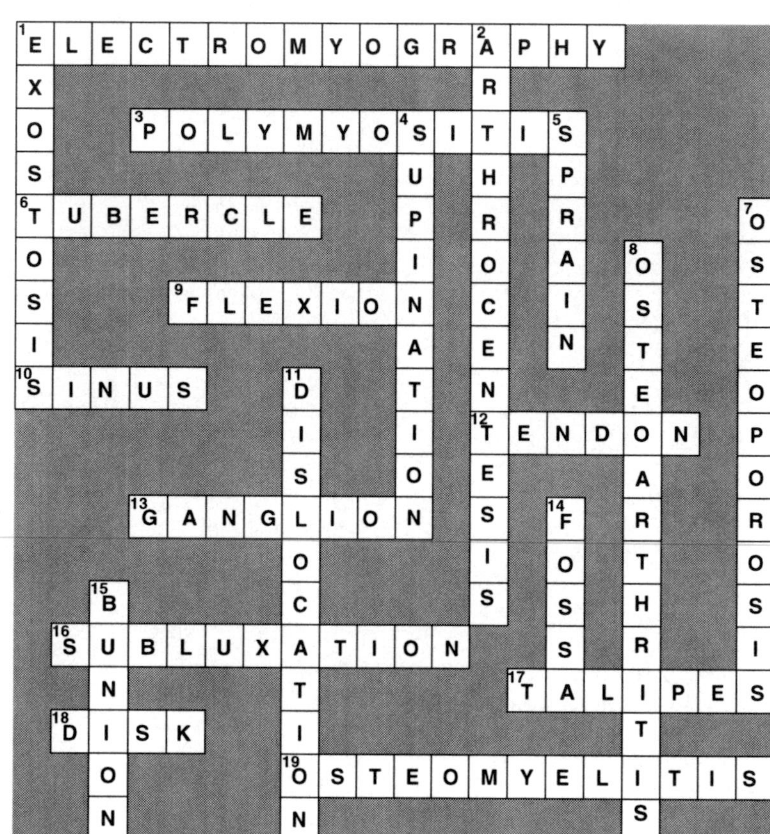

Practical Applications

A

1. D
2. B
3. A
4. C

B

1. D
2. A

Chapter Fifteen
Answers to Terminology Section

Terminology	Meaning

Bones—General Terms (textbook pages 594–598)

hypercalcemia	Excessive calcium in the bloodstream.
decalcification	Removal of calcium from bones.
kyphosis	Abnormal posterior curvature of the thoracic vertebrae.
laminectomy	Removal of a lamina to relieve the symptoms of a ruptured intervertebral disk (disc).
lordosis	Abnormal anterior curvature of the backbones in the lumbar region.
lumbar	Pertaining to the loins or lower back (near the waist) region.
lumbosacral	Pertaining to the lower back and the sacrum.
myelopoiesis	Formation of bone marrow.
orthopedics	The specialty of medicine dealing with bones and bone diseases. Orthopedists originally straightened (orth/o) the bones of children (ped/o).
osteitis	Inflammation of bones.
osteodystrophy	Poor development of bones.
osteogenesis	Formation of bone.
scoliosis	Abnormal condition of lateral curvature of the spine.
spondylosis	Abnormal condition of vertebrae.
vertebroplasty	Repair of a fractured vertebra.

Suffixes

osteoblast	Immature bone cell.
osteoclast	Large cell found in the bone marrow of growing bones; absorbs and removes unwanted bone tissue.
spondylolisthesis	Forward displacement of a vertebra over a lower segment.
osteomalacia	Softening of bone.
epiphysis	End of a long bone.
pubic symphysis	Junction of the pubic bones on the midline in front of the body.
osteoporosis	Condition of increased porosity of bone with loss of bony tissue and decrease in bone mass.
osteotome	Instrument to cut bone.

Specific Bones

acetabular	Pertaining to the acetabulum (hip socket).
calcaneal	Pertaining to the calcaneus (heel bone).
carpal	Pertaining to the wrist bones.
supraclavicular	Pertaining to above the collarbone.
subcostal	Pertaining to below the ribs.
chondrocostal	Pertaining to the cartilage attached to the ribs.
craniotomy	Incision of the skull.
craniotome	Instrument to cut the skull.
femoral	Pertaining to the thigh bone (femur).
fibular	Pertaining to the smaller of the two lower leg bones (fibula).
humeral	Pertaining to the upper arm bone (humerus).

iliac	Pertaining to the ilium (upper portion of the hip bone).
ischial	Pertaining to the ischium (lower and posterior part of the hip bone).
malleolar	Pertaining to the malleolus (process on each side of the ankle).
mandibular	Pertaining to the lower jaw bone.
maxillary	Pertaining to the upper jaw bone.
metacarpectomy	Removal of hand bones.
metatarsalgia	Pain of the foot bones.
olecranal	Pertaining to the elbow.
patellar	Pertaining to the kneecap.
pelvimetry	Measurement of the proportions of the pelvic bone (before childbirth).
peroneal	Pertaining to the fibula.
phalangeal	Pertaining to the finger or toe bones.
pubic	Pertaining to the pubis (anterior portion of the hip bone).
radial	Pertaining to the lateral lower arm bone.
scapular	Pertaining to the shoulder bone.
sternal	Pertaining to the breast bone.
tarsectomy	Removal of ankle bones.
tibial	Pertaining to the tibia, the larger and inner of the two lower leg bones.
ulnar	Pertaining to the medial lower arm bone.

Joints (textbook pages 604–605)

ankylosis	Abnormal stiffening and immobility of a joint.
arthroplasty	Surgical repair of a joint.
arthrotomy	Incision of a joint.
hemarthrosis	Abnormal condition of blood in a joint.
hydrarthrosis	Abnormal accumulation of fluid in a joint.
polyarthritis	Inflammation of many joints.
articular cartilage	The cartilage surrounding the bones in a joint.
bursitis	Inflammation of a bursa.
achondroplasia	Improper cartilage formation in development of bones (leads to a type of dwarfism).
chondroma	Tumor (benign) of cartilage.
chondromalacia	Abnormal softening of cartilage.
ligamentous	Pertaining to a ligament.
rheumatologist	Specialist in treatment of joint disorders.
synovitis	Inflammation of a synovial membrane.
tenorrhaphy	Suture of a tendon.
tenosynovitis	Inflammation of a tendon and its sheath.
tendinitis	Inflammation of a tendon; also spelled tendonitis.
arthrodesis	Binding together (surgical fusion) of a joint.
spinal stenosis	Narrowing of the neural canal or nerve root canals in the lumbar spine.

Muscles (textbook pages 615–617)

fasciotomy	Incision of fascia.
fibromyalgia	Pain of fibrous connective tissue and muscle.
leiomyoma	Tumor (benign) of a smooth muscle.
leiomyosarcoma	Tumor (malignant) of a smooth muscle.
myalgia	Pain of a muscle.

electromyography	Process of recording the electricity in muscle.
myopathy	Disease of muscles.
myocardial	Pertaining to heart muscle.
myositis	Inflammation of muscle.
plantar flexion	Bending downward of the sole of the foot.
rhabdomyoma	Tumor (benign) of a skeletal muscle.
rhabdomyosarcoma	Tumor (malignant) of skeletal muscle.
sarcopenia	Loss of muscle mass and strength associated with aging.
myasthenia gravis	Condition of muscle weakness caused by a failure in transmission of nervous impulses from a nerve to muscle cell.
atrophy	Decrease in size of a normally developed organ or tissue; wasting of tissue.
hypertrophy	Excessive development (increase in cell size).
amyotrophic	Pertaining to loss of muscle development (in amyotrophic lateral sclerosis muscles can't move because of degeneration of nerve cells in the brain and spinal cord).
abduction	Process of carrying away (muscle is pulled away from the midline of the body).
adduction	Process of carrying toward (muscle is pulled toward the midline of the body).
dorsiflexion	Bending of the foot backward and upward.
polymyalgia	Pain of many muscles.

Chapter 16

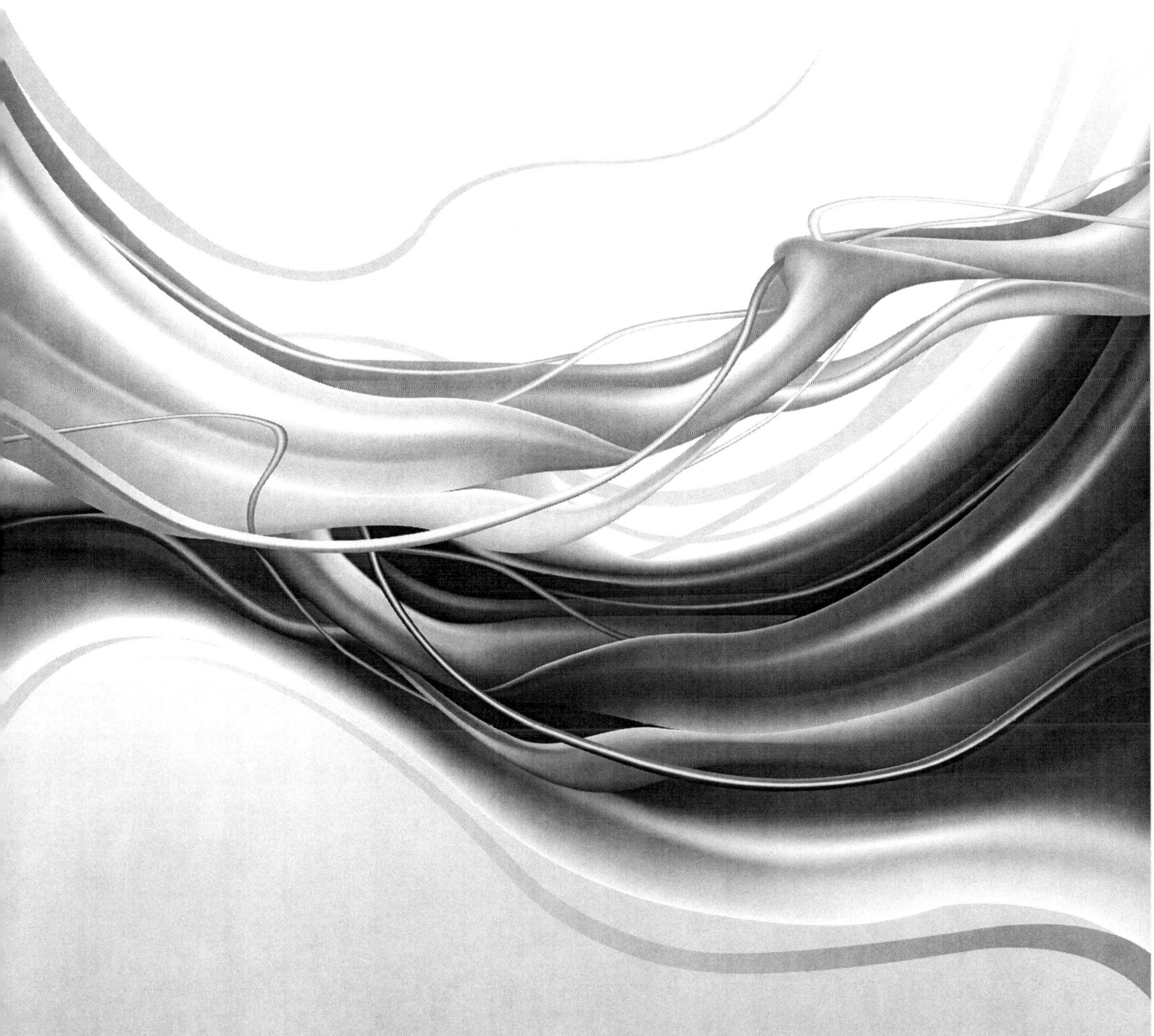

Chapter Sixteen

MULTIPLE CHOICE QUIZ

Name: ______________________

In the box write the letter of the choice that is the definition of the term or best answers the question. There is only one correct answer for each question.

1. A type of epithelial cell in the epidermis is a: ☐
A. Adipocyte
B. Neuron
C. Chondrocyte
D. Histiocyte
E. Squamous cell

2. Dermis: ☐
A. Basal layer of skin
B. Middle layer of skin
C. Epithelial layer
D. Above the epidermis
E. Subcutaneous tissue

3. A hard protein material found in the epidermis: ☐
A. Melanin
B. Sebum
C. Keratin
D. Collagen
E. Cerumen

4. Structural protein found in skin and connective tissue: ☐
A. Cartilage
B. Collagen
C. Cerumen
D. Melanin
E. Sebum

5. Xer/o means: ☐
A. Dry
B. Scaly
C. Thick
D. Yellow
E. White

6. Pertaining to under a nail: ☐
A. Hypodermic
B. Hypoglossal
C. Epidermis
D. Subcutaneous
E. Subungual

7. What is a combining form meaning skin? ☐
A. Ichthy/o
B. Adip/o
C. Cutane/o
D. Pachy/o
E. Xanth/o

8. Absence of pigment in skin: ☐
A. Erythroderma
B. Melanism
C. Xanthoderma
D. Dermatitis
E. Albinism

9. Inflammation of the soft tissue around a nail: ☐
A. Onychomycosis
B. Erythema
C. Epidermolysis
D. Paronychia
E. Dermatitis

10. Profuse sweating: ☐
A. Anhidrosis
B. Diaphoresis
C. Hidradenitis
D. Seborrhea
E. Keratosis

11. Fungal infection: ☐
A. Leukoderma
B. Keratosis
C. Erythema
D. Trichomycosis
E. Seborrhea

12. Fatty mass within a sebaceous gland: ☐
A. Steatoma
B. Lipoma
C. Pilosebaceous
D. Onychophagia
E. Verrucae

13. A wheal is a/an: ....
A. Macule
B. Wart
C. Polyp
D. Ulcer
E. Hive

14. Bullae: ....
A. Papules
B. Macules
C. Fissures
D. Large blisters
E. Nodules

15. Pustule: ....
A. Cyst
B. Pruritus
C. Urticaria
D. Small abscess
E. Ecchymoses

16. Itching: ....
A. Pruritis
B. Petechiae
C. Alopecia
D. Purpura
E. Pruritus

17. Keloid: ....
A. Thickened scar
B. Leukoplakia
C. Comedo
D. Callus
E. Wart

18. Inflammatory disease of the joints and collagen of the skin; can affect other organs of the body: ....
A. Impetigo
B. Systemic lupus erythematosus
C. Mycosis fungoides
D. Actinic keratosis
E. Eczema

19. Moles that can develop into malignant melanoma: ....
A. Basal cell carcinomas
B. Squamous cell carcinomas
C. Verrucae
D. Dysplastic nevi
E. Polyps

20. Bed sore; break in continuity of skin: ....
A. Leukoplakia
B. Psoriasis
C. Tinea
D. Decubitus ulcer
E. Scleroderma

21. Chronic recurrent dermatosis with silvery gray scales covering red patches in skin: ....
A. Leukoplakia
B. Psoriasis
C. Tinea
D. Decubitus ulcer
E. Scleroderma

22. A dermatomycosis: ....
A. Leukoplakia
B. Psoriasis
C. Tinea
D. Decubitus ulcer
E. Scleroderma

23. White patches on a mucous membrane of tongue or cheek: ....
A. Leukoplakia
B. Psoriasis
C. Tinea
D. Decubitus ulcer
E. Scleroderma

24. Connective tissue in the skin hardens: ....
A. Leukoplakia
B. Psoriasis
C. Tinea
D. Decubitus ulcer
E. Scleroderma

25. Layers of growth are removed and examined microscopically: ....
A. Fungal test
B. Scratch test
C. Mohs surgery
D. Cryosurgery
E. Punch biopsy

Chapter Sixteen
VOCABULARY QUIZ

Name: ______________________

A. Match the following terms with their meanings below:

albino
apocrine sweat gland
basal layer
collagen
cuticle
dermis
eccrine sweat gland
epidermis
epithelium
hair follicle

1. Structural protein found in the skin and connective tissue ______________________
2. Middle layer of the skin ______________________
3. Layer of skin cells forming the outer and inner surfaces of the body ______________________
4. Sac within which each hair grows ______________________
5. Person with skin deficient in pigment (melanin) ______________________
6. Band of epidermis at the base and sides of the nail plate ______________________
7. Most numerous of sweat producing glands in the skin ______________________
8. Deepest region of the epidermis; it gives rise to all the epidermal cells ______________________
9. Large dermal exocrine gland; located in axilla and genitals ______________________
10. Outermost layer of the skin ______________________

B. Match the following terms with their meanings below:

adipocyte
integumentary system
keratin
lunula
melanin
paronychium
pore
sebaceous gland
sebum
squamous epithelium
stratified
stratum corneum
subcutaneous layer

1. Fat cell ______________________
2. Tiny opening on the surface of the skin ______________________
3. Oily substance secreted by sebaceous glands ______________________
4. Half-moon–shaped white area at the base of a nail ______________________
5. Soft tissue surrounding the nail border ______________________
6. Arranged in layers ______________________
7. Flat scale-like cells comprising the epidermis ______________________
8. Major skin pigment ______________________
9. Hard protein material found in the epidermis, hair, and nails ______________________
10. Innermost layer of the skin, containing fatty tissue ______________________
11. The skin and its accessory structures, such as hair and nails ______________________
12. Outermost layer of the epidermis; consists of flattened keratinized cells ______________________
13. Oil-secreting gland in the dermis; associated with hair follicles ______________________

Chapter Sixteen

TERMINOLOGY QUIZ

Name: ______________________________

A. Using the following word parts, create or complete terms based on the following definitions:

adip/o	cutane/o	-itis	-plasty
albin/o	derm/o, dermat/o	-lysis	epi-
caus/o	diaphor/o	-ose	sub-
cauter/o	-algia	-ous	

1. Burning pain: ______________________________
2. Scraping away skin (to treat acne or fine wrinkles): ______________________________ abrasion
3. Pertaining to under the skin: ______________________________
4. Pertaining to fat: ______________________________
5. Uppermost (outermost) layer of the skin: ______________________________ dermis
6. Specialist in the study of skin: ______________________________ logist
7. Genetic tendency to have allergic inflammation of the skin: atopic ______________________________
8. Condition of little or no skin pigment: ______________________________ ism
9. Instrument used to burn tissue: electro ______________________________ y
10. Surgical repair of the skin: ______________________________
11. Loosening of the outer layer of skin: ______________________________
12. Condition of sweating: ______________________________ esis

B. Using the following word parts, create or complete terms based on the following definitions:

erythem/o	kerat/o	myc/o	-oma
erythemat/o	leuk/o	onych/o	-osis
hidr/o	lip/o	-cyte	
ichthy/o	melan/o	-ia	

1. Overgrowth and thickening of stratum corneum: ______________________________ osis
2. Benign tumor of fat tissue: ______________________________
3. Condition of lack of sweating: an ______________________________
4. Redness of the skin: ______________________________ a
5. White plaques on the skin or mucous membranes: ______________________________ plakia
6. Dark, pigmented cell in the skin: ______________________________
7. Dry, scaly skin: ______________________________ osis
8. Removal of subcutaneous fat tissue: ______________________________ suction
9. Malignant tumor of pigmented cells in the skin: ______________________________

10. Abnormal condition of fungal infection: ______________________
11. Separation of the nail (plate) from the nail bed: ______________________ lysis
12. Abnormal condition of fungal infection in a nail: ______________________ osis
13. Swelling and infection of soft tissue around a nail: par ______________________

C. Using the following word parts, create or complete terms based on the following definitions:

phyt/o	seb/o	ungu/o	-ectomy
pil/o	squam/o	xanth/o	-oma
py/o	steat/o	xer/o	hyper-
rhytid/o	trich/o	-al	sub-

1. Removal of wrinkles: ______________________
2. Pertaining to under a nail: ______________________
3. Collection of fatty material in a cyst: ______________________ oma
4. Pus within the skin: ______________________ derma
5. Very dry skin: ______________________ osis
6. Nodules of lipid (yellowish) material develop under the skin: ______________________ oma
7. Excessive amount of hair growth ______________________ osis
8. Pertaining to skin cells that are scale-like: ______________________ ous epithelium
9. Excessive secretion from sebaceous glands: ______________________ orrhea
10. Abnormal condition of fungal infection of the skin: dermato ______________________ osis
11. Pertaining to hair follicles and glands that secrete sebum: ______________________ sebaceous

D. Match the following combining forms for colors with their meanings below (HINT: some combining forms will have the same meanings).

albin/o	cyan/o	leuk/o	xanth/o
anthrac/o	eosin/o	lute/o	
chlor/o	erythr/o	melan/o	
cirrh/o	jaund/o	poli/o	

1. gray ______________________
2. blue ______________________
3. black ______________________
4. green ______________________
5. white ______________________
6. rosy ______________________
7. yellow ______________________
8. tawny yellow ______________________
9. red ______________________

Chapter Sixteen
PATHOLOGY QUIZ

Name: ______________________________

A. Match the following cutaneous lesions with their descriptions below:

crust	fissure	papule	ulcer
cyst	macule	polyp	vesicle
erosion	nodule	pustule	wheal

1. Small collection of clear fluid (serum); blister ______________________________
2. Growth extending from the surface of a mucous membrane ______________________________
3. Thick-walled, closed sac containing fluid or semisolid material ______________________________
4. Flat lesion, measuring less than 1 cm in diameter: freckle ______________________________
5. Collection of dried serum and cellular debris ______________________________
6. Smooth edematous area that is redder and paler than surrounding skin ______________________________
7. Solid, round or oval elevated lesion equal to or more than 1 cm in diameter ______________________________
8. Groove or crack-like sore ______________________________
9. Small (less than 1 cm in diameter), solid elevation of the skin ______________________________
10. Papule containing pus ______________________________
11. Wearing away or loss of epidermis ______________________________
12. Open sore on the skin or mucous membranes (deeper than an erosion) ______________________________

B. Match the following pathologic terminology with descriptions given below:

acne	cellulitis	exanthematous viral diseases	urticaria
alopecia	eczema	petechiae	
burns	ecchymoses	pruritus	

1. Acute allergic reaction in which red, round wheals develop on the skin ______________________________
2. Itching ______________________________
3. Chronic papular and pustular eruption of the skin with increased sebum production ______________________________
4. Absence of hair from areas where it normally grows ______________________________
5. Small pinpoint hemorrhages ______________________________
6. Diffuse, acute infection of the skin marked by local heat, redness, pain, and swelling ______________________________

7. Injury to tissue caused by heat contact ______________________

8. Bluish black (purplish large lesions) on the skin ______________________

9. Rubella, rubeola, and varicella are examples ______________________

10. Inflammatory skin disease with erythematous, papulovesicular lesions (atopic dermatitis is an example) ______________________

C. Match the following pathologic terminology with descriptions given below:

callus	keloid	scleroderma	vitiligo
gangrene	psoriasis	systemic lupus erythematosus	
impetigo	scabies	tinea	

1. Chronic autoimmune inflammatory disease of collagen in skin, joints, and internal organs (butterfly erythematous rash is characteristic) ______________________

2. Infection of the skin caused by a fungus ______________________

3. Hypertrophied, thickened scar occurring after trauma or surgical incision ______________________

4. Loss of pigmentation in areas of the skin ______________________

5. Chronic, progressive disease of skin and internal organs with hardening and shrinking of connective tissue ______________________

6. Chronic, recurrent dermatosis marked by itchy, scaly red patches covered by silvery gray scales ______________________

7. Death of tissue associated with loss of blood supply ______________________

8. Contagious parasitic infection of the skin with intense pruritus ______________________

9. Increased growth of cells in the keratin layer of the epidermis caused by pressure or friction ______________________

10. Bacterial inflammatory skin disease marked by vesicles, pustules, and crusted-over lesions ______________________

D. Match the following pathologic terminology with descriptions given below:

basal cell carcinoma	leukoplakia	squamous cell carcinoma
Kaposi sarcoma	malignant melanoma	urticaria (hives)
keratosis	nevus	verruca

1. Pigmented lesion of the skin; a mole ______________________

2. Thickened and rough lesion of the epidermis; associated with aging or skin damage ______________________

3. Epidermal growth (wart) caused by a virus ______________________

4. Malignant tumor of the basal cell layer of the epidermis ______________________

5. Malignant, vascular, neoplastic growth characterized by cutaneous nodules ______________________

6. White, thickened patches on mucous membrane tissue of the tongue or cheek ______________________

7. Malignant tumor of squamous epithelial cells in the epidermis ______________________

8. Cancerous growth composed of melanocytes ______________________

9. Acute allergic reaction in which red, round wheals develop on the skin ______________________

Chapter Sixteen

LABORATORY TESTS AND CLINICAL PROCEDURES QUIZ

Name: ______________________________

Match the names for the following laboratory tests and clinical procedures with their descriptions below:

bacterial analyses	electrodesiccation	skin biopsy
cryosurgery	fungal tests	skin testing
curettage	Mohs micrographic surgery	

1. Use of subfreezing temperatures (liquid nitrogen application) to destroy tissue ______________________
2. Suspected malignant lesions are removed and examined microscopically in a pathology laboratory ______________________
3. Tissue is destroyed by burning with an electric spark ______________________
4. Samples of skin are examined for presence of microorganisms ______________________
5. Substances are injected intradermally or applied to the skin and results are observed ______________________
6. Thin layers of malignant tissue are removed and each is examined microscopically ______________________
7. Scrapings from skin lesions, hair specimens, or nail clippings are sent to a laboratory for culture and microscopic examination (KOH test may be used) ______________________
8. Use of a sharp dermal instrument (shaped like a spoon) to scrape away a lesion ______________________

Chapter Sixteen

ABBREVIATIONS QUIZ

Name: ______________________________

On the line provided, give meanings for the following abbreviations, then write each abbreviation next to its explanation below:

1. ABCDE ______________________________
2. bx ______________________________
3. Derm. ______________________________
4. DLE ______________________________
5. PPD ______________________________
6. PUVA ______________________________
7. SC ______________________________
8. SLE ______________________________

a. __________ Treatment for psoriasis and other skin conditions

b. __________ Photo-sensitive scaling, plaque-like, superficial eruption of the skin

c. __________ Study of the skin

d. __________ Under the skin

e. __________ Skin test for tuberculosis

f. __________ Characteristics associated with melanoma

g. __________ Autoimmune inflammatory disease of collagen in skin, joints, and internal organs

h. __________ Removal of tissue and microscopic examination

Chapter Sixteen
EXERCISE QUIZ

Name: ______________________________

A. Select from the following to complete the sentences below:

adipocyte	cuticle	lunula	stratum corneum
basal layer	dermis	melanin	
collagen	keratin	sebum	

1. A fat cell is a ______________________________
2. The half-moon–shaped white area at the base of a nail is called the ______________________________
3. A structural protein found in skin and connective tissue is ______________________________
4. A black pigment found in the epidermis is ______________________________
5. The deepest region of the epidermis is the ______________________________
6. The outermost layer of the epidermis, consisting of flattened keratinized cells is the ______________________________
7. An oily substance secreted by sebaceous glands is ______________________________
8. The middle layer of the skin is the corium or ______________________________
9. A hard protein material found in epidermis, hair, and nails is ______________________________
10. A band of epidermis at the base and side of the nail plate is the ______________________________

B. Complete the following terms from their meanings given below:

11. The outermost layer of skin: epi ______________________________
12. Profuse sweating: dia ______________________________
13. Excessive secretion from sebaceous glands: sebo ______________________________
14. Inflammation and swelling of soft tissue around a nail: par ______________________________
15. Fungal infection of hands and feet: dermato ______________________________
16. Burning sensation (pain) in the skin: caus ______________________________

C. Build medical terms from the definitions and word parts given:

17. surgical repair of the skin: dermato ______________________________
18. pertaining to under the skin: sub ______________________________
19. abnormal condition of lack of sweat: an ______________________________
20. abnormal condition of proliferation of keratinized cells: kerat ______________________________
21. abnormal condition of dry, scaly (fish-like) skin: ______________________________ osis
22. loosening of the epidermis: epidermo ______________________________

23. yellow tumor (nodule under the skin): ______________________ oma
24. under the nail: sub ______________________
25. abnormal condition of nail fungus: onycho ______________________

D. Match the cutaneous lesion with its meaning below.

cyst	macule	papule	pustule	vesicle
fissure	nodule	polyp	ulcer	wheal

26. circumscribed collection of clear fluid (blister) ______________________
27. smooth, slightly elevated edematous area (hive) ______________________
28. discolored, flat lesion (freckle or patch) ______________________
29. groove or crack-like sore ______________________
30. mushroom-like growth extending from the surface of a mucous membrane ______________________
31. circumscribed collection of pus ______________________
32. closed sac containing fluid or semisolid material ______________________
33. open sore or erosion of skin ______________________
34. solid elevation of the skin (pimple) ______________________
35. larger than 1 cm solid elevation of the skin ______________________

E. Give medical terms for the following:

36. baldness ______________________
37. itching ______________________
38. blackhead ______________________
39. purplish, macular patch ______________________
40. loss of pigment in skin ______________________
41. small pinpoint hemorrhages ______________________

F. Give the term that fits the definition (some letters or word parts are given):

42. contagious parasitic infection with intense pruritus: sc ______________________
43. white patches on mucous membrane of tongue or cheek: leuko ______________________
44. characterized by a rash: ex ______________________
45. colored pigmentation of the skin (mole): n ______________________
46. acute, allergic reaction in which hives develop: u ______________________
47. large blisters: b ______________________
48. raised, thickened scar: k ______________________
49. sac of fluid and hair over the sacral region of the back: p ______________________ cyst
50. chickenpox: v ______________________

G. Match the pathologic skin condition with its description below:

acne	gangrene	psoriasis	tinea
decubitus ulcer	impetigo	scleroderma	
eczema	malignant melanoma	systemic lupus erythematosus	

51. Buildup of sebum and keratin in pores of the skin leading to papular and pustular eruptions ____________________

52. Fungal skin infection ____________________

53. Chronic hardening and shrinking of connective tissue ____________________

54. Bedsore ____________________

55. Necrosis of skin tissue resulting from ischemia ____________________

56. Contagious, infectious pyoderma ____________________

57. Chronic, recurrent dermatosis marked by silvery gray scales covering red patches on the skin ____________________

58. Cancerous tumor composed of melanocytes ____________________

59. Widespread inflammatory disease of joints and collagen of the skin with "butterfly" rash on the face ____________________

60. Chronic or acute inflammatory skin disease with erythematous, pustular, or papular lesions ____________________

H. Give short answers for the following:

61. Two skin tests for allergy are ____________________ and ____________________

62. A surgical procedure to core out a disk of skin for microscopic analysis is a ____________________

63. The procedure in which thin layers of malignant growth are removed and each is microscopically analyzed is ____________________

64. Moles that do not form properly and may progress to form melanomas are called ____________________

65. Destruction of tissue by intensely cold temperatures is called ____________________

Chapter Sixteen

DICTATION AND COMPREHENSION QUIZ: VOCABULARY, COMBINING FORMS, AND SUFFIXES

Name: ______________________________

A. Dictation of Terms

1.	____________	11.	____________
2.	____________	12.	____________
3.	____________	13.	____________
4.	____________	14.	____________
5.	____________	15.	____________
6.	____________	16.	____________
7.	____________	17.	____________
8.	____________	18.	____________
9.	____________	19.	____________
10.	____________	20.	____________

B. Comprehension of Terms: Match number of the above term with its meaning below.

______ Tumor of fatty tissue
______ Half-moon–shaped white area at the base of a nail
______ Condition of absence of pigment in the skin
______ Pigment that gives the skin color
______ Band of epidermis at the base and sides of the nail plate
______ Intensely unpleasant burning sensation in skin
______ Scraping away of skin (to remove tattoos or fine wrinkles)
______ Pertaining to redness of the skin
______ Condition of absence of sweating
______ Baldness
______ Condition of white plaques (spots or patches) on the tongue or cheek
______ Separation of the nail plate from the nail bed
______ Inflammation of skin with yellow or brown-gray greasy scales (dandruff)
______ Pertaining to under a nail
______ Inflammation and swelling of the soft tissue around the nail
______ Dry skin
______ Pertaining to hair and glands that secrete sebum
______ Abnormal condition of thickened area of the epidermis
______ Abnormal condition of a fungal infection of the skin
______ Structural protein found in the skin and connective tissue

Chapter Sixteen

DICTATION AND COMPREHENSION QUIZ: PATHOLOGY

Name: ______________________________

A. Dictation of Terms

1.	______________________________	11.	______________________________
2.	______________________________	12.	______________________________
3.	______________________________	13.	______________________________
4.	______________________________	14.	______________________________
5.	______________________________	15.	______________________________
6.	______________________________	16.	______________________________
7.	______________________________	17.	______________________________
8.	______________________________	18.	______________________________
9.	______________________________	19.	______________________________
10.	______________________________	20.	______________________________

B. Comprehension of Terms: Match number of the above term with its meaning below.

______ Infection of the skin caused by a fungus
______ Increased growth of cells in the horny (keratinized) layer of the epidermis
______ Hypertrophied, thickened scar that occurs after trauma or surgical incision
______ Normal scar left by a healed wound
______ Bacterial inflammatory skin disease; a contagious pyoderma
______ Papular and pustular eruption of the skin; comedones occur
______ Chronic, recurrent dermatosis marked by itchy, scaly, red patches covered by silvery gray scales
______ Inflammatory skin disease with erythematous, papulovesicular lesions; common allergic reaction in children and adults
______ Loss of pigment in areas of the skin
______ Itching
______ Bluish black marks on the skin caused by hemorrhages into the skin
______ Large areas of bleeding under the skin
______ Death of tissue associated with loss of blood supply
______ A small solid elevation of the skin (pimple)
______ A smooth slightly elevated edematous area that is redder or paler than the surrounding skin
______ An acute allergic reaction of the skin with hives and itching
______ Bedsore
______ Malignant tumor of cells in the epidermal layer of the skin
______ An exanthematous viral disease; German measles
______ Large vesicles

Chapter Sixteen
SPELLING QUIZ

Name: ______________________________

A. Circle the term that is spelled correctly and write its meaning in the space provided:

1.	paroncyhia	paronychia ______________________
2.	pilosebaceous	pillosebaecous ______________________
3.	subungwnal	subungual ______________________
4.	xanthoma	xanantoma ______________________
5.	dermatophytosis	dermatophitosis ______________________
6.	wheel	wheal ______________________
7.	verruca	veruca ______________________
8.	callis	callus ______________________
9.	keratosis	carrotosis ______________________
10.	tinnea	tinea ______________________

B. Circle the term that is spelled correctly. The meaning of each term is given.

11.	Inflammatory skin disease	ezcema	eksema	eczema
12.	Itching..	pruritis	purtritis	pruritus
13.	Red, round wheals (hives)	urticaria	urtakaria	urtikaria
14.	Malignant tumor of pigmented skin cells	melenoma	melonoma	melanoma
15.	Mole..	nevus	nevas	nevis
16.	Blackhead..	komedo	comedo	comeddo
17.	Absence of skin pigment	albinism	allbinism	albenism
18.	Chronic recurrent dermatosis with itchy, scaly patches...........................	psoriesis	psoraisis	psoriasis
19.	Structural protein found in skin and connective tissue	collegen	kollagen	collagen
20.	Profuse sweating.......................................	diaphoresis	diaforesis	diaphoriesis

Chapter Sixteen
PRONUNCIATION QUIZ

Name: ______________________________

A. Underline the accented syllable in the following terms:

1. impetigo
2. erythema
3. eczema
4. pilonidal cyst
5. dermatomycosis
6. steatoma
7. vitiligo
8. sebaceous gland
9. epithelium
10. albinism

B. Match the term in Column I with its meaning in Column II:

Column I		Column II
1. adipose	_______	A. A collection of pigmented cells on the skin surface
2. dermis	_______	B. Layer of skin cells on outer and inner surfaces on the body
3. epithelium	_______	C. Pertaining to fat
4. urticaria	_______	D. Hard protein material found in the skin, hair, and nails
5. paronychia	_______	E. Structural protein found in the skin and connective tissue
6. tinea	_______	F. Hives
7. melanin	_______	G. A black pigment formed by cells in the skin
8. nevus	_______	H. Fungal infection of the skin
9. keratin	_______	I. The middle layer of the skin; corium
10. collagen	_______	J. Inflammation of soft tissue around the skin

C. Complete the following terms using the definitions given:

1. epidermo ____________________	Loosening of the epidermis
2. ____________________ itis	Inflammation of sweat glands
3. ____________________ cyte	Fat cell
4. ____________________ esis	Excessive or profuse sweating
5. ____________________ ous	Pertaining to under the skin
6. ____________________ o	A blackhead
7. ____________________ osis	A purplish patch on the skin caused by hemorrhage
8. ____________________ous	Pertaining to hair and oil glands
9. ____________________ oid	Hypertrophied, thickened scar
10. ____________________a	Fungal infection of the skin

Chapter Sixteen
DIAGRAM QUIZ 1

Name: ______________________________

Label the diagram below using the terms listed below:

Fissure	Nodule
Crust	Papule
Cyst	Wheal
Erosion	Ulcer
Polyp	Vesicle
Macule	Pustule

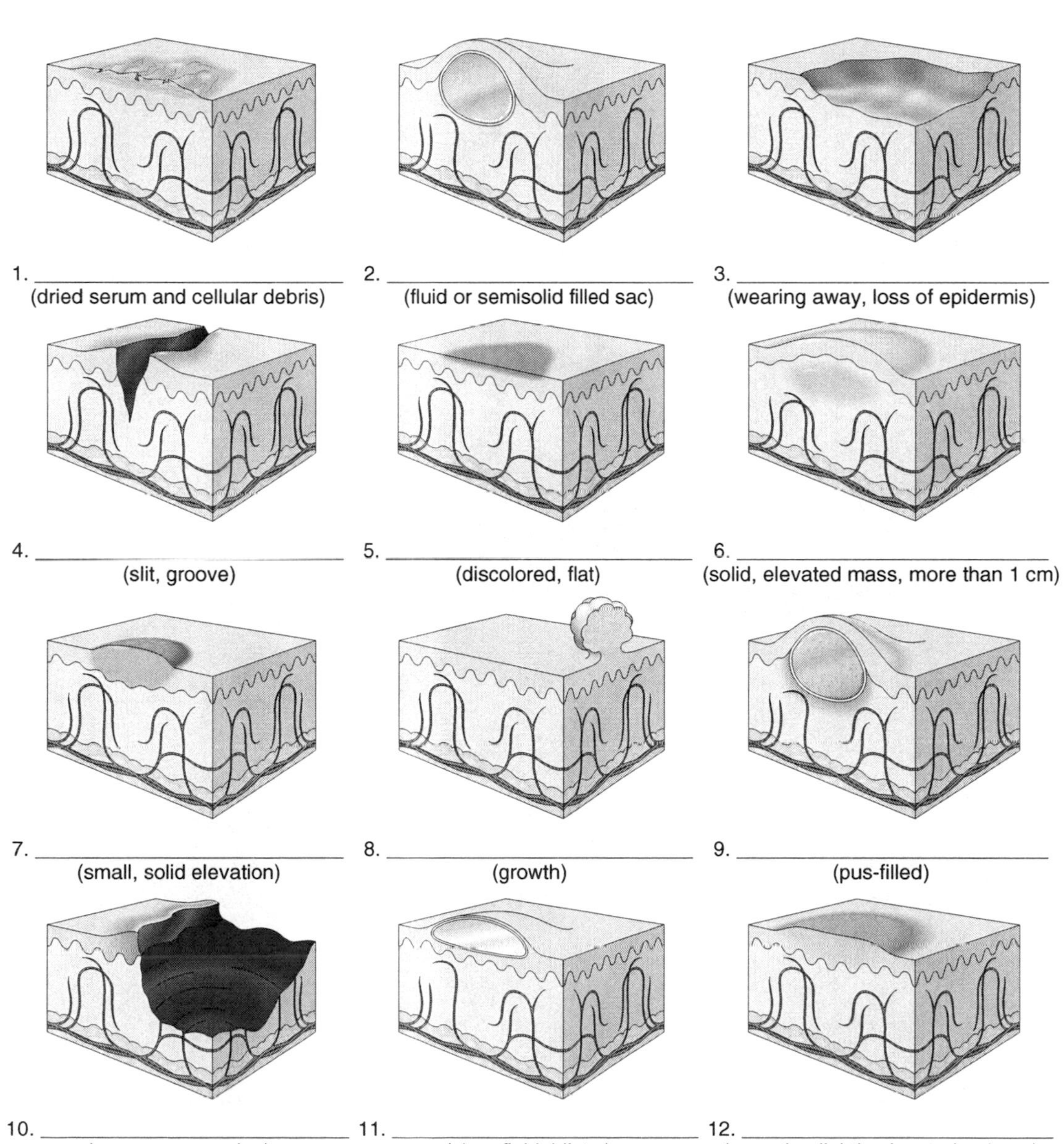

Chapter Sixteen
DIAGRAM QUIZ 2

Name: ______________________________

Label the diagram below using the terms listed below:

basal layer
dermis
epidermis
melanocytes
stratum corneum
subcutaneous layer

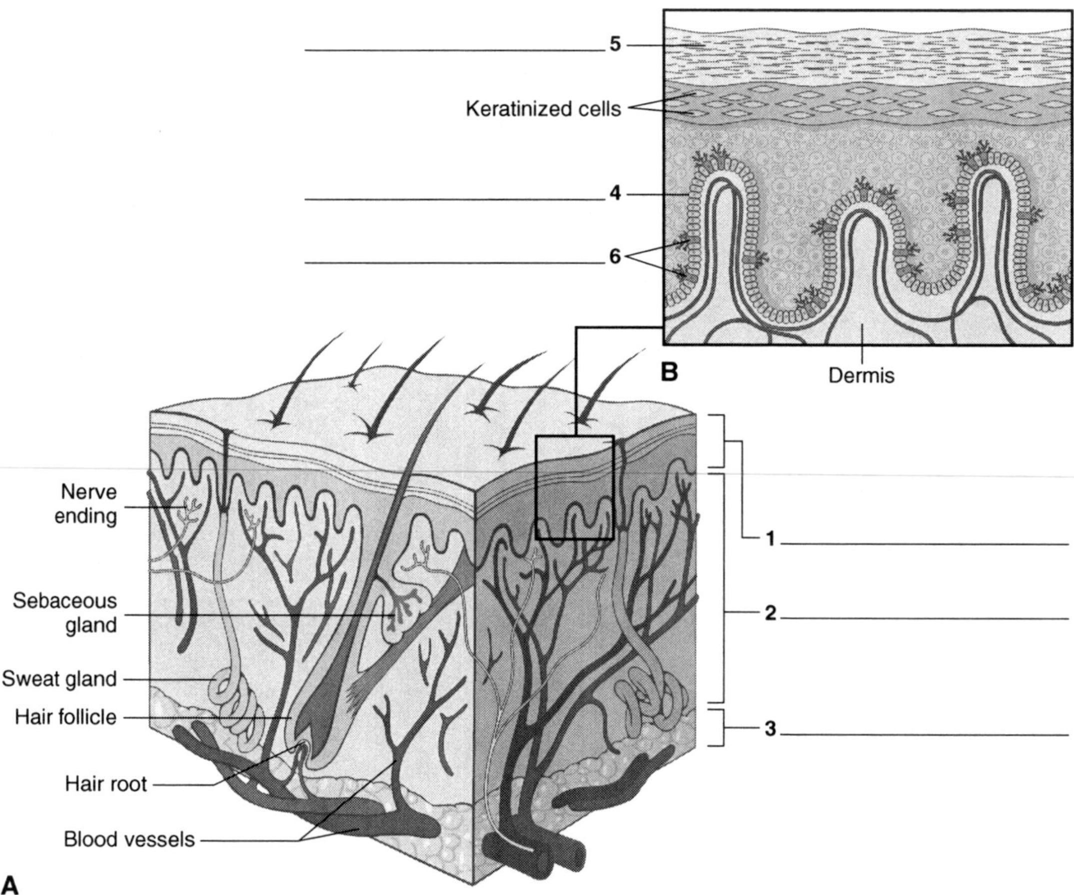

Chapter Sixteen
REVIEW SHEET QUIZ

Name: ______________________________

A. Give meanings for the following combining forms:

1. adip/o ____________________
2. albin/o ____________________
3. caus/o ____________________
4. cutane/o ____________________
5. dermat/o ____________________
6. diaphor/o ____________________
7. erythem/o ____________________
8. hidr/o ____________________
9. hydr/o ____________________
10. trich/o ____________________
11. onych/o ____________________
12. myc/o ____________________
13. ungu/o ____________________
14. lip/o ____________________
15. pil/o ____________________

B. Give combining forms for the following meanings:

1. pus ____________________
2. black ____________________
3. dry ____________________
4. yellow ____________________
5. wrinkle ____________________
6. scaly, fish-like ____________________

C. Give meanings for the following suffixes:

1. -algia ____________________
2. -derma ____________________
3. -lysis ____________________
4. -osis ____________________
5. -ous ____________________
6. -plakia ____________________
7. -plasty ____________________
8. -rrhea ____________________

Chapter Sixteen
MEDICAL SCRAMBLE

Name: ______________________

Unscramble the letters to form dermatologic terms from the clues. Use the letters in the squares to complete the bonus term.

1. *Clue:* Small skin elevation containing pus

   __ __ __ ☐ __ __ ☐ U P E S L U T

2. *Clue:* Contagious, parasitic infection with intense pruritus

   __ __ ☐ __ __ ☐ __ I B S A C E S

3. *Clue:* Epidermal growth caused by a virus

   __ __ ☐ __ ☐ ☐ __ C R E R A V U

4. *Clue:* Loss of pigmentation

   __ __ ☐ __ __ __ ☐ __ I G I L O V T I

BONUS TERM: *Clue:* Procedure using a sharp instrument to scrape away skin lesions

☐ ☐ ☐ ☐ ☐ ☐ ☐ ☐ ☐

Chapter Sixteen
CROSSWORD PUZZLE

Name: ____________________

Fill in the crossword puzzle below using the clues listed underneath it.

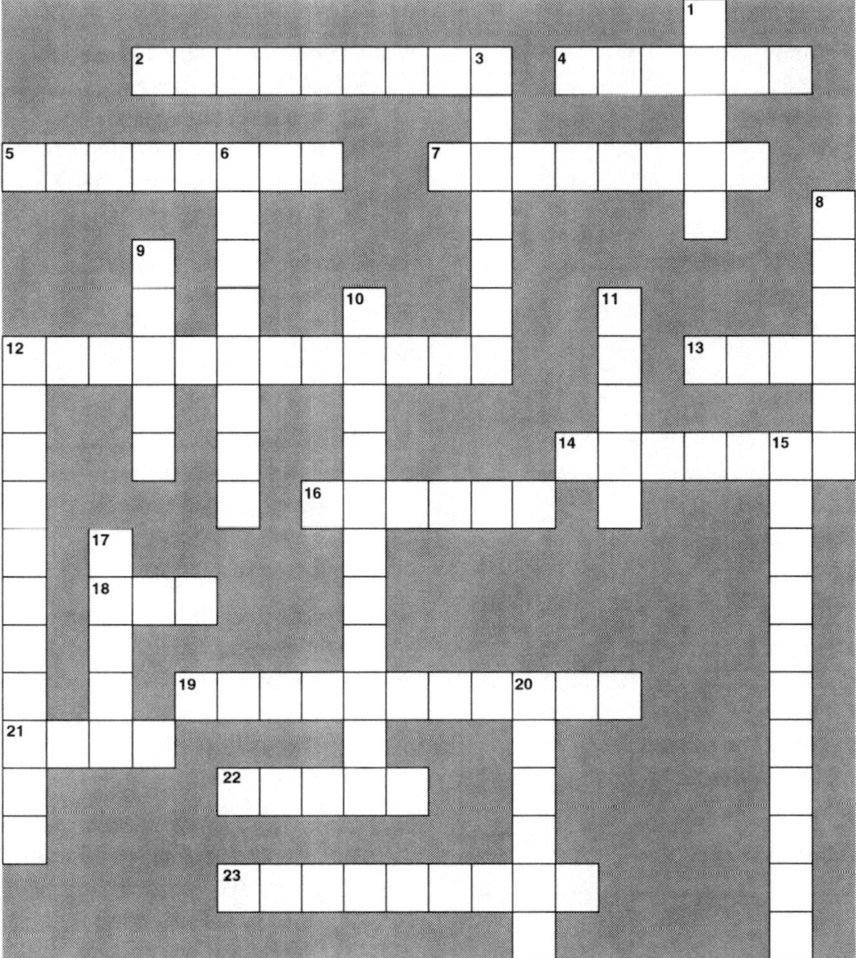

Across Clues

2. Chronic recurrent dermatosis marked by itchy, scaly, red patches covered by silvery scales.
4. Small, solid elevation of the skin.
5. Depigmentation in areas of the skin.
7. Death of tissue from loss of blood supply.
12. Innermost layer of the skin (under the skin).
13. Papular and pustular eruption of the skin.
14. Wart.
16. Increased growth of cells in the horny layer of the epidermis due to pressure or friction.
18. Outer layer of the skin:_____ dermis.
19. White, thickened patches on mucous membrane tissue of the tongue or cheek.
21. A "butterfly_____"; as in SLE.
22. A mushroom-like growth extending on a stalk from the surface of a mucous membrane.
23. Thickened area of the epidermis; actinic and seborrheic are types.

Down Clues

1. Injuries to tissue caused by heat contact.
3. A contagious, parasitic infection of the skin with intense pruritus.
6. Bacterial, inflammatory, contagious skin disease characterized by vesicles and pustules.
8. Inflammatory skin disease with erythematous papulovesicular lesions.
9. An open sore or erosion of the skin.
10. Study of the skin.
11. Infection of the skin caused by a fungus.
12. A chronic disease of the skin with hardening and shrinking of connective tissue.
15. Tissue is destroyed by the application of intensely cold liquid nitrogen.
17. Colored (pigmented) lesion of the skin; a mole.
20. An enlarged, thickened scar after trauma or surgery.

Chapter Sixteen

PRACTICAL APPLICATIONS

Name: ____________________

The following questions can be used with the Disease Descriptions on page 664 of the text:

1. **Which condition is caused by a fungal infection? ....** ☐
   A. Mycosis fungoides
   B. Candidiasis
   C. Cellulitis
   D. Both A and B

2. **Which condition is cancerous? ....** ☐
   A. Mycosis fungoides
   B. Candidiasis
   C. Cellulitis
   D. Both B and C

3. **Which condition is caused by a bacterial infection? ....** ☐
   A. Mycosis fungoides
   B. Candidiasis
   C. Cellulitis
   D. Both A and C

4. **What is a common location for candidiasis? ....** ☐
   A. Soles of the feet
   B. Lumbar area of the spine
   C. Mouth and genital area
   D. Underarm

5. **Paronychial lesions occur around the: ....** ☐
   A. Nails
   B. Hair follicles
   C. Groin
   D. Armpit

6. **Thrush can occur in the: ....** ☐
   A. Mouth
   B. Vagina
   C. Between the fingers
   D. A and B

7. **Cellulitis is a nonsuppurative infection. This means: ....** ☐
   A. It is not contagious
   B. It is caused by a virus
   C. It affects the epidermis
   D. It is not purulent

8. **Edematous skin means: ....** ☐
   A. Swollen tissue
   B. Reddish brown
   C. White plaques
   D. Skin ulcer

9. **Streptococci are: ....** ☐
   A. Berry-shaped bacteria in clusters
   B. Berry-shaped bacteria in twisted chains
   C. A type of fungus
   D. A type of bacillus

10. **Mycosis fungoides involves malignant: ....** ☐
    A. Erythrocytes
    B. Leukocytes
    C. Thrombocytes
    D. Neutrophils

11. **Generalized erythroderma means: ....** ☐
    A. Lymph nodes are involved
    B. Tumor has invaded the spleen
    C. Widespread red skin
    D. Ulcerations are present

12. **Treatment for mycosis fungoides includes: ....** ☐
    A. Surgery
    B. Dermatologic chemotherapy
    C. Radiotherapy
    D. Both B and C

Chapter Sixteen
ANSWERS TO THE QUIZZES

Multiple Choice Quiz

1. E
2. B
3. C
4. B
5. A
6. E
7. C
8. E
9. D
10. B
11. D
12. A
13. E
14. D
15. D
16. E
17. A
18. B
19. D
20. D
21. B
22. C
23. A
24. E
25. C

Vocabulary Quiz

A

1. collagen
2. dermis
3. epithelium
4. hair follicle
5. albino
6. cuticle
7. eccrine sweat gland
8. basal layer
9. apocrine sweat gland
10. epidermis

B

1. adipocyte
2. pore
3. sebum
4. lunula
5. paronychium
6. stratified
7. squamous epithelium
8. melanin
9. keratin
10. subcutaneous layer
11. integumentary system
12. stratum corneum
13. sebaceous gland

Terminology Quiz

A

1. causalgia
2. dermabrasion
3. subcutaneous
4. adipose
5. epidermis
6. dermatologist
7. atopic dermatitis
8. albinism
9. electrocautery
10. dermatoplasty
11. epidermolysis
12. diaphoresis

B

1. keratosis
2. lipoma
3. anhidrosis
4. erythema
5. leukoplakia
6. melanocyte
7. ichthyosis
8. liposuction
9. melanoma
10. mycosis
11. onycholysis
12. onychomycosis
13. paronychia

C

1. rhytidectomy
2. subungual
3. steatoma
4. pyoderma
5. xerosis
6. xanthoma
7. hypertrichosis
8. squamous epithelium
9. seborrhea
10. dermatophytosis
11. pilosebaceous

D

1. poli/o
2. cyan/o
3. anthrac/o, melan/o,
4. chlor/o
5. albin/o, leuk/o
6. eosin/o
7. jaund/o, lute/o, xanth/o
8. cirrh/o
9. erythr/o

Pathology Quiz

A

1. vesicle
2. polyp
3. cyst
4. macule
5. crust
6. wheal
7. nodule
8. fissure
9. papule
10. pustule
11. erosion
12. ulcer

B

1. urticaria
2. pruritus
3. acne
4. alopecia
5. petechiae
6. cellulitis
7. burns
8. ecchymoses
9. exanthematous viral diseases
10. eczema

C

1. systemic lupus erythematosus
2. tinea
3. keloid
4. vitiligo
5. scleroderma
6. psoriasis
7. gangrene
8. scabies
9. callus
10. impetigo

D

1. nevus
2. keratosis
3. verruca
4. basal cell carcinoma
5. Kaposi sarcoma
6. leukoplakia
7. squamous cell carcinoma
8. malignant melanoma
9. urticaria (hives)

Laboratory Tests and Clinical Procedures Quiz

1. cryosurgery
2. skin biopsy
3. electrodesiccation
4. bacterial analyses
5. skin testing
6. Mohs micrographic surgery
7. fungal tests
8. curettage

Abbreviations Quiz

1. asymmetry (of shape), border (irregularity), color (variation within one lesion), diameter (greater than 6 mm), evolution (change)
2. biopsy
3. dermatology
4. discoid lupus erythematosus
5. purified protein derivative
6. psoralen–ultraviolet A light therapy
7. subcutaneous
8. systemic lupus erythematosus

a. PUVA
b. DLE
c. Derm.
d. SC
e. PPD
f. ABCDE
g. SLE
h. bx

Exercise Quiz

A

1. adipocyte
2. lunula
3. collagen
4. melanin
5. basal layer
6. stratum corneum
7. sebum
8. dermis
9. keratin
10. cuticle

B

11. epidermis
12. diaphoresis
13. seborrhea
14. paronychia
15. dermatomycosis
16. causalgia

C

17. dermatoplasty
18. subcutaneous
19. anhidrosis
20. keratosis
21. ichthyosis
22. epidermolysis
23. xanthoma
24. subungual
25. onychomycosis

D

26. vesicle
27. wheal
28. macule
29. fissure
30. polyp
31. pustule
32. cyst
33. ulcer
34. papule
35. nodule

E

36. alopecia
37. pruritus
38. comedo
39. purpura
40. albinism
41. petechiae

F

42. scabies
43. leukoplakia
44. exanthematous
45. nevus
46. urticaria
47. bullae
48. keloid
49. pilonidal cyst
50. varicella

G

51. acne
52. tinea
53. scleroderma
54. decubitus ulcer
55. gangrene
56. impetigo
57. psoriasis
58. malignant melanoma
59. systemic lupus erythematosus
60. eczema

H

61. patch and scratch
62. punch biopsy
63. Mohs surgery
64. dysplastic nevi
65. cryosurgery

Dictation and Comprehension: Vocabulary, Combining Forms, and Suffixes

A

1. albinism
2. alopecia
3. anhidrosis
4. causalgia
5. collagen
6. cuticle
7. dermabrasion
8. dermatomycosis
9. erythematous
10. keratosis
11. leukoplakia
12. lipoma
13. lunula
14. melanin
15. onycholysis
16. paronychia
17. pilosebaceous
18. seborrheic dermatitis
19. subungual
20. xerosis

B

12 Tumor of fatty tissue
13 Half-moon–shaped white area at the base of a nail
1 Condition of absence of pigment in the skin
14 Pigment that gives the skin color
6 Band of epidermis at the base and sides of the nail plate
4 Intensely unpleasant burning sensation in skin
7 Scraping away of skin (to remove tattoos or fine wrinkles)
9 Pertaining to redness of the skin
3 Condition of absence of sweating
2 Baldness
11 Condition of white plaques (spots or patches) on the tongue or cheek
15 Separation of the nail plate from the nail bed
18 Inflammation of skin with yellow or brown-gray greasy scales (dandruff)
19 Pertaining to under a nail
16 Inflammation and swelling of the soft tissue around the nail
20 Dry skin
17 Pertaining to hair and glands that secrete sebum
10 Abnormal condition of thickened area of the epidermis
8 Abnormal condition of a fungal infection of the skin
5 Structural protein found in the skin and connective tissue

Dictation and Comprehension: Pathology

A

1. acne
2. basal cell carcinoma
3. bullae
4. callus

5. cicatrix
6. decubitus ulcer
7. ecchymoses
8. eczema
9. gangrene
10. impetigo
11. keloid
12. papule
13. pruritus
14. psoriasis
15. purpura
16. rubella
17. tinea
18. urticaria
19. vitiligo
20. wheal

B

17 Infection of the skin caused by a fungus
4 Increased growth of cells in the horny (keratinized) layer of the epidermis
11 Hypertrophied, thickened scar that occurs after trauma or surgical incision
5 Normal scar left by a healed wound
10 Bacterial inflammatory skin disease; a contagious pyoderma
1 Papular and pustular eruption of the skin; comedones occur
14 Chronic, recurrent dermatosis marked by itchy, scaly, red patches covered by silvery gray scales
8 Inflammatory skin disease with erythematous, papulovesicular lesions; common allergic reaction in children and adults
19 Loss of pigment in areas of the skin
13 Itching
7 Bluish black marks on the skin caused by hemorrhages into the skin
15 Large areas of bleeding under the skin
9 Death of tissue associated with loss of blood supply
12 A small solid elevation of the skin (pimple)
20 A smooth slightly elevated edematous area that is redder or paler than the surrounding skin
18 An acute allergic reaction of the skin with hives and itching
6 Bedsore
2 malignant tumor of cells in the epidermal layer of the skin
16 An exanthematous viral disease; German measles
3 Large vesicles

Spelling Quiz

A

1. paronychia—infection of the nail bed
2. pilosebaceous—pertaining to hair and sebaceous gland
3. subungual—pertaining to under a nail
4. xanthoma—lipid collection under the skin
5. dermatophytosis—abnormal condition of fungal infection of the skin
6. wheal—smooth, slightly elevated swollen area
7. verruca—wart
8. callus—increased growth in epidermis due to pressure
9. keratosis—thickened area of the epidermis
10. tinea—fungal infection of the skin

B

11. eczema
12. pruritus
13. urticaria
14. melanoma
15. nevus
16. comedo
17. albinism
18. psoriasis
19. collagen
20. diaphoresis

Pronunciation Quiz

A

1. impetigo
2. erythema
3. eczema
4. pilonidal cyst
5. dermatomycosis
6. steatoma
7. vitiligo
8. sebaceous gland
9. epithelium
10. albinism

B

1. C
2. I
3. B
4. F
5. J
6. H
7. G
8. A
9. D
10. E

C

1. epidermolysis
2. hidradenitis
3. adipocyte
4. diaphoresis
5. subcutaneous
6. comedo
7. ecchymosis
8. pilosebaceous
9. keloid
10. tinea

Diagram Quiz 1

1. Crust
2. Cyst
3. Erosion
4. Fissure
5. Macule
6. Nodule
7. Papule
8. Polyp
9. Pustule
10. Ulcer
11. Vesicle
12. Wheal

Diagram Quiz 2

1. epidermis
2. dermis
3. subcutaneous layer
4. basal layer
5. stratum corneum
6. melanocytes

Review Sheet Quiz

A

1. fat
2. white
3. burn, burning
4. skin
5. skin
6. profuse sweating
7. redness
8. sweat
9. water
10. hair
11. nail
12. fungus
13. nail

14. fat
15. hair

B

1. py/o
2. melan/o
3. xer/o
4. xanth/o
5. rhytid/o
6. ichyth/o

C

1. pain
2. skin
3. separation, breakdown
4. condition, abnormal condition
5. pertaining to
6. plaque
7. surgical repair
8. flow, discharge

Medical Scramble

1. PUSTULE
2. SCABIES
3. VERRUCA
4. VITILIGO

BONUS TERM: CURETTAGE

Crossword Puzzle

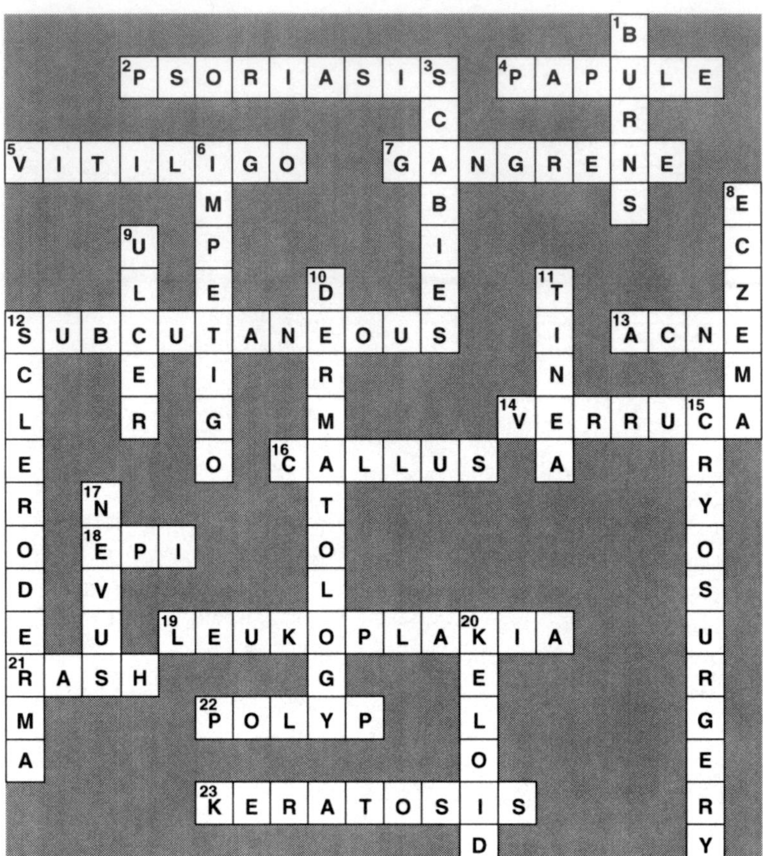

Practical Applications

1. B
2. A
3. C
4. C
5. A
6. D
7. D
8. A
9. B
10. B
11. C
12. D

Chapter Sixteen
Answers to Terminology Section

(textbook pages 658–661)

Terminology	Meaning
Combining Forms	
adipose	Pertaining to fat.
albinism	Condition of no pigment in skin, hair, and eyes (white skin).
causalgia	Intense burning sensation in the skin (due to nerve damage).
electrocautery	Wires used during surgery to burn through tissue.
subcutaneous	Pertaining to beneath the skin.
epidermis	Outermost layer of skin.
dermatitis	Inflammation of skin.
dermatoplasty	Surgical repair of the skin.
dermatologist	Specialist in diseases of the skin.
dermabrasion	A surgical procedure to remove acne scars, tattoos, and fine wrinkles. Skin is scraped away; sandpaper or mechanical methods are used on frozen skin.
epidermolysis	Loosening of the skin.
diaphoresis	Condition of profuse sweating.
erythema	Condition of redness of the skin (flushing).
anhidrosis	Condition of lack of sweat.
ichthyosis	Abnormal condition of dry, scaly skin (fish-like skin).
keratosis	Abnormal condition of thickened areas of the skin (horny cells accumulate).
leukoplakia	Condition of white plaques on the skin.
lipoma	Tumor (benign) of fat tissue.
liposuction	Removal of subcutaneous fat tissue with a blunt-tipped cannula (tube) through which suction (aspiration) is applied.
melanocyte	Cell that forms melanin and is found in the epidermis of the skin.
melanoma	Tumor (malignant) of melanocytes.
mycosis	Any disease caused by fungus.
onycholysis	Separation of nail plate from the nail bed in fungal infections or after trauma.
onychomycosis	Abnormal condition of fungal infection of nails.
paronychia	Condition of inflammation and swelling (infection) of the tissue around the nail.
dermatophytosis	Abnormal condition of fungus (plant) infection in the skin.
pilosebaceous	Pertaining to a sebaceous gland and hair.
pyoderma	Condition of pus infection within the skin.
rhytidectomy	Removal of wrinkles.
seborrhea	"Flow of sebum"; disturbance of sebaceous glands marked by increase in the flow of sebum.
squamous epithelium	Pertaining to scale-like cells that cover the outside of the body (epidermis) and line the inner tubes of the body.
steatoma	Fatty mass arising from sebaceous glands; sebaceous cyst.
hypertrichosis	Excessive amount of hair growth.
subungual	Pertaining to under a nail.
xanthoma	Flat, slightly elevated, rounded plaque or nodule usually found on the eyelids.
xerosis	Abnormal condition of dry, rough skin.

Chapter 17

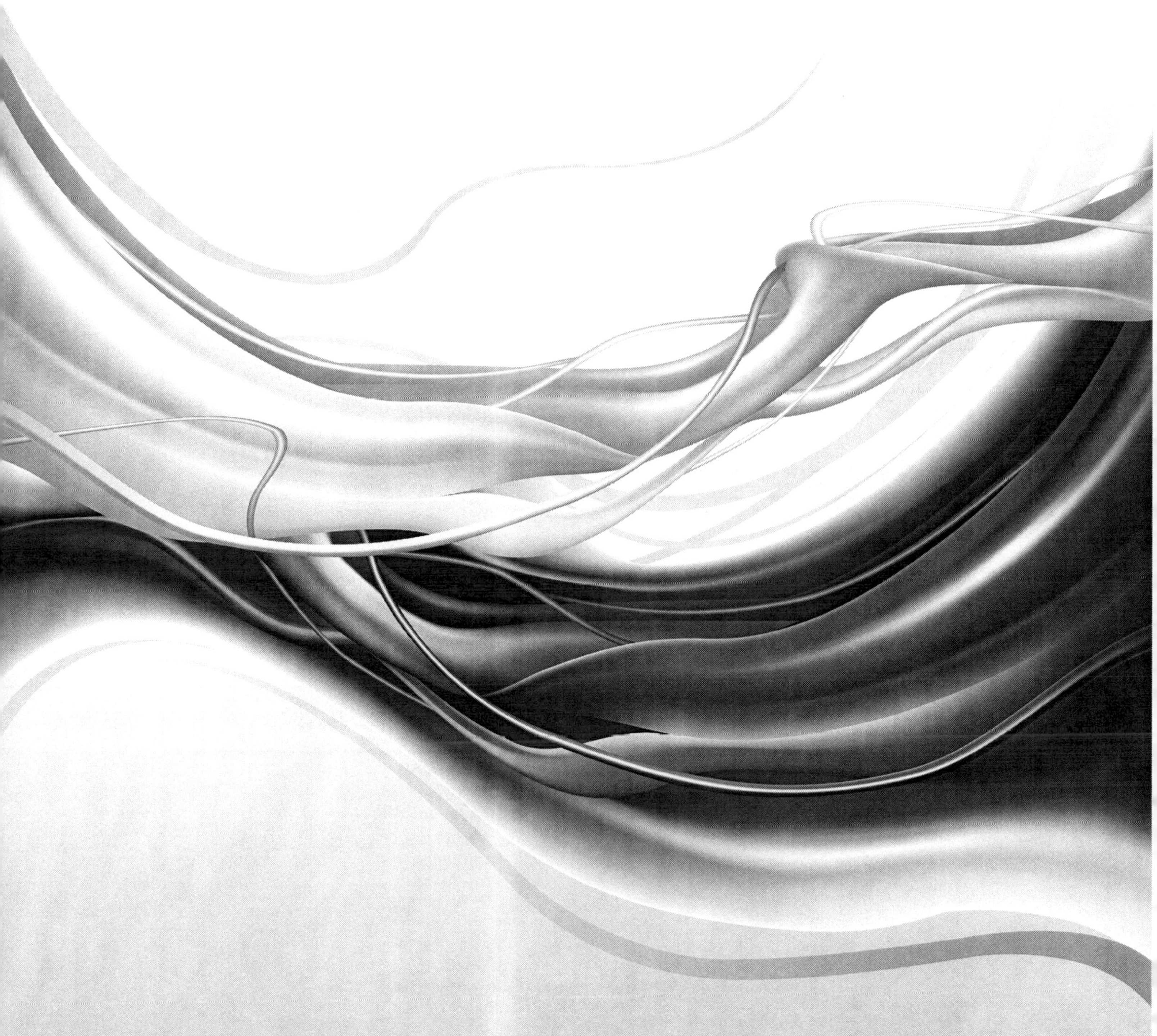

Chapter Seventeen

MULTIPLE CHOICE QUIZ

Name: ______________________________

In the box write the letter of the choice that is the definition of the term or best answers the question. There is only one correct answer for each question.

1. Fibrous layer of clear tissue that extends over the anterior portion of the eye and is continuous with the white of the eye: ☐

A. Fundus
B. Ciliary body
C. Pupil
D. Cornea
E. Iris

2. Yellowish region in the retina; contains the fovea centralis: ☐

A. Optic disc
B. Posterior chamber
C. Macula lutea
D. Sclera
E. Choroid

3. What eye structure is transparent, biconvex, and focuses light on the retina? ☐

A. Conjunctiva
B. Lens
C. Vitreous body
D. Aqueous humor
E. Sclera

4. Place where optic nerve fibers cross in the brain: ☐

A. Optic disc
B. Optic chiasma
C. Retina
D. Olfactory lobe
E. Cerebral cortex

5. Adjustment of the lens by the ciliary body: ☐

A. Accommodation
B. Refraction
C. Binocular vision
D. Photophobia
E. Amblyopia

6. Photosensitive receptor cells of the retina; make the perception of color possible: ☐

A. Rods
B. Cones
C. Megakaryocyte
D. Optic disc
E. Optic chiasm

7. The combining form for cornea is: ☐

A. Ocul/o
B. Opt/o
C. Scler/o
D. Choroid/o
E. Kerat/o

8. The combining form for the ciliary body is: ☐

A. Phak/o
B. Lacrim/o
C. Irid/o
D. Cycl/o
E. Dacry/o

9. The meaning of palpebr/o is: ☐

A. Eyelid
B. Cornea
C. Tear gland
D. Lens of the eye
E. Optic disc

10. An eye inflammation commonly called "pinkeye" is: ☐

A. Iritis
B. Conjunctivitis
C. Dacryoadenitis
D. Scleritis
E. Uveitis

11. Impairment of vision due to old age: ☐

A. Emmetropia
B. Diplopia
C. Esotropia
D. Presbyopia
E. Anisocoria

12. **Myopia:** ☐
   A. Nearsightedness
   B. Farsightedness
   C. Astigmatism
   D. Strabismus
   E. Glaucoma

13. **Astigmatism:** ☐
   A. Localized purulent infection of the eye
   B. Atrophy of the retina
   C. Esotropia
   D. Exotropia
   E. Defective curvature of the cornea or lens

14. **Glaucoma is primarily diagnosed by:** ☐
   A. Tonometry
   B. Ophthalmoscopy
   C. Slit-lamp biomicroscopy
   D. Fluorescein angiography
   E. Visual field exam

15. **A blind spot; area of depressed vision surrounded by an area of normal vision:** ☐
   A. Nyctalopia
   B. Exotropia
   C. Scotoma
   D. Esotropia
   E. Strabismus

16. **Macular degeneration produces:** ☐
   A. Loss of central vision
   B. Hemianopia
   C. Retinal detachment
   D. Nystagmus
   E. Cataracts

17. **Small hard mass on the eyelid; formed from a sebaceous gland enlargement:** ☐
   A. Scleral buckle
   B. Blepharochalasis
   C. Chalazion
   D. Cataract
   E. Steatoma

18. **Snail-shaped, spirally wound tube in the inner ear is the:** ☐
   A. Auricle
   B. Cochlea
   C. Auditory meatus
   D. Utricle
   E. Pinna

19. **Channel between the middle ear and the nasopharynx:** ☐
   A. Organ of Corti
   B. Semicircular canal
   C. Labyrinth
   D. Eustachian tube
   E. Oval window

20. **Myring/o means:** ☐
   A. Cerumen
   B. Tympanic membrane
   C. Stapes
   D. Auditory canal
   E. Semicircular canals

21. **Bacterial infection of the middle ear:** ☐
   A. Serous otitis media
   B. Cholesteatoma
   C. Mastoiditis
   D. Barotitis
   E. Suppurative otitis media

22. **Tinnitus:** ☐
   A. Hearing loss occurring with old age
   B. Dizziness associated with nausea and sensations of whirling motion
   C. Ringing sound in ears
   D. Dysphonia
   E. Aural discharge

23. **Visual examination of the ear:** ☐
   A. Audiometry
   B. Otoscopy
   C. Tympanometry
   D. Tuning fork test
   E. Ophthalmoscopy

24. **Nerve deafness occurring with aging:** ☐
   A. Vertigo
   B. Ménière disease
   C. Acoustic neuroma
   D. Presbycusis
   E. Otopyorrhea

25. **Fungal infection of the ear:** ☐
   A. Macrotia
   B. Salpingitis
   C. Otomycosis
   D. Cholesteatoma
   E. Labyrinthitis

Chapter Seventeen

VOCABULARY QUIZ: THE EYE

Name: ______________________________

A. Match the following terms with their meanings below:

accommodation	choroid	cornea
anterior chamber	ciliary body	fovea centralis
aqueous humor	cone	rod
biconvex	conjunctiva	vitreous humor

1. Fluid produced by the ciliary body and found in the anterior chamber of the eye ______________________________
2. Photoreceptor cell in the retina; responsible for color and central vision ______________________________
3. Middle, vascular layer of the eye, between the retina and the sclera ______________________________
4. Normal adjustment of the eye to focus on objects from far to near ______________________________
5. Tiny pit or depression in the retina that is the region of clearest vision ______________________________
6. Area behind the cornea and in front of the lens and iris ______________________________
7. Having two sides that are rounded, elevated, and curved evenly; characteristic of the lens of the eye ______________________________
8. Delicate membrane under the surface of the eyelids and covering the anterior eyeball ______________________________
9. Fibrous transparent layer of clear tissue that extends over the anterior portion of the eyeball ______________________________
10. Structure surrounding the lens that connects the choroid and iris; it alters the shape of the lens ______________________________
11. Soft jelly-like material behind the lens; maintains the shape of the eyeball ______________________________
12. Photoreceptor cell essential for vision in dim light and for peripheral vision ______________________________

B. Match the following terms with their meanings below:

fundus of the eye	optic chiasm	refraction
iris	optic disc	retina
lens	optic nerve	sclera
macula	pupil	thalamus

1. Colored, pigmented layer that opens or closes to allow more or less light into the eye ______________________
2. Light-sensitive nerve cell layer containing photoreceptor cells (rods and cones) ______________________
3. Central opening of the eye ______________________
4. Yellowish region on the retina, slightly below the optic disc; contains the fovea centralis ______________________
5. Point at which optic nerve fibers cross in the brain ______________________
6. Bending of light rays by the cornea, lens, and fluids of the eye to bring them into focus on the retina ______________________
7. Region at the back of the eye where the optic nerve meets the retina ______________________
8. Cranial nerve carrying impulses from the retina to the brain (cerebral cortex) ______________________
9. Transparent, biconvex body behind the pupil; it bends light rays to focus them on the retina ______________________
10. Posterior, inner portion of the eye ______________________
11. Tough, white outer coat of the eyeball ______________________
12. Relay center of the brain; optic nerve fibers pass through the thalamus on their way to the cerebral cortex ______________________

Chapter Seventeen

TERMINOLOGY QUIZ: THE EYE

Name: ______________________________

A. Using the following word parts, create or complete terms based on the following definitions:

aden/o	cor/o	ir/o, irid/o	-plegic
aque/o	corne/o	-ectomy	-ptosis
blephar/o	cycl/o	-ia	
conjunctiv/o	dacry/o	-itis	

1. Pertaining to a rubbing away or scratching of the cornea: ____________________ al abrasion
2. Prolapse of an eyelid: ______________________________
3. Fluid (water) found in the anterior chamber of the eye: ____________________ ous humor
4. Inflammation of tear glands: ______________________________
5. Inflammation of an eyelid: ______________________________
6. Pertaining to paralysis of the ciliary body of the eye: ______________________________
7. Inflammation of the iris of the eye: ______________________________
8. Condition of unequal size of pupils: aniso ______________________________
9. Inflammation of the membrane lining the undersurface of the eyelids: ____________________
10. Removal (a portion) of the iris: ______________________________

B. Using the following word parts, create or complete terms based on the following definitions:

kerat/o	ophthalm/o	-itis	intra-
lacrim/o	opt/o, optic/o	-logist	
ocul/o	palpebr/o	-plegia	

1. Pertaining to within the eye: ______________________________ar
2. Paralysis of the eye: ophthalmo ______________________________
3. Inflammation of the cornea: ______________________________
4. Process of tearing: ______________________________ ation
5. Specialist in examining eyes and prescribing corrective lenses: ____________________ metrist
6. Pertaining to an eyelid: ______________________________ al
7. A medical doctor who specializes in treating disorders of the eye: ____________________
8. Pertaining to tears: ______________________________ al
9. Nonmedical professional who grinds lenses and fits glasses: ____________________ ian
10. Pertaining to vision: ______________________________ ic

C. Using the following word parts, create or complete terms based on the following definitions:

corne/o	pupill/o	uve/o	-itis
papill/o	retin/o	vitre/o	-pathy
phac/o, phak/o	scler/o	-ia	

1. Pertaining to the cornea and the sclera: ______________________ al
2. Soft jelly-like material behind the lens: ______________________ ous humor
3. Pertaining to the central area surrounded by the iris: ______________________ ary
4. Swelling in the region of the optic disc: ______________________ edema
5. Inflammation of the vascular layer of the eye: ______________________
6. Disease of the retina of the eye: ______________________
7. Use of ultrasonic vibrations to fragment the lens and remove it from the eye:

   ______________________ emulsification
8. Inflammation of the white of eye: ______________________
9. Condition of absence of a lens: a ______________________
10. Inflammation of the retina: ______________________

D. Using the following word parts, create or complete terms based on the following definitions:

ambly/o	nyct/o	xer/o	-tropia
dipl/o	phot/o	-osis	an-
glauc/o	presby/o	-opia	eso-
mi/o	scot/o	-phobia	hemi-
mydr/o			

1. Contraction of the pupil: ______________________
2. Condition of double vision: ______________________
3. Night blindness: ______________________
4. Condition of dull, dim vision (reduction in visual acuity): ______________________
5. Impairment of vision in old age: ______________________
6. Condition of dry eyes: ______________________ ophthalmia
7. Increased intraocular pressure leads to retinal and optic nerve damage: ______________________ oma
8. Enlargement of pupils: ______________________ iasis
9. Sensitivity to light: ______________________
10. Area of depressed vision surrounded by an area of normal vision: ______________________ oma
11. Absence of vision in half of the visual field: ______________________ opsia
12. Abnormal inward turning of an eye: ______________________

Chapter Seventeen

PATHOLOGY QUIZ: THE EYE—ERRORS OF REFRACTION

Name: ______________________________

Match the following abnormal conditions or symptoms with their descriptions below:

astigmatism
cataract
chalazion
diabetic retinopathy
glaucoma
hordeolum
hyperopia
macular degeneration
myopia
nystagmus
presbyopia
retinal detachment
strabismus

1. Progressive damage to the macula of the eye ______________________________
2. Clouding of the lens causing decreased vision ______________________________
3. Nearsightedness ______________________________
4. Farsightedness ______________________________
5. Small, hard cystic mass on the eyelid ______________________________
6. Increased intraocular pressure resulting in damage to the retina and optic nerve ______________
7. Repetitive rhythmic movements of one or both eyes ______________________________
8. Localized purulent bacterial infection of the sebaceous gland in the eyelid; stye ______________
9. Retinal microaneurysms, hemorrhages, or new vascular growth within the retina ______________
10. Defective curvature of the cornea or lens of the eye ______________________________
11. Abnormal deviation of the eye; esotropia and exotropia ______________________________
12. Impairment of vision due to old age ______________________________
13. Separation of retinal layers ______________________________

Chapter Seventeen

CLINICAL PROCEDURES QUIZ: THE EYE

Name: ______________________

Match the following clinical procedures with their descriptions below:

enucleation	LASIK	slit-lamp microscopy
fluorescein angiography	ophthalmoscopy	visual acuity test
keratoplasty	phacoemulsification	visual field test
laser photocoagulation	scleral buckle	vitrectomy

1. Suture of a silicone band to the sclera over a detached portion of the retina: ______________________
2. Surgical repair of the cornea (corneal transplant): ______________________
3. Visual examination of the interior of the eye: ______________________
4. Measurement of the area (peripheral and central) within which objects are seen: ______________________
5. Intravenous injection of a dye followed by serial photographs of the retina: ______________________
6. Removal of the vitreous humor: ______________________
7. Use of an excimer laser to correct errors of refraction: ______________________
8. Clarity of vision is assessed: ______________________
9. Ultrasonic vibrations break up the lens, which then is aspirated through the ultrasonic probe: ______________________
10. Removal of the entire eyeball: ______________________
11. Intense, precisely focused light beam creates an inflammatory reaction that seals retinal tears and leaky retinal blood vessels: ______________________
12. Examination of anterior ocular structures under microscopic magnification: ______________________

Chapter Seventeen

VOCABULARY QUIZ: THE EAR

Name: ______________________________

A. Match the following terms with their meanings below:

auditory canal	cochlea	incus
auditory nerve fibers	endolymph	labyrinth
auricle	eustachian tube	malleus
cerumen		

1. Snail-shaped spirally wound tube in the inner ear; contains hearing sensitive receptor cells ______________________________
2. Carry impulses from the inner ear to the brain (cerebral cortex) ______________________________
3. Waxy substance secreted by the external ear; ear wax ______________________________
4. Second little bone of the middle ear; shaped like an anvil ______________________________
5. Channel between the middle ear and the nasopharynx; auditory tube ______________________________
6. Flap of the ear ______________________________
7. First little bone of the middle ear; shaped like a hammer ______________________________
8. Fluid within the labyrinth of the ear ______________________________
9. Maze-like series of canals within the inner ear ______________________________
10. Channel that leads from the auricle to the eardrum; auditory meatus ______________________________

B. Match the following terms with their meanings below:

organ of Corti	perilymph	stapes
ossicle	pinna	tympanic membrane
oval window	semicircular canals	vestibule

1. Third small bone of the middle ear; shaped like a stirrup ______________________________
2. Flap of the ear; auricle ______________________________
3. Central cavity of the labyrinth, connecting the semicircular canals and the cochlea ______________________________
4. Eardrum ______________________________
5. Membrane between the middle and inner ear ______________________________
6. Sensitive auditory receptive area in the cochlea of the inner ear ______________________________
7. Passages in the inner ear associated with maintenance of equilibrium ______________________________
8. Small bone ______________________________
9. Fluid contained in the labyrinth of the inner ear ______________________________

Chapter Seventeen

TERMINOLOGY QUIZ: THE EAR

Name: ______________________________

A. *Use the following word parts to create or complete the terms from the definitions below:*

acous/o	aur/o, auricul/o	ossicul/o	-logist
audi/o	cochle/o	-itis	-plasty
audit/o	mastoid/o	-gram	

1. Pertaining to the ear: ______________________________al
2. Pertaining to hearing: ______________________________ory
3. Pertaining to hearing: ______________________________tic
4. Surgical repair of a small bone in the ear: ______________________________
5. Pertaining to the snail-shaped spirally wound tube in the inner ear: ____________________ ar
6. Inflammation of the posterior portion of the temporal bone: ______________________________
7. Record of hearing: ______________________________
8. Pertaining to behind the ear: post ______________________________ ar
9. Inflammation of the eardrum: ______________________________
10. Nonmedical specialist in hearing: ______________________________

B. *Use the following word parts to create or complete the terms from the definitions below:*

audi/o	pharyng/o	vestibul/o	-otia
laryng/o	py/o	-acusis, -cusis	-plasty
myc/o	salping/o	-logist	-rrhea
ot/o	tympan/o	-meter	

1. Condition of fungal infection in the ear: ______________________________ osis
2. Specialist in the study of the ear and voice box (region of): ______________________________
3. Discharge of pus from the ear: ______________________________
4. Instrument to measure hearing: ______________________________
5. Surgical repair of the eardrum: ______________________________
6. Nerve deafness that occurs with old age: presby ______________________________
7. Abnormally large ears: macr ______________________________
8. Pertaining to the eustachian tube and the throat: ______________________________ eal
9. Pertaining to the central cavity of the labyrinth of the ear and the cochlea:

   ______________________________ cochlear
10. Abnormally acute hearing: hyper ______________________________

Chapter Seventeen
PATHOLOGY QUIZ: THE EAR

Name: ______________________________

Match the following abnormal conditions or symptoms with their descriptions below:

acoustic neuroma	Ménière disease	tinnitus
cholesteatoma	otitis media	vertigo
deafness	otosclerosis	

1. Hardening of the bony tissue of the middle ear: ______________________________
2. Sensation of irregular or whirling motion, either of oneself or of external objects: ______________________________
3. Inflammation of the middle ear: ______________________________
4. Collection of skin cells and cholesterol in a sac within the middle ear: ______________________________
5. Disorder of the labyrinth of the inner ear (with accumulation of fluid): ______________________________
6. Benign tumor arising from the 8th cranial nerve: ______________________________
7. Loss of the ability to hear: ______________________________
8. Sensation of noises (ringing, buzzing) in the ears: ______________________________

Chapter Seventeen
CLINICAL PROCEDURES AND QUIZ: THE EAR

Name: ____________________

Match the following procedures or abbreviations with their descriptions below:

AD	cochlear implant	PE tube
AOM	ear thermometry	tuning fork test
audiometry	ENG	
AS	otoscopy	

1. Measurement of the temperature of the tympanic membrane by detection of infrared radiation from the eardrum ____________________
2. Testing the sense of hearing: ____________________
3. Left ear ____________________
4. Right ear ____________________
5. Surgically implanted device allows sensorineural hearing-impaired persons to understand speech: ____________________
6. Test of balance mechanism of the inner ear by assessing eye movements (electronystagmography): ____________________
7. Type of inflammation of the middle ear: ____________________
8. Test of ear conduction using vibration source (Rinne and Weber tests): ____________________
9. Visual examination of the ear canal: ____________________
10. Ventilating tube placed in the eardrum to treat recurrent otitis media: ____________________

Chapter Seventeen

ABBREVIATIONS QUIZ: EYE AND EAR

Name: ____________________

On the line provided, give meanings for the following abbreviations, then write each abbreviation next to its explanation below:

1. IOL ______________________________
2. AOM ______________________________
3. ENG ______________________________
4. VA ______________________________
5. IOP ______________________________
6. ENT ______________________________
7. PERRLA ______________________________
8. AMD ______________________________
9. VF ______________________________
10. PE tube ______________________________

a. __________ Patient reads from a Snellen chart to test clarity of vision

b. __________ Helps relieve chronic middle ear infection and inflammation

c. __________ Area within which objects are seen when the eyes are fixed, looking straight ahead

d. __________ Measure of fluid buildup in the anterior portion of the eye and associated with glaucoma

e. __________ Severe inflammation of the middle portion of the ear

f. __________ Loss of central vision occurring with old age

g. __________ Normal result when the dark opening of the eye is examined

h. __________ Artificial part inserted during cataract surgery

i. __________ Specialty of an otorhinolaryngologist

j. __________Test of the balance mechanism of the inner ear by assessing rapidly twitching eye movements

Chapter Seventeen
EXERCISE QUIZ

Name: ______________________________

EYE

A. Match the structure of the eye with its description below:

choroid	conjunctiva	iris	pupil	sclera
ciliary body	cornea	lens	retina	vitreous humor

1. Contains sensitive cells (rods and cones) that transmit light energy to nervous impulses ______________________________
2. Contains muscles that control the shape of the lens and secrete aqueous humor ______________________________
3. Transparent body behind the iris and in front of the vitreous humor; refracts light rays to bring them into focus on the retina ______________________________
4. Jelly-like material behind the lens; helps to maintain the shape of the eyeball ______________________________
5. Dark center of the eye through which light rays enter ______________________________
6. Vascular layer of the eyeball that is continuous with the iris ______________________________
7. Delicate membrane lining the eyelids and covering the anterior eyeball ______________________________
8. Fibrous layer of clear tissue that extends over the anterior portion of the eyeball ______________________________
9. Colored portion of the eye; surrounds the pupil ______________________________
10. Tough, white outer coat of the eyeball ______________________________

B. Supply the term to complete the following:

11. Region at the back of the eye where the retina meets the optic nerve is ______________________________
12. The normal adjustment of the lens to bring an object into focus is ______________________________
13. A yellowish region on the retina lateral to the optic disc is ______________________________
14. Bending of light rays by the cornea, lens, and fluids of the eye is ______________________________
15. Photosensitive receptor cells in the retina that make color perception possible are ______________________________
16. Photosensitive receptor cells that make vision in dim light possible are ______________________________

C. Give meanings for the following terms:

17. anisocoria ______________________________
18. papilledema ______________________________
19. photophobia ______________________________
20. scotoma ______________________________

D. Complete the medical term from its definition and word parts given:

21. inflammation of an eyelid: ______________________________ itis
22. inflammation of the cornea: ______________________________ itis
23. inflammation of the iris: ______________________________ itis
24. inflammation of the conjunctiva: ______________________________ itis
25. pertaining to within the eye: intra ______________________________

E. Match the following terms with their meanings below:

aphakia	exotropia	uveitis
esotropia	hemianopsia	xerophthalmia

26. Inflammation of the vascular layer of the eye ______________________________
27. Condition of dry eyes ______________________________
28. Outward deviation of the eye ______________________________
29. Inward deviation of the eye ______________________________
30. Absence of the lens of the eye ______________________________
31. Absence of vision in half of the visual field ______________________________

F. Describe the following visual conditions:

32. presbyopia ______________________________
33. myopia ______________________________
34. diplopia ______________________________
35. amblyopia ______________________________
36. hyperopia ______________________________
37. emmetropia ______________________________

G. Match the following abnormal conditions of the eye with their meanings below:

cataract	glaucoma	macular degeneration
diabetic retinopathy	hordeolum (stye)	strabismus

38. Abnormal deviations of the eye ______________________

39. Increased intraocular pressure results in retinal and optic nerve damage ______________________

40. Localized purulent infection of a sebaceous gland in the eyelid ______________________

41. Clouding of the lens causes decreased vision ______________________

42. Retinal microaneurysms, hemorrhages occur secondary to an endocrine condition ______________________

43. Deterioration of the macula lutea of the retina ______________________

H. Give the meanings for the following abbreviations:

44. OU ______________________

45. OD ______________________

46. OS ______________________

47. PERRLA ______________________

48. c. gl. ______________________

49. VF ______________________

50. s. gl. ______________________

Chapter Seventeen
EXERCISE QUIZ

Name: ______________________________

EAR

A. Arrange the following in the correct order to indicate their sequence in the transmission of sound waves to the brain from the outer ear:

auditory liquids and receptors
auditory nerve fibers
cerebral cortex
cochlea
external auditory canal
incus
malleus
oval window
pinna
stapes
tympanic membrane

1. ______________________________
2. ______________________________
3. ______________________________
4. ______________________________
5. ______________________________
6. ______________________________
7. ______________________________
8. ______________________________
9. ______________________________
10. ______________________________
11. ______________________________

B. Give the meanings for the following medical terms:

12. semicircular canals ______________________________
13. cerumen ______________________________
14. perilymph and endolymph ______________________________
15. tympanic membrane ______________________________

C. Complete the following medical terms from their definitions given:

16. removal of the third bone of the middle ear: ______________________________ ectomy
17. instrument to measure hearing: ______________________________ meter
18. deafness due to old age: ______________________________ cusis
19. inflammation of the middle ear: ot ______________________________
20. surgical repair of the eardrum: ______________________________ plasty

D. Give the meanings for the following medical terms:

21. vertigo ______________________________
22. otosclerosis ______________________________
23. tinnitus ______________________________
24. labyrinthitis ______________________________
25. myringitis ______________________________
26. suppurative otitis media ______________________________
27. mastoiditis ______________________________
28. Ménière disease ______________________________
29. acoustic neuroma ______________________________
30. cholesteatoma ______________________________

E. Give the meanings for the following abbreviations:

31. AS ______________________________
32. ENG ______________________________
33. EENT ______________________________
34. AD ______________________________
35. ENT ______________________________

Chapter Seventeen

DICTATION AND COMPREHENSION QUIZ: EYE

Name: ______________________

A. Dictation of Terms

1. ______________________ 11. ______________________
2. ______________________ 12. ______________________
3. ______________________ 13. ______________________
4. ______________________ 14. ______________________
5. ______________________ 15. ______________________
6. ______________________ 16. ______________________
7. ______________________ 17. ______________________
8. ______________________ 18. ______________________
9. ______________________ 19. ______________________
10. ______________________ 20. ______________________

B. Comprehension of Terms: Match the number of the above term with its meaning below.

_____ Visual examination of the eye
_____ White portion of the eye
_____ Fluid produced by the ciliary body; circulates through the anterior chamber of the eye
_____ Pupils are of unequal size
_____ Delicate membrane lining the eyelids and covering the anterior eyeball
_____ Inflammation of the cornea
_____ Paralysis of the ciliary muscles of the eye
_____ Double vision
_____ Clouding of the lens, causing decreased vision
_____ Abnormal deviation of the eye (esotropia and exotropia)
_____ Defective curvature of the cornea or lens of the eye
_____ Small, hard cystic mass on the eyelid
_____ Impairment of vision due to old age
_____ Nearsightedness
_____ Inflammation of the iris
_____ Loss of vision in one half of the visual field
_____ Swelling in the region of the optic disc
_____ Process of recording blood vessels in the back of the eye after IV injection of a dye
_____ Progressive damage to the yellowish region on the retina (lateral to and slightly below the optic disc)
_____ Absence of the lens of the eye

Chapter Seventeen

DICTATION AND COMPREHENSION QUIZ: EAR

Name: ______________________________

A. Dictation of Terms

1.	______________	11.	______________
2.	______________	12.	______________
3.	______________	13.	______________
4.	______________	14.	______________
5.	______________	15.	______________
6.	______________	16.	______________
7.	______________	17.	______________
8.	______________	18.	______________
9.	______________	19.	______________
10.	______________	20.	______________

B. Comprehension of Terms: Match the number of the above term with its meaning below.

______ Fluid contained in the inner part of the ear
______ Maze-like series of canals of the inner ear
______ The outer flap of the ear; auricle
______ Channel between the middle ear and the nasopharynx
______ Waxy substance secreted by the external ear
______ Collection of skin cells and cholesterol in a sac within the middle ear
______ Incision of the eardrum
______ Hardening of bony tissue in the inner ear; ankylosis of the stapes may occur
______ Passages in the inner ear that are associated with maintaining equilibrium
______ Specialist in the study of the ear and voice box
______ Sensation of noises (ringing, buzzing, whistling) in the ears
______ Sensation of irregular or whirling motion either of oneself or of external objects
______ Surgical repair of a small bone in the middle ear
______ Instrument to measure hearing
______ Fungal infection of the ear
______ Channel leading from the outer ear flap to the eardrum
______ Benign tumor arising from the 8th cranial nerve in the brain
______ Snail-shaped spirally wound tube in the inner ear; contains hearing-sensitive cells
______ Surgical repair of the eardrum
______ Inflammation of the middle ear with pus formation

Chapter Seventeen
SPELLING QUIZ

Name: ____________________

A. Circle the term that is spelled correctly and write its meaning in the space provided:

1. anisocoria — anisocorea ____________________
2. acqueous humer — aqueous humor ____________________
3. blepharitis — blepheritis ____________________
4. cateract — cataract ____________________
5. conjuntivia — conjunctiva ____________________
6. cornea — kornea ____________________
7. cilliary body — ciliary body ____________________
8. dacryorhea — dacryorrhea ____________________
9. glaucoma — glaukoma ____________________
10. opthalmologist — ophthalmologist ____________________

B. Circle the term that is spelled correctly. The meaning of each term is given.

11. Pertaining to sound	acoustic	acustic	akustic
12. Outer flap of the ear	pina	penna	pinna
13. Fungal ear condition	otomicosis	automycosis	otomycosis
14. Ringing in the ears	tinnitis	tinitus	tinnitus
15. Surgical repair of the eardrum	tympanoplasty	tinpanoplasty	timpanoplasty
16. Incision of the eardrum	myringotomy	myringetomy	miringotomy
17. Waxy discharge from the ear	ceremen	serumen	cerumen
18. Dizziness	virtigo	vertigo	vertego
19. Hearing impairment due to old age	presbycussis	presbicusis	presbycusis
20. Removal of a middle ear bone	stapedectomy	stapidectomy	stapidectomy

Chapter Seventeen
PRONUNCIATION QUIZ

Name: ______________________________

A. Underline the accented syllable in the following words:

1. prosthesis
2. corneoscleral
3. audiometer
4. malleus
5. palpebral
6. presbycusis
7. mydriatic
8. blepharitis
9. retinopathy
10. macrotia

B. Match the term in Column I with its meaning in Column II:

Column I		Column II
1. cerumen	_______	A. Clouding of the lens
2. cochlea	_______	B. Small bone in the middle ear
3. cornea	_______	C. Abnormal deviation of the eye caused by muscle weakness
4. chalazion	_______	D. Wax found in the outer ear
5. cataract	_______	E. Clear tissue that covers the front portion of the eyeball
6. pinna	_______	F. Ringing sound in the ears
7. eustachian tube	_______	G. The flap, or outside part, of the ear
8. stapes	_______	H. A snail-shaped spirally wound tube in the inner ear
9. tinnitus	_______	I. Small hard mass on the eyelid
10. strabismus	_______	J. Tube connecting the middle ear to the throat

C. Complete the following medical terms from their definitions:

1.	____________________ opia	Impairment of vision due to old age
2.	____________________ oplasty	Surgical repair of the eardrum
3.	__________ o__________	Paralysis of the eye
4.	____________________ eal	Pertaining to the eustachian tube and the throat
5.	hemi ____________________	Loss of one half of the visual field
6.	____________________ itis	Inflammation of the vascular layer of the eye
7.	a ____________________	Condition of the absence of the lens
8.	oto ____________________	Hardening of the bony tissue in the inner ear

Chapter Seventeen

DIAGRAM QUIZ—EYE

Name: ______________________________

Label the diagram below using the following terms:

EYE

Anterior chamber
Choroid
Ciliary body
Conjunctiva
Cornea
Fovea centralis
Iris
Lens
Macula
Optic disc
Optic nerve
Pupil
Retina
Sclera
Vitreous humor

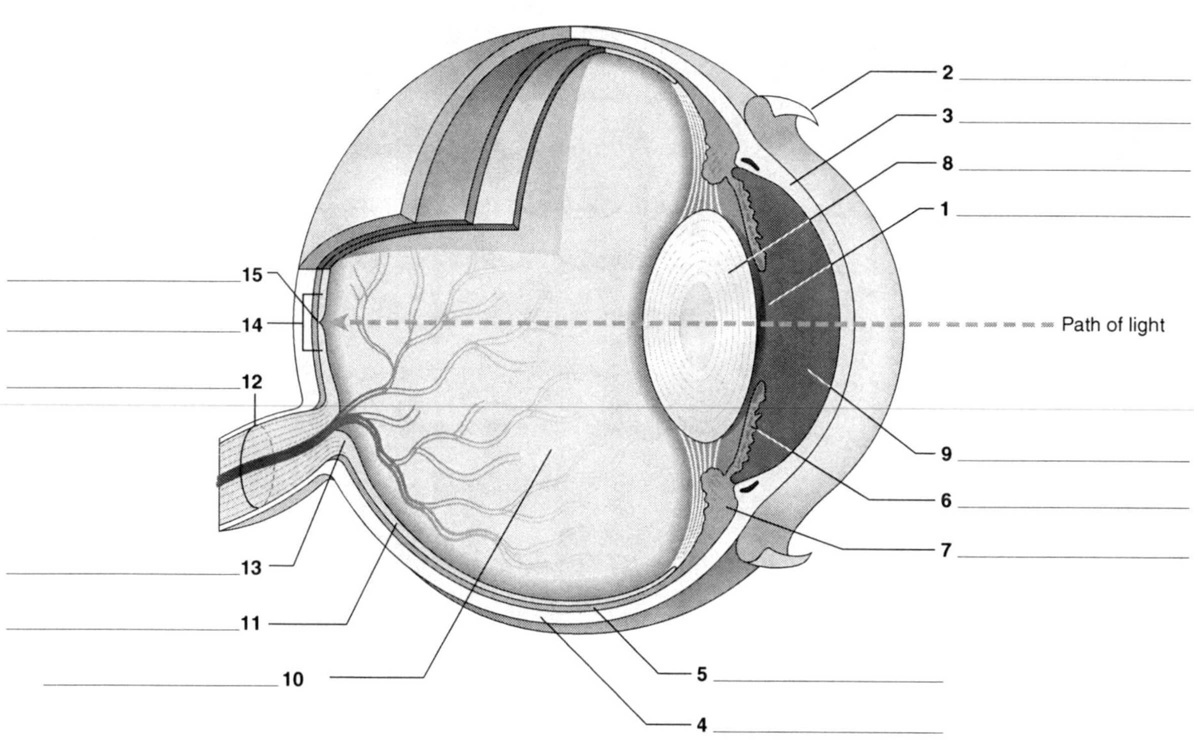

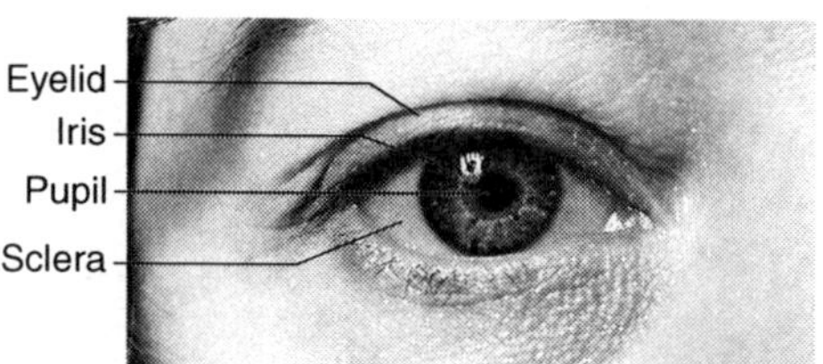

Chapter Seventeen
FLOW CHART QUIZ—EYE

Name: ______________________________

Label the flow chart below using the following terms:

anterior chamber and aqueous humor
cerebral cortex (occipital lobe)
cornea
lens
optic chiasm
optic nerve fibers
pupil
retina (robs & cones)
thalamus
vitreous chamber and vitreous humor

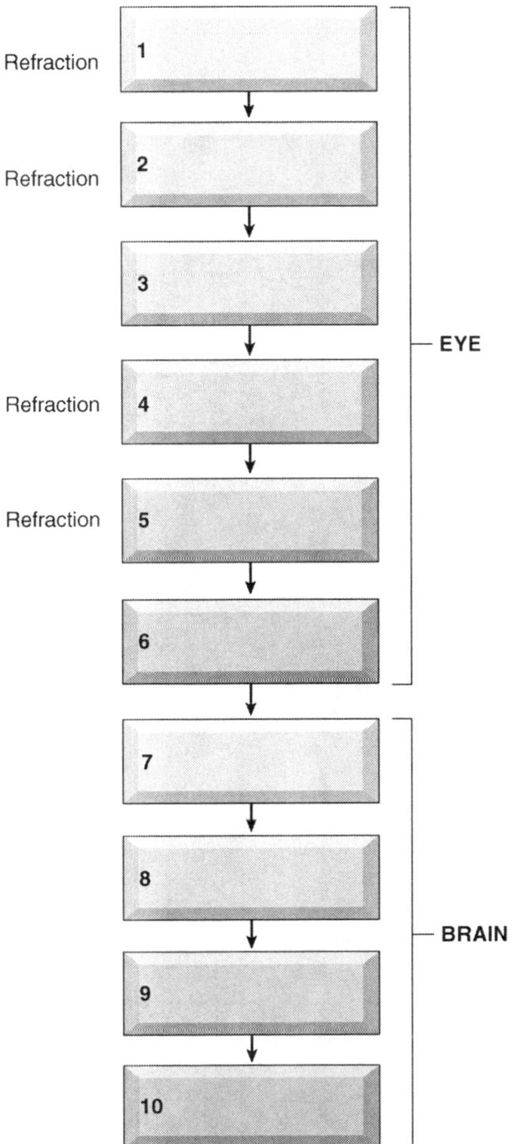

Chapter Seventeen
DIAGRAM QUIZ—EAR

Name: ______________________

Label the diagram below using the terms listed below:

EAR

Auditory nerve fibers
Cochlea
Eustachian (auditory) tube
External auditory meatus
Incus
Malleus
Oval window
Pinna (auricle)
Semicircular canals
Stapes
Tympanic membrane
Vestibule

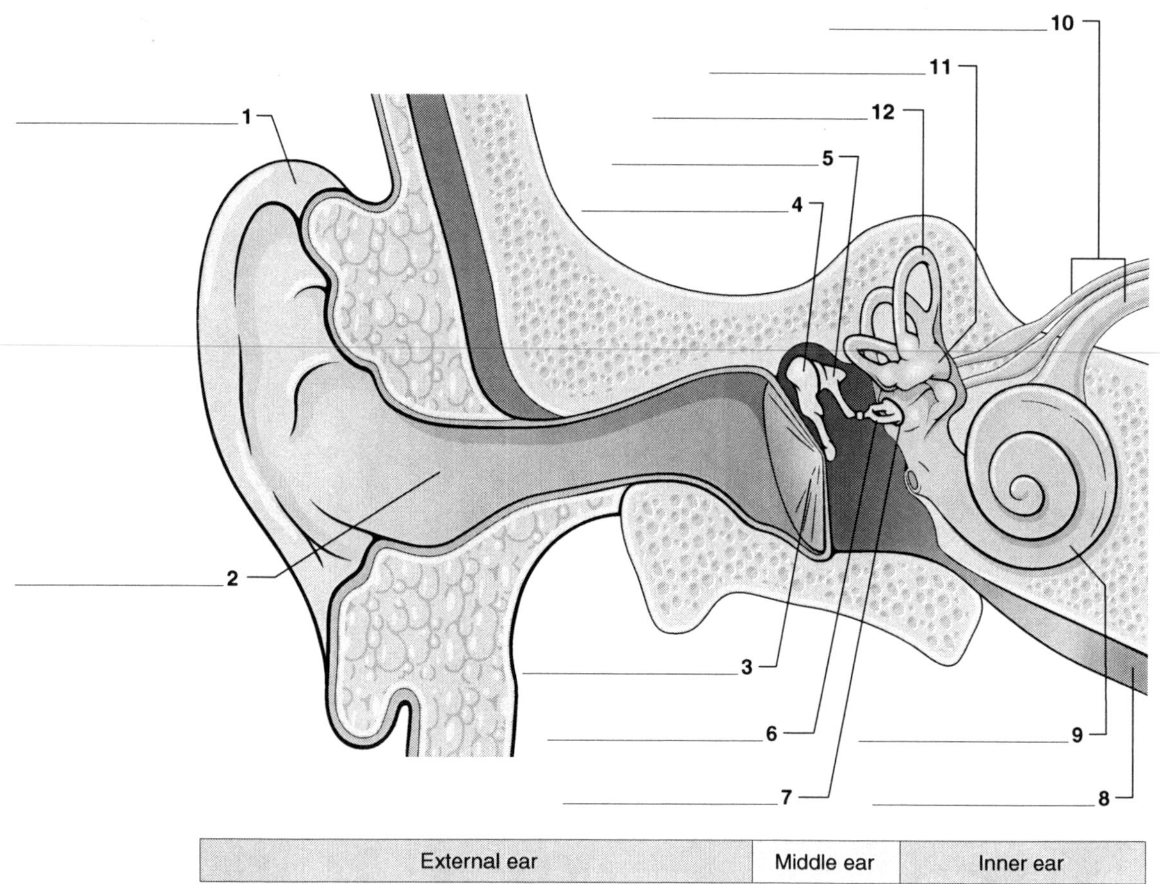

Chapter Seventeen
FLOW CHART QUIZ—EAR

Name: ______________________________

Label the flow chart below using the following terms:

auditory liquids and receptors in the organ of Corti
auditory nerve fibers
cerebral cortex
cochlea
external auditory canal
incus
malleus
oval window
pinna
stapes
tympanic membrane

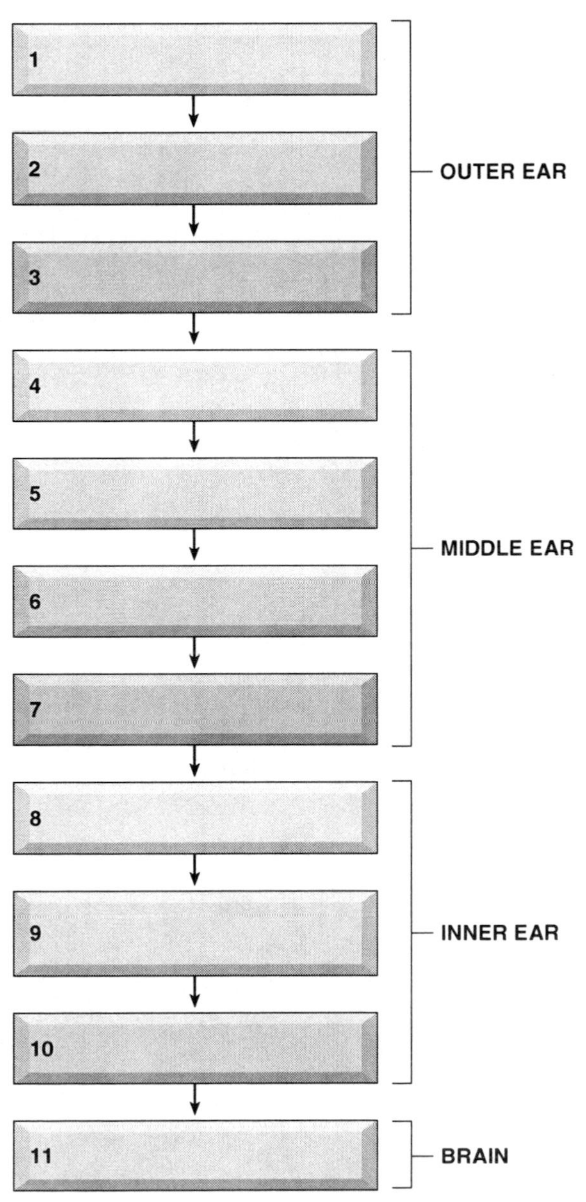

Chapter Seventeen
REVIEW SHEET QUIZ

Name: ______________________

A. Give meanings for the following combining forms:

1. acous/o ______________
2. ambyl/o ______________
3. anis/o ______________
4. aque/o ______________
5. audit/o ______________
6. aur/o ______________
7. blephar/o ______________
8. cochle/o ______________
9. conjunctiv/o ______________
10. cor/o ______________

B. Give meanings for the following combining forms

1. corne/o ______________
2. cycl/o ______________
3. dacry/o ______________
4. dipl/o ______________
5. glauc/o ______________
6. ir/o ______________
7. kerat/o ______________
8. lacrim/o ______________
9. mi/o ______________
10. mydr/o ______________

C. Give meanings for the following combining forms

1. myring/o ______________
2. nyct/o ______________
3. ocul/o ______________
4. ophthalm/o ______________
5. opt/o ______________
6. ossicul/o ______________
7. ot/o ______________
8. palpebr/o ______________
9. papill/o ______________
10. phac/o ______________
11. phot/o ______________
12. presby/o ______________

D. Give meanings for the following combining forms:

1. pupill/o ____________________
2. retin/o ____________________
3. salping/o ____________________
4. scler/o ____________________
5. scot/o ____________________
6. staped/o ____________________
7. tympan/o ____________________
8. uve/o ____________________
9. vitre/o ____________________
10. xer/o ____________________

E. Give meanings for the following suffixes:

1. -cusis ____________________
2. -opia ____________________
3. -otia ____________________
4. -meter ____________________
5. -metry ____________________
6. -phobia ____________________
7. -plegia ____________________
8. -tropia ____________________

Chapter Seventeen
MEDICAL SCRAMBLE

Name: ______________________________

Unscramble the letters to form terms relating to eye or ear abnormalities from the clues. Use the letters in the squares to complete the bonus term.

1. *Clue:* The lens appears cloudy

   ☐ ___ ___ ___ ___ ☐ ___ ___ A T C R T A C A

2. *Clue:* Increased intraocular pressure

   ___ ☐ ___ ☐ ___ ___ ___ ☐ A U G M O L A C

3. *Clue:* The eardrum is inflamed

   ☐ ___ ___ ___ ___ ___ ___ ___ ___ ___ Y S I M I G R T N I

4. *Clue:* You feel as if objects are whirling around you

   ___ ___ ☐ ___ ___ ___ ___ O V T E G I R

BONUS TERM: *Clue:* Age-related, gradual loss of central vision is ________ degeneration

☐ ☐ ☐ ☐ ☐ ☐ ☐

Chapter Seventeen
CROSSWORD PUZZLE

Name: ______________________

Fill in the crossword puzzle below using the clues listed underneath it.

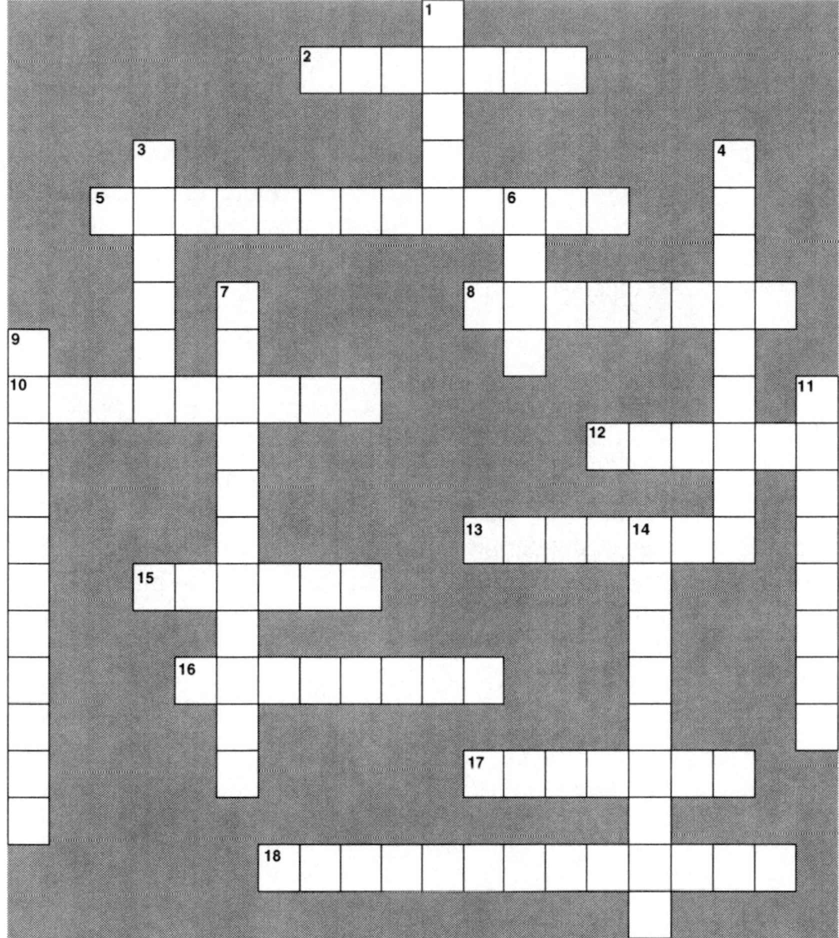

Across Clues

2. Small bone.
5. Normal adjustment of the lens by the ciliary muscle.
8. Having two sides that are rounded, elevated, and curved evenly.
10. Pertaining to the sense of smell. From the Latin, *olfacoro*, meaning "to smell".
12. Nearsightedness.
13. A snail-shaped spirally wound tube in the inner ear.
15. One of the tiny bones in the middle ear; stirrups.
16. Ringing sound in the ear; means "tinkling" in Latin.
17. Sensation of irregular or whirling motion either of oneself or of external objects.
18. Collection of skin cells and cholesterol in a sac within the middle ear.

Down Clues

1. Auricle; ear flap.
3. Tough, white, outer coat of the eyeball.
4. Farsightedness.
6. Colored portion of the eye.
7. Defective curvature of the cornea or lens of the eye.
9. Delicate membrane lining the eyelids and covering the exposed surfaces of the sclera.
11. Clouding of the lens, causing decreased vision.
14. Maze-like series of canals in the inner ear.

Chapter Seventeen

PRACTICAL APPLICATIONS

Name: ______________________

A. Questions for Operative Report (page 727)

1. **What was the patient's diagnosis before surgery?..................................** ☐
   A. Inflammation of the right eye and ear
   B. Inflammation of the left ear, adenoids, and tonsils
   C. Inflammation of both ears with tonsillar and adenoidal inflammation
   D. Eardrum was perforated; inflamed tonsils and adenoids

2. **What operation was performed?..........** ☐
   A. Removal of adenoids and tonsils
   B. Incision of the eardrums and placement of PE tubes; removal of adenoids and tonsils
   C. Removal of tonsils and adenoids and tube placement in left ear
   D. Removal of tonsils and placement of tubes in right ear

B. Chart Note

This 36-year-old woman presents with the complaint of dacryorrhea and irritation OS for about 48 hours. She has a thick mucous discharge that sticks the lids together overnight. Vision seems fine except for blurring by mucus. She denies trauma or ocular pathology. No symptoms of URI or allergy. She has no photophobia and has not been around anyone with pinkeye.

The conjunctiva (OS) is diffusely hyperemic, and there is chemosis (edema of the conjunctiva) and moderate lid edema. Traces of mucopurulent discharge are evident on the lid. Exam with Pontocaine (local anesthetic) and fluorescein reveals no corneal abrasions or ulceration. No foreign bodies are noted on the palpebral conjunctiva. PERRLA. Ocular fundus is normal. Slit-lamp examination shows no pathology in the cornea, anterior chamber, or lens. Tonometry is deferred. Far point vision testing with the Snellen chart is 20/20 in each eye.

Diagnosis is acute bacterial conjunctivitis OS.

1. **What are the patient's main symptoms?..** ☐
   A. Blurred vision and itchy eyes
   B. Right eye irritation and excessive tearing
   C. Left eye irritation and excessive tearing
   D. Both eyes are tearing and irritated

2. **Where is the eye problem? ....** ☐
   A. In the cornea of the right eye
   B. Under the eyelids of both eyes
   C. In the cornea of the left eye
   D. The conjunctiva and lid of the left eye

3. **Hyperemic means:.............................** ☐
   A. Not enough blood is flowing to the area
   B. Too much blood is flowing to an area
   C. There is blood and pus in the area
   D. The conjunctiva is purulent

4. **What is the condition of the patient's pupils? ....** ☐
   A. Pupils were not tested
   B. No foreign bodies were found in the pupils
   C. No abrasions or ulcerations noticed
   D. Pupils equal, round, reactive to light and accommodation

Chapter Seventeen
ANSWERS TO THE QUIZZES

Multiple Choice Quiz

1. D
2. C
3. B
4. B
5. A
6. B
7. E
8. D
9. A
10. B
11. D
12. A
13. E
14. A
15. C
16. A
17. C
18. B
19. D
20. B
21. E
22. C
23. B
24. D
25. C

Vocabulary Quiz: The Eye

A

1. aqueous humor
2. cone
3. choroid
4. accommodation
5. fovea centralis
6. anterior chamber
7. biconvex
8. conjunctiva
9. cornea
10. ciliary body
11. vitreous humor
12. rod

B

1. iris
2. retina
3. pupil
4. macula
5. optic chiasm
6. refraction
7. optic disc
8. optic nerve
9. lens
10. fundus of the eye
11. sclera
12. thalamus

Terminology Quiz: The Eye

A

1. corneal abrasion
2. blepharoptosis
3. aqueous humor
4. dacryoadenitis
5. blepharitis
6. cycloplegic
7. iritis
8. anisocoria
9. conjunctivitis
10. iridectomy

B

1. intraocular
2. ophthalmoplegia
3. keratitis
4. lacrimation
5. optometrist
6. palpebral
7. ophthalmologist
8. lacrimal
9. optician
10. optic

C

1. corneoscleral
2. vitreous humor
3. pupillary
4. papilledema
5. uveitis
6. retinopathy
7. phacoemulsification
8. scleritis
9. aphakia
10. retinitis

D

1. miosis
2. diplopia
3. nyctalopia
4. amblyopia
5. presbyopia
6. xerophthalmia
7. glaucoma
8. mydriasis
9. photophobia
10. scotoma
11. hemianopsia
12. esotropia

Pathology Quiz: The Eye–Errors of Refraction

1. macular degeneration
2. cataract
3. myopia
4. hyperopia
5. chalazion
6. glaucoma
7. nystagmus
8. hordeolum
9. diabetic retinopathy
10. astigmatism
11. strabismus
12. presbyopia
13. retinal detachment

Clinical Procedures Quiz: The Eye

1. scleral buckle
2. keratoplasty
3. ophthalmoscopy
4. visual field test
5. fluorescein angiography
6. vitrectomy
7. LASIK
8. visual acuity test
9. phacoemulsification
10. enucleation
11. laser photocoagulation
12. slit-lamp microscopy

Vocabulary Quiz: The Ear

A

1. cochlea
2. auditory nerve fibers
3. cerumen
4. incus
5. eustachian tube
6. auricle
7. malleus
8. endolymph
9. labyrinth
10. auditory canal

B

1. stapes
2. pinna
3. vestibule
4. tympanic membrane
5. oval window
6. organ of Corti
7. semicircular canals
8. ossicle
9. perilymph

Terminology Quiz: The Ear

A

1. aural
2. auditory
3. acoustic
4. myringoplasty
5. cochlear
6. mastoiditis
7. audiogram
8. postauricular
9. myringitis
10. audiologist

B

1. otomycosis
2. otolaryngologist
3. otopyorrhea
4. audiogram
5. tympanoplasty
6. presbycusis
7. macrotia
8. salpingopharyngeal
9. vestibulocochlear
10. hyperacusis

Pathology Quiz: The Ear

1. otosclerosis
2. vertigo
3. otitis media
4. cholesteatoma
5. Ménière disease
6. acoustic neuroma
7. deafness
8. tinnitus

Clinical Procedures and Abbreviations Quiz: The Ear

1. ear thermometry
2. audiometry
3. AS
4. AD
5. cochlear implant
6. ENG
7. AOM
8. tuning fork test
9. otoscopy
10. PE tube

Abbreviations Quiz: Eye and Ear

1. intraocular lens
2. acute otitis media
3. electronystagmography
4. visual acuity
5. intraocular pressure
6. ear, nose and throat
7. pupils equal, round, reactive to light and accommodation
8. age-related macular degeneration
9. visual field
10. pressure equalizing tube

a. VA
b. PE tube
c. VF
d. IOP
e. AOM
f. AMD
g. PERRLA
h. IOL
i. ENT
j. ENG

Exercise Quiz

EYE

A

1. retina
2. ciliary body
3. lens
4. vitreous humor
5. pupil
6. choroid
7. conjunctiva
8. cornea
9. iris
10. sclera

B

11. optic disc (disk)
12. accommodation
13. macula lutea
14. refraction
15. cones
16. rods

C

17. pupils are unequal in size
18. swelling; fluid accumulation in the back of the eye
19. sensitivity to light
20. blind spot

D

21. blepharitis
22. keratitis
23. iritis
24. conjunctivitis
25. intraocular

E

26. uveitis
27. xerophthalmia
28. exotropia
29. esotropia
30. aphakia
31. hemianopsia

F

32. decreased vision in old age
33. nearsightedness
34. double vision
35. dim vision; lazy eye
36. farsightedness
37. normal vision

G

38. strabismus
39. glaucoma
40. hordeolum (stye)
41. cataract
42. diabetic retinopathy
43. macular degeneration

H

44. both eyes
45. right eye
46. left eye
47. pupils equal, round, reactive to light and accommodation
48. with glasses
49. visual field
50. without glasses

EAR

A

1. pinna
2. external auditory canal
3. tympanic membrane
4. malleus
5. incus
6. stapes
7. oval window
8. cochlea
9. auditory liquids and receptors
10. auditory nerve fibers
11. cerebral cortex

B

12. passages in the inner ear associated with equilibrium
13. waxy substance secreted by the external ear
14. auditory fluids in the labyrinth of the inner ear
15. eardrum

C

16. stapedectomy
17. audiometer

18. presbycusis
19. otitis media
20. tympanoplasty

D

21. sensation of irregular or whirling motion; dizziness
22. hardening of bony tissue in the labyrinth of the ear
23. noise sound (ringing) in the ears
24. inflammation of the inner ear (labyrinth)
25. inflammation of the eardrum
26. inflammation of middle ear with pus formation
27. inflammation of the mastoid bone near the ear
28. labyrinth disorder with elevated endolymph pressure in the cochlea
29. benign tumor of the acoustic nerve in the brain
30. collection of skin cells and cholesterol in a sac within the middle ear

E

31. left ear
32. electronystagmography
33. eyes, ears, nose, and throat
34. right ear
35. ear, nose, and throat

Dictation and Comprehension Quiz: Eye

A

1. anisocoria
2. aphakia
3. aqueous humor
4. astigmatism
5. cataract
6. chalazion
7. conjunctiva
8. cycloplegia
9. diplopia
10. fluorescein angiography
11. hemianopsia
12. iritis
13. keratitis
14. macular degeneration
15. myopia
16. ophthalmoscopy
17. papilledema
18. presbyopia
19. sclera
20. strabismus

B

16 Visual examination of the eye
19 White portion of the eye
3 Fluid produced by the ciliary body; circulates through the anterior chamber of the eye
1 Pupils are of unequal size
7 Delicate membrane lining the eyelids and covering the anterior eyeball
13 Inflammation of the cornea
8 Paralysis of the ciliary muscles of the eye
9 Double vision
5 Clouding of the lens, causing decreased vision
20 Abnormal deviation of the eye (esotropia and exotropia)
4 Defective curvature of the cornea or lens of the eye
6 Small, hard cystic mass on the eyelid
18 Impairment of vision due to old age
15 Nearsightedness
12 Inflammation of the iris
11 Loss of vision in one half of the visual field
17 Swelling in the region of the optic disc
10 Process of recording blood vessels in the back of the eye after IV injection of a dye
14 Progressive damage to the yellowish region on the retina (lateral to and slightly below the optic disc)
2 Absence of the lens of the eye

Dictation and Comprehension Quiz: Ear

A

1. acoustic neuroma
2. audiometer
3. auditory meatus
4. cerumen
5. cholesteatoma
6. cochlea
7. eustachian tube
8. labyrinth
9. myringotomy
10. ossiculoplasty
11. otolaryngologist
12. otomycosis
13. otosclerosis
14. perilymph
15. pinna
16. semicircular canals
17. suppurative otitis media
18. tinnitus
19. tympanoplasty
20. vertigo

B

14 Fluid contained in the inner part of the ear
8 Maze-like series of canals of the inner ear
15 The outer flap of the ear; auricle
7 Channel between the middle ear and the nasopharynx
4 Waxy substance secreted by the external ear
5 Collection of skin cells and cholesterol in a sac within the middle ear
9 Incision of the eardrum
13 Hardening of bony tissue in the inner ear; ankylosis of the stapes may occur
16 Passages in the inner ear that are associated with maintaining equilibrium
11 Specialist in the study of the ear and voice box
18 Sensation of noises (ringing, buzzing, whistling) in the ears
20 Sensation of irregular or whirling motion either of oneself or of external objects
10 Surgical repair of a small bone in the middle ear
2 Instrument to measure hearing
12 Fungal infection of the ear
3 Channel leading from the outer ear flap to the eardrum
1 Benign tumor arising from the 8th cranial nerve in the brain
6 A snail-shaped, spirally wound tube in the inner ear; contains hearing-sensitive cells
19 Surgical repair of the eardrum
17 Inflammation of the middle ear with pus formation

Spelling Quiz

A

1. anisocoria—pupils are unequal size
2. aqueous humor—fluid in the anterior and posterior chambers of the eye
3. blepharitis—inflammation of the eyelid

4. cataract—clouding of the lens, causing decreased vision
5. conjunctiva—delicate membrane lining the eyelids and covering the anterior eyeball
6. cornea—fibrous, transparent layer of clear tissue over the anterior of the eyeball
7. ciliary body—on each side of the lens to control the shape of lens
8. dacryorrhea—excessive flow of tears
9. glaucoma—increased intraocular pressure
10. ophthalmologist—doctor who examines the eye and treats eye disorders

B

11. acoustic
12. pinna
13. otomycosis
14. tinnitus
15. tympanoplasty
16. myringotomy
17. cerumen
18. vertigo
19. presbycusis
20. stapedectomy

Pronunciation Quiz

A

1. prosthesis
2. corneoscleral
3. audiometer
4. malleus
5. palpebral
6. presbycusis
7. mydriatic
8. blepharitis
9. retinopathy
10. macrotia

B

1. D
2. H
3. E
4. I
5. A
6. G
7. J
8. B
9. F
10. C

C

1. presbyopia
2. tympanoplasty
3. ophthalmoplegia
4. salpingopharyngeal
5. hemianopsia
6. uveitis
7. aphakia
8. otosclerosis

Diagram Quiz—Eye

1. Pupil
2. Conjunctiva
3. Cornea
4. Sclera
5. Choroid
6. Iris
7. Ciliary body
8. Lens
9. Anterior chamber
10. Vitreous humor
11. Retina
12. Optic nerve
13. Optic disc
14. Macula
15. Fovea centralis

Flow Chart Quiz—Eye

1. cornea
2. anterior chamber and aqueous humor
3. pupil
4. lens
5. vitreous chamber and vitreous humor
6. retina (rods & cones)
7. optic nerve fibers
8. optic chiasm
9. thalamus
10. cerebral cortex (occipital lobe)

Diagram Quiz—Ear

1. Pinna (auricle)
2. External auditory meatus (auditory canal)
3. Tympanic membrane (eardrum)
4. Malleus
5. Incus
6. Stapes
7. Oval window
8. Eustachian (auditory) tube
9. Cochlea
10. Auditory nerve fibers
11. Vestibule
12. Semicircular canals

Flow Chart Quiz—Ear

1. pinna
2. external auditory canal
3. tympanic membrane
4. malleus
5. incus
6. stapes
7. oval window
8. cochlea
9. auditory liquids and receptors in the organ of Corti
10. auditory nerve fibers
11. cerebral cortex

Review Sheet Quiz

A

1. hearing
2. dull, dim
3. unequal
4. water
5. hearing
6. ear
7. eyelid
8. cochlea
9. conjunctiva
10. pupil

B

1. cornea
2. ciliary body
3. tears; tear duct
4. double
5. gray
6. iris
7. cornea
8. tears
9. smaller, less
10. widen, enlarge

C

1. eardrum
2. night
3. eye
4. eye
5. eye, vision
6. ossicle (small bone)
7. ear
8. eyelid
9. optic disc
10. lens
11. light
12. old age

D

1. pupil
2. retina
3. eustachian tube, auditory tube
4. sclera
5. darkness
6. stapes
7. eardrum, tympanic membrane
8. uvea (vascular layer of the eye)
9. glassy
10. dry

E

1. hearing
2. vision
3. ear condition
4. instrument to measure
5. process of measurement
6. fear
7. paralysis
8. to turn

Medical Scramble

1. CATARACT
2. GLAUCOMA
3. MYRINGITIS
4. VERTIGO

BONUS TERM: MACULAR

Practical Applications

A

1. C
2. B

B

1. C
2. D
3. B
4. D

Crossword Puzzle

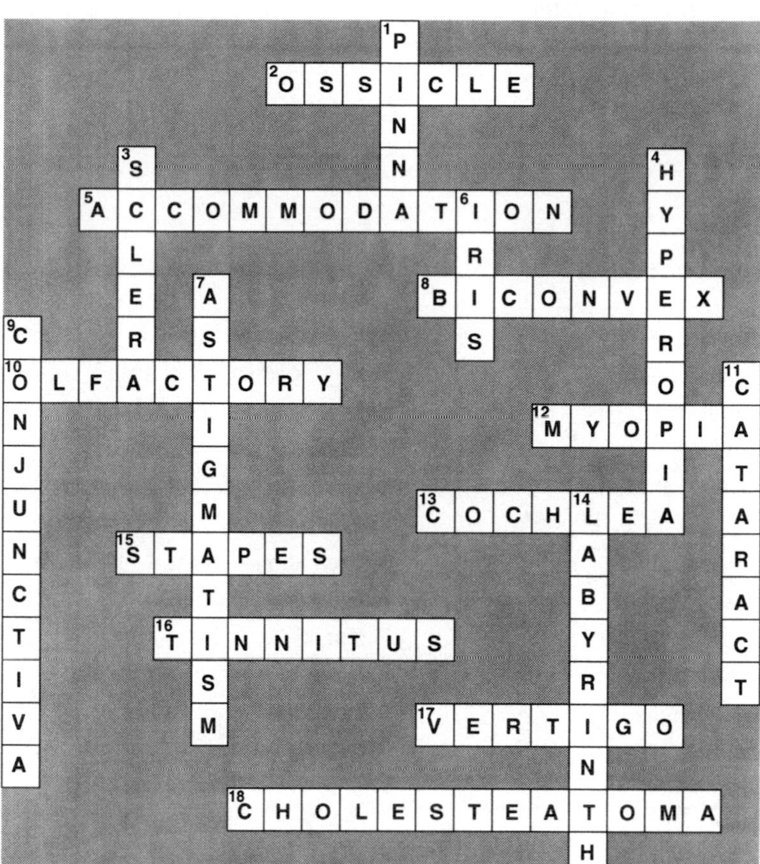

Chapter Seventeen
Answers to Terminology Section

Terminology	Meaning

EYE (textbook pages 702–706)

Structures and Fluids

aqueous humor	Watery fluid that circulates through the posterior and anterior chambers of the eye.
blepharitis	Inflammation of an eyelid.
blepharoptosis	Prolapse (sagging) of an eyelid.
conjunctivitis	Inflammation of the conjunctiva.
anisocoria	Pupils are of unequal size.
corneal abrasion	Defect in the surface of the cornea.
cycloplegic	Pertaining to paralysis of the ciliary muscle (causing paralysis of accommodation).
dacryoadenitis	Inflammation of a lacrimal (tear) gland.
iritis	Inflammation of the iris.
iridic	Pertaining to the iris.
iridectomy	Removal of (a portion of) the iris.
keratitis	Inflammation of the cornea.
lacrimal	Pertaining to tears.
lacrimation	The process of forming tears.
intraocular	Pertaining to within the eye.
ophthalmologist	One who specializes in the study of the eye, its disorders and treatment.
ophthalmic	Pertaining to the eye.
ophthalmoplegia	Paralysis of the eye (muscles).
optic	Pertaining to the eye or to vision.
optometrist	One who "measures" (examines) eyes and prescribes lenses.
optician	One who grinds lenses and fits glasses.
palpebral	Pertaining to the eyelid.
papilledema	Swelling of the optic disc (associated with increased intracranial pressure) and hyperemia (increased blood flow).
phacoemulsification	Technique of cataract extraction using high-frequency ultrasonic vibrations to remove the clouded lens.
aphakia	Absence of the lens of the eye.
pupillary	Pertaining to the pupil.
retinitis	Inflammation of the retina.
hypertensive retinopathy	Disease of the retina associated with (secondary to) high blood pressure.
corneoscleral	Pertaining to the cornea and scleral layers of the eye.
scleritis	Inflammation of the sclera.
uveitis	Inflammation of the uvea (vascular layer of the eye).
vitreous humor	Clear, watery fluid filling the jelly-like mass (vitreous body) that fills the cavity of the eyeball.

Conditions

amblyopia	Dullness of vision (can be caused by poor nutrition, trauma to the eye, or suppression of vision in one eye to avoid diplopia).

diplopia	Double vision (the perception of two images of a single object).
glaucoma	Disease of the eye marked by increased intraocular pressure.
miosis	Condition of contraction of the pupils.
mydriasis	Condition of enlargement of the pupils.
nyctalopia	Condition of night blindness.
photophobia	Condition of sensitivity to light.
presbyopia	Condition of defective vision with advancing age; loss of accommodation.
scotoma	Area of depressed vision surrounded by area of normal vision (blind spot).
xerophthalmia	Condition of dry eyes.

Suffixes

hyperopia	Farsightedness.
hemianopsia	Condition of absence of vision in half of a visual field.
esotropia	Condition in which the eyes turn inward.

EAR (textbook pages 720–721)

acoustic	Pertaining to hearing or sound.
audiogram	Record of hearing as taken by an audiometer.
audiologist	Health care professional specializing in the evaluation and rehabilitation of people with hearing loss.
auditory	Pertaining to hearing.
aural	Pertaining to the ear.
postauricular	Pertaining to behind the ear.
cochlear	Pertaining to the cochlea (spiral-shaped tube in the inner ear).
mastoiditis	Inflammation of the mastoid process (behind the ear).
myringotomy	Incision of the eardrum.
myringitis	Inflammation of the eardrum.
ossiculoplasty	Surgical repair of a middle ear bone.
otic	Pertaining to the ear.
otomycosis	Abnormal condition of a fungal infection in the ear.
otopyorrhea	Discharge of pus from the ear.
otolaryngologist	Specialist in the ear and larynx (upper respiratory region).
salpingopharyngeal	Pertaining to the eustachian tube and the throat.
stapedectomy	Removal of the stapes bone (middle ear bone).
tympanoplasty	Surgical repair of the eardrum.
vestibulocochlear	Pertaining to the vestibule and cochlea of the inner ear. This is the 8th cranial nerve (acoustic nerve).
hyperacusis	Abnormally acute sensitivity to sounds.
presbycusis	Progressive, bilateral hearing loss occurring with age.
audiometer	Instrument to measure the sharpness of hearing.
macrotia	Condition of large ears.

Chapter 18

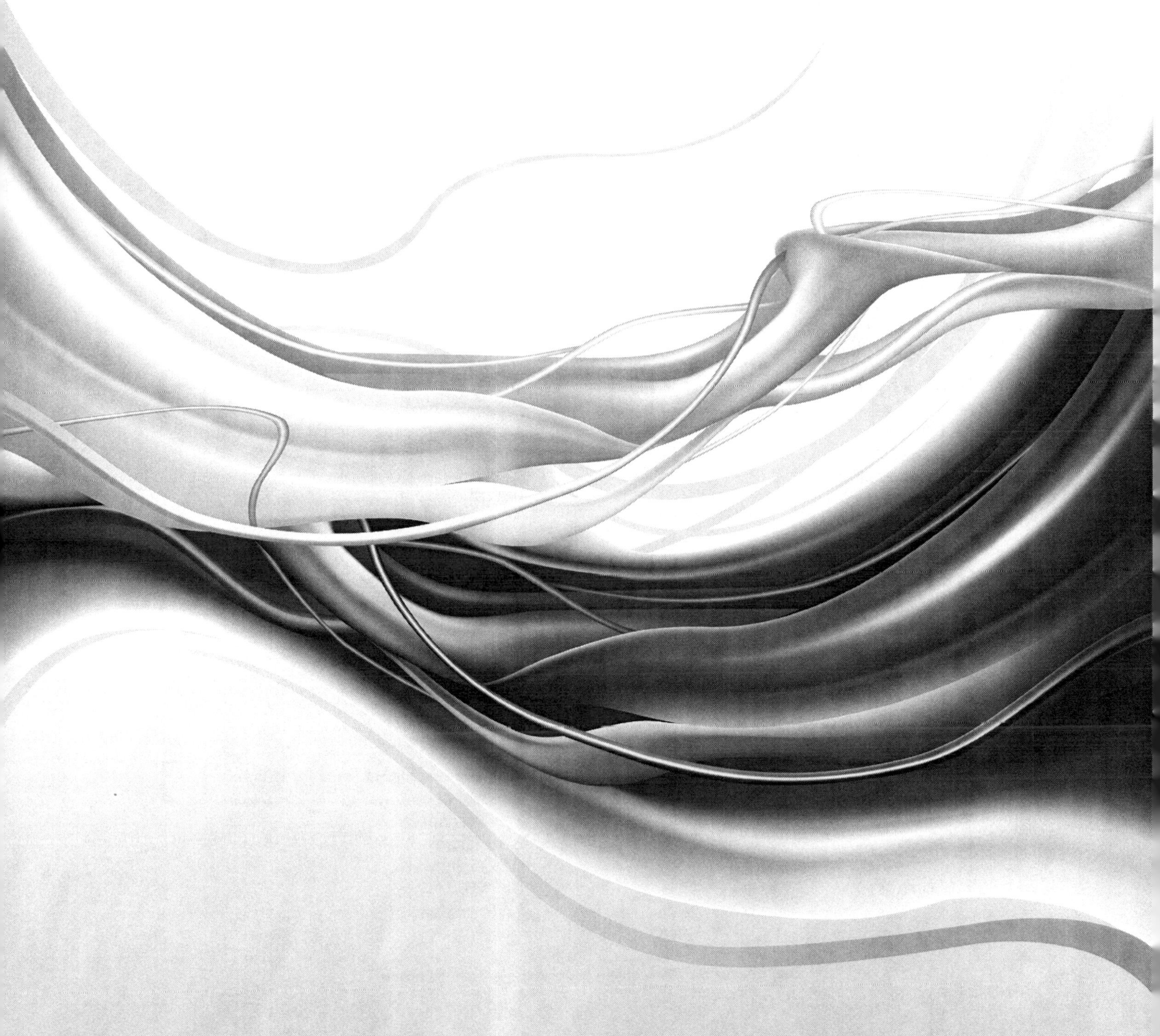

Chapter Eighteen
MULTIPLE CHOICE QUIZ

Name: ______________________________

In the box write the letter of the choice that is the definition of the term or best answers the question. There is only one correct answer for each question.

1. **Which is a function of the thyroid gland?** .... ☐
   A. Secretes immunologic substances
   B. Secretes thymosin
   C. Secretes corticosteroids
   D. Secretes thyroid-stimulating hormone
   E. Secretes thyroxine

2. **What is another name for the anterior lobe of the pituitary gland?** .... ☐
   A. Hypophysis
   B. Hypothalamus
   C. Adenohypophysis
   D. Neurohypophysis
   E. Thalamus

3. **Which of the following secretes cortisol?** .... ☐
   A. Testes
   B. Ovaries
   C. Adrenal medulla
   D. Adrenal cortex
   E. Pituitary gland

4. **Which is a hormone secreted by the pancreas?** .... ☐
   A. Estrogen
   B. Insulin
   C. Vasopressin
   D. Epinephrine
   E. Glucose

5. **Which hormone regulates calcium in the blood and bones?** .... ☐
   A. Parathyroid hormone
   B. Thyroxine
   C. Thyroid-stimulating hormone
   D. Prolactin
   E. Prostaglandins

6. **Which hormone stimulates the adrenal cortex to secrete hormones?** .... ☐
   A. Growth hormone
   B. ADH
   C. ACTH
   D. Cortisone
   E. Secretin

7. **Which is an example of an electrolyte?** .... ☐
   A. Insulin
   B. Sodium
   C. Renin
   D. Glucagon
   E. Steroid

8. **Which is an element that is present in thyroxine?** .... ☐
   A. Iron
   B. Calcium
   C. Vitamin D
   D. Glucose
   E. Iodine

9. **Which is a hormone secreted by the ovary and adrenal cortex?** .... ☐
   A. Follicle-stimulating hormone
   B. Luteinizing hormone
   C. Androgen
   D. Estrogen
   E. Oxytocin

10. **Which is a description of gonadotropins?** .... ☐
    A. Secreted by the anterior lobe of the pituitary gland
    B. Stimulate the growth of long bones
    C. Stimulate glucose uptake in cells
    D. Secreted by the testes
    E. Stimulate the secretion of milk

11. **What is the term for excessive development of mammary tissue in a male?** .... ☐
    A. Homeostasis
    B. Hypogonadism
    C. Galactorrhea
    D. Gynecomastia
    E. Hypernatremia

12. **Kal/i is a combining form for which substance?** .... ☐
    A. Phosphorus
    B. Sodium
    C. Calcium
    D. Milk
    E. Potassium

13. Insulin deficiency or resistance leads to hyperglycemia and ketoacidosis:...... ☐
A. Graves disease
B. Diabetes mellitus
C. Cushing syndrome
D. Acromegaly
E. Myxedema

14. A group of symptoms produced by excess of cortisol from the adrenal cortex:.. ☐
A. Graves disease
B. Diabetes mellitus
C. Cushing syndrome
D. Acromegaly
E. Myxedema

15. Advanced hypothyroidism in adulthood:.. ☐
A. Graves disease
B. Diabetes mellitus
C. Cushing syndrome
D. Acromegaly
E. Myxedema

16. Post-puberty hypersecretion of growth hormone from the anterior pituitary gland:... ☐
A. Graves disease
B. Diabetes mellitus
C. Cushing syndrome
D. Acromegaly
E. Myxedema

17. Thyrotoxicosis; hypersecretion of the thyroid gland:................................... ☐
A. Graves disease
B. Diabetes mellitus
C. Cushing syndrome
D. Acromegaly
E. Myxedema

18. Which term means enlargement of the thyroid gland? .... ☐
A. Hypergonadism
B. Euthyroid
C. Goiter
D. Hypophyseal enlargement
E. Tetany

19. Exophthalmos is a symptom of which endocrine disorder? .... ☐
A. Endemic goiter
B. Thyroid carcinoma
C. Graves disease
D. Nodular goiter
E. Pituitary gland hypertrophy

20. Which is a description of tetany? .... ☐
A. Constant muscle contraction
B. Increased bone growth
C. Hypercalcemia
D. Hypokalemia
E. Hypernatremia

21. Natr/o is the combining form for which substance? .... ☐
A. Sugar
B. Milk
C. Sodium
D. Iodine
E. Potassium

22. Characteristic of type 1 diabetes mellitus? .... ☐
A. Gradual onset; patient is asymptomatic
B. Ketoacidosis seldom occurs
C. Treatment is diet and oral hypoglycemic agents
D. Little or no insulin produced
E. Usually occurs after age 30

23. Which of the following is associated with neuropathy, nephropathy, and retinopathy? .... ☐
A. Hyperthyroidism
B. Deficient ADH secretion
C. Secondary complications of diabetes mellitus
D. Hypergonadism
E. Panhypopituitarism

24. Which is a description of achondroplasia?................................ ☐
A. Enlargement of extremities
B. Defective cartilage formation that affects bone growth
C. Tumor of the sella turcica
D. Abnormal formation of cartilage in an adult
E. Hyperfunctioning of pituitary gland

25. Which is a description of a thyroid scan?... ☐
A. CT image of thyroid gland
B. Radioimmunoassay of thyroxine in the bloodstream
C. Ultrasound image of the neck
D. Skull x-ray of the brain
E. Administration of radioactive compound and visualization with a scanner to detect tumors or nodules

Chapter Eighteen
VOCABULARY QUIZ

Name: ______________________________

A. Match the following glands with their descriptions below:

adrenal cortex	pancreas	testes
adrenal medulla	parathyroid glands	thyroid gland
ovaries	pituitary gland	

1. Two glands enclosed in the scrotal sac of a male ______________________________
2. Located behind the stomach; alpha and beta islet cells secrete hormones ______________
3. Located in the neck on either side of the trachea; secretes thyroxine ______________
4. Inner section of a gland above each kidney; secretes epinephrine ______________
5. Located at the base of the brain in the sella turcica; hypophysis ______________
6. Outer section of a gland above each kidney: secretes cortisol, aldosterone, and sex hormones ______________________________
7. Located in the lower abdomen of a female; responsible for egg cell production and estrogen secretion ______________________________
8. Four small glands on the posterior side of the thyroid gland ______________________

B. Match the following hormones with their descriptions below:

adrenaline (epinephrine)	antidiuretic hormone (ADH)	estradiol
adrenocorticotropic hormone (ACTH)	calcitonin	follicle-stimulating hormone
aldosterone	cortisol	glucagon
androgen		

1. Male hormone secreted by the testes ______________________________
2. Female hormone secreted by the ovaries ______________________________
3. Secreted by the posterior lobe of the pituitary gland; vasopressin ______________
4. Secreted by the adrenal medulla; increases heart rate and blood pressure ______________
5. Secreted by the thyroid gland; decreases blood calcium levels ______________
6. Secreted by the adrenal cortex; increases salt reabsorption ______________
7. Secreted by the anterior lobe of the pituitary gland; stimulates hormone secretion and egg production by the ovaries ______________________________
8. Secreted by the pancreas; increases blood sugar by conversion of glycogen to glucose ______________________________

9. Secreted by the anterior lobe of the pituitary gland; stimulates secretions of the adrenal cortex ____________________

10. Secreted by the adrenal cortex; increases blood sugar ____________________

C. *Match the following hormones with their descriptions below:*

growth hormone (somatotropin)	oxytocin	testosterone
insulin	parathormone	thyroid-stimulating hormone
luteinizing hormone	prolactin	progesterone
		thyroxine

1. Secreted by the ovaries; prepares the uterus for pregnancy ____________________
2. Secreted by beta islet cells of the pancreas; lowers blood sugar ____________________
3. Secreted by the anterior lobe of the pituitary gland; promotes milk secretion ____________________
4. Secreted by the anterior lobe of the pituitary gland; stimulates secretion by the thyroid gland ____________________
5. Male hormone secreted by the testes ____________________
6. Secreted by the posterior lobe of the pituitary gland; stimulates contraction of the uterus during childbirth ____________________
7. Secreted by the thyroid gland; increases metabolism in cells; T4 ____________________
8. Secreted by the anterior lobe of the pituitary gland; stimulates ovulation ____________________
9. Secreted by the anterior lobe of the pituitary gland; stimulates growth of bones and soft tissues ____________________
10. Secreted by the parathyroid glands; increases blood calcium ____________________

D. Match the following terms with their descriptions below:

catecholamines	hypothalamus	sella turcica
corticosteroids	glucocorticoid	sympathomimetic
electrolyte	mineralocorticoid	target tissue
homeostasis		

1. Region of the brain lying below the thalamus; secretes factors and hormones that affect the pituitary gland ______________________
2. Cavity in the skull that contains the pituitary gland ______________________
3. Tendency of an organism to maintain a constant internal environment ______________________
4. Mimicking or copying the effect of the sympathetic nervous system; adrenaline is an example ______________________
5. Mineral salt found in the blood and tissues and necessary for proper functioning of cells; potassium is an example ______________________
6. Hormones derived from an amino acid and secreted by the adrenal medulla ______________________
7. Cells of an organ that are affected or stimulated by specific hormones ______________________
8. Steroid hormone secreted by the adrenal cortex; regulates mineral salts and water balance ______________________
9. Steroid hormones secreted by the adrenal cortex; cortisol, aldosterone, and sex hormones are examples ______________________
10. Steroid hormone secreted by the adrenal cortex; regulates glucose, fat, and protein metabolism ______________________

Chapter Eighteen
TERMINOLOGY QUIZ

Name: ______________________________

A. Using the following word parts, create or complete terms based on the following definitions:

aden/o	pituitar/o	-pathy	hypo-
adrenal/o	thyr/o	-tropic	poly-
gonad/o	thyroid/o	-tropin	
pancreat/o	-ectomy	-uria	
parathyroid/o	-itis	hyper-	

1. Removal of a gland behind the thyroid gland: ______________________________
2. A hormone that stimulates the thyroid gland: ______________________________ hormone
3. Removal of one of the glands above the kidney: ______________________________
4. Condition of decreased secretion of the master gland: ______________________________ ism
5. Inflammation of the thyroid gland: ______________________________
6. Resection of an endocrine gland below the stomach: ______________________________
7. Removal of a gland: ______________________________
8. Condition of excessive urination: ______________________________
9. Deficiency (in growth and secretions) of the sex glands: ______________________________ ism
10. Any hormone that stimulates the sex glands: ______________________________

B. Using the following word parts, create or complete terms based on the following definitions:

andr/o	dips/o	-emia
calc/o, calci/o	estr/o	hyper-
cortic/o	gluc/o	hypo-
crin/o	glyc/o	

1. High levels of sugar in the blood: ______________________________
2. Excessive thirst: ______________________________ ia
3. Low levels of calcium in the blood: ______________________________
4. A hormone secreted by the adrenal cortex: ______________________________ steroid
5. Pertaining to sugar in the blood: ______________________________ emic
6. High levels of calcium in the urine: ______________________________
7. Male hormone (producing male characteristics): ______________________________ gen
8. Pertaining to producing female characteristics: ______________________________ genic
9. High levels of calcium in the blood: ______________________________
10. Animal starch: ______________________________ gen

C. Using the following word parts, create or complete terms based on the following definitions:

home/o	natr/o	toxic/o	-osis
hormon/o	phys/o	-ectomy	anti-
kal/i	somat/o	-emia	hypo-
lact/o	ster/o	-in, ine	
myx/o	toc/o		

1. Removal of the pituitary gland: hypo ________________
2. A hormone that promotes rapid labor and delivery: oxy________________in
3. Low levels of sodium in the blood: ________________
4. Hormone that stimulates milk secretion: pro ________________in
5. Chemical that promotes water loss in urine: ________________diuretic hormone
6. Abnormal condition of mucus-like material under the skin: ________________ edema
7. Abnormal condition of oversecretion from the thyroid gland: thyro ________________
8. Low levels of potassium in the blood: ________________
9. Growth hormone: ________________ tropin
10. Many hormones are examples of this solid, ring-shaped molecule: ________________ oid

D. Using the following word parts, create or complete terms based on the following definitions:

glycos/o	-emia	hyper-
glyc/o	-in, ine	hypo-
kal/i	-tropin	pan-
pituitar/o	-uria	tetra-
-agon	eu-	tri-

1. Decrease of all hormones secreted by the pituitary gland: ________________ ism
2. Condition of sugar in urine: ________________
3. Low levels of sugar in the blood: ________________
4. High levels of potassium in the blood: ________________
5. Thyroid gland hormone (T_4): ________________ iodothyron ________________ine
6. Hormone secreted by the pituitary gland to stimulate the adrenal cortex:

   adrenocortico ________________
7. Normal thyroid function: ________________ thyroid
8. Deficient secretion of insulin by the pancreas: ________________ insulinism
9. Hormone secreted by the adrenal medulla: epinephr ________________
10. Hormone secreted by the pancreas to increase blood sugar levels: gluc ________________

Chapter Eighteen
PATHOLOGY QUIZ

Name: ______________________

A. Match the following abnormal conditions with their descriptions below:

Addison disease	hyperparathyroidism	pheochromocytoma
adrenal virilism	hyperthyroidism	thyroid carcinoma
cretinism	hypoparathyroidism	
Cushing syndrome	myxedema	

1. Cancer of the thyroid gland (papillary and follicular are types) ______________
2. Advanced hypothyroidism in adulthood ______________
3. Deficient production of parathyroid hormone (tetany results) ______________
4. Excessive secretion of adrenal gland androgens ______________
5. Hypofunctioning of the adrenal cortex ______________
6. Excessive production of parathormone ______________
7. Extreme hypothyroidism during infancy and childhood ______________
8. Overactivity of the thyroid gland (thyrotoxicosis) ______________
9. Group of signs and symptoms produced by excess cortisol from the adrenal cortex ______________
10. Benign tumor of the adrenal medulla ______________

B. Match the following abnormal conditions with their descriptions below:

acromegaly	dwarfism	panhypopituitarism
diabetes insipidus	gigantism	syndrome of inappropriate ADH
diabetes mellitus	hyperinsulinism	

1. Insufficient secretion of antidiuretic hormone (vasopressin) ______________
2. Congenital hyposecretion of growth hormone ______________
3. Hypersecretion of the anterior pituitary gland beginning after puberty ______________
4. Hypersecretion of growth hormone from the anterior pituitary beginning before puberty ______________
5. Deficiency of all pituitary hormones ______________
6. Lack of insulin secretion or resistance of insulin to promote sugar, starch and fat (carbohydrate) metabolism in cells ______________
7. Excess secretion of insulin leads to hypoglycemia ______________
8. Excess secretion of antidiuretic hormone ______________

Chapter Eighteen

LABORATORY TESTS AND CLINICAL PROCEDURES QUIZ

Name: ______________________________

Match the following tests and procedures with their descriptions below:

exophthalmometry	serum and urine tests
fasting plasma glucose	thyroid function tests
radioactive iodine uptake scan	thyroid scan

1. Measurement of eyeball protrusion (sign of Graves disease): ______________________________
2. Device detects radioactivity and visualizes the thyroid gland after IV administration of radioactive technetium compound: ______________________________
3. Measurement of T_3, T_4, and TSH in the bloodstream: ______________________________
4. Measures circulating glucose level in a patient who as fasted at least 8 hours: ______________________________
5. Radioactive iodine is given orally and its uptake by the thyroid gland is imaged: ______________________________
6. Hormones, electrolytes, glucose and other substances are measured in blood and urine: ______________________________

Chapter Eighteen

ABBREVIATIONS QUIZ

Name: ______________________________

On the line provided, give meanings for the following abbreviations, then write each abbreviation next to its explanation below:

1. TSH ____________________
2. RAI ____________________
3. Na^+ ____________________
4. GH ____________________
5. T_4 ____________________
6. GTT ____________________
7. ACTH ____________________
8. TFT ____________________
9. DM ____________________
10. DI ____________________

a. __________ Type 1 and type 2 are forms of this condition

b. __________ This is an electrolyte

c. __________ This test assesses the function of an endocrine gland in the neck

d. __________ Secretion of this hormone stimulates an endocrine gland above the kidney

e. __________ Secretion of this hormone from the anterior pituitary gland stimulates an endocrine gland in the neck

f. __________ Hormone secreted from the thyroid gland

g. __________ Treatment for Graves disease to destroy an overactive thyroid gland

h. __________ Posterior pituitary gland fails to release vasopressin

i. __________ Somatotropin

j. __________ Test to assess the sugar levels in the blood

Chapter Eighteen
EXERCISE QUIZ

Name: ______________________

A. Name the endocrine organs that produce the following hormones:

1. insulin ______________________
2. cortisol ______________________
3. epinephrine ______________________
4. follicle-stimulating hormone ____________
5. thyroxine ______________________
6. aldosterone ______________________
7. vasopressin ______________________
8. estradiol ______________________
9. growth hormone ______________________
10. progesterone ______________________

B. Give the meaning of the following abbreviations for hormones:

11. ACTH ______________________
12. ADH ______________________
13. TSH ______________________
14. PTH ______________________
15. T_4 ______________________
16. T_3 ______________________
17. LH ______________________
18. GH ______________________

C. Match the following hormones with their actions:

ACTH	epinephrine	testosterone
ADH	estradiol	thyroxine
aldosterone	insulin	
cortisol	parathyroid hormone	

19. sympathomimetic; elevates heart rate, blood pressure ______________________
20. promotes growth and maintenance of male sex characteristics ______________________
21. stimulates water reabsorption by kidney tubules; decreases urine ______________________
22. increases metabolism in body cells ______________________
23. raises blood calcium ______________________
24. increases reabsorption of sodium by kidney tubules ______________________
25. stimulates secretion of hormones from adrenal cortex ______________________
26. increases blood sugar ______________________
27. helps transport glucose to cells and decreases blood sugar ______________________
28. develops and maintains female sex characteristics ______________________

D. *Build medical terms from their definitions and word parts given:*

29. abnormal condition (hypersecretion) of the thyroid gland: thyro ______________________
30. removal of the pancreas: ______________________ ectomy
31. condition of deficiency or underdevelopment of sex organs: hypo ______________________
32. pertaining to producing female characteristics: ______________________ genic
33. removal of the pituitary gland: ______________________ ectomy
34. deficiency of calcium in the blood: hypo ______________________
35. excessive sugar in the blood: ______________________ emia

E. *Indicate whether the following are related to hypo- or hypersecretion, and name the endocrine gland involved:*

	hypo- or hyper-	gland
36. acromegaly	____________	____________
37. tetany	____________	____________
38. diabetes mellitus	____________	____________
39. Graves disease	____________	____________
40. myxedema	____________	____________
41. Cushing syndrome	____________	____________
42. cretinism	____________	____________

F. *Give the meanings for the following conditions:*

43. hyponatremia ______________________
44. polydipsia ______________________
45. glycosuria ______________________
46. euthyroid ______________________

G. *Give the meanings for the following terms or abbreviations related to diabetes mellitus:*

47. type 1 ______________________
48. diabetic neuropathy ______________________
49. ketoacidosis ______________________
50. type 2 ______________________

Chapter Eighteen

DICTATION AND COMPREHENSION QUIZ: VOCABULARY AND TERMINOLOGY

Name: ______________________

A. Dictation of Terms

1. ______________________ 11. ______________________
2. ______________________ 12. ______________________
3. ______________________ 13. ______________________
4. ______________________ 14. ______________________
5. ______________________ 15. ______________________
6. ______________________ 16. ______________________
7. ______________________ 17. ______________________
8. ______________________ 18. ______________________
9. ______________________ 19. ______________________
10. ______________________ 20. ______________________

B. Comprehension of Terms: Match number of the above term with its meaning below.

_______ Hormone secreted by the posterior part of the pituitary gland; increases reabsorption of water
_______ Hormone secreted by the adrenal cortex; increases salt (sodium) reabsorption by the kidney
_______ A mineral salt found in the blood and tissues; potassium is an example
_______ excessive thirst
_______ Hormone secreted by the thyroid gland; lowers blood calcium
_______ Resection of a gland near and behind the stomach
_______ Hormone secreted by the posterior pituitary gland; stimulates contraction of the uterus during labor
_______ Sugar present in the urine
_______ Hormone secreted by the thyroid gland; thyroxine
_______ Tendency of an organism to maintain a constant internal environment
_______ Blood condition of deficient sodium
_______ Type of hormone secreted by the adrenal cortex; necessary for the use of sugars, fats, and proteins
_______ Anterior lobe of the pituitary gland
_______ Resection of four small glands in the neck region
_______ Hormone secreted by the ovaries
_______ Blood condition of deficient potassium
_______ Region of the brain that produces factors to stimulate the pituitary gland
_______ Hormone secreted by the anterior lobe of the pituitary gland; stimulates the adrenal cortex
_______ Condition of sugar in the blood
_______ Hormone derived from an amino acid and secreted by the adrenal medulla; epinephrine is an example

Chapter Eighteen

DICTATION AND COMPREHENSION QUIZ: ABNORMAL CONDITIONS, LABORATORY TESTS, PROCEDURES

Name: ______________________________

A. Dictation of Terms

1. ______________________ 11. ______________________
2. ______________________ 12. ______________________
3. ______________________ 13. ______________________
4. ______________________ 14. ______________________
5. ______________________ 15. ______________________
6. ______________________ 16. ______________________
7. ______________________ 17. ______________________
8. ______________________ 18. ______________________
9. ______________________ 19. ______________________
10. ______________________ 20. ______________________

B. Comprehension of Terms: Match number of the above term with its meaning below.

______ Test that measures hormone levels in plasma
______ Test that measures levels of sugar in the blood
______ Radioactive compound is given and localizes in the thyroid gland
______ Enlargement of extremities caused by excessive growth hormone after puberty
______ Insufficient secretion of antidiuretic hormone produces this condition
______ Malignant tumor of an endocrine gland in the neck
______ Extreme hypothyroidism during infancy and childhood produces this condition
______ Advanced hypothyroidism in adulthood produces this condition
______ Enlargement and bulging of the eyeballs caused by hyperthyroidism
______ Excessive hair on the face and body of adult women
______ Group of symptoms produced by excess of cortisol from the adrenal cortex
______ Enlargement of the thyroid gland
______ Overactivity of the thyroid gland (Graves disease)
______ Benign tumor of the adrenal medulla
______ Lack of insulin secretion or resistance of insulin to promoting sugar, starch, and fat metabolism in cells
______ Constant muscle contraction
______ Fats are improperly burned, leading to accumulation of ketones in the body
______ Hypofunctioning of the adrenal cortex

Chapter Eighteen
SPELLING QUIZ

Name: ______________________________

A. Circle the term that is spelled correctly and write its meaning in the space provided.

1. courtisol — cortisol ______________________
2. goiter — goyter ______________________
3. estrogen — estrogin ______________________
4. pitiutary gland — pituitary gland ______________________
5. gonadotrophan — gonadotropin ______________________
6. uthyroid — euthyroid ______________________
7. hypocalemia — hypokalemia ______________________
8. hypophysectomy — hypophisectomy ______________________
9. pancrease — pancreas ______________________
10. corticosteroid — cortikosteroid ______________________

B. Circle the term that is spelled correctly. The meaning of each term is given.

11. Hormone secreted by the thyroid gland	thyroixine	thiroxine	thyroxine
12. Condition of eyeballs that protrude outward	exopthalmos	exophthmalmos	exophthalmos
13. Hormone secreted by the ovary	progesterone	projesterone	progesteron
14. Constant muscle contraction	tetany	teteny	tettany
15. Hormone secreted by the islet cells of Langerhans	insalin	insulin	insulen
16. State of equilibrium or constancy	homeiostasis	homostasis	homeostasis
17. Part of the brain that controls the secretions of the pituitary gland	hypothalmus	hypothalmis	hypothalamus
18. Excessive thirst	polydipsea	pollydipsia	polydipsia
19. Enlargement of extremities due to hypersecretion of growth hormone	acromegaly	accromegaly	acromeagaly
20. Hyposecretion of the thyroid gland in adulthood	mixadema	myxedema	myxademae

Chapter Eighteen
PRONUNCIATION QUIZ

Name: ____________________

A. Underline the accented syllable in the following terms:

1. glucagon
2. parathormone
3. adenohypophysis
4. testosterone
5. sella turcica
6. goiter
7. exophthalmos
8. homeostasis
9. mineralocorticoid
10. gonadotropin

B. Match the term in Column I with its meaning in Column II:

Column I		Column II
1. aldosterone	_______	A. Starch; storage form of sugar
2. diabetes insipidus	_______	B. A mineral salt found in the blood and in tissues
3. diabetes mellitus	_______	C. Hormone secreted by the adrenal cortex
4. progesterone	_______	D. Hormone secreted by the adrenal medulla
5. glycogen	_______	E. Hormone secreted by the ovary
6. cretinism	_______	F. Disease condition due to malfunction of the posterior lobe of the pituitary gland
7. epinephrine	_______	G. Extreme hypothyroidism in childhood
8. thyroxine	_______	H. Disease condition due to malfunction of cells in the pancreas
9. electrolyte	_______	I. Hormone secreted by anterior lobe of pituitary gland
10. prolactin	_______	J. Hormone secreted by thyroid gland

C. Complete the following terms from their definitions below:

1. hyper ____________________	Excessive amount of calcium in the blood
2. hypo ____________________	Deficient amount of potassium in the blood
3. hypo ____________________	Deficient sodium in the blood
4. ____________________ ectomy	Removal of the pancreas
5. glyc- ____________________	Pertaining to sugar in the blood
6. poly ____________________	Excessive thirst
7. ____________________ thyroid	Normal thyroid function
8. tri ____________________	Hormone secreted by the thyroid gland

Chapter Eighteen
DIAGRAM QUIZ

Name: ____________________

Label the diagram below using the terms listed below:

Adrenal glands
Ovaries
Pancreas
Parathyroid glands
Pineal gland
Pituitary gland
Testes
Thyroid gland

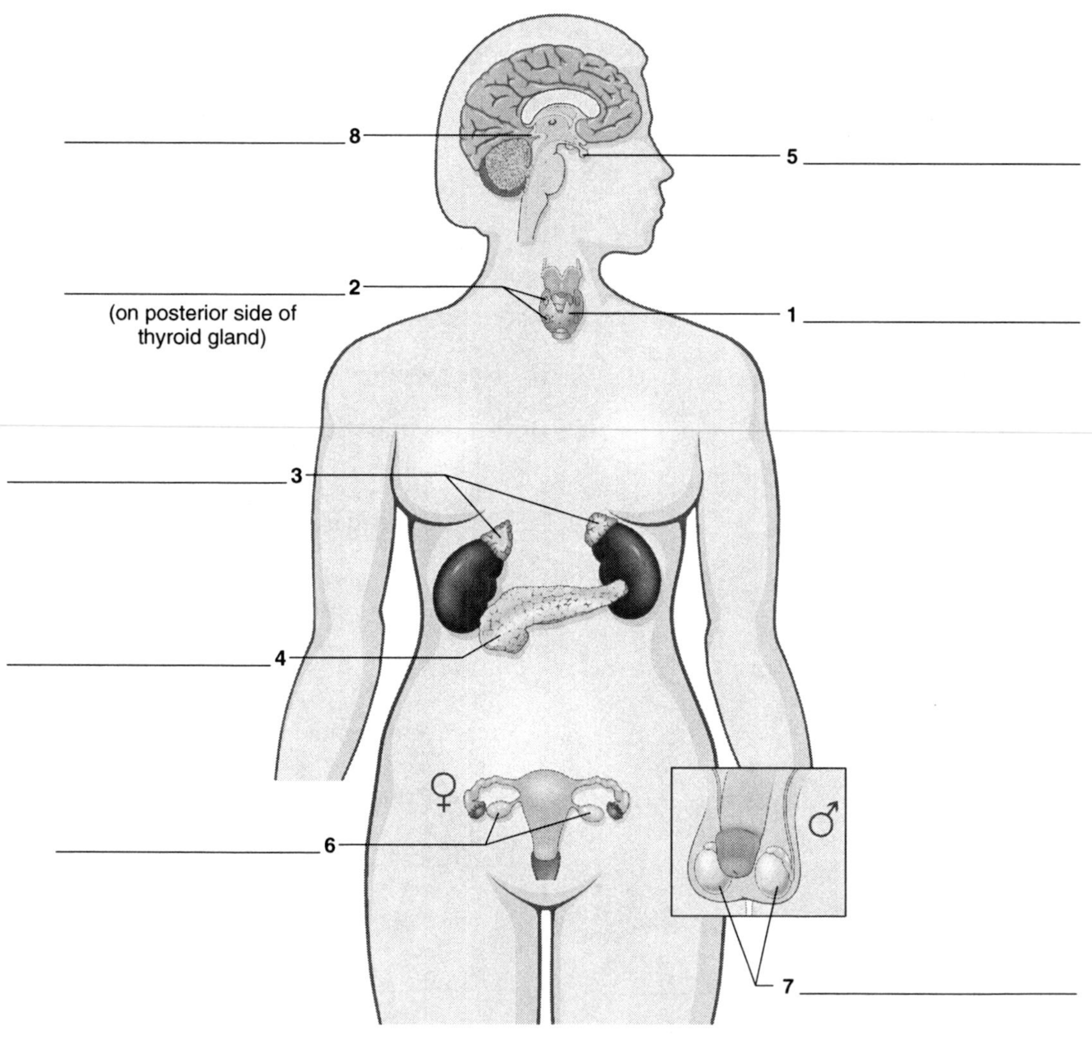

Chapter Eighteen
REVIEW SHEET QUIZ

Name: ______________________

A. Give meanings for the following combining forms:

1. aden/o ______________________
2. adrenal/o ______________________
3. andr/o ______________________
4. calc/o ______________________
5. cortic/o ______________________
6. dips/o ______________________
7. estr/o ______________________
8. gluc/o ______________________
9. glyc/o ______________________
10. gonad/o ______________________

B. Give meanings for the following combining forms:

1. kal/i ______________________
2. lact/o ______________________
3. myx/o ______________________
4. natr/o ______________________
5. pancreat/o ______________________
6. somat/o ______________________
7. thyr/o ______________________
8. toxic/o ______________________
9. ur/o ______________________
10. home/o ______________________

C. Give meanings for the following suffixes and prefixes:

1. -agon ______________________
2. -ectomy ______________________
3. -emia ______________________
4. -genic ______________________
5. -tropin ______________________
6. -uria ______________________
7. -megaly ______________________
8. hyper- ______________________
9. hypo- ______________________
10. pan- ______________________
11. tetra- ______________________
12. poly- ______________________
13. tri- ______________________
14. eu- ______________________

Chapter Eighteen
MEDICAL SCRAMBLE

Name: ______________________________

Unscramble the letters to form endocrine system–related terms from the clues. Use the letters in the squares to complete the bonus term.

1. *Clue:* Condition caused by increased growth hormone after puberty

☐ ___ ___ ___ ☐ ___ ___ ___ ___ ___ E C G Y A R L A O M

2. *Clue:* Hormone stimulating childbirth

___ ☐ ☐ ___ ___ ___ ___ ___ I T C X O N Y O

3. *Clue:* The "flight or fight" hormone

___ ☐ ___ ☐ ___ ___ ___ ___ ___ ☐ E L E A N D I R N A

4. *Clue:* Inner portion of the gland above the kidney

☐ ___ ___ ___ ___ ___ ___ U A M L E L D

BONUS TERM: *Clue:* A condition caused by deficiency of thyroid hormone in an adult

☐ ☐ ☐ ☐ ☐ ☐ ☐ ☐

Chapter Eighteen

CROSSWORD PUZZLE

Name: ______________________

Fill in the crossword puzzle below using the clues listed underneath it.

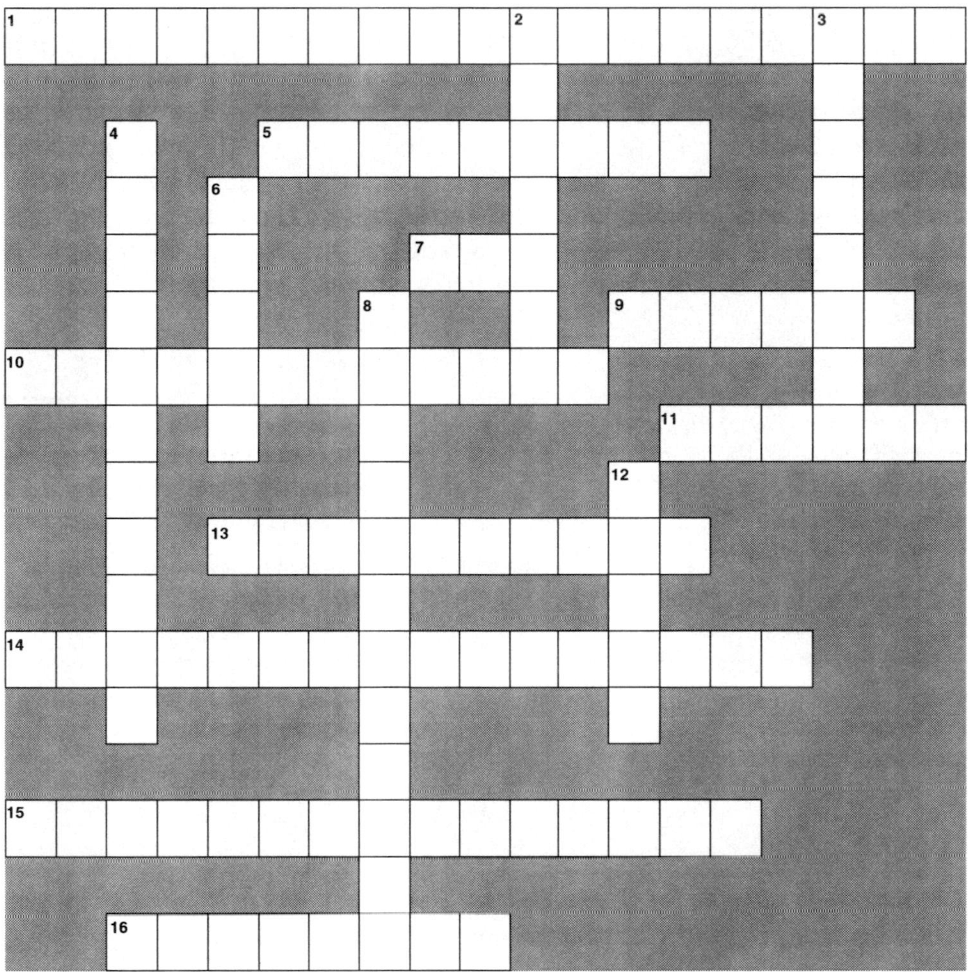

Across Clues

1. ACTH.
5. Kal/i means ____________________.
7. Pan- means ____________________.
9. Two endocrine glands in the scrotal sac of a male.
10. A hormone produced by the ovaries.
11. Toxic/o means ____________________.
13. Enlargement of the extremities; pituitary gland.
14. T_3.
15. Pertaining to mimicking or copying the effect of the sympathetic nervous system.
16. Home/o means ____________________.

Down Clues

2. Produced by the islet cells of the pancreas.
3. Endocrine gland behind the stomach.
4. Tendency in an organism to return to an. equilibrium or constant, stable state.
6. Tri- means ____________________.
8. A male hormone produced by the testes.
12. Aden/o means ____________________.

Chapter Eighteen

PRACTICAL APPLICATIONS

Name: ______________________

A. Cushing Syndrome

Hypertension, both systolic and diastolic, is a common feature of Cushing syndrome. Other clinical features are likely to attract more attention than the hypertension: obesity with "buffalo hump" and "moon face," muscular weakness, scattered bruises, and osteoporosis. The excessive secretion of adrenocortical steroids that is responsible for the syndrome is frequently due to primary disease of the adrenals, either hyperplasia or discrete tumors. However, the hyperactivity of the adrenal cortex may be secondary to a tumor or malfunction of the pituitary or a neoplasm secreting an ACTH-like substance elsewhere in the body. Appropriate x-ray studies, including arteriograms or retrograde venograms of the adrenals, may disclose a tumor in the adrenals, hypophysis, or elsewhere.

1. **Which is a common clinical feature of Cushing syndrome?......................** ☐
   - A. Decreased blood flow to the heart
   - B. Abnormal sounds in the heart
   - C. Peripheral edema
   - D. High blood pressure when the heart is contracting and relaxing
2. **Cushing syndrome is associated with which of the following?......................** ☐
   - A. Tendency to accumulate fat in tissues
   - B. Tetany
   - C. Bone tumors
   - D. Low blood pressure
3. **What is a probable etiology of Cushing syndrome?...........................** ☐
   - A. Excessive porosity of bones
   - B. Decreased secretion of adrenal hormones
   - C. Decreased secretion of pituitary hormones
   - D. Tumor or disease of the adrenal cortex
4. **What is a likely secondary cause of Cushing syndrome?...........................** ☐
   - A. Decreased secretion of ACTH
   - B. Blocked artery in the kidney
   - C. Tumor of the adenohypophysis
   - D. Muscular weakness

B. Chart Note

A 26-year-old woman is referred for Graves disease. The patient was first found to be hyperthyroid shortly after she became pregnant. She has a tremor in her hands, a sensation of being hot, insomnia, weakness in her legs, and exophthalmos.

Physical examination reveals thyromegaly; the gland is rather mushy and soft. No nodules were noted. T_3 and T_4 levels were ordered and an appointment was made to have an uptake scan.

1. **What is the cause of Graves disease?...** ☐
   - A. The thyroid gland is slow to function
   - B. The pancreas is hyperfunctioning
   - C. The thyroid gland is oversecreting
   - D. Hyperactive ovarian function
2. **Why were T_3 and T_4 levels ordered?.....** ☐
   - A. To measure the extent of eyelid prolapse
   - B. To assess the function of the thyroid gland
   - C. To measure the size of the thyroid gland
   - D. To assess heart function

Chapter Eighteen
ANSWERS TO THE QUIZZES

Multiple Choice Quiz

1. E
2. C
3. D
4. B
5. A
6. C
7. B
8. E
9. D
10. A
11. D
12. E
13. B
14. C
15. E
16. D
17. A
18. C
19. C
20. A
21. C
22. D
23. C
24. B
25. E

Vocabulary Quiz

A

1. testes
2. pancreas
3. thyroid gland
4. adrenal medulla
5. pituitary gland
6. adrenal cortex
7. ovaries
9. parathyroid glands

B

1. androgen
2. estradiol
3. antidiuretic hormone (ADH)
4. adrenaline (epinephrine)
5. calcitonin
6. aldosterone
7. follicle-stimulating hormone
8. glucagon
9. adrenocorticotropic hormone (ACTH)
10. cortisol

C

1. progesterone
2. insulin
3. prolactin
4. thyroid-stimulating hormone
5. testosterone
6. oxytocin
7. thyroxine
8. luteinizing hormone
9. growth hormone (somatotropin)
10. parathormone

D

1. hypothalamus
2. sella turcica
3. homeostasis
4. sympathomimetic
5. electrolyte
6. catecholamines
7. target tissue
8. mineralocorticoid
9. corticosteroids
10. glucocorticoid

Terminology Quiz

A

1. parathyroidectomy
2. thyrotropic hormone
3. adrenalectomy
4. hypopituitarism
5. throiditis
6. pancreatectomy
7. adenectomy
8. polyuria
9. hypogonadism
10. gonadotropin

B

1. hyperglycemia
2. polydipsia
3. hypocalcemia
4. corticosteroid
5. glycemic
6. hypercalciuria
7. androgen
8. estrogenic
9. hypercalcemia
10. glycogen

C

1. hypophysectomy
2. oxytocin
3. hyponatremia
4. prolactin
5. antidiuretic hormone
6. myxedema
7. thyrotoxicosis
8. hypokalemia
9. somatotrophin
10. steroid

D

1. panhypopituitarism
2. glycosuria
3. hypoglycemia
4. hyperkalemia
5. tetraiodothyronine
6. adrenocorticotropin
7. euthyroid
8. hypoinsulinism
9. epinephrine
10. glucagon

Pathology Quiz

A

1. thyroid carcinoma
2. myxedema
3. hypoparathyroidism
4. adrenal virilism
5. Addison disease
6. hyperparathyroidism
7. cretinism
8. hyperthyroidism
9. Cushing syndrome
10. pheochromocytoma

B

1. diabetes insipidus
2. dwarfism
3. acromegaly
4. gigantism
5. panhypopituitarism
6. diabetes mellitus
7. hyperinsulinism
8. syndrome of inappropriate ADH

Laboratory Tests and Clinical Procedures Quiz

1. exophthalmometry
2. thyroid scan
3. thyroid function tests
4. fasting plasma glucose
5. radioactive iodine uptake scan
6. serum and urine tests

Abbreviations Quiz

1. thyroid-stimulating hormone
2. radioactive iodine
3. sodium
4. growth hormone
5. thyroxine
6. glucose tolerance test
7. adrenocorticotropic hormone
8. thyroid function test
9. diabetes mellitus
10. diabetes insipidus

a. DM
b. Na^+
c. TFT
d. ACTH
e. TSH
f. T_4
g. RAI
h. DI
i. GH
j. GTT

Exercise Quiz

A

1. pancreas
2. adrenal cortex
3. adrenal medulla
4. ovary
5. thyroid gland
6. adrenal cortex
7. posterior pituitary gland
8. ovary; adrenal cortex
9. anterior pituitary gland
10. ovary

B

11. adrenocorticotropic hormone
12. antidiuretic hormone
13. thyroid-stimulating hormone
14. parathyroid hormone; parathormone
15. tetraiodothyronine (thyroxine)
16. triiodothyronine
17. luteinizing hormone
18. growth hormone

C

19. epinephrine
20. testosterone
21. ADH
22. thyroxine
23. parathyroid hormone
24. aldosterone
25. ACTH
26. cortisol
27. insulin
28. estradiol

D

29. thyrotoxicosis
30. pancreatectomy
31. hypogonadism
32. estrogenic
33. hypophysectomy
34. hypocalcemia
35. hyperglycemia

E

36. hyper/adenohypophysis
37. hypo/parathyroid
38. hypo/pancreas
39. hyper/thyroid
40. hypo/thyroid
41. hyper/adrenal cortex
42. hypo/thyroid

F

43. low levels of sodium in the blood
44. excessive thirst
45. sugar in the urine
46. normal thyroid function

G

47. insulin-dependent diabetes mellitus
48. disease of nerves secondary to diabetes mellitus
49. abnormal condition of ketones in the blood (acid-forming); complication of diabetes mellitus
50. non–insulin-dependent diabetes mellitus

Dictation and Comprehension Quiz: Vocabulary and Terminology

A

1. adenohypophysis
2. adrenocorticotropin
3. aldosterone
4. calcitonin
5. catecholamine
6. electrolyte
7. glucocorticoid
8. glycemia
9. glycosuria
10. homeostasis
11. hypokalemia
12. hyponatremia
13. hypothalamus
14. oxytocin
15. pancreatectomy
16. parathyroidectomy
17. polydipsia
18. progesterone
19. tetraiodothyronine
20. vasopressin

B

20 Hormone secreted by the posterior part of the pituitary gland; increases reabsorption of water
3 Hormone secreted by the adrenal cortex; increases salt (sodium) reabsorption by the kidney
6 A mineral salt found in the blood and tissues; potassium is an example
17 Excessive thirst
4 Hormone secreted by the thyroid gland; lowers blood calcium
15 Resection of a gland near and behind the stomach
14 Hormone secreted by the posterior pituitary gland; stimulates contraction of the uterus during labor
9 Sugar present in the urine
19 Hormone secreted by the thyroid gland; thyroxine
10 Tendency of an organism to maintain a constant internal environment
12 Blood condition of deficient sodium
7 Type of hormone secreted by the adrenal cortex; necessary for the use of sugars, fats, and proteins
1 Anterior lobe of the pituitary gland
16 Resection of four small glands in the neck region
18 Hormone secreted by the ovaries
11 Blood condition of deficient potassium
13 Region of the brain that produces factors to stimulate the pituitary gland
2 Hormone secreted by the anterior lobe of the pituitary gland; stimulates the adrenal cortex
8 Condition of sugar in the blood
5 Hormone derived from an amino acid and secreted by the adrenal medulla; epinephrine is an example

Dictation and Comprehension Quiz: Abnormal Conditions, Laboratory Tests, Procedures

A

1. acromegaly
2. Addison disease
3. cretinism
4. Cushing syndrome
5. diabetes insipidus
6. diabetes mellitus
7. exophthalmos
8. glucose tolerance test
9. goiter

10. hirsutism
11. ketoacidosis
12. myxedema
13. pheochromocytoma
14. radioimmunoassay
15. tetany
16. thyroid carcinoma
17. thyroid scan
18. thyrotoxicosis

B

14 Test that measures hormone levels in plasma
8 Test that measures levels of sugar in the blood
17 Radioactive compound is given and localizes in the thyroid gland
1 Enlargement of extremities caused by excessive growth hormone after puberty
5 Insufficient secretion of antidiuretic hormone produces this condition
16 Malignant tumor of an endocrine gland in the neck
3 Extreme hypothyroidism during infancy and childhood produces this condition
12 Advanced hypothyroidism in adulthood produces this condition
7 Enlargement and bulging of the eyeballs caused by hyperthyroidism
10 Excessive hair on the face and body of adult women
4 Group of symptoms produced by excess of cortisol from the adrenal cortex
9 Enlargement of the thyroid gland
18 Overactivity of the thyroid gland (Graves disease)
13 Benign tumor of the adrenal medulla
6 Lack of insulin secretion or resistance of insulin to promoting sugar, starch, and fat metabolism in cells
15 Constant muscle contraction
11 Fats are improperly burned, leading to accumulation of ketones in the body
2 Hypofunctioning of the adrenal cortex

Spelling Quiz

A

1. cortisol—hormone secreted by the adrenal cortex
2. goiter—enlargement of the thyroid gland
3. estrogen—hormone secreted by the ovaries
4. pituitary gland—located at the base of the brain
5. gonadotropin—hormone secreted by the pituitary gland
6. euthyroid—normal thyroid function
7. hypokalemia—low potassium in the blood
8. hypophysectomy—removal of the pituitary gland
9. pancreas—endocrine gland behind the stomach
10. corticosteroid—type of hormone secreted by the adrenal cortex

B

11. thyroxine
12. exophthalmos
13. progesterone
14. tetany
15. insulin
16. homeostasis
17. hypothalamus
18. polydipsia
19. acromegaly
20. myxedema

Pronunciation Quiz

A

1. glucagon
2. parathormone
3. adenohypophysis
4. testosterone
5. sella turcica
6. goiter
7. exophthalmos
8. homeostasis
9. mineralocorticoid
10. gonadotropin

B

1. C
2. F
3. H
4. E
5. A
6. G
7. D
8. J
9. B
10. I

C

1. hypercalcemia
2. hypokalemia
3. hyponatremia
4. pancreatectomy
5. glycemic
6. polydipsia
7. euthyroid
8. triiodothyronine

Diagram Quiz

1. Thyroid gland
2. Parathyroid glands
3. Adrenal glands
4. Pancreas
5. Pituitary gland
6. Ovaries
7. Testes
8. Pineal gland

Review Sheet Quiz

A

1. gland
2. adrenal gland
3. male
4. calcium
5. cortex; outer area
6. thirst
7. female
8. sugar
9. sugar
10. sex glands; gonads (organs that produce sex cells or gametes)

B

1. potassium
2. milk
3. mucus
4. sodium
5. pancreas
6. body
7. thyroid gland
8. poison
9. urine
10. sameness

C

1. assemble, gather together
2. removal, excision, resection
3. blood condition
4. pertaining to producing
5. stimulating the function of
6. urine condition
7. enlargement
8. excessive, above
9. deficient, below
10. all
11. four
12. many, much
13. three
14. good, normal

Medical Scramble

1. ACROMEGALY
2. OXYTOCIN
3. ADRENALINE
4. MEDULLA

BONUS TERM: MYXEDEMA

Crossword Puzzle

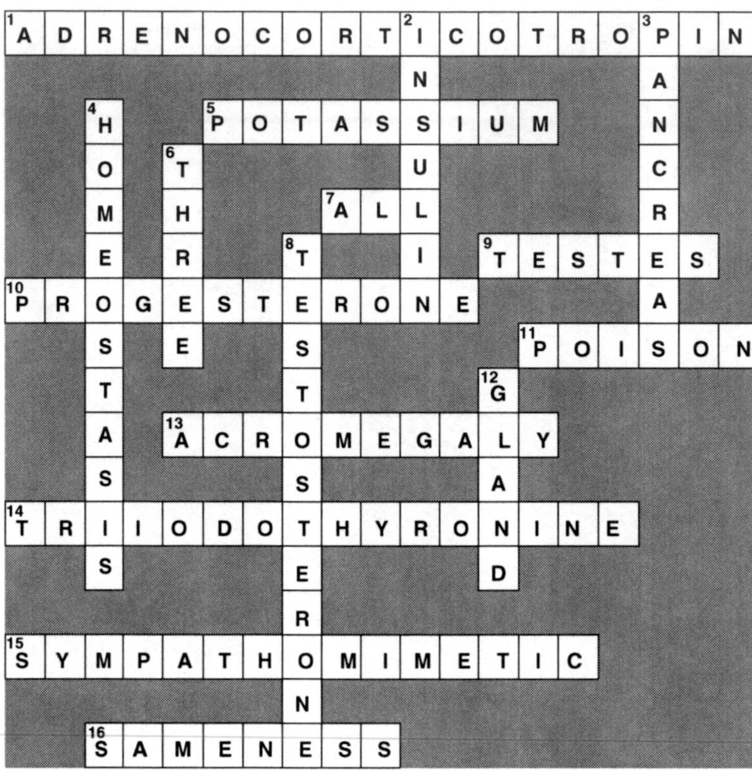

Practical Applications

A

1. D
2. A
3. D
4. C

B

1. C
2. B

Chapter Eighteen

Answers to Terminology Section

(textbook pages 762–765)

Terminology	Meaning
adenectomy	Removal of a gland.
adrenalectomy	Removal of an adrenal gland.
gonadotropin	Hormone that is secreted from the pituitary gland and acts on the gonads (ovaries and testes).
hypogonadism	Condition of decreased function of the gonads, with decreased growth and sexual development.
pancreatectomy	Removal of the pancreas.
parathyroidectomy	Removal of the parathyroid glands.
hypopituitarism	Condition resulting from decreased secretion by the pituitary gland.
thyrotropic hormone	Hormone secreted by the anterior pituitary gland that acts on the thyroid gland (TSH or thyroid-stimulating hormone).
thyroiditis	Inflammation of the thyroid gland.
androgen	Hormone producing or stimulating male characteristics (e.g., testosterone).
hypercalcemia	Increased calcium in the blood.
hypercalciuria	High levels of calcium in urine.
hypocalcemia	Decreased calcium in the blood.
corticosteroid	Any of the hormones produced by the adrenal cortex.
endocrinologist	Specialist in diagnosis and treatment of endocrine gland disorders.
polydipsia	Condition of excessive thirst.
estrogenic	Pertaining to having properties similar to estrogen (producing estrogen-like effects).
glucagon	Hormone from the pancreas that causes sugar to be released into the bloodstream when blood sugar levels are low.
hyperglycemia	Blood condition of increased sugar.
glycemic	Pertains to sugar in the blood.
glycogen	An animal starch; produced from sugar by the liver.
homeostasis	State of equilibrium (constancy) of the body's internal environment.
hormonal	Pertaining to hormones.
hypokalemia	Low levels of potassium in the blood.
prolactin	Hormone secreted by the anterior pituitary that promotes the growth of breast tissue and stimulates milk production.
myxedema	Condition of mucous-like swelling of the face and soft tissues; due to hyposecretion of the thyroid gland in adults.
hyponatremia	Blood condition of deficiency of sodium.
hypophysectomy	Removal of the pituitary gland.
somatotropin	Hormone secreted by the anterior pituitary gland; stimulates growth of bones and tissues (growth hormone).
steroid	An organic (containing carbon) compound with a ring structure; bile acids, vitamin D, certain hormones.
oxytocin	Hormone secreted by the posterior lobe of the pituitary gland; stimulates childbirth.
thyrotoxicosis	Condition of increased secretion from the thyroid gland with symptoms such as sweating, rapid pulse, tremors, and exophthalmos.
antidiuretic hormone	Secreted by the posterior lobe of the pituitary gland; causes water to be retained in the body.

Suffixes

glucagon	Hormone from the pancreas that "assembles" sugar from starch and increases blood sugar when it is low.
hypoglycemia	Low levels of sugar in blood.
epinephrine	Hormone secreted by the adrenal medulla; raises blood pressure.
adrenocorticotropin	Hormone secreted by the anterior lobe of the pituitary gland; stimulates the adrenal cortex to release its hormones.
glycosuria	Condition of sugar in the urine.

Prefixes

euthyroid	Normal thyroid function.
hyperkalemia	High levels of potassium in blood.
hypoinsulinism	Low levels of insulin.
oxytocin	Hormone from the neurohypophysis that stimulates childbirth.
panhypopituitarism	Condition of deficient secretion of all hormones from the pituitary gland.
polyuria	Excessive urine production.
tetraiodothyronine (T_4)	Thyroid gland hormone containing 4 atoms of iodine; thyroxine.
triiodothyronine (T_3)	Thyroid gland hormone containing 3 atoms of iodine.

Chapter 19

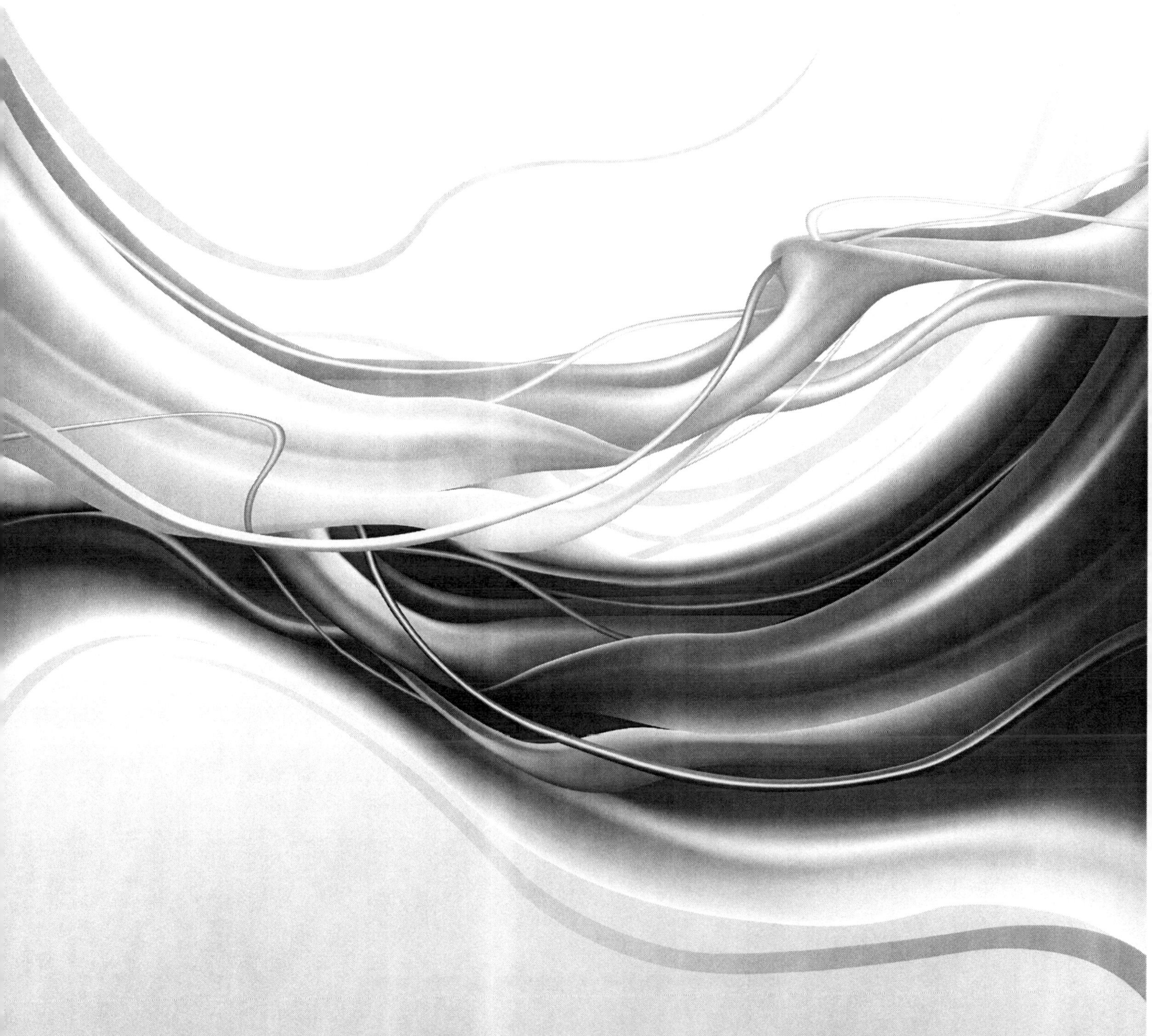

Chapter Nineteen
MULTIPLE CHOICE QUIZ

Name: ______________________________

In the box write the letter of the choice that is the definition of the term or best answers the question. There is only one correct answer for each question.

1. **Which term describes the spread of malignant tumors to a distant location?** ☐
   A. Metastasis
   B. Anaplasia
   C. Infiltration
   D. Invasion
   E. Encapsulation

2. **Which is an example of a solid tumor derived from epithelial tissue?** ☐
   A. Leiomyoma
   B. Rhabdomyoma
   C. Chondrosarcoma
   D. Adenocarcinoma of the lung
   E. Ewing sarcoma

3. **Which is a description of a fungating tumor?** ☐
   A. Open, exposed surface on the tumor
   B. Containing dead tissue
   C. Characterized by inflammation
   D. Large, soft, flesh tumor
   E. Mushrooming pattern of growth as tumor cells pile on top of each other

4. **Which term includes sessile and pedunculated types of growths?** ☐
   A. Polypoid
   B. Cystic
   C. Medullary
   D. Verrucous
   E. Necrotic

5. **What term describes localized tumor growth?** ☐
   A. Metastasis
   B. Carcinoma in situ
   C. Pleomorphic
   D. Anaplastic
   E. Sarcoma

6. **Which is a description of scirrhous-type tumors?** ☐
   A. Form small nipple-like projections
   B. Form microscopic glandular-type sacs
   C. Hard densely packed tumor cells
   D. Resemble squamous epithelial cells
   E. Contain a variety of tumor cells

7. **What does staging a tumor mean?** ☐
   A. Assessing the degree of differentiation
   B. Analyzing the microscopic appearance of tumor cells
   C. The tumor has spread
   D. Assessing the extent of tumor spread
   E. Treatment involves radiotherapy

8. **What does mutagenic mean?** ☐
   A. Producing a change in the DNA of a cell
   B. Increased cell growth
   C. New growth in numbers of cells
   D. Tumors are large and fleshy
   E. Cells are very differentiated

9. **What does the notation T1N2M0 mean?** ☐
   A. Tumor is localized and no lymph nodes are involved
   B. Tumor cannot be assessed
   C. Lymph nodes are not demonstrably abnormal
   D. Tumor is present with palpable regional lymph nodes and no metastases
   E. Metastasis to distant lymph nodes is detectable

10. **What is the definition of a mutation?** ☐
    A. Inheritable change in a cell
    B. Specialization of cells
    C. Plan for treatment of an illness
    D. Cell division
    E. Giving radiation in small doses

11. **Which is an example of genetic material that causes cancer?** ....
   A. Vinyl chloride
   B. Hydrocarbons
   C. Diethylstilbestrol
   D. Alkylating agents
   E. Oncogenes

12. **Which is a description of exenteration?** ....
   A. Malignant tissue is frozen
   B. Cells are scraped from region
   C. Tumors are burned
   D. Wide resection of tumor and removal of surrounding tissue
   E. Material is taken from the vagina or cervix and analyzed microscopically

13. **What is the meaning of fulguration?** ...
   A. Destruction of tissue by electric sparks
   B. Treatment with drugs
   C. Treatment with radiation
   D. Tumor is removed by surgical excision
   E. Aspiration biopsy technique

14. **Which is an example of a known type of inherited cancer?** ....
   A. Bone cancer
   B. Lung cancer
   C. Retinoblastoma
   D. Basal cell carcinoma
   E. Adenocarcinoma of the cervix

15. **What is a definition of modality?** ....
   A. Method of treatment
   B. Damage to normal tissue
   C. Change in genetic material
   D. Description of the diagnosis
   E. Death of cells

16. **Which is a definition of a radioresistant tumor?** ....
   A. Tumor is completely eradicated by chemical therapy
   B. Tumor requires large doses of radiation to produce death of cells
   C. Tumor in which irradiation causes death of cancer cells without damage to surrounding tissue
   D. Tumor is not significantly affected by drug treatment
   E. Tumor is resistant to surgical intervention

17. **Which is a description of cauterization?** ....
   A. Treating a tumor with freezing temperatures
   B. Treating tissue with heat
   C. Drying tissue electrically
   D. Surgical puncture to remove fluid
   E. Removing cells by scraping the walls of an organ

18. **What is apoptosis?** ....
   A. Type of ionizing radiation
   B. Programmed cell death
   C. Prolapse of an eyelid
   D. Use of drugs to increase the sensitivity of tumors to x-rays
   E. Abnormal growth of cells

19. **What term means assisting or aiding?** ....
   A. Lethal
   B. Fractionation
   C. Aspiration
   D. Adjuvant
   E. Grading

20. **Which term is used in treatment of tumors with radiation?** ....
   A. Steroid
   B. Antibiotic
   C. Antimetabolite
   D. Linear accelerator
   E. Plant alkaloid

21. **Which is a description of an estrogen receptor assay?** ....
   A. Tests for the presence of carcinoembryonic antigen in the blood
   B. Tests for a portion of human chorionic gonadotropin in serum of patients
   C. Tests the presence of a protein antigen in serum of liver and testicular cancer patients
   D. Tests the concentration of hormone receptor sites in cells of breast cancer patients
   E. Tests for the amount of carcinogenic hormones in the bloodstream of cancer patients

22. Which best describes a wide surgical incision of the abdomen to detect disease? ☐

A. Staging laparotomy
B. Liver and spleen scan
C. Peritoneoscopy
D. Bone marrow biopsy
E. Laparoscopy

23. What best describes interferon? ☐

A. Carcinogen
B. Molecularly targeted drug
C. Alkylating agent used for chemotherapy
D. Type of electron beam
E. Biological response modifier

24. What term means return of symptoms of disease? ☐

A. Remission
B. Mutation
C. Metastasis
D. Relapse
E. Differentiation

25. Which term means cancerous tumor derived from bone? ☐

A. Adenocarcinoma
B. Osteogenic sarcoma
C. Osteoma
D. Chondrosarcoma
E. Wilms tumor

26. A side effect of radiation therapy (redness of skin): ☐

A. Alopecia
B. Myelosuppression
C. Mucositis
D. Fibrosis
E. Erythema

27. A side effect of chemotherapy or radiotherapy (hair loss): ☐

A. Alopecia
B Myelosuppression
C. Mucositis
D. Fibrosis
E. Erythema

28. A side effect of radiation therapy to the lungs (abnormal growth of connective tissue): ☐

A. Alopecia
B. Myelosuppression
C. Mucositis
D. Fibrosis
E. Erythema

29. Hypoplasia of bone marrow: ☐

A. Alopecia
B. Myelosuppression
C. Mucositis
D. Fibrosis
E. Erythema

30. Inflammation of the inner lining of an organ: ☐

A. Alopecia
B. Myelosuppression
C. Mucositis
D. Fibrosis
E. Erythema

Chapter Nineteen
VOCABULARY QUIZ

Name: ______________________________

A. Match the following terms with their meanings below:

adjuvant therapy	angiogenesis	benign tumor
alkylating agents	antimetabolites	biologic response modifiers
anaplasia	antimitotics	
antibiotics	apoptosis	

1. Substances produced by normal cells that either directly block tumor growth or stimulate the immune system to fight cancer ______________________________
2. Synthetic chemicals containing alkyl groups that interfere with DNA synthesis ______________________________
3. Loss of differentiation of cells ______________________________
4. Programmed cell death ______________________________
5. Chemicals that prevent cell division by inhibiting formation of substances necessary to make DNA ______________________________
6. Process of forming new blood vessels ______________________________
7. Noncancerous growth ______________________________
8. Chemical substances, produced by bacteria or primitive plants; inhibit the growth of cells in cancer chemotherapy ______________________________
9. Drugs that block mitosis (cell division) ______________________________
10. Assisting primary treatment ______________________________

B. Match the following terms with their meanings below:

biological therapy	chemotherapy	differentiating agents
carcinogens	dedifferentiation	differentiation
carcinoma	deoxyribonucleic acid (DNA)	electron beams
cellular oncogenes		

1. Treatment with drugs ______________________________
2. Genetic material within the nucleus of a cell ______________________________
3. Cancerous tumor ______________________________
4. Drugs that promote tumor cells to differentiate, stop growing, and die ______________________________
5. Pieces of DNA that can cause a normal cell to become malignant ______________________________

6. Loss of differentiation of cells; reversion to a more primitive type; anaplasia ______________
7. Agents that cause cancer; chemicals, drugs, radiation, viruses ______________
8. Use of the body's own defenses to destroy tumor cells ______________
9. Low-energy beams of radiation for treatment of skin or surface tumors ______________
10. Specialization of cells ______________

C. Match the following terms with their meanings below:

external beam radiation	gray (Gy)	mitosis
fractionation	irradiation	modality
genetic screening	metastasis	morbidity
grading of tumors		

1. Unit of absorbed radiation dose ______________
2. Exposure to any form of radiant energy such as light, heat, or x-rays ______________
3. Evaluation of the degree of maturity of tumor cells ______________
4. Giving radiation in small, repeated doses ______________
5. Replication of cells; two identical cells from a parent cell ______________
6. Spread of a malignant tumor to a secondary site ______________
7. Condition of being diseased ______________
8. Family members are tested to determine whether they have inherited a cancer-causing gene ______________
9. Radiation applied to a tumor from a distant source ______________
10. Method of treatment, such as surgery, chemotherapy, or radiation ______________

D. Match the following terms with their meanings listed below:

mucinous	oncogene	protocol
mutation	palliative	proton therapy
neoplasm	pedunculated	radiation
nucleotide		

1. Energy carried by a stream of particles ______________
2. Unit of DNA composed of a sugar, phosphate, and a base ______________
3. Possessing a stem or stalk (peduncle) ______________
4. Subatomic particles produced by a cyclotron deposit an absorbed dose of radiation at a focused point in the body ______________
5. New growth (tumor) ______________
6. Detailed plan for treatment ______________

7. Region of DNA in tumor cells or in viruses that cause cancer ____________________
8. Change in genetic material (DNA) of a cell ____________________
9. Relieving, but not curing symptoms ____________________
10. Containing mucus ____________________

E. Match the following terms with their meanings listed below:

radiocurable tumor	radiotherapy	sarcoma
radioresistant tumor	relapse	simulation
radiosensitive tumor	remission	steroids
radiosensitizers	ribonucleic acid (RNA)	stereotactic radiosurgery

1. Study using CT scan or MRI to map treatment prior to radiation treatment ____________________
2. Return of symptoms of disease ____________________
3. Treatment of tumors using radiation; radiation oncology ____________________
4. Dose of radiation delivered under highly precise guidance (Gamma Knife surgery) ____________________
5. Tumor cells that are destroyed by radiation therapy ____________________
6. Partial or complete disappearance of symptoms of disease ____________________
7. Tumor cells that require large doses of radiation to be destroyed ____________________
8. Cellular substance that along with DNA plays an important role in protein synthesis ____________________
9. Drugs that increase the sensitivity of tumors to x-rays ____________________
10. Complex, naturally occurring chemicals (such as hormones) that are used in cancer chemotherapy ____________________
11. Cancerous tumor derived from connective or flesh tissue ____________________
12. Tumor in which radiation can cause the death of cells without serious damage to surrounding tissue ____________________

Chapter Nineteen
TERMINOLOGY QUIZ

Name: ______________________________

A. Use the following word parts to create or complete the terms from the definitions below:

alveol/o	cry/o	fung/i
cac/o	cyst/o	sarc/o
carcin/o	electr/o	-ic
cauter/o	fibr/o	-oma
chem/o	follicul/o	-therapy

1. Localized cancer; confined to the site of origin: ______________________ in situ
2. Surgery with using cold temperatures: ______________________ surgery
3. General ill health and malnutrition: ______________________ hexia.
4. Pertaining to small glandular sacs, as seen under the microscope: ______________ ar
5. Treatment with drugs: ______________________
6. Malignant tumor of fibrous tissue: ______________________
7. Pertaining to tumor cells arranged in small sacs, as seen under a microscope: __________ ar
8. Burning tissue using electricity: ______________________ ization.
9. Pertaining to a tumor with large open spaces filled with fluid: ______________ tumor
10. Mushrooming pattern of tumor growth: ______________________ ating tumor

B. Use the following word parts to create or complete the terms from the definitions below:

fibromat/o	necr/o	plas/o	-tic
medull/o	neur/o	ple/o	dys-
mucos/o	onc/o	-itis	
mut/a	papill/o	-logy	
mutagen/o	pharmac/o	-osis	

1. Pertaining to a tumor containing dead tissue: ______________________ tumor
2. Inflammation of a mucous membrane: ______________________
3. Pertaining to causing genetic change: ______________________ ic
4. Forming small finger-like or nipple-like projection of cells as seen under a microscope: ______________________ ary
5. Change in the genetic material (DNA) of a cell: ______________________ ation
6. Study of tumors: ______________________.
7. Tumor cells forming a variety of cells, as seen under a microscope: ______________ morphic

8. Tumors of fibrous tissue surrounding nerves (a genetic disorder): ____________________

9. Abnormal-appearing (but not clearly cancerous) cells as seen under a microscope: __________ tic

10. Pertaining to a large, soft, fleshy tumor: ______________________________ ary tumor

C. Use the following word parts to create or complete the terms from the definitions below:

aden/o	polyp/o	xer/o
angi/o	radi/o	-blastoma
carcin/o	retin/o	-genesis
neur/o	sarc/o	-ous
oste/o	scirrh/o	-plasia

1. Densely packed tumor cells, as seen under a microscope: ____________________

2. Use of radioactive substances in the diagnosis and treatment of disease: ______________ ation

3. Formation of blood vessels: ______________________________

4. Growths that are like projections extending outward from a base: ______________ oid tumor

5. Childhood cancer arising from immature cells in the posterior, light-sensitive area of the

   eye: ______________________________

6. Childhood cancer that arises in immature cells of the autonomic

   nervous system: ______________________________

7. Condition of dry mouth: ______________________________ stomia

8. Malignant tumor of bone: ______________________________ oma

9. Malignant tumor of glandular tissue: ______________________________ oma

10. Condition of excessive formation of cells: hyper ______________________________

D. Use the following word parts to create or complete the terms from the definitions below:

derm/o	-plasm	-therapy	epi-
myel/o	-ptosis	ana-	meta-
prot/o	-stasis	apo-	neo-
radi/o	-suppression	brachy-	tele-

1. Treatment using ionizing radiation to destroy tumor cells: ____________________.

2. Written plan detailing the procedures to be followed in research

   or treatment: ______________________________ col.

3. Spread of a malignant tumor to a distant or secondary site: ____________________.

4. Radiation treatment delivered via a distant source

   (external beam radiation): ______________________________

5. Condition of loss of differentiation of cells (reversion to a more primitive formation):

   ______________________________ plasia

6. Programmed cell death: ______________________________

7. Cells that resemble epithelial cells, as seen under the microscope: ______________ oid

8. Abnormal transformation of differentiated cells to differentiated tissue of another kind: ______________________________ plasia

9. Bone marrow activity is decreased (side effect of chemotherapy): ______________

10. Radiation delivered in close range to a tumor site: ______________________

11. New formation (growth): ______________________________ plasm

Chapter Nineteen

LABORATORY TESTS AND CLINICAL PROCEDURES QUIZ

Name: ______________________________

Match the following laboratory tests and clinical procedures with their descriptions below:

bone marrow biopsy
bone marrow or stem cell transplant
core needle biopsy
cytogenetic analysis
exfoliative cytology
fiberoptic colonoscopy
immunohistochemistry
laparoscopy
mammography
PET/CT scan
protein marker tests
radionuclide scans

1. X-ray examination of the breast to detect breast cancer ______________________________
2. Aspiration of bone marrow tissue and examination under a microscope ____________________
3. Visual examination of the abdominal cavity using small incisions and an endoscope ______________________________
4. Radioactive substances are injected intravenously and images of organs are obtained ______________________________
5. Cells are scraped from the region of suspected disease and examined under a microscope ______________________________
6. Cells that give rise to blood cells are infused intravenously into a patient ____________________
7. Visual examination of the colon ______________________________
8. Localizing antigens or proteins in tissues using labeled antibodies ____________________
9. CA-125, PSA, beta-hCG, and CEA are detected in the blood or on the surface of tumor cells ______________________________
10. Insertion of a large-bore needle into tissue to remove cells for microscopic examination ______________________________
11. Chromosomes of normal or tumor cells are examined for breaks, translocations, or deletions of DNA ______________________________
12. Combination of two machines; one to examine chemical reactions and one to examine physical structure ______________________________

Chapter Nineteen
ABBREVIATIONS QUIZ

Name: ______________________________

On the line provided, give meanings for the following abbreviations, then write each abbreviation next to its explanation below:

1. BMT ______________________________
2. bx ______________________________
3. CEA ______________________________
4. cGY ______________________________
5. ER ______________________________
6. EPO ______________________________
7. mets ______________________________
8. TNM ______________________________
9. VEGF ______________________________
10. XRT ______________________________

a. __________ Protein marker found on breast cancer cells

b. __________ Treatment with irradiation

c. __________ Dose of radiation

d. __________ Staging system for malignant tumors

e. __________ Removal of tissue and examination under a microscope

f. __________ Healthy blood-forming tissue is transferred from a donor to a recipient

g. __________ Hormone made in the kidney to stimulate the formation of red blood cells

h. __________ Spreading of malignant tumor to a distant location

i. __________ Protein that promotes the formation of blood vessels

j. __________ Protein that appears in the blood (marker) of patients with colorectal, pancreatic, and other cancers

Chapter Nineteen
EXERCISE QUIZ

Name: ______________________________

A. Identify the following characteristics of malignant tumors from their definitions below. Word parts are given as clues.

1. Loss of differentiation of cells and reversion to a more primitive cell type: ana ______________________________
2. Extending beyond the normal tissue boundaries: in ______________________________
3. Having the ability to enter and destroy surrounding tissue: in ______________________________
4. Spreading to a secondary site: meta ______________________________

B. Match the following terms or abbreviations with their meanings below:

chemical carcinogen	mitosis	oncogene	RNA	virus
DNA	mutation	radiation	ultraviolet radiation	

5. Replication of cells; two identical cells are produced from a parent cell ______________________________
6. Cellular substance (ribonucleic acid) that is important in protein synthesis ______________________________
7. Infectious agent that reproduces by entering a host cell and using the host's genetic material to make copies of itself ______________________________
8. Rays given off by the sun ______________________________
9. An agent (hydrocarbon, insecticide, hormone) that causes cancer ______________________________
10. Genetic material within the nucleus that controls replication and protein synthesis ______________________________
11. Region of genetic material that causes cancer; found in tumor cells or viruses ______________________________
12. Change in the genetic material of a cell ______________________________
13. Energy carried by a stream of particles ______________________________

C. Give meanings for the following terms:

14. adenocarcinoma ______________________________
15. osteosarcoma ______________________________
16. benign ______________________________
17. differentiation ______________________________
18. neoplasm ______________________________

D. Name the terms that describe microscopic tumor growth. Definitions and word parts are given.

19. forming small nipple-like projections: papill ____________________
20. abnormal formation of cells: dys ____________________
21. localized growth of cells: carcin ____________________
22. densely packed; containing fibrous connective tissue: ____________________ ous
23. patterns resembling microscopic sacs: alveol ____________________
24. small gland-type sacs: foll ____________________
25. lacking structures typical of mature cells: un ____________________

E. Match the following gross descriptions of tumors with their meanings:

cystic	inflammatory	necrotic	ulcerating
fungating	medullary	polypoid	verrucous

26. characterized by redness, swelling, and heat ____________________
27. tumors are large, soft, fleshy ____________________
28. containing dead tissue ____________________
29. mushrooming pattern of growth ____________________
30. characterized by large, open, exposed surfaces ____________________
31. tumors form large, open spaces filled with fluid ____________________
32. tumors resemble wart-like growths ____________________
33. growths are projections from a base (sessile and pedunculated) ____________________

F. Match the surgical procedure in Column I with its meaning in Column II.

Column I		Column II
34. fulguration	_______	A. Removal of tumor and a margin of abnormal tissue for diagnosis and possible cure for small tumors
35. en bloc resection	_______	B. Removal of entire tumor with large area of surrounding tissue and lymph nodes
36. incisional biopsy	_______	C. Burning a lesion
37. excisional biopsy	_______	D. Destruction of tissue using heat
38. cryosurgery	_______	E. Cutting into tumor and removing a piece to establish diagnosis
39. cauterization	_______	F. Freezing a lesion
40. pelvic exenteration	_______	G. Wide resection involving tumor, organ of origin, and surrounding tissue in the area of the hip

G. Give meanings for the following terms:

41. relapse ______________________________
42. morbidity ______________________________
43. protocol ______________________________
44. modality ______________________________
45. remission ______________________________
46. adjuvant therapy ______________________________

H. Match the test or procedure with its description below:

beta-hCG test	CEA test	exfoliative cytology	staging laparotomy
bone marrow biopsy	core needle biopsy	laparoscopy	
CA-125	estrogen receptor assay	PSA test	

47. Test for the presence of a portion of human chorionic gonadotropin hormone (a marker for testicular cancer) ______________________________
48. Incision of the abdomen to determine extent of disease ______________________________
49. Protein marker test to detect ovarian cancer cells in blood ______________________________
50. Visual examination of the abdominal cavity; peritoneoscopy ______________________________
51. Test for the presence of a hormone receptor on breast cancer cells ______________________________
52. Removal and microscopic examination of bone marrow tissue ______________________________
53. Obtaining a plug of tissue for microscopic examination ______________________________
54. Blood test for the presence of an antigen related to prostate cancer ______________________________
55. Blood test for carcinoembryonic antigen (marker for GI cancer) ______________________________
56. Cells are scraped off tissue and microscopically examined ______________________________

Chapter Nineteen

DICTATION AND COMPREHENSION QUIZ

Name: ______________________________

A. Dictation of Terms

1.	______________________	11.	______________________
2.	______________________	12.	______________________
3.	______________________	13.	______________________
4.	______________________	14.	______________________
5.	______________________	15.	______________________
6.	______________________	16.	______________________
7.	______________________	17.	______________________
8.	______________________	18.	______________________
9.	______________________	19.	______________________
10.	______________________	20.	______________________

B. Comprehension of Terms: Match number of the above term with its meaning below.

______ Programmed cell death
______ Specialization of cells
______ Giving radiation therapy in small, repeated doses
______ Spread of a malignant tumor to a secondary site
______ Condition of being diseased
______ Drug that increases the sensitivity of tumors to radiation therapy
______ Loss of specialization of cells; reversion to a more primitive type
______ Malignant tumor of connective tissue
______ Possessing a stem or stalk; characteristic of some polypoid tumors
______ Formation of blood vessels
______ Region of DNA found in tumor cells; examples are *abl, ras, src*
______ Synthetic chemicals containing groups that interfere with DNA synthesis
______ Visual examination of the abdomen using small incisions and an endoscope
______ Removal of tumor along with a large area of surrounding tissue and lymph nodes
______ Microscopic description of tumors possessing a variety of cells
______ Localized cancer; confined to the site of origin
______ Malnutrition associated with chronic disease (such as malignancy) and ill health
______ Malignant tumor of epithelial tissue (glandular cells)
______ Cells are scraped from an area of suspected disease and examined microscopically
______ Pertaining to producing change in cells

Chapter Nineteen
SPELLING QUIZ

Name: ______________________________

A. Circle the term that is spelled correctly and write its meaning in the space provided.

1.	retinoblastoma	retinoblasoma	______________
2.	metastasis	matestasis	______________
3.	bengine	benign	______________
4.	chemotherapy	chemotheraphy	______________
5.	oncology	onkocology	______________
6.	malignent	malignant	______________
7.	carsinoma in situ	carcinoma in situ	______________
8.	hyperplasia	hyperplayzea	______________
9.	displastic	dysplastic	______________
10.	polypoid	polipoid	______________

B. Circle the term that is spelled correctly. The meaning of each term is given.

11.	Malignant tumor of fibrous tissue	fibrosacroma	fibrosarcoma	fibrosarkoma
12.	Additional treatment	adjuvant therapy	adjivent theraphy	adjuvent therapy
13.	Replication of cells	miteosis	mitosis	meiosis
14.	Specialization of cells	differentiation	differantiation	differentsheation
15.	Return of disease symptoms	relaspe	relapse	relapze
16.	Plan for treatment	protocal	protokol	protocol
17.	Densely packed tumors	scirrhous	skirrus	scirrhus
18.	Complex, naturally occurring chemicals	steroids	stairoids	steriods
19.	Pertaining to tumors filled with mucus	mucinous	mucanous	musinous
20.	Condition of being diseased	morbitity	morbidity	morbitidy

Chapter Nineteen
PRONUNCIATION QUIZ

Name: ______________________

A. Underline the accented syllable in the following terms:

1. papillary tumor
2. exenteration
3. cauterization
4. laparoscopy
5. anaplasia
6. alkylating
7. adjuvant
8. neurofibromatosis
9. antimetabolites
10. mucinous

B. Match the term in Column I with its meaning in Column II:

Column I		Column II
1. benign	______	A. In glass; an experiment performed in a laboratory with chemicals
2. neoplasm	______	B. Harmless; not cancerous
3. morbidity	______	C. Production of two identical cells from a parent cell
4. protocol	______	D. Plan for treatment
5. in vitro	______	E. To remove substances from a cavity using suction
6. in vivo	______	F. In life; an experiment performed in a living animal
7. lethal	______	G. The condition of being diseased
8. mitosis	______	H. A new growth; tumor
9. carcinogen	______	I. A substance that produces cancer
10. aspiration	______	J. Pertaining to producing death

C. Complete the following medical terms from their definitions:

1. cach ______________________	Malnutrition associated with cancer
2. ______________________oma	Cancerous tumor of a gland
3. ______________________oma	Tumor of embryonic retinal cells
4. meta ______________________	Beyond control; spreading of a cancer tumor to secondary origin
5. angio ______________________	Formation of blood vessels
6. in ______________________	Extending beyond normal boundaries; local invasion of tissue
7. chemo ______________________	Treatment using drugs
8. ped______________________	Possessing a stem or stalk
9. dif ______________________	Specialization of cells

Chapter Nineteen

REVIEW SHEET QUIZ

Name: ______________________________

A. Give meanings for the following combining forms:

1. aden/o ____________________
2. cac/o ____________________
3. carcin/o ____________________
4. cauter/o ____________________
5. chem./o ____________________
6. cry/o ____________________
7. cyst/o ____________________
8. fibr/o ____________________
9. follicul/o ____________________
10. fung/i ____________________

B. Give meanings for the following combining forms:

1. medull/o ____________________
2. mucos/o ____________________
3. mut/a ____________________
4. necr/o ____________________
5. neur/o __________ __________
6. onc/o ____________________
7. papill/o ____________________
8. pharmac/o ____________________
9. plas/o ____________________
10. ple/o ____________________
11. polyp/o ____________________
12. radi/o ____________________
13. sarc/o ____________________
14. scirrh/o ____________________
15. xer/o ____________________

C. Give meanings for the following suffixes and prefixes:

1. -blastoma ____________________
2. -oid ____________________
3. -oma ____________________
4. -plasia ____________________
5. -plasm ____________________
6. -ptosis ____________________
7. -stasis ____________________
8. -genesis ____________________
9. -suppression ____________________
10. -therapy ____________________
11. ana- ____________________
12. anti- ____________________
13. apo- ____________________
14. brachy- ____________________
15. dys- ____________________
16. meta- ____________________
17. tele- ____________________
18. epi- ____________________

Chapter Nineteen

MEDICAL SCRAMBLE

Name: ____________________

Unscramble the letters to form cancer-related terms from the clues. Use the letters in the squares to complete the bonus term.

1. *Clue:* Partial or complete disappearance of symptoms of disease

   ___ ☐ ☐ ___ ___ ___ ___ ___ ☐ S N E M I I R S O

2. *Clue:* Spread of a cancerous tumor to another site or secondary location

   ☐ ___ ___ ☐ ___ ___ ___ ___ ___ ☐ T T A E A I S S S M

3. *Clue:* Pertaining to abnormal formation or development of cells; not clearly malignant

   ___ ☐ ___ ___ ___ ___ ___ ___ ___ ☐ C L Y A S S P T I D

4. *Clue:* Increased growth in numbers of normal cells

   ☐ ___ ___ ☐ ___ ___ ☐ ___ ___ ___ ___ S P E R I A Y P H A L

BONUS TERM: *Clue:* Pertaining to embryonic connective tissue from which connective tissue tumors (sarcomas) arise

☐ ☐ ☐ ☐ ☐ ☐ ☐ ☐ ☐ ☐ ☐

Chapter Nineteen
CROSSWORD PUZZLE

Name: ______________________________

Fill in the crossword puzzle below using the clues listed underneath it.

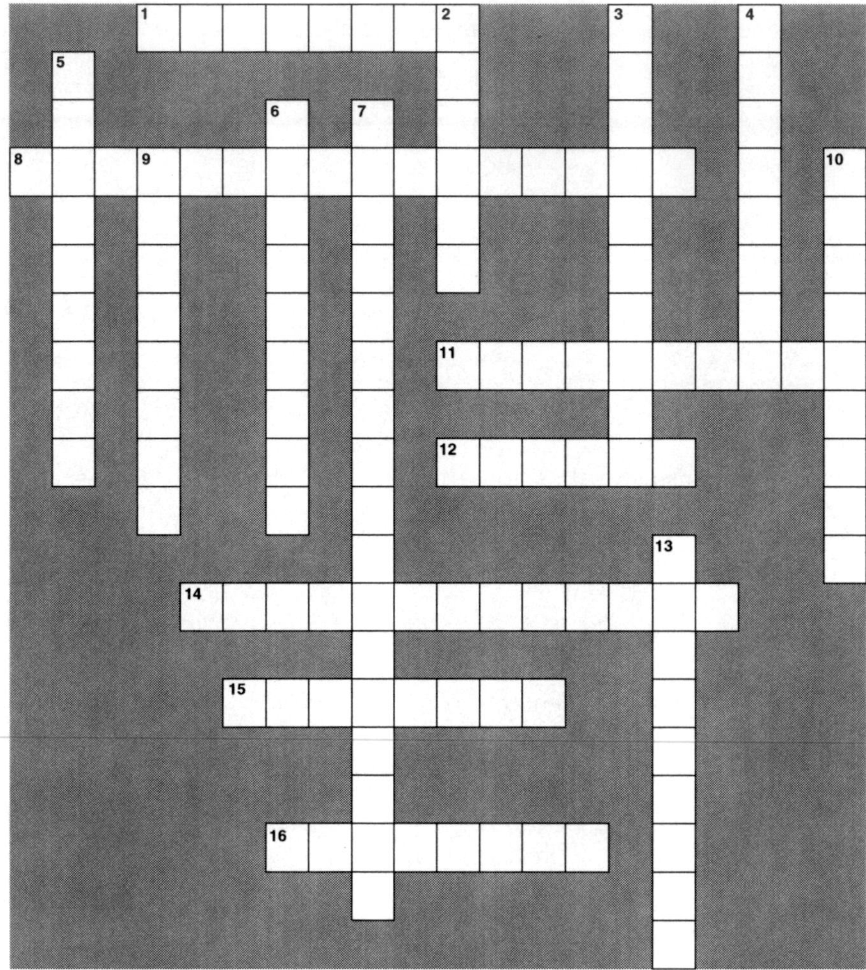

Across Clues

1. Containing dead tissue.
8. Lacking microscopic structures typical of normal, fully matured cells.
11. Forming microscopic gland-type sacs.
12. Noncancerous, not harmful.
14. Giving radiation in small, repeated doses.
15. Method of treatment, such as surgery, chemotherapy, or radiation.
16. New growth.

Down Clues

2. Forming large open sacs filled with fluid.
3. Characterizing an open, exposed surface resulting from death of overlying tissue.
4. An explicit detailed plan for treatment.
5. Mushrooming pattern of growth.
6. Resembling a wart-like growth.
7. Loss of differentiation cells.
9. Having the ability to enter and destroy surrounding tissue.
10. Hard, densely packed tumors, overgrown with fibrous tissue.
13. Damage to normal tissue; state of being diseased.

Chapter Nineteen
PRACTICAL APPLICATIONS

Name: ______________________

A. Case Study

The patient is a 63-year-old woman with a history (10 years ago) of squamous cell carcinoma in situ of the cervix, which was treated with a total abdominal hysterectomy. Three years ago a pelvic mass was palpated, and exploratory laparotomy revealed a multinodular solid cystic mass of 10 to 12 cm. The mass arose from the right ovary and was adherent to the right pelvic wall. The patient underwent resection of the mass, and the pathology revealed squamous cell carcinoma of the ovary. She subsequently had combined modality treatment with chemotherapy (cisplatin and 5-fluorouracil) and radiation therapy to the pelvis. The latest CT scan of the abdomen revealed a new right retroperitoneal lymph node. CT-guided fine needle aspiration was consistent with metastatic ovarian squamous cell carcinoma.

1. **What best describes the patient's original diagnosis?..............................** ☐
   A. Endometrial and cervical carcinoma
   B. Localized cancer of the lower portion of the uterus
   C. Cervical cancer that spread to the abdomen
   D. Ovarian cancer

2. **What was the initial primary treatment?..** ☐
   A. Drug treatment
   B. Radiation treatment
   C. Drug and radiation treatment
   D. Surgical removal of the entire uterus

3. **What procedure identified the new pelvic mass?......................................** ☐
   A. Incision of the abdomen
   B. Radiation therapy
   C. Total abdominal hysterectomy
   D. CT scan of the abdomen

4. **Which treatment modalities were used for the patient's ovarian carcinoma?.......................................** ☐
   A. Computed tomography of the abdomen
   B. Fine-needle aspiration of the ovary
   C. Drug and radiation therapy in addition to surgical removal
   D. Surgical resection of the mass

5. **How would you characterize the disease in the patient's retroperitoneal lymph node?....................................** ☐
   A. Cancer of the lymphatic system
   B. Cervical cancer that had spread
   C. Primary ovarian cancer
   D. Ovarian cancer that had spread

B. Research Report

In a recent trial comparing the antiemetics ondansetron (Zofran) and metoclopramide (Reglan), ondansetron was more effective and produced less severe side effects. The trial involved 24 medical centers and 307 cancer patients receiving high doses of cisplatin.

1. **What type of drug is ondansetron?.....................................** ☐
   A. Chemotherapeutic
   B. Antipsychotic medication
   C. Antibiotic
   D. Antinauseant

2. **When is ondansetron prescribed?..** ☐
   A. After cancer surgery
   B. In conjunction with metoclopramide
   C. When patients are receiving high-dose chemotherapy for cancer
   D. Before cancer surgery

C. Chart Note

Pt with metastatic squamous cell carcinoma of the tongue. Toward the end of XRT, the pt complained of some intermittent costal and low vertebral pain. The pt presented to the ER when pain control was no longer achieved using Percocet. CT scan and MRI were performed, revealing a number of vertebral bodies involved with tumor in the upper lumbar and lower thoracic regions. Preliminary reading suggests no evidence of cord compression, yet there is evidence of disk protrusion at T6-T7. We are consulted for palliative XRT of the spine lesions for purpose of pain control.

1. What was probably causing the patient's pain? .... ☐
A. Tuberculosis of the spine
B. Pressure on the spinal cord
C. Tumor of the oral cavity
D. Metastatic tumor in the backbones

2. What does costal mean? .... ☐
A. Pertaining to ribs
B. Pertaining to spinal cord
C. Pertaining to the back
D. Pertaining to the breast bone

3. What is palliative XRT? .... ☐
A. Diagnostic workup for malignancy
B. Chemotherapy for painful cancer treatment
C. Radiotherapy to relieve symptoms but not to cure
D. Surgery to relieve pain

4. What type of doctor wrote this report? .... ☐
A. Radiologist
B. Radiation oncologist
C. Nuclear medicine specialist
D. Orthopedist

D. Tests and Their Uses in Oncology

Match the following tests with their uses:

Bone density (DEXA) test	Mammogram
CA-125	MRI
Chest x-ray	Pap test (smear)
Colonoscopy	PET scan
CT	Pelvic ultrasound

1. This test would reveal osteoporosis ____________
2. Test that shows thoracic viscera in PA or LAT views ____________
3. A test used to specifically diagnose abnormalities in breast tissue ____________
4. This test uses magnetic waves to show soft tissue lesions ____________
5. Blood test that reveals levels of protein marker associated with ovarian cancer ____________
6. Test to identify lesions in the large bowel ____________
7. In this test, tissue is removed and examined to detect vaginal and cervical cancer ____________
8. Sound waves can show areas of abnormality in region of the hip ____________
9. Radiopharmaceutical is injected and traced to organs to detect tumors ____________
10. X-rays primarily in axial plane show bony and organ tissue abnormalities ____________

Chapter Nineteen
ANSWERS TO THE QUIZZES

Multiple Choice Quiz

1. A
2. D
3. E
4. A
5. B
6. C
7. D
8. A
9. D
10. A
11. E
12. D
13. A
14. C
15. A
16. B
17. B
18. B
19. D
20. D
21. D
22. A
23. E
24. D
25. B
26. E
27. A
28. D
29. B
30. C

Vocabulary Quiz

A

1. biologic response modifiers
2. alkylating agents
3. anaplasia
4. apoptosis
5. antimetabolites
6. angiogenesis
7. benign tumor
8. antibiotics
9. antimitotics
10. adjuvant therapy

B

1. chemotherapy
2. deoxyribonucleic acid (DNA)
3. carcinoma
4. differentiating agents
5. cellular oncogenes
6. dedifferentiation
7. carcinogens
8. biological therapy
9. electron beams
10. differentiation

C

1. gray (Gy)
2. irradiation
3. grading of tumors
4. fractionation
5. mitosis
6. metastasis
7. morbidity
8. genetic screening
9. external beam radiation
10. modality

D

1. radiation
2. nucleotide
3. pedunculated
4. proton therapy
5. neoplasm
6. protocol
7. oncogene
8. mutation
9. palliative
10. mucinous

E

1. simulation
2. relapse
3. radiotherapy
4. stereotactic radiosurgery
5. radiocurable tumor
6. remission
7. radioresistant tumor
8. ribonucleic acid (RNA)
9. radiosensitizers
10. steroids
11. sarcoma
12. radiosensitive tumor

Terminology Quiz

A

1. carcinoma in situ
2. cryosurgery
3. cachexia
4. follicular
5. chemotherapy
6. fibrosarcoma
7. alveolar
8. electrocauterization
9. cystic tumor
10. fungating tumor

B

1. necrotic tumor
2. mucositis
3. mutagenic
4. papillary
5. mutation
6. oncology
7. pleomorphic
8. neurofibromatosis
9. dysplastic
10. medullary tumor

C

1. scirrhous
2. radiation
3. angiogenesis
4. polypoid tumor
5. retinoblastoma
6. neuroblastoma
7. xerostomia
8. osteosarcoma
9. adenocarcinoma
10. hyperplasia

D

1. radiotherapy
2. protocol
3. metastasis
4. teletherapy
5. anaplasia
6. apoptosis
7. epidermoid
8. metaplasia
9. myelosuppression
10. brachytherapy
11. neoplasm

Laboratory Tests and Clinical Procedures Quiz

1. mammography
2. bone marrow biopsy
3. laparoscopy
4. radionuclide scans
5. exfoliative cytology
6. bone marrow or stem cell transplant
7. fiberoptic colonoscopy
8. immunohistochemistry
9. protein marker tests
10. core needle biopsy
11. cytogenetic analysis
12. PET/CT scan

Abbreviations Quiz

1. bone marrow transplantation
2. biopsy
3. CEA carcinoembryonic antigen
4. centigray
5. estrogen receptor
6. erythropoietin
7. metastases
8. tumor, nodes, metastases
9. vascular endothelial growth factor
10. radiation therapy

a. ER
b. XRT
c. cGY
d. TNM
e. bx
f. BMT
g. EPO
h. mets
i. VEGF
j. CEA

Exercise Quiz

A

1. anaplasia
2. infiltrative
3. invasive
4. metastasis

B

5. mitosis
6. RNA
7. virus
8. ultraviolet radiation
9. chemical carcinogen
10. DNA
11. oncogene
12. mutation
13. radiation

C

14. cancerous tumor of glandular tissue
15. cancerous tumor of bone
16. harmless; not cancerous
17. specialization of cells
18. new growth; tumor

D

19. papillary
20. dysplastic
21. carcinoma in situ
22. scirrhous
23. alveolar
24. follicular
25. undifferentiated

E

26. inflammatory
27. medullary
28. necrotic
29. fungating
30. ulcerating
31. cystic
32. verrucous
33. polypoid

F

34. D
35. B
36. E
37. A
38. F
39. C
40. G

G

41. return of symptoms of disease
42. the condition of being diseased
43. an explicit, detailed plan for treatment
44. method of treatment
45. absence of symptoms of disease
46. assisting primary treatment

H

47. beta-hCG test
48. staging laparotomy
49. CA-125
50. laparoscopy
51. estrogen receptor assay
52. bone marrow biopsy
53. core needle biopsy
54. PSA test
55. CEA test
56. exfoliative cytology

Dictation and Comprehension Quiz

A

1. adenocarcinoma
2. alkylating agents
3. anaplasia
4. angiogenesis
5. apoptosis
6. cachexia
7. carcinoma in situ
8. differentiation
9. en bloc resection
10. exfoliative cytology
11. fibrosarcoma
12. fractionation
13. laparoscopy
14. metastasis
15. morbidity
16. mutagenic
17. oncogene
18. pedunculated
19. pleomorphic
20. radiosensitizer

B

5 Programmed cell death
8 Specialization of cells
12 Giving radiation therapy in small, repeated doses
14 Spread of a malignant tumor to a secondary site
15 Condition of being diseased
20 Drug that increases the sensitivity of tumors to radiation therapy
3 Loss of specialization of cells; reversion to a more primitive type
11 Malignant tumor of connective tissue
18 Possessing a stem or stalk; characteristic of some polypoid tumors
4 Formation of blood vessels
17 Region of DNA found in tumor cells; examples are *abl*, *ras*, *src*
2 Synthetic chemicals containing groups that interfere with DNA synthesis
13 Visual examination of the abdomen using small incisions and an endoscope
9 Removal of tumor along with a large area of surrounding tissue and lymph nodes
19 Microscopic description of tumors possessing a variety of cells
7 Localized cancer; confined to the site of origin
6 Malnutrition associated with chronic disease (such as malignancy) and ill health
1 Malignant tumor of epithelial tissue (glandular cells)
10 Cells are scraped from an area of suspected disease and examined microscopically
16 Pertaining to producing change in cells

Spelling Quiz

A

1. retinoblastoma—malignant tumor of the eye (inherited)
2. metastasis—spread of a malignant tumor
3. benign—harmless; not cancerous
4. chemotherapy—cancer treatment with drugs
5. oncology—the study of malignant tumors
6. malignant—harmful, cancerous
7. carcinoma in situ—localized cancer
8. hyperplasia—increased growth in numbers of cells
9. dysplastic—pertaining to abnormal formation of cells
10. polypoid—growths that are projections from a base

B

11. fibrosarcoma
12. adjuvant therapy
13. mitosis
14. differentiation
15. relapse
16. protocol
17. scirrhous
18. steroids
19. mucinous
20. morbidity

Pronunciation Quiz

A

1. papillary tumor
2. exenteration
3. cauterization
4. laparoscopy
5. anaplasia
6. alkylating
7. adjuvant
8. neurofibromatosis
9. antimetabolites
10. mucinous

B

1. B
2. H
3. G
4. D
5. A
6. F
7. J
8. C
9. I
10. E

C

1. cachexia
2. adenocarcinoma
3. retinoblastoma
4. metastasis
5. angiogenesis
6. infiltrative
7. chemotherapy
8. pedunculated
9. differentiation

Review Sheet Quiz

A

1. gland
2. bad
3. cancer, cancerous
4. burn, heat
5. chemical, drug
6. cold
7. sac of fluid
8. fibers
9. small glandular sacs
10. fungus, mushroom

B

1. soft, inner part
2. mucous membrane
3. genetic change
4. death
5. nerve
6. tumor
7. nipple-like
8. chemical, drug
9. formation
10. many, more
11. polyp
12. rays, x-rays
13. flesh, connective tissue
14. hard
15. dry

C

1. immature tumor
2. resembling, derived from
3. mass, tumor
4. formation, growth
5. formation, growth
6. falling, prolapse
7. stop, control
8. formation
9. to stop
10. treatment
11. backward
12. against
13. off, away
14. short (distance)
15. painful, difficult, abnormal
16. beyond, change
17. far
18. upon

Medical Scramble

1. REMISSION
2. METASTASIS
3. DYSPLASTIC
4. HYPERPLASIA

BONUS TERM: MESENCHYMAL

Crossword Puzzle

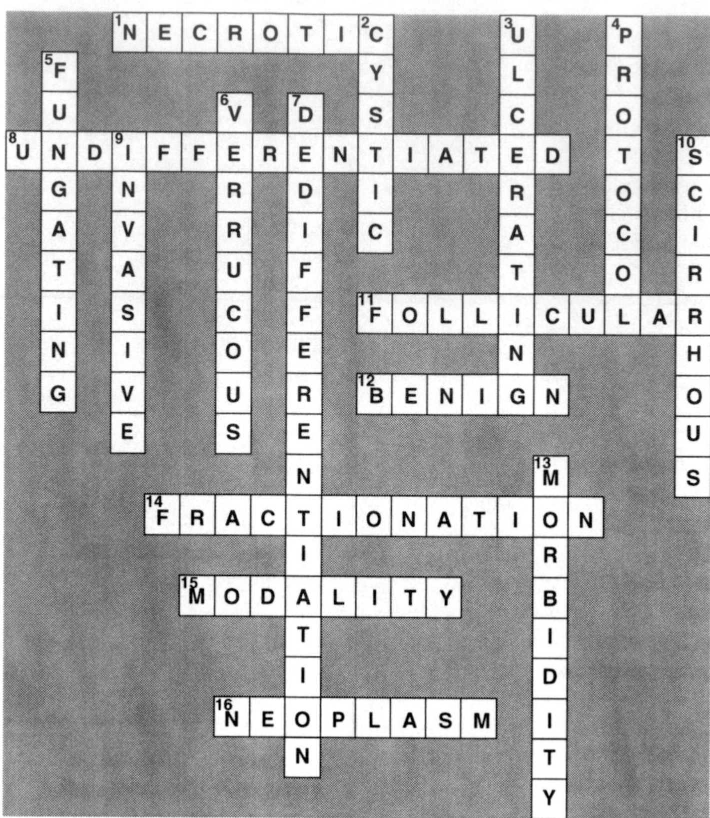

Practical Applications

A

1. B
2. D
3. A
4. C
5. D

B

1. D
2. C

C

1. D
2. A
3. C
4. B

D

1. bone density (DEXA) test
2. chest x-ray
3. mammogram
4. MRI
5. CA-125
6. colonoscopy
7. Pap test (smear)
8. pelvic ultrasound
9. PET scan
10. CT

Chapter Nineteen

Answers to Terminology Section

(textbook pages 821–823)

Terminology	Meaning
alveolar	Pertaining to tumor growth in small microscopic sacs (descriptive of connective tissue tumors—sarcomas).
cachexia	General ill health and malnutrition associated with chronic disease such as cancer.
carcinoma in situ	Localized tumor growth.
electrocauterization	Burning tissue to destroy it (using electricity).
chemotherapy	Treatment using drugs.
cryosurgery	Destruction of tissue using cold temperatures.
cystic tumor	Tumor forms with large open spaces filled with fluid.
fibrosarcoma	Malignant tumor of fiber-producing cells (flesh or connective tissue origin).
follicular	Pertaining to microscopic description of tumor growth in small gland-type sacs.
fungating tumor	Mushrooming pattern of growth in which tumor cells pile one on top of another and project from the tissue surface.
medullary tumor	Large, soft, fleshy tumor.
mucositis	Inflammation of mucous membranes.
mutation	Change in the genetic material of a cell.
mutagenic	Pertaining to producing mutation.
necrotic	Tumor containing dead cells.
neurofibromatosis	Tumors of fibrous connective tissue surrounding nerve cells (neurofibromas). This is a genetic disorder.
oncology	Study of tumors.
papillary	Pertaining to tumors that grow in small nipple-like or finger-like pattern.
dysplastic	Pertaining to abnormal growth of cells but not clearly cancerous.
pleomorphic	Pertaining to tumors that contain a variety of cell types.
protocol	Detailed plan for treatment of illness.
polypoid tumor	Tumors that grow as projections extending outward from a base.
radiation	Use of radioactive substances in the diagnosis and treatment of disease.
osteosarcoma	Malignant tumor (flesh tissue) of bone.
scirrhous	Pertaining to hard, densely packed tumors, overgrown with fibrous tissue.
xerostomia	Conditions of dry mouth.
retinoblastoma	Tumor of the retina of the eye (embryonic cells); congenital and hereditary tumor.
neuroblastoma	Cancerous tumor of embryonic nervous tissue; a sarcoma composed of neuroblasts and affecting infants and children up to 10 years of age. The tumor usually arises in the autonomic nervous system.
angiogenesis	Formation of blood vessels.
adenocarcinoma	Cancerous tumor of glandular tissue.
hyperplasia	Condition of increased growth of cells (in numbers).
neoplasm	New growth (tumor).
myelosuppression	Stopping or inhibiting the growth of bone marrow tissue. This means that blood cells (leukocytes, erythrocytes, and platelets), normally formed in bone marrow, are not produced.
radiotherapy	Ionizing radiation used to treat malignancies.
anaplasia	Reversion of cells to a more embryonic type (as happens in malignancy).

apoptosis	Programmed cell death.
brachytherapy	Implantation of small sealed containers or seeds of radioactive material directly or near tumors.
epidermoid	Resembling epidermal tissue (tumors that arise from aberrant epidermal cells).
metastasis	The spread of a malignant tumor from its original location to a distant site.
metaplasia	Abnormal transformation of adult differentiated cells to differentiated tissue of another kind.
teletherapy	Radiation therapy using high-energy beams from a distant (tele-) source, such as a linear accelerator or cyclotron (proton therapy).

Chapter 20

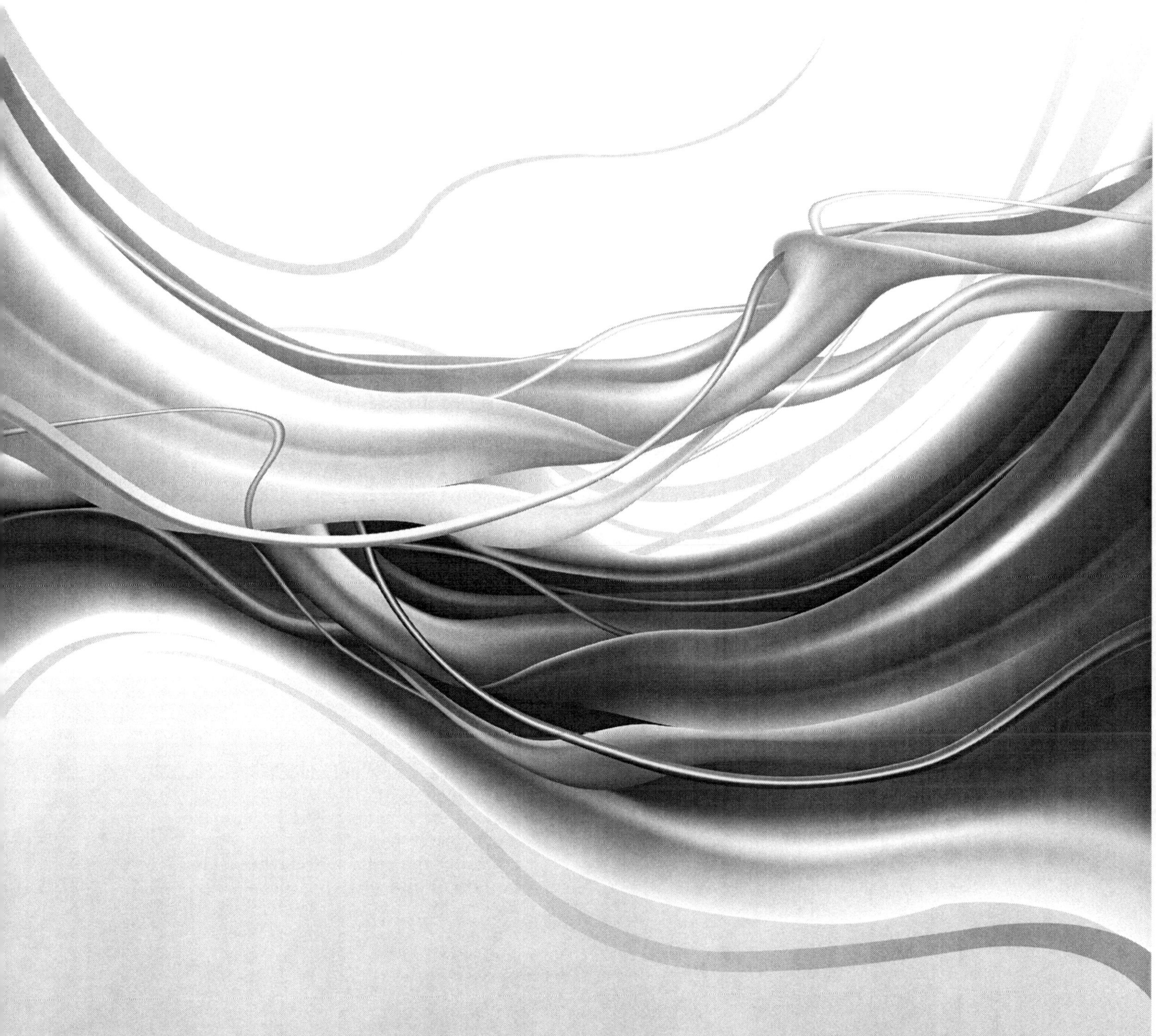

Chapter Twenty

MULTIPLE CHOICE QUIZ

Name: ______________________

In the box write the letter of the choice that is the definition of the term or best answers the question. There is only one correct answer for each question.

1. **What is the medical specialty that studies the characteristics and uses of radioactive substances in diagnosis of disease?..........** ☐
   A. Radiology
   B. Nuclear medicine
   C. Radiation oncology

2. **What does a radiologist do?..........** ☐
   A. Treats malignancy with radiation
   B. Aids a physician in administering x-ray procedures
   C. Specializes in the practice of administering diagnostic nuclear medicine procedures
   D. Specializes diagnostic techniques such as ultrasound, MRI and CT scans

3. **Which of the following is true of a radiopaque substance?..........** ☐
   A. Absorbs most of the x-rays it is exposed to
   B. Lung tissue is an example
   C. Is an air-containing structure
   D. Permits the passage of most x-rays

4. **Which best describes a barium enema?..........** ☐
   A. Iodine compound is given and x-rays are taken of the intestinal tract
   B. A fluorescent screen is used instead of a photographic plate to visualize images
   C. Metallic powder is introduced to the large intestine and x-rays are taken
   D. Radioactive substance is given and x-rays are taken

5. **X-ray of the renal pelvis and urinary tract after injecting dye into a vein:.....** ☐
   A. Venogram
   B. IVP
   C. RP
   D. Intravenous cholangiogram

6. **Myelogram: ....** ☐
   A. X-ray of lymphatic vessels
   B. X-ray of muscle
   C. X-ray of the bone marrow
   D. X-ray of the spinal cord

7. **Which is an x-ray of a joint? ....** ☐
   A. Pneumoencephalogram
   B. Arthroscopy
   C. Arthrogram
   D. Digital subtraction angiography

8. **Which term describes an x-ray test to show an organ in depth?..........** ☐
   A. Lymphoscintigraphy
   B. Tomography
   C. Ultrasonography
   D. Arteriography

9. **What best characterizes a CT scan?.....** ☐
   A. Uses radioactive substances to produce an x-ray image
   B. Gives a vertical front-to-back image of the body organs
   C. Magnetic and radio waves are used to create image
   D. Uses ionizing x-rays and a computer to produce transverse and other images of body organs

10. **What best characterizes an MRI? ....** ☐
    A. Sagittal, frontal, and cross-sectional images are produced using magnetic and radio waves
    B. Sound images are produced in addition to magnetic images
    C. X-rays and a contrast medium are used
    D. Radioactive matter enhances x-rays

11. **In which x-ray view is the patient upright with the back to the x-ray machine and the film to the chest? .....** ☐
    A. Oblique x-ray view
    B. Lateral x-ray view
    C. AP view
    D. PA view

12. **What is the meaning of adduction? .....** ☐
    A. Bending a part of the body
    B. Moving the part of the body toward the midline of the body
    C. Moving the part away from the midline
    D. Turning inward

13. What is a substance that gives off high-energy particles or rays? .... ☐
A. Scintillation scanner
B. Half-life
C. Barium
D. Radioisotope

14. In which test is a radiopharmaceutical injected intravenously and traced within the vessels of the lung? .... ☐
A. Chest x-ray of the lung
B. CT scan of the thoracic cavity
C. Perfusion study of the lung
D. Ventilation scan of the lung

15. What is an in vivo test? .... ☐
A. Experiments are performed in a laboratory
B. Radiopharmaceuticals are used
C. Radionuclide is incorporated into a chemical substance
D. Experiments are performed in a living organism

16. What can liver and spleen scans detect? .... ☐
A. Cirrhosis and splenomegaly due to abscess or tumor
B. Blood flow through the heart and large vessels
C. Areas of metabolic deficiency in the brain
D. Thyroid carcinoma

17. Interventional radiologists perform all of the following except .... ☐
A. Administration of radiation therapy
B. Placement of drainage catheters
C. Occlusion of bleeding vessels
D. Instillation of antibiotics or chemotherapy via catheters

18. What is thallium-201? .... ☐
A. Gamma camera
B. Contrast material
C. Fluorescent material
D. Radionuclide

19. In which procedure is a transducer used? .... ☐
A. MRI
B. Ultrasound
C. Bone scan
D. CT Scan

20. PACS is a .... ☐
A. Radiopharmaceutical used in a PET scan
B. Protocol for transmission between imaging devices
C. Technique using a radioactive substance and a computer to create three-dimensional images
D. System to replace traditional films with digital equivalents

21. FDG is a .... ☐
A. Radiopharmaceutical used in a PET scan
B. Protocol for transmission between imaging devices
C. Technique using a radioactive substance and a computer to create three-dimensional images
D. System to replace traditional films with digital equivalents

22. DICOM is a .... ☐
A. Radiopharmaceutical used in a PET scan
B. Protocol for transmission between imaging devices
C. Technique using a radioactive substance and a computer to create three-dimensional images
D. System to replace traditional films with digital equivalents

23. SPECT is a: .... ☐
A. Radiopharmaceutical used in a PET scan
B. Protocol for transmission between imaging devices
C. Technique using a radioactive substance and a computer to create three-dimensional images
D. System to replace traditional films with digital equivalents

Chapter Twenty
VOCABULARY QUIZ

Name: ______________________________

A. Match the following terms with their meanings below:

computed tomography (CT)
contrast studies
gamma camera
gamma rays
half-life
interventional radiology
ionization

1. Time required for a radioactive substance to lose half its radioactivity by disintegration ______________________________
2. High-energy rays emitted by radioactive substances ______________________________
3. Therapeutic procedures performed by a radiologist ______________________________
4. Transformation of electrically neutral substances into electrically charged particles ______________________________
5. Diagnostic x-ray procedure whereby a cross-sectional and other images of a specific body segment are produced ______________________________
6. Materials are injected to obtain contrast with surrounding tissue when shown on x-ray film______________________________
7. Machine to detect gamma rays emitted from radiopharmaceuticals during scanning for diagnostic purposes ______________________________

B. Match the following terms with their meanings below:

in vitro
in vivo
labeled compound
magnetic resonance (MR)
nuclear medicine
positron emission tomography (PET)
radioimmunoassay
radioisotope
radiology
radiolucent

1. Permitting the passage of x-rays ______________________________
2. Process, test, or procedure performed, measured, or observed in a living organism ______________________________
3. Radioactive substance is given intravenously and a cross-sectional image is created of cellular metabolism based on local concentration of the radioactive substance ______________________________
4. Process, test, or procedure performed, measured, or observed outside a living organism ______________________________

5. Medical specialty that studies the uses of radioactive substances in diagnosis of disease ______________________

6. Magnetic field and radio waves produce images of the body in three planes (coronal, sagittal, and axial) ______________________

7. Radiopharmaceutical used in nuclear medicine studies ______________________

8. Test that combines radioactive chemicals and antibodies to detect minute quantities of substances in a patient's blood ______________________

9. Radioactive form of an element; radionuclide ______________________

10. Medical specialty concerned with the study of x-rays and their use in the diagnosis of disease. ______________________

C. Match the following terms with their meanings below:

radiopaque	single photon emission computed tomography	ultrasound transducer
radiopharmaceutical	tagging	uptake
scan		ventilation-perfusion studies
scintigraphy		

1. Rate of absorption of a radionuclide into an organ or tissue ______________________

2. Image of an area, organ, or tissue obtained from ultrasound, radioactive tracer studies, computed tomography, or magnetic resonance imaging ______________________

3. Handheld device that sends and receives ultrasound signals ______________________

4. Attaching a radionuclide to a chemical and following its path in the body ______________________

5. Radiopharmaceutical is inhaled and injected intravenously followed by imaging its passage through the respiratory tract ______________________

6. Obstructing the passage of x-rays ______________________

7. Diagnostic nuclear medicine test using radiopharmaceuticals and gamma cameras to create images ______________________

8. Radioactive tracer is injected intravenously and a computer reconstructs a three-dimensional image based on a composite of many views ______________________

9. Radioactive drug (radionuclide plus chemical) that is administered for diagnostic and therapeutic purposes ______________________

Chapter Twenty
TERMINOLOGY QUIZ

Name: ______________________________

A. Using the following word parts, build or complete medical terms from the definitions below:

angi/o	pyel/o	vitr/o
hyster/o	radi/o	viv/o
is/o	son/o	-gram
pharmaceut/o	therapeut/o	

1. X-ray record of blood vessels: ______________________________
2. One who records x-rays: ______________________________grapher
3. Ultrasound record of the uterus: ______________________________
4. Procedure performed outside the living organism: in ______________________________
5. Pertaining to a radioactive compound used in diagnosis or treatment: ____________________ ical
6. Procedure performed within a living organism: in ______________________________
7. X-ray record of the renal pelvis: ______________________________
8. Pertaining to treatment: ______________________________ ic
9. An unstable form of an element that emits radioactivity: ______________________________ tope
10. Study of x-rays: ______________________________ logy

B. Using the following word parts, build or complete medical terms from the definitions below:

cardi/o	tom/o	-opaque
hyster/o	-gram	echo-
salping/o	-graphy	ultra-
son/o	-lucent	

1. Obstructing the passage of x-rays: radi ______________________________
2. Permitting the passage of x-rays: radio ______________________________
3. X-ray record of the uterus and fallopian tubes: ______________________________
4. Process of recording ultrasound images of the heart: ______________________________
5. Process of recording cross-sectional and other views of the body

   using x-rays: computed ______________________________
6. Process of recording sound waves as they bounce off organs of the body: ____________________

Chapter Twenty
ABBREVIATIONS QUIZ

Name: ______________________

A. On the line provided, give meanings for the following abbreviations, then write each abbreviation next to its explanation below:

1. angio ______________________
2. AP ______________________
3. Ba ______________________
4. CT ______________________
5. CXR ______________________
6. Decub ______________________
7. 18F FDG ______________________
8. Gd ______________________
9. I-123 ______________________
10. KUB ______________________

a. __________ Lying down

b. __________ Lungs are typically seen in this x-ray film

c. __________ Radiopharmaceutical used in PET scanning

d. __________ Contrast is injected into arteries for visualization via x-ray

e. __________ Contrast medium used in upper and lower GI series

f. __________ Front and back x-ray views

g. __________ Urinary tract is visualized without contrast

h. __________ MRI contrast agent

i. __________ Cross-sectional and other views obtained via multiple x-ray images

j. __________ Radioisotope used in thyroid studies

B. On the line provided, give meanings for the following abbreviations, then write each abbreviation next to its explanation below:

1. LAT ______________________________
2. MDCT ______________________________
3. MRI ______________________________
4. PACS ______________________________
5. PET ______________________________
6. RFA ______________________________
7. Tc-99m ______________________________
8. T-spine ______________________________
9. UGI ______________________________
10. US ______________________________
11. V/Q scan ______________________________

a. __________ Radioisotope used in heart, brain, thyroid, liver, bone, and lung scans

b. __________ Use of magnetic waves to create images of soft tissues in the body

c. __________ X-ray views of the backbone in the region of the chest

d. __________ Used to assess lung function

e. __________ Side view

f. __________ Replacement of traditional films with digital equivalents that can be accessed from several places and retrieved more rapidly

g. __________ Barium swallow

h. __________ Radioactive substance and a computer are used to create images to show function of tissues

i. __________ Interventional radiologists use this procedure to destroy abnormal tissue

j. __________ Sound waves create images of organs and tissues

k. __________ State of the art scanner that produces multiple (e.g., 64-slice) images

Chapter Twenty
EXERCISE QUIZ

Name: ______________________________

A. Name the medical term from its definition and word parts given:

1. obstructing the passage of x-rays: radio ______________________________
2. permitting the passage of x-rays: radio ______________________________
3. aids physicians in performing ultrasound procedures: ______________________ grapher
4. radioactive element that gives off energy in the form of radiation: radio ____________
5. radioactive drug administered for diagnostic purposes: radio ______________________
6. transformation of stable substances into charged particles: ______________________ization
7. a physician who specializes in diagnostic radiology: radi ______________________
8. study of uses of radioactive substances in the diagnosis of disease: ______________ medicine

B. Match the special diagnostic technique below with its definition:

computed tomography	interventional radiology	positron emission tomography
contrast studies	magnetic resonance imaging	ultrasonography

9. Radiopaque substances are given and x-rays taken ______________________________
10. Radioactive substance is given intravenously and a cross-sectional image is created of cellular metabolism based on local concentration of the radioactive substance ______________________
11. Echoes of high-frequency sound waves are used to diagnose disease ______________________
12. A magnetic field and radio waves are used to form images of the body ______________________
13. X-ray pictures are taken circularly around an area of the body and a computer synthesizes the information into a composite axial picture ______________________________
14. Therapeutic procedures are performed by a radiologist under the guidance of fluoroscopy or ultrasound ______________________________

C. Give the meanings for the following medical terms:

15. in vitro ______________________________
16. in vivo ______________________________
17. radiopharmaceutical ______________________________
18. bone scan ______________________________

D. Match the diagnostic test in Column I with the part of the body that is imaged in Column II:

Column I		Column II
19. myelography	________	A. Lymphatic system
20. pyelography	________	B. Spinal cord
21. angiography	________	C. Uterus and fallopian tubes
22. lymphoscintigraphy	________	D. Blood vessels
23. upper GI series	________	E. Esophagus, stomach, and small intestine
24. cholangiography	________	F. Lower gastrointestinal tract
25. barium enema	________	G. Renal pelvis of kidney and urinary tract
26. hysterosalpingography	________	H. Bile vessels (ducts)

E. Give meanings for the following abbreviations:

27. MRI ____________________
28. IVP ____________________
29. CXR ____________________
30. U/S ____________________
31. PA ____________________
32. PET ____________________
33. PACS ____________________
34. DICOM ____________________
35. AP ____________________
36. KUB ____________________
37. LAT ____________________
38. I-131 ____________________

Chapter Twenty
DICTATION AND COMPREHENSION QUIZ

Name: ______________________________

A. Dictation of Terms

1. ______________________________ 10. ______________________________
2. ______________________________ 11. ______________________________
3. ______________________________ 12. ______________________________
4. ______________________________ 13. ______________________________
5. ______________________________ 14. ______________________________
6. ______________________________ 15. ______________________________
7. ______________________________ 16. ______________________________
8. ______________________________ 17. ______________________________
9. ______________________________ 18. ______________________________

B. Comprehension of Terms: Match number of the above term with its meaning below.

______ Turning outward
______ Measurement or observation within a living organism
______ Permitting the passage of most x-rays
______ Rate of absorption of a radionuclide into an organ or tissue
______ A procedure in which something is measured or observed outside a living organism
______ A radioactive form of a substance
______ Process (two dimensional) used to detect radioactivity emitted in diagnostic imaging
______ X-ray record of the uterus and fallopian tubes
______ Movement toward the midline of the body
______ Radioactive substances produce cross-sectional images of regions of the body
______ Radioactive drug (radionuclide plus chemical) that is administered for diagnostic or therapeutic purposes
______ Pertaining to treatment
______ Obstructing the passage of x-rays
______ Diagnostic x-ray procedure in which cross-sectional images are made of specific body segments
______ X-ray record of the renal pelvis
______ Process of recording x-ray images of bile vessels
______ X-ray position; lying down and on one's side
______ Process of recording sound waves in order to produce an image of the heart

Chapter Twenty
SPELLING QUIZ

Name: ______________________

A. Circle the term that is spelled correctly and write its meaning in the space provided:

1.	en vivo	in vivo ______________
2.	therapeutic	therapreutic ______________
3.	colangiography	cholangiography ______________
4.	radionuclide	radioneuclide ______________
5.	radiolucent	radiolucant ______________
6.	anterioposterior	anteroposterior ______________
7.	transducer	transduser ______________
8.	radiopharmaceutical	radiopharmaseutical ______________
9.	traser studies	tracer studies ______________
10.	in vetro	in vitro ______________

B. Circle the term that is spelled correctly. The meaning of each term is given.

11.	X-ray record of the spinal cord .... myleogram	myelogram	mielogram
12.	Moving toward the midline .... abduction	adduckshun	adduction
13.	Lying down position .... rekumbent	recumbant	recumbent
14.	Lying on the back .... supine	soupine	suppine
15.	Obstructing the passage of x-rays .... radiopaquie	radiopaque	radioopaque
16.	X-ray of the renal pelvis .... pyleogram	pyelogram	pyilogram
17.	X-ray record of vessels .... anjiogram	angeiogram	angiogram
18.	Radioactive form of a substance .... radioisotope	radioiceotope	radioisotop
19.	Lying on the belly .... prone	proone	pron

Chapter Twenty
PRONUNCIATION QUIZ

Name: ______________________________

A. Underline the accented syllable in the following terms:

1. radioisotope
2. ultrasonography
3. angiography
4. supine
5. recumbent
6. echocardiography
7. ionization
8. scintigraphy
9. lateral decubitus

B. Match the term in Column I with its meaning in Column II:

Column I		Column II
1. flexion	________	A. Turning outward
2. extension	________	B. Lying on one's belly; face down
3. prone	________	C. Bending a part of the body
4. abduction	________	D. Lying on one's back
5. supine	________	E. Radionuclides are used as tags attached to chemicals and followed throughout the body
6. eversion	________	F. Test of blood flow to heart muscle
7. oblique	________	G. Lengthening or straightening a flexed limb
8. ^{99m}technetium sestamibi scan	________	H. Carrying a limb away from the body
9. tracer studies	________	I. Positioned at an angle

C. Complete the following medical terms from their definitions:

1. ______________________ gram — X-ray record of the urinary tract
2. ______________________ gram — X-ray record of the bile vessels
3. radio ______________________ — A radioactive drug used in diagnosis of disease
4. ______________________ gram — X-ray record of the uterus and the fallopian tubes
5. ______________________ ology — Study of x-rays
6. radio ______________________ — Permitting the passage of x-rays

Chapter Twenty
REVIEW SHEET QUIZ

Name: ______________________________

Give meanings for the following combining forms, suffixes and prefixes:

1. therapeut/o ____________________
2. is/o ____________________
3. pharmaceut/o ____________________
4. radi/o ____________________
5. son/o ____________________
6. viv/o ____________________
7. vitr/o ____________________
8. echo- ____________________
9. -gram ____________________
10. -graphy ____________________
11. -lucent ____________________
12. -opaque ____________________
13. ultra- ____________________

Chapter Twenty
MEDICAL SCRAMBLE

Name: ______________________________

Unscramble the letters to form radiology and nuclear medicine terms from the clues. Use the letters in the squares to complete the bonus term.

1. *Clue:* Movement toward the midline of the body

   ___ ☐ ___ ___ ___ ☐ ___ ___ ___ C I D T N O U D A

2. *Clue:* Obstructing the passage of x-rays

   ___ ☐ ___ ___ ___ ___ ___ ___ ☐ ___ P U R D O Q E I A A

3. *Clue:* Lying on one's back

   ☐ ___ ___ ___ ___ ☐ N E S I P U

4. *Clue:* X-ray image of blood vessels after injecting contrast material into the vessels

   ___ ☐ ___ ___ ___ ☐ ___ ___ ___ M A G A G O R N I

5. *Clue:* Permitting the passage of x-rays

   ☐ ___ ___ ___ ___ ___ ___ ☐ ___ ___ ___ C U T L E D A I R O N

BONUS TERM: *Clue:* Handheld device that sends and receives ultrasound signals

☐ ☐ ☐ ☐ ☐ ☐ ☐ ☐ ☐ ☐

Chapter Twenty

CROSSWORD PUZZLE

Name: ______________________

Fill in the crossword puzzle below using the clues listed underneath it.

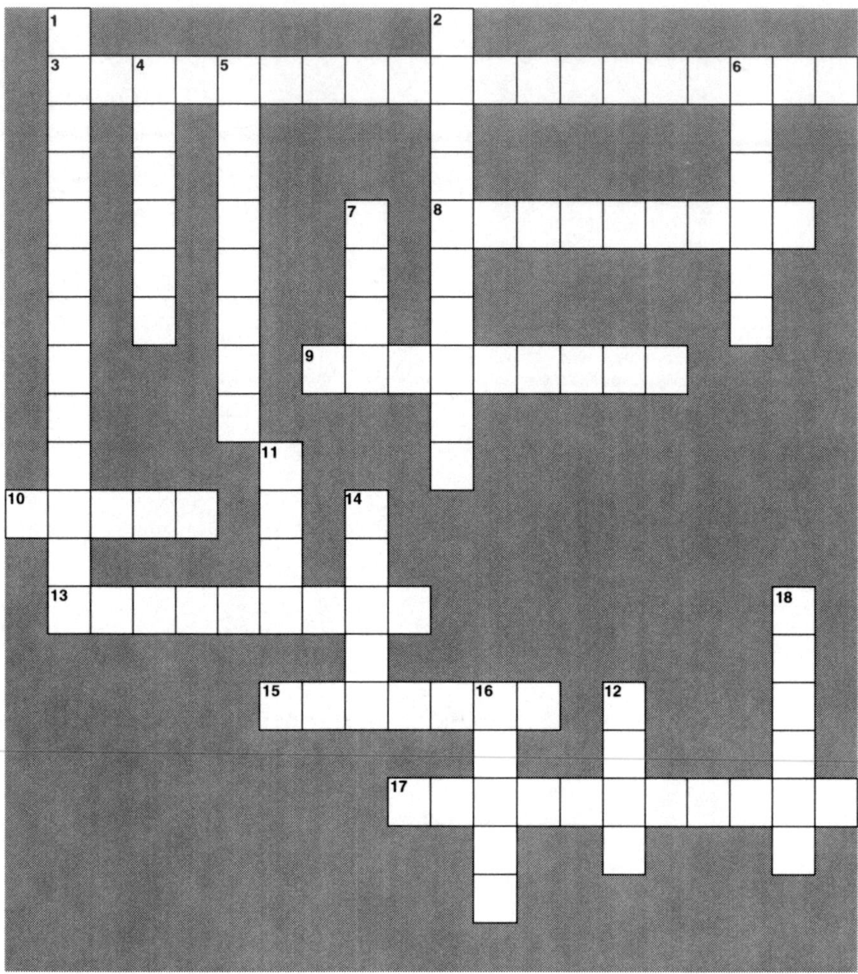

Across Clues

3. An x-ray record of the uterus and fallopian tubes to determine patency.
8. Moving a part of the body away from the midline.
9. Lying down; synonym of decubitus.
10. Lying on the belly.
13. An x-ray recording of the spinal cord.
15. -opaque means ________.
17. Permitting the passage of most x-rays.

Down Clues

1. An x-ray recording of the bile vessels.
2. Handheld device that projects high frequency sound waves is a/an ________ transducer.
4. Lying on the back.
5. Turning outward.
6. -gram means ________.
7. Viv/o means ________.
11. Pharmaceut/o means ________.
12. Cholangiography detects ________ duct abnormality.
14. Vitr/o means ________.
16. The combining form meaning x-rays.
18. Ultra- means ________.

Chapter Twenty
PRACTICAL APPLICATIONS

Name: ______________________

A. Radiology Report

Mass Adjacent to Thyroid—Lt side on US done 5/5/10
EXAM: NECK W/WOUT CONTRAST
5/9/10

Initially scans were obtained throughout the neck without IV contrast. Following this, a bolus of IV contrast was given and rapid scans obtained through the region of interest in the neck, related to the left lobe of the thyroid. As demonstrated on the recent ultrasound, there is a well-defined oblong mass in the left neck measuring 2.2 × 3 × 1.8 cm in size. This lies posterolateral to the left thyroid lobe and is predominantly between the left common carotid artery, which is displaced posteromedially, and the left internal jugular vein, which is displaced laterally. No other adenopathy, and the remainder of the thyroid appears unremarkable.

IMPRESSION: The mass appears to be extrinsic to the thyroid, possible even within the carotid sheath. The lesion appears to be relatively avascular. The differential diagnosis would include an unusually enlarged lymph node, a very atypical thyroid nodule, or a soft tissue tumor. The lesion is very easily accessible to needle biopsy and this would certainly be the easiest method of obtaining positive confirmation. This could be done using US guidance.

1. **What type of radiologic test is described here?**................................. ☐
   A. Ultrasound
   B. CT scans
   C. Pyelogram
   D. PET scan

2. **Where is the mass located?**................. ☐
   A. Within the left lobe of the thyroid gland
   B. Between the left and right carotid arteries
   C. Behind and to the side of the left lobe of the thyroid gland
   D. In front and to the side of the thyroid gland

3. **Which of the following is not a possible diagnosis?**............................ ☐
   A. An unusual mass on the thyroid gland
   B. Lymphadenopathy
   C. Tumor mass adjacent to the thyroid gland
   D. Lesion composed of many blood vessels

4. **What procedure will help determine the diagnosis?** .... ☐
   A. Aspiration of tissue and pathologic examination
   B. Removal of the thyroid gland
   C. Removal of thyroid tissue for biopsy
   D. Further scans with ultrasound guidance

B. Chart Note

The pt underwent a bone scan, which revealed irregular foci of tracer in lower T spine (T11-T12) consistent with compression fracture. There was also increased tracer in the posterior/lateral right ribs. On physical exam she was diffusely tender and in pain throughout her chest/ribs and spine. The pt also underwent chest CT, which demonstrated extensive parenchymal and pleural disease encasing the entire chest and involving vessels and bronchi. Her adrenals and liver, vertebral bodies, and R scapula were also involved with metastatic disease.

1. What type of test is a bone scan?......... ☐

A. Chest x-ray of ribs and bones of back
B. MRI of the skeleton
C. Dye is injected and traced in blood vessels
D. Radioisotope is injected and traced in bones

2. What type of doctor administers this test?.. ☐

A. Diagnostic radiologist
B. Nuclear medicine specialist
C. Radiation oncologist
D. Medical oncologist

3. Extensive parenchymal and pleural disease means: .... ☐

A. Tumor is in the spinal cord
B. Tumor is in the backbones
C. Tumor is in the lungs and membranes around the lungs
D. Tumor is in the abdominal, pelvic, and chest regions

4. The bone scan revealed: .... ☐

A. Disease in the lungs
B. Areas of tumor in the lower chest region and ribs
C. Disease in the adrenals and liver
D. Metastatic disease in the right shoulder bone

Chapter Twenty

ANSWERS TO THE QUIZZES

Multiple Choice Quiz

1. B
2. D
3. A
4. C
5. B
6. D
7. C
8. B
9. D
10. A
11. D
12. B
13. D
14. C
15. D
16. A
17. A
18. D
19. B
20. D
21. A
22. B
23. C

Vocabulary Quiz

A

1. half-life
2. gamma rays
3. interventional radiology
4. ionization
5. computed tomography (CT)
6. contrast studies
7. gamma camera

B

1. radiolucent
2. in vivo
3. positron emission tomography (PET)
4. in vitro
5. nuclear medicine
6. magnetic resonance (MR)
7. labeled compound
8. radioimmunoassay
9. radioisotope
10. radiology

C

1. uptake
2. scan
3. ultrasound transducer
4. tagging
5. ventilation-perfusion studies
6. radiopaque
7. scintigraphy
8. single photon emission computed tomography
9. radiopharmaceutical

Terminology Quiz

A

1. angiogram
2. radiographer
3. hysterosonogram
4. in vitro
5. radiopharmaceutical
6. in vivo
7. pyelogram
8. therapeutic
9. radioisotope
10. radiology

B

1. radiopaque
2. radiolucent
3. hysterosalpingogram
4. echocardiography
5. computed tomography
6. ultrasonography

Abbreviations Quiz

A

1. angiography
2. anteroposterior
3. barium
4. computed tomography
5. chest x-ray (film)
6. decubitus
7. fluorodeoxyglucose
8. gadolinium
9. isotope of radioactive iodine
10. kidneys, ureters, bladder

a. Decub
b. CXR
c. 18F FDG
d. angio
e. Ba
f. AP
g. KUB
h. GD
i. CT
j. I-123

B

1. lateral
2. multidetector CT scanner
3. magnetic resonance imaging
4. picture archival and communications system
5. positron emission tomography
6. radiofrequency ablation
7. radioactive technetium
8. thoracic spine
9. upper gastrointestinal (series)
10. ultrasound
11. ventilation-perfusion scan

a. Tc-99m
b. MRI
c. T-spine
d. V/Q scan
e. LAT
f. PACS
g. UGI
h. PET
i. RFA
j. US
k. MDCT

Exercise Quiz

A

1. radiopaque
2. radiolucent
3. sonographer
4. radionuclide or radioisotope
5. radiopharmaceutical
6. ionization
7. radiologist
8. nuclear

B

9. contrast studies
10. positron emission tomography
11. ultrasonography
12. magnetic resonance imaging
13. computed tomography
14. interventional radiology

C

15. a test in which something is measured or observed outside a living organism
16. a test in which something is measured or observed in a living organism
17. a radioactive drug that is given safely for diagnostic and therapeutic purposes
18. radioisotope is administered and traced within the bones

D

19. B
20. G

21. D
22. A
23. E
24. H
25. F
26. C

E

27. magnetic resonance imaging
28. intravenous pyelogram
29. chest x-ray
30. ultrasound
31. posteroanterior
32. positron emission tomography
33. picture archival and communications system
34. digital image communication in medicine
35. anteroposterior
36. kidneys, ureters, bladder
37. lateral
38. radioactive iodine

Dictation and Comprehension

A

1. adduction
2. cholangiography
3. uptake
4. computed tomography
5. echocardiography
6. eversion
7. therapeutic
8. hysterosalpingogram
9. in vitro
10. in vivo
11. lateral decubitus
12. intravenous pyelogram
13. positron emission tomography
14. radioisotope
15. radiolucent
16. radiopaque
17. radiopharmaceutical
18. scintigraphy

B

6 Turning outward
10 Measurement or observation within a living organism
15 Permitting the passage of most x-rays
3 Rate of absorption of a radionuclide into an organ or tissue
9 A procedure in which something is measured or observed outside a living organism
14 A radioactive form of a substance
18 Process (two dimensional) used to detect radioactivity emitted in diagnostic imaging
8 X-ray record of the uterus and fallopian tubes
1 Movement toward the midline of the body
13 Radioactive substances produce cross-sectional images of regions of the body
17 Radioactive drug (radionuclide plus chemical) that is administered for diagnostic or therapeutic purposes
7 Pertaining to treatment
16 Obstructing the passage of x-rays
4 Diagnostic x-ray procedure in which cross-sectional images are made of specific body segments
12 X-ray record of the renal pelvis
2 Process of recording x-ray images of bile vessels
11 X-ray position; lying down and on one's side
5 Process of recording sound waves in order to produce an image of the heart

Spelling Quiz

A

1. in vivo—tests are done within a living organism
2. therapeutic—pertaining to treatment
3. cholangiography—x-ray record of the bile vessels
4. radionuclide—radioactive chemical that gives off energy in the form of radiation; radioisotope
5. radiolucent—permitting the passage of most x-rays
6. anteroposterior—pertaining to the front and back
7. transducer—device that sends and receives ultrasound signals
8. radiopharmaceutical—a radioactive drug that is given for diagnostic or therapeutic purposes
9. tracer studies—radionuclides are used as labels and traced within the body
10. in vitro—tests are done outside a living organism

B

11. myelogram
12. adduction
13. recumbent
14. supine
15. radiopaque
16. pyelogram
17. angiogram
18. radioisotope
19. prone

Pronunciation Quiz

A

1. radioisotope
2. ultrasonography
3. angiography
4. supine
5. recumbent
6. echocardiography
7. ionization
8. scintigraphy
9. lateral decubitus

B

1. C
2. G
3. B
4. H
5. D
6. A
7. I
8. F
9. E

C

1. urogram
2. cholangiogram
3. radiopharmaceutical
4. hysterosalpingogram
5. radiology
6. radiolucent

Review Sheet Quiz

A

1. treatment
2. same
3. drug
4. x-rays
5. sound
6. life
7. glass
8. a repeated sound
9. record
10. process of recording
11. to shine
12. obscure
13. beyond

Medical Scramble

1. ADDUCTION
2. RADIOPAQUE
3. SUPINE
4. ANGIOGRAM
5. RADIOLUCENT

BONUS TERM: TRANSDUCER

Crossword Puzzle

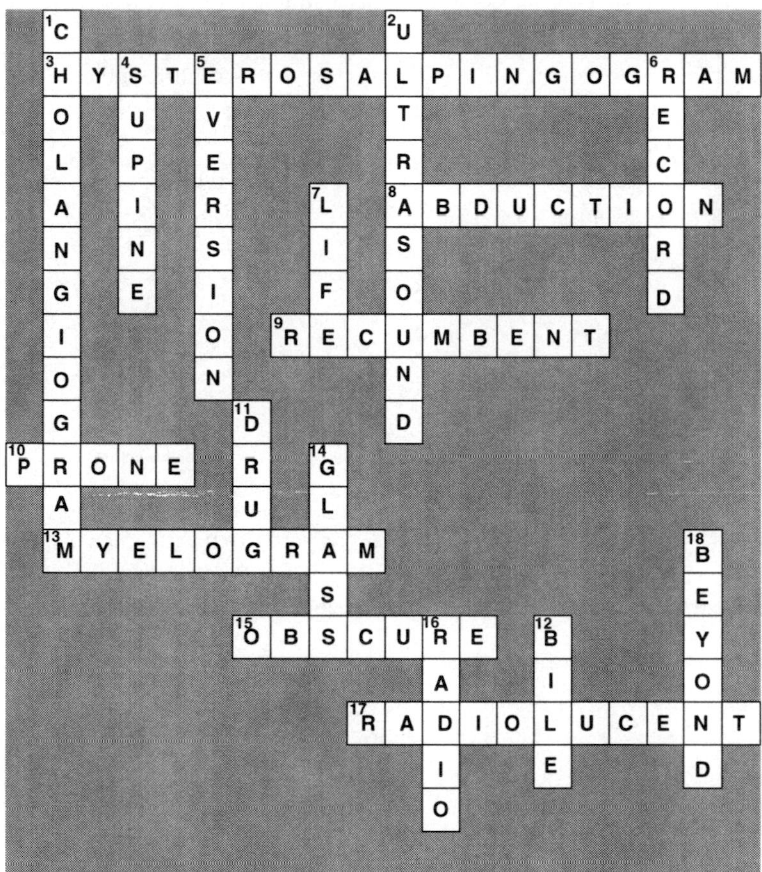

Practical Applications

A

1. B
2. C
3. D
4. A

B

1. D
2. B
3. C
4. B

Chapter Twenty
Answers to Terminology Section

(textbook pages 866–876)

Terminology	Meaning
radioisotope	A radioactive form of an element (radioisotopes of an element have similar structure but with different weights and charges).
radiopharmaceutical	Pertaining to the combination of a radioisotope and a drug.
radiographer	Aids physicians in administering diagnostic x-ray procedures.
hysterosonogram	Record of sound waves within the uterus (after injection of fluid to distend the uterine cavity).
therapeutic	Pertaining to treatment (therapy).
in vitro	Experiments performed in a test tube (glass); outside of a living organism.
in vivo	Experiments performed within a living organism.
angiogram	Record (x-ray) of blood vessels.
hysterosalpingogram	Record (x-ray) of the uterus and fallopian tubes.
pyelogram	Record (x-ray) of the renal pelvis of the kidney.
computed tomography	Process of recording x-ray images of the body in a cross-sectional view; a computer is used and images taken all around a section of the body.
radiolucent	Permitting the passage of x-rays (rays shine through).
radiopaque	Obscuring or obstructing the passage of x-rays.
echocardiography	Process of recording sound waves (echoes) as they bounce off the heart; a picture is produced that shows the sound waves as they are reflected from tissues of different densities.
ultrasonography	Process of using ultrasound waves in the body to produce sound echoes that are recorded as an image.

Chapter 21

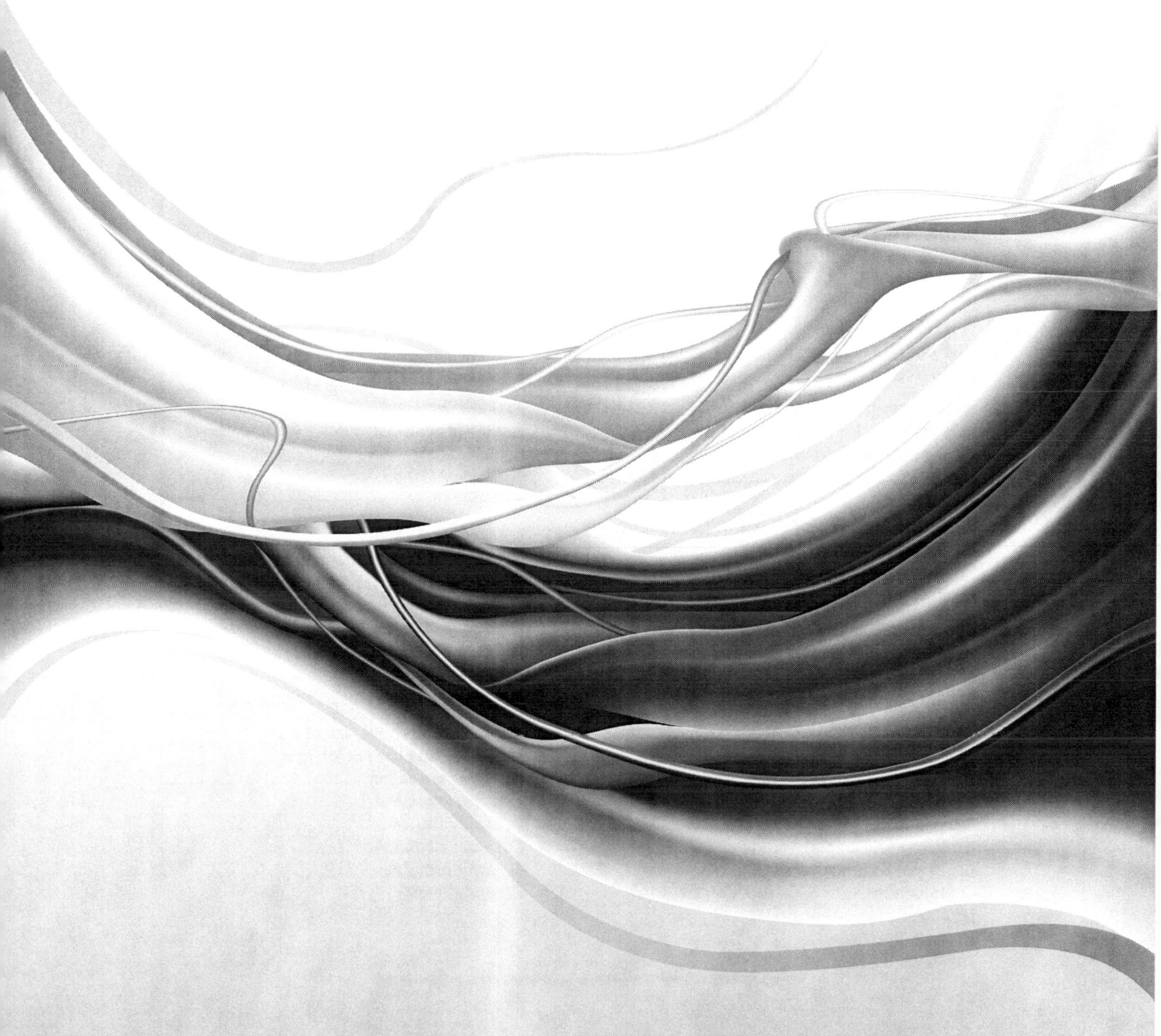

Chapter Twenty-One
MULTIPLE CHOICE QUIZ

Name: ______________________

In the box write the letter of the choice that is the definition of the term or best answers the question. There is only one correct answer for each question.

1. **Study of the interaction of drugs and subcellular entities such as enzymes and DNA is called: ....** ☐
   A. Medicinal chemistry
   B. Pharmacodynamics
   C. Chemotherapy
   D. Molecular pharmacology
   E. Pharmacokinetics

2. **Finding proper antidotes to the harmful effects of drugs is part of the specialty of: ....** ☐
   A. Molecular pharmacology
   B. Toxicology
   C. Medicinal chemistry
   D. Pharmacodynamics
   E. Pharmacokinetics

3. **Which of the following is a drug generic name? ....** ☐
   A. Omnipen
   B. ampicillin
   C. aminopenicillanic acid
   D. Polycillin
   E. Principen

4. **Which agency holds the legal responsibility for deciding whether a drug may be distributed and sold?..** ☐
   A. PDR
   B. United States Pharmacopeia
   C. National Institutes of Health
   D. Hospital Formulary
   E. FDA

5. **The combination of two drugs can cause an effect that is greater than the sum of the individual effects of each:..........** ☐
   A. Iatrogenic
   B. Additive action
   C. Tolerance
   D. Synergism
   E. Idiosyncrasy

6. **Suppositories are inserted: ....** ☐
   A. Parenteral administration
   B. Rectal administration
   C. Inhalation
   D. Topical
   E. Oral

7. **Drugs are swallowed and absorbed through the intestinal tract:................** ☐
   A. Parenteral administration
   B. Rectal administration
   C. Inhalation
   D. Topical
   E. Oral

8. **Drugs are injected through a syringe into a muscle, vein, or body cavity: ....** ☐
   A. Parenteral administration
   B. Rectal administration
   C. Inhalation
   D. Topical
   E. Oral

9. **Aerosols are administered in this way:..** ☐
   A. Parenteral administration
   B. Rectal administration
   C. Inhalation
   D. Topical
   E. Oral

10. **Drugs are applied on the skin: ....** ☐
   A. Parenteral administration
   B. Rectal administration
   C. Inhalation
   D. Topical
   E. Oral

11. **What is anaphylaxis? ....** ☐
   A. A type of hypersensitivity reaction
   B. Factors in the patient's condition that make the use of a drug dangerous
   C. A condition produced by the treatment
   D. Toxic effects that routinely result from use of a drug
   E. An antipruritic and antiseptic drug

12. **Drugs that block release of a substance that causes allergic reactions are called: ....** ☐
   A. Anticoagulants
   B. Antidiabetics
   C. Anticonvulsants
   D. Antihistamines
   E. Anesthetics

13. **Morphine:..** ☐
 A. Endocrine drug
 B. Cardiovascular drug
 C. Analgesic drug
 D. Stimulant drug
 E. Anticoagulant drug

14. **Beta-blocker:.....................................** ☐
 A. Endocrine drug
 B. Cardiovascular drug
 C. Analgesic drug
 D. Stimulant drug
 E. Anticoagulant drug

15. **Heparin:...** ☐
 A. Endocrine drug
 B. Cardiovascular drug
 C. Analgesic drug
 D. Stimulant drug
 E. Anticoagulant drug

16. **Estrogen:..** ☐
 A. Endocrine drug
 B. Cardiovascular drug
 C. Analgesic drug
 D. Stimulant drug
 E. Anticoagulant drug

17. **Amphetamine and caffeine:.................** ☐
 A. Endocrine drug
 B. Cardiovascular drug
 C. Analgesic drug
 D. Stimulant drug
 E. Anticoagulant drug

18. **What is the effect of a diuretic?...........** ☐
 A. Lowers blood pressure by promoting fluid excretion from the kidney
 B. Widens blood vessels
 C. Stops blood clotting
 D. Lowers cholesterol
 E. Increases blood pressure by holding water in the body

19. **Penicillin is an example of which type of drug? ....** ☐
 A. Antihistamine
 B. Analgesic
 C. Antiemetic
 D. Antibiotic
 E. Hypnotic

20. **A drug that works against fever is:......** ☐
 A. Antipruritic
 B. Antipyretic
 C. Anesthetic
 D. Anticoagulant
 E. Hypnotic

21. **Drugs that control anxiety and severe disturbances of behavior:....................** ☐
 A. Sedatives
 B. Anticonvulsants
 C. Analgesics
 D. Tranquilizers
 E. Anesthetics

22. **Drugs that relax without necessarily producing sleep: ....** ☐
 A. Sedatives
 B. Anticonvulsants
 C. Analgesics
 D. Tranquilizers
 E. Anesthetics

23. **Drugs used to relieve pain, induce sleep, and suppress cough: ....** ☐
 A. Sedatives
 B. Anticonvulsants
 C. Analgesics
 D. Tranquilizers
 E. Anesthetics

24. **Drugs that produce loss of sensation throughout the entire body: ....** ☐
 A. Sedatives
 B. Anticonvulsants
 C. Analgesics
 D. Tranquilizers
 E. Anesthetics

25. **Drugs used to treat epilepsy:...............** ☐
 A. Sedatives
 B. Anticonvulsants
 C. Analgesics
 D. Tranquilizers
 E. Anesthetics

Chapter Twenty-One
VOCABULARY QUIZ

Name: ______________________________

A. Match the following terms with their descriptions below:

addiction	antagonistic action	chemical name
additive action	antidote	contraindication
aerosol	brand name	generic name
anaphylaxis		

1. Commercial name for a drug; trademark or trade name ______________________
2. Exaggerated hypersensitivity reaction to a previously encountered drug or foreign protein ______________________
3. Physical and psychological dependence on and craving for a drug ______________________
4. Particles of a drug suspended in air ______________________
5. Chemical formula for a drug ______________________
6. Factor in the patient's condition that prevents the use of a particular drug or treatment ______________________
7. Legal, noncommercial name for a drug ______________________
8. Combination of two drugs gives less than an additive effect ______________________
9. Agent given to counteract an unwanted effect of a drug ______________________
10. Drug action in which the combination of two similar drugs is equal to the sum of the effects of each ______________________

B. Match the following terms with their descriptions below:

iatrogenic	molecular pharmacology	pharmacist
idiosyncrasy	oral administration	pharmacy
inhalation	parenteral administration	pharmacodynamics
medicinal chemistry		

1. Study of new drug synthesis; relationship between chemical structure and biological effects ______________________
2. Condition caused by treatment given by physicians or medical personnel ______________________
3. Drugs are given by mouth ______________________
4. Administration of drugs in gaseous or vapor form through the nose or mouth ______________________
5. Drugs are given by injection into the skin, muscles, or veins ______________________
6. Study of interaction of drugs and their target molecules, enzymes, or cell surface receptors ______________________

7. Location for preparing and dispensing drugs ______________________
8. Specialist in preparing and dispensing drugs ______________________
9. Unexpected effect produced in a particularly sensitive individual but not seen in most patients ______________________
10. Study of the effects and strength of a drug within the body ______________________

C. Match the following terms with their descriptions below:

Food and Drug Administration (FDA)	receptor	sublingual administration
pharmacokinetics	rectal administration	synergism
pharmacology	side effect	syringe
Physicians' Desk Reference (PDR)		

1. Drugs are inserted through the anus into the rectum ______________________
2. Study of the preparation, properties, uses, and actions of drugs ______________________
3. Target substance with which a drug interacts in the body ______________________
4. Instrument for introducing or withdrawing fluids from the body ______________________
5. Combination of two drugs causes an effect that is greater than the sum of the individual effects of each drug alone ______________________
6. Drug products are listed and described in this book ______________________
7. Study of drug absorption, distribution, metabolism, and excretion over a period of time ______________________
8. Governmental agency having the legal responsibility for enforcing proper drug manufacture and clinical use ______________________
9. Drugs are given by placement under the tongue ______________________
10. Adverse reaction that routinely results from use of a drug ______________________

D. Match the following terms with their descriptions below:

ACE inhibitor	antacid	toxicity
amphetamine	tolerance	toxicology
analgesic	topical application	vitamin
anesthetic		

1. Drug that relieves pain ______________________
2. Substance found in foods and essential in small quantities for growth and good health ______________________
3. Harmful effects of a drug ______________________
4. Larger and larger drug doses must be given to achieve the desired effect ______________________

5. Study of harmful chemicals and their effects on the body ______________________
6. Central nervous system stimulant ______________________
7. Drug that reduces or eliminates sensation ______________________
8. Drug that lowers blood pressure ______________________
9. Drug that neutralizes acid in the stomach ______________________
10. Drugs are applied locally on the skin or mucous membranes of the body ______________________

E. Match the following terms with their descriptions below:

antibiotic	calcium channel blocker	emetic
beta-blocker	cathartic	glucocorticoid
bisphosphonate	diuretic	hypnotic
caffeine		

1. Drug that promotes vomiting ______________________
2. Drug that produces sleep or a trance-like state ______________________
3. Drug that prevents bone loss and osteopenia ______________________
4. Drug that relieves constipation ______________________
5. Drug that is antiarrhythmic, antihypertensive, and antianginal; blocks receptors in blood vessels ______________________
6. Hormone from the adrenal cortex that raises blood sugar and reduces inflammation ______________________
7. Drug that increases production of urine and thus reduces the volume of blood in the body; lowers blood pressure ______________________
8. Central nervous system stimulant ______________________
9. Drug produced by a plant or microorganism, which has the ability to inhibit or destroy foreign organisms ______________________
10. Drug that blocks the entrance of calcium into heart muscle and lining of blood vessels; antihypertensive, antiarrhythmic, and antianginal drug ______________________

F. Match the following terms with their meanings below:

antihistamine	progestin	stimulant
antiplatelet	purgative	thyroid hormone
aromatase inhibitor	sedative	tranquilizer
narcotic		

1. Reduces estrogen in the blood by blocking an enzyme ____________________
2. Reduces the ability of thrombocytes to stick together and form a clot ____________________
3. Drug that excites and promotes activity; caffeine and amphetamines are examples ____________________
4. Drug that controls anxiety and severe disturbances of behavior ____________________
5. Drug that relieves constipation; strong cathartic and laxative ____________________
6. Habit-forming drug that relieves pain by producing stupor or insensibility; morphine and opium are examples ____________________
7. Secretion from an endocrine gland in the neck; stimulates cellular metabolism ____________________
8. Female hormone that stimulates the uterine lining during pregnancy ____________________
9. A mildly hypnotic drug that relaxes without necessarily producing sleep ____________________
10. Drug that is effective in preventing symptoms of allergy ____________________

Chapter Twenty-One
TERMINOLOGY QUIZ

Name: ______________________________

A. Use the following word parts to create or complete the terms from the definitions below:

aer/o	chem/o	esthes/o	-ia	-y
alges/o	cras/o	hist/o	-ism	anti-
bronch/o	cutane/o	hypn/o	-ous	
	erg/o	iatr/o	-therapy	

1. Condition of lack of feeling or sensation: an ______________________
2. Treatment using drugs: ______________________
3. Pertaining to under the skin: sub ______________________
4. A drug that widens bronchial tubes: ______________________ dilator
5. Effect of combination of two drugs is greater than each drug alone: syn ______________________
6. Pertaining to sleep: ______________________ tic
7. Unexpected effect of a drug (peculiar to an individual): idiosyn ______________________
8. Particles of drug suspended in air: ______________________ sol
9. Blocks the action of a substance produced in tissues (activated in allergic responses):

   ______________________ amine
10. Adverse effect related to being produced by a treatment: ______________________ genic

B. Use the following word parts to create or complete the terms from the definitions below:

derm/o	narc/o	pyret/o	-ic
erythr/o	or/o	thec/o	-logy
lingu/o	pharmac/o	tox/o	anti-
myc/o	prurit/o	-al	intra-

1. Pertaining to under the tongue: sub ______________________
2. Pertaining to under the skin: hypo ______________________
3. Pertaining to a stupor: ______________________ tic
4. Study of drugs: ______________________
5. Antibiotic drug produced from a red mold: ______________________ in
6. Pertaining to the mouth: ______________________
7. Pertaining to against fever: ______________________ ic
8. Pertaining to within the sheath (of the brain and spinal cord): ______________________.
9. Pertaining to against itching: ______________________ ic
10. Pertaining to a poison: ______________________ ic

C. Use the following word parts to create or complete the terms from the definitions below:

bi/o	vit/o	anti-	syn-
toxic/o	-logy	contra-	
vas/o	-ous	intra-	
ven/o	ana-	par-	

1. Pertaining to a drug that is against life (bacterial life): ________________ tic
2. Pertaining to other than through the intestine: ________________ enteral
3. Exaggerated hypersensitivity reaction: ________________ phylaxis
4. Pertaining to when the effect of two drugs is greater than either alone: ________________ ergistic
5. Pertaining to within a vein: ________________
6. A factor that prevents the use of a drug or treatment: ________________ indication
7. A drug that widens a blood vessel: ________________ dilator
8. Agent given to counteract an unwanted effect of a drug: ________________ dote
9. Study of poisons: ________________
10. Substance found in foods that is necessary for good health and life: ________________ amin

Chapter Twenty-One
EXERCISE QUIZ

Name: ______________________________

A. Match the pharmacologic specialty with its description below:

chemotherapy
molecular pharmacology
pharmacodynamics
pharmacokinetics
toxicology

1. Study of how drugs interact with subcellular parts ______________________________
2. Use of drugs in the treatment of disease ______________________________
3. Study of the harmful effects of drugs ______________________________
4. Study of drug effects in the body ______________________________
5. Study of drug absorption, distribution, metabolism, and excretion over a period of time ______________________________

B. Name the route of drug administration from its description below:

6. Drug is administered via suppository or fluid into the anus ______________________________
7. Drug is administered via vapor or gas into the nose or mouth ______________________________
8. Drug is administered under the tongue ______________________________
9. Drug is applied locally on skin or mucous membrane ______________________________
10. Drug is given by mouth and absorbed through the stomach or intestine ______________________________
11. Drug is injected via syringe under the skin, into a vein, muscle, or cavity ______________________________

C. Give meanings for the following terms:

12. antipruritic ______________________________
13. intrathecal ______________________________
14. antiseptic ______________________________
15. aerosol ______________________________
16. subcutaneous ______________________________

D. Give the meaning for the following terms:

17. cathartic ______________________________
18. antiemetic ______________________________
19. narcotic ______________________________
20. beta-blocker ______________________________
21. bronchodilator ______________________________

E. Match the term in Column I with an associated term in Column II:

Column I		Column II
22. antihistamine	_______	A. Relieves allergic symptoms
23. analgesic	_______	B. Penicillin or erythromycin
24. stimulant	_______	C. Barbiturate
25. sedative	_______	D. Nonsteroidal anti-inflammatory drug
26. tranquilizer	_______	E. Phenothiazines
27. antidiabetic	_______	F. Caffeine or amphetamines
28. antibiotic	_______	G. Insulin

F. Select from the following terms to complete the definitions below:

antianginal	cholesterol-lowering drug	vasoconstrictor
anticoagulant	digoxin	vasodilator
antihypertensive	diuretic	

29. drug that widens blood vessels ______________________________
30. drug that reduces blood pressure ______________________________
31. drug that strengthens the force and efficiency of the heartbeat ______________________________
32. drug that narrows blood vessels ______________________________
33. drug that prevents chest pain due to ischemia ______________________________
34. drug that reduces lipids in blood ______________________________
35. drug that promotes excretion of urine, lowering blood pressure ______________________________

G. Match the drug or type of drug in Column I with the condition it treats in Column II:

Column I		Column II
36. anticonvulsant	_______	A. Myalgia
37. anticoagulant	_______	B. Epilepsy
38. antacid	_______	C. Epigastric discomfort
39. antibiotic	_______	D. Thrombosis
40. tranquilizer	_______	E. Bacterial pneumonia
41. analgesic	_______	F. Congestive heart failure
42. digoxin	_______	G. High blood pressure
43. antihistamine	_______	H. Abnormal uterine bleeding due to hormonal imbalance
44. antihypertensive	_______	I. Severe behavior disturbances and anxiety
45. progestins	_______	J. Anaphylaxis

Chapter Twenty-One

DICTATION AND COMPREHENSION QUIZ

Name: ______________________________

A. Dictation of Terms

1. ______________________________ 11. ______________________________
2. ______________________________ 12. ______________________________
3. ______________________________ 13. ______________________________
4. ______________________________ 14. ______________________________
5. ______________________________ 15. ______________________________
6. ______________________________ 16. ______________________________
7. ______________________________ 17. ______________________________
8. ______________________________ 18. ______________________________
9. ______________________________ 19. ______________________________
10. ______________________________ 20. ______________________________

B. Comprehension of Terms: Match number of the above term with its meaning below.

______ An unexpected effect produced in a sensitive individual, but not seen in most patients
______ An agent given to counteract an unwanted effect of a drug
______ Harmful effects of a drug
______ Drug action in which the combination of two drugs causes an effect that is greater than the sum of the individual effects of each drug alone
______ A central nervous system stimulant
______ Drug that relieves constipation
______ Drug that stops the action of epinephrine at sites on receptors of heart muscle cells
______ Drug that lowers body temperature
______ An antibiotic substance
______ Pertaining to delivery of a drug within the membranes lining the spinal cord
______ A factor in the patient's condition that prevents the use of a drug or treatment
______ Drug that acts as a sedative
______ Pertaining to killing microorganisms
______ Drug that prevents abnormal brain activity
______ Drug that opens airways
______ Particles of drug suspended in air
______ Tube for introducing or withdrawing fluids
______ Drug that prevents vomiting and nausea
______ Pertaining to giving a drug by injection into the skin, muscles, or veins
______ Drug that blocks the action of histamine and helps prevent symptoms of allergy

Chapter Twenty-One
SPELLING QUIZ

Name: ______________________________

A. Circle the term that is spelled correctly and write its meaning in the space provided.

1. areolsol aerosol ______________________________
2. antacid antiacid ______________________________
3. antedote antidote ______________________________
4. antipyretic antepyretic ______________________________
5. cartharic cathartic ______________________________
6. hypnotic hipnotic ______________________________
7. iatrogenic iatragenic ______________________________
8. caffiene caffeine ______________________________
9. syringe syrinje ______________________________
10. tolerence tolerance ______________________________

B. Circle the term that is spelled correctly. The meaning of each term is given.

11. Agent that excites and promotes activity .... stimulent stimulant stimolent
12. Drug that promotes vomiting .... emetic enemetic emetik
13. Drug that relieves chest pain .... anteanginal anteanjinal antianginal
14. Hypersensitivity reaction .... anaphilaxis anaphylaxis antiphylaxis
15. Drug that is given by injection .... parenteral parinteral parentarol
16. Legal, noncommercial name for a drug .... genareic generic jeneric
17. Harmful effects of a drug .... toxcitity toxicity toxicitiy
18. Drug that relieves pain .... analjesic anesthetic analgesic
19. Drugs that are applied locally on the skin .... topical typoical typical
20. Drug that restores heart to a regular cycle .... antirhhytmic antiarrhythmic antiarryhthmic

Chapter Twenty-One
PRONUNCIATION QUIZ

Name: ______________________________

A. Underline the accented syllable in the following words:

1. antiarrhythmic
2. anaphylaxis
3. idiosyncrasy
4. synergistic
5. pharmacokinetics
6. antihistamine
7. cathartic
8. antidote
9. intrathecal
10. generic name

B. Match the term in Column I with its meaning in Column II:

Column I		Column II
1. amphetamine	_______	A. The combination of two similar drugs is equal to the sum of the effects of each
2. antiemetic	_______	B. An agent that lowers blood pressure by increasing the release of urine
3. diuretic	_______	C. A habit-forming drug that produces sleep and stupor
4. narcotic	_______	D. A central nervous system stimulant
5. hypodermic	_______	E. A drug that relieves pain
6. erythromycin	_______	F. Pertaining to under the skin
7. laxative	_______	G. A drug that relieves constipation
8. analgesic	_______	H. An agent that acts against vomiting
9. toxicity	_______	I. Harmful effects of a drug
10. additive action	_______	J. An antibiotic

C. Complete the following medical terms from their definitions:

1. anti ______________________	Pertaining to an agent that reduces fever
2. anti ______________________	An agent that prevents or delays blood clotting
3. par ______________________	Administration of drugs other than through the intestinal tract, such as into the skin, muscles, or veins
4. gluco ______________________	Hormone from the adrenal cortex that raises blood sugar
5. anti ______________________	Agent that lowers blood pressure
6. ______________________ ology	Study of poisonous effects of drugs
7. intra ______________________	Pertaining to within a sheath or within the membranes surrounding the spinal cord

Chapter Twenty-One
REVIEW SHEET QUIZ

Name: ______________________________

A. Give meanings for the following combining forms:

1. aer/o ______________________
2. alges/o ______________________
3. bronch/o ______________________
4. chem./o ______________________
5. cras/o ______________________
6. cutane/o ______________________
7. derm/o ______________________
8. enter/o ______________________
9. erg/o ______________________
10. esthesi/o ______________________

B. Give meanings for the following combining forms:

1. hist/o ______________________
2. hypn/o ______________________
3. iatr/o ______________________
4. lingu/o ______________________
5. myc/o ______________________
6. narc/o ______________________
7. or/o ______________________
8. pharmac/o ______________________
9. prurit/o ______________________
10. pyret/o ______________________
11. thec/o ______________________

C. Give meanings for the following combining forms, suffixes and prefixes:

1. tox/o ______________________
2. vas/o ______________________
3. ven/o ______________________
4. vit/o ______________________
5. -dote ______________________
6. -genic ______________________
7. -in ______________________
8. -phylaxis ______________________
9. ana- ______________________
10. anti- ______________________
11. contra- ______________________
12. syn- ______________________
13. par- ______________________

Chapter Twenty-One

MEDICAL SCRAMBLE

Name: ______________________

Unscramble the letters to form pharmacology terms from the clues. Use the letters in the squares to complete the bonus term.

1. *Clue:* Drug that acts against viruses such as the herpesvirus and HIV.

   ___ ☐ ___ ___ ___ ___ ___ ☐ ___ RATVALINI

2. *Clue:* Movement of a drug across a cell membrane into body cells.

   ___ ___ ☐ ___ ___ ___ ___ ___ ___ PONRRTTAS

3. *Clue:* Pertaining to under the skin.

   ___ ___ ___ ___ ___ ☐ ___ ___ ___ ☐ MYOPRICHED

4. *Clue:* Pertaining to a condition that is produced by a physician or treatment.

   ☐ ___ ___ ___ ___ ☐ ___ ___ ___ ___ CANIETORIG

5. *Clue:* Pertaining to under the tongue.

   ☐ ___ ___ ___ ___ ___ ___ ___ ___ ☐ BUGINLLUSA

BONUS TERM: ***Clue:*** Drug that relieves pain

☐ ☐ ☐ ☐ ☐ ☐ ☐ ☐ ☐

Chapter Twenty-One
CROSSWORD PUZZLE

Name: ______________________________

Fill in the crossword puzzle below using the clues listed below it.

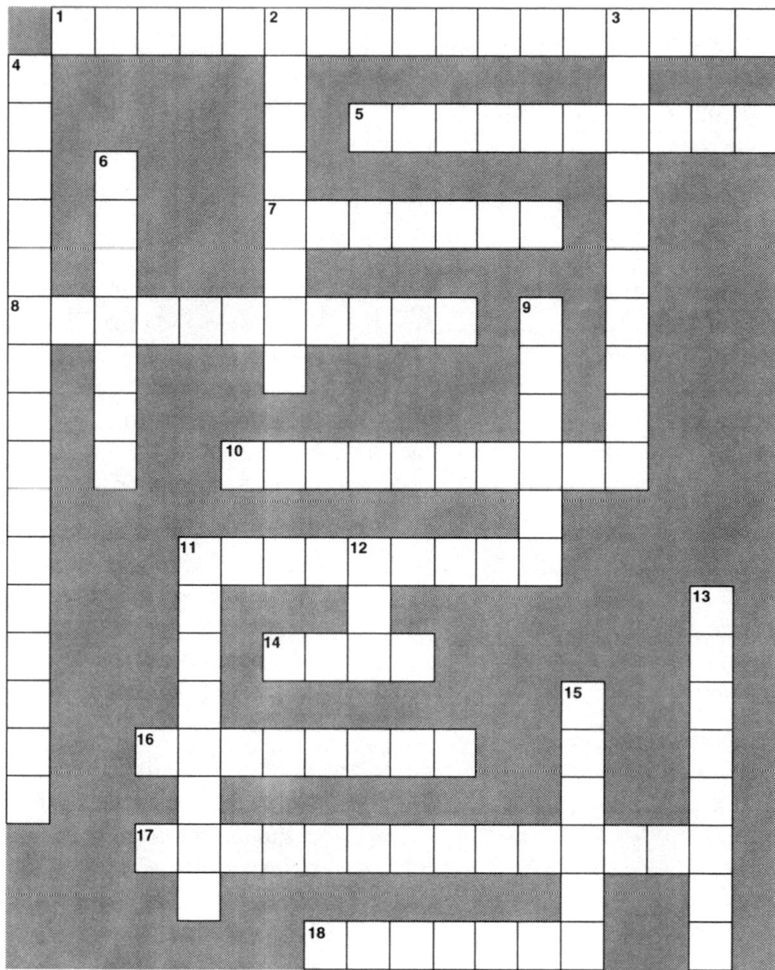

Across Clues

1. Factors in the patient's condition that prevent the use of a particular drug or treatment.
5. Administration of drugs in gaseous or vapor form through the nose or mouth.
7. Instrument for introducing or withdrawing fluids from the body.
8. Hypersensitive reaction of the body to a drug or foreign organism.
10. Drug that reduces or eliminates sensation.
11. Drug that relieves constipation.
14. Erg/o means _____; as in syn<u>erg</u>ism.
16. Mildly hypnotic drug that relaxes without necessarily producing sleep.
17. Type of drug that prevents convulsions.
18. Cras/o means _____; as in blood dys<u>cras</u>ia.

Down Clues

2. Particles of drug suspended in the air.
3. Any adverse condition in a patient resulting from treatment by a physician.
4. Study of drug absorption, distribution, metabolism, and excretion over a period of time.
6. Substance found in foods and essential in small quantities for growth and good health.
9. Drug that promotes vomiting.
11. Central nervous system stimulant; found in coffee.
12. Aer/o means _____.
13. An agent that produces sleep; from the Greek *hypnos* meaning sleep.
15. Hist/o means _____; as in anti<u>hist</u>amine.

Chapter Twenty-One

PRACTICAL APPLICATIONS

Name: ______________________

A. The following questions are based on the prescription information given below:

Fluoxetine (Prozac) 20 mg p.o. b.i.d.

Dimenhydrinate (Dramamine) 10 mg 2 tab q 4-6h

Ondansetron (Zofran) 4 mg 1 tab/caps t.i.d. p.r.n. for nausea

Ranitidine (Zantac) 300 mg 1 tab p.c. daily

Pseudoephedrine (Sudafed) 60 mg 1 caps q.i.d. for 15 days

Acetaminophen (300 mg) & codeine (30 mg) 1 tab q.i.d. p.r.n. for pain

1. **Which drug is given after meals to relieve the pain of ulcers?................** ☐
   A. Fluoxetine
   B. Dimenhydrinate
   C. Acetaminophen
   D. Ranitidine

2. **Which drug is an antiemetic and prescribed three times a day as necessary?......................................** ☐
   A. Ranitidine
   B. Pseudoephedrine
   C. Ondansetron
   D. Dimenhydrinate

3. **Which drug is an analgesic and prescribed four times a day as needed?..** ☐
   A. Fluoxetine
   B. Acetaminophen and codeine
   C. Dimenhydrinate
   D. Ranitidine

4. **Which drug is used to treat depression and prescribed twice a day orally?...............................** ☐
   A. Ondansetron
   B. Pseudoephedrine
   C. Fluoxetine
   D. Acetaminophen

5. **Which drug is an antihistamine, bronchodilator, and decongestant and prescribed four times a day for an extended period?............................** ☐
   A. Pseudoephedrine
   B. Dimenhydrinate
   C. Fluoxetine
   D. Acetaminophen

6. **Which drug is an antihistamine and antinauseant, used to prevent motion sickness, and prescribed every few hours (up to six times a day)?.............** ☐
   A. Ranitidine
   B. Dimenhydrinate
   C. Pseudoephedrine
   D. Ondansetron

B. FYI

Drugs taken by a mother during pregnancy may have harmful effects on the fetus or newborn. Some examples are analgesics (heroin, morphine) that produce respiratory depression, addiction, and neonatal mortality; anesthetics that produce fetal bradycardia; anticoagulants that lead to hemorrhage and fetal death; hormones (androgens and estrogens) that produce masculinization or clitoromegaly.

1. **What drug can produce slow heartbeat in the fetus?.....................** ☐
   A. Testosterone
   B. Morphine
   C. Anesthetic
   D. Anticoagulant

2. **What drug, taken by the mother, puts the fetus at risk for bleeding? ....** ☐
   A. Estrogen
   B. Anticoagulant
   C. Heroin
   D. Anesthetic

C. Drug Identifications

Match the following drugs with a description that fits it below. Write the name of the drug in the space provided.

Bactrim (trimethoprim/sulfamethoxazole)
Benadryl (diphenhydramine)
BuSpar (buspirone)
Fosamax (alendronate sodium)
Lasix (furosemide)
Lovenox (enoxaparin sodium)
Motrin (ibuprofen)
Nolvadex (tamoxifen)
Prevacid (lansoprazole)
Vasotec (enalapril)

1. This is a nonsteroidal antiestrogen medication indicated for the treatment of breast cancer in postmenopausal women. It is used when tumor cells are estrogen-receptor positive. It can be used to prevent breast cancer in women at high risk. ____________________
2. This is a potent diuretic to treat edema associated with congestive heart failure. ____________________
3. This is a nonsteroidal anti-inflammatory drug (NSAID) used to relieve the pain and inflammation of arthritis. It is also indicated for use to treat fever, dysmenorrhea, and mild to moderate pain. ____________________
4. This is a nonprescription antihistamine often used for severe allergic reactions (bee stings or poison ivy) and nasal allergy symptoms. It may also be used as an antipruritic (cream or lotion), sleep aid, or cough suppressant. ____________________
5. This antibiotic medication is prescribed to treat urinary tract infections, acute otitis media, and respiratory infections. ____________________
6. This medication is indicated for the treatment and prevention of osteoporosis in postmenopausal women. It increases bone mass to help reduce the incidence of fractures, such as in the wrist and spine. ____________________
7. This tranquilizer is prescribed for a patient with diagnosed general anxiety disorder. ____________________
8. This medication is commonly prescribed to treat duodenal and gastric ulcers. ____________________
9. This angiotensin-converting enzyme (ACE) inhibitor is indicated for the treatment of hypertension, heart failure, and in patients after MI, when the function of the left ventricle of the heart has been affected. ____________________
10. This is a low-molecular-weight heparin, indicated for the prevention of deep vein thrombosis, which may lead to pulmonary embolism in patients undergoing surgery (e.g., hip or knee replacement). It is usually administered by injection. ____________________

Chapter Twenty-One

ANSWERS TO THE QUIZZES

Multiple Choice Quiz

1. D	4. E	7. E	10. D	13. C	16. A	19. D	22. A	25. B
2. B	5. D	8. A	11. A	14. B	17. D	20. B	23. C	
3. B	6. B	9. C	12. D	15. E	18. A	21. D	24. E	

Vocabulary Quiz

A

1. brand name
2. anaphylaxis
3. addiction
4. aerosol
5. chemical name
6. contraindication
7. generic name
8. antagonistic action
9. antidote
10. additive effect

B

1. medicinal chemistry
2. iatrogenic
3. oral administration
4. inhalation
5. parenteral administration
6. molecular pharmacology
7. pharmacy
8. pharmacist
9. idiosyncrasy
10. pharmacodynamics

C

1. rectal administration
2. pharmacology
3. receptor
4. syringe
5. synergism
6. *Physicians' Desk Reference* (PDR)
7. pharmacokinetics
8. Food and Drug Administration (FDA)
9. sublingual administration
10. side effect

D

1. analgesic
2. vitamin
3. toxicity
4. tolerance
5. toxicology
6. amphetamine
7. anesthetic
8. ACE inhibitor
9. antacid
10. topical application

E

1. emetic
2. hypnotic
3. bisphosphonate
4. cathartic
5. beta-blocker
6. glucocorticoid
7. diuretic
8. caffeine
9. antibiotic
10. calcium channel blocker

F

1. aromatase inhibitor
2. antiplatelet
3. stimulant
4. tranquilizer
5. purgative
6. narcotic
7. thyroid hormone
8. progestin
9. sedative
10. antihistamine

Terminology Quiz

A

1. anesthesia
2. chemotherapy
3. subcutaneous
4. bronchodilator
5. synergism
6. hypnotic
7. idiosyncrasy
8. aerosol
9. antihistamine
10. iatrogenic

B

1. subungual
2. hypodermic
3. narcotic
4. pharmacology
5. erythromycin
6. oral
7. antipyretic
8. intrathecal
9. pruritic
10. toxic

C

1. antibiotic
2. parenteral
3. anaphylaxis
4. synergistic
5. intravenous
6. contraindication
7. vasodilator
8. antidote
9. toxicology
10. vitamin

Exercise Quiz

A

1. molecular pharmacology
2. chemotherapy
3. toxicology
4. pharmacodynamics
5. pharmacokinetics

B

6. rectal
7. inhalation
8. sublingual
9. topical
10. oral
11. parenteral

C

12. against itching
13. within the membranes around the spinal cord
14. against infection
15. particles suspended in air
16. under the skin

D

17. drug that relieves constipation
18. drug that prevents nausea and vomiting
19. potent analgesic that relieves pain
20. drug that lowers blood pressure, restores heart rhythm
21. drug that opens bronchial tubes

E

22. A
23. D
24. F
25. C
26. E
27. G
28. B

F

29. vasodilator
30. antihypertensive
31. digoxin
32. vasoconstrictor
33. antianginal
34. cholesterol-lowering drug
35. diuretic

G

36. B
37. D
38. C
39. E
40. I
41. A
42. F
43. J
44. G
45. H

Dictation and Comprehension Quiz

A

1. aerosol
2. amphetamine
3. anticonvulsant
4. antidote
5. antihistamine
6. antinauseant
7. antipyretic
8. bactericidal
9. benzodiazepine
10. beta-blocker
11. bronchodilator
12. cathartic
13. contraindication
14. erythromycin
15. idiosyncrasy
16. intrathecal
17. parenteral
18. synergism
19. syringe
20. toxicity

B

15 An unexpected effect produced in a sensitive individual, but not seen in most patients
4 An agent given to counteract an unwanted effect of a drug
20 Harmful effects of a drug
18 Drug action in which the combination of two drugs causes an effect that is greater than the sum of the individual effects of each drug alone
2 A central nervous system stimulant
12 Drug that relieves constipation
10 Drug that stops the action of epinephrine at sites on receptors of heart muscle cells
7 Drug that lowers body temperature
14 An antibiotic substance
16 Pertaining to delivery of a drug within the membranes lining the spinal cord
13 A factor in the patient's condition that prevents the use of a drug or treatment
9 Drug that acts as a sedative
8 Pertaining to killing microorganisms
3 Drug that prevents abnormal brain activity (as in epilepsy)
11 Drug that opens airways
1 Particles of drug suspended in air
19 Tube for introducing or withdrawing fluids
6 Drug that prevents vomiting and nausea
17 Pertaining to giving a drug by injection into the skin, muscles, or veins
5 Drug that blocks the action of histamine and helps prevent symptoms of allergy

Spelling Quiz

A

1. aerosol—particles of drug suspended in air
2. antacid—drug that neutralizes acid in the stomach
3. antidote—agent given to counteract an unwanted effect of a drug
4. antipyretic—drug given against fever
5. cathartic—drug that relieves constipation
6. hypnotic—agent that produces sleep
7. iatrogenic—an effect that is produced as a result of mistakes in drug use or of individual sensitivity to a drug
8. caffeine—central nervous system stimulant
9. syringe—instrument for introducing or withdrawing fluid
10. tolerance—drug action in which larger and larger doses must be given to achieve the desired effect

B

11. stimulant
12. emetic
13. antianginal
14. anaphylaxis
15. parenteral
16. generic
17. toxicity
18. analgesic
19. topical
20. antiarrhythmic

Pronunciation Quiz

A

1. antiarrhythmic
2. anaphylaxis
3. idiosyncrasy
4. synergistic
5. pharmacokinetics
6. antihistamine
7. cathartic
8. antidote
9. intrathecal
10. generic name

B

1. D
2. H
3. B
4. C
5. F
6. J
7. G
8. E
9. I
10. A

C

1. antipyretic
2. anticoagulant
3. parenteral
4. glucocorticoid
5. antihypertensive
6. toxicology
7. intrathecal

Review Sheet Quiz

A

1. air
2. sensitivity to pain
3. bronchial tube
4. drug
5. mixture
6. skin
7. skin
8. work
9. feeling, sensation

B

1. tissue
2. sleep
3. physician, treatment
4. tongue
5. mold, fungus
6. stupor
7. mouth
8. drug
9. itching
10. fever
11. sheath (of brain and spinal cord)

C

1. poison
2. vessel
3. vein
4. life
5. what is given
6. pertaining to producing
7. substance
8. protection
9. upward, excessive, again
10. against
11. against, opposite
12. together, with
13. other than, apart from

Medical Scramble

1. ANTIVIRAL
2. TRANSPORT
3. HYPODERMIC
4. IATROGENIC
5. SUBLINGUAL

BONUS TERM: ANALGESIC

Crossword Puzzle

	1 C	O	N	T	R	2 A	I	N	D	I	C	A	T	3 I	O	N	S
4 P						E								A			
H						R		5 I	N	H	A	L	A	T	I	O	N
A		6 V				O								R			
R		I				7 S	Y	R	I	N	G	E		O			
M		T				O								G			
8 A	N	A	P	H	Y	L	A	X	I	S		9 E		E			
C		M				S						M		N			
O		I										E		I			
K		N			10 A	N	E	S	T	H	E	T	I	C			
I												I					
N				11 C	A	T	H	12 A	R	T	I	C					
E				A				I								13 H	
T				F		14 W	O	R	K							Y	
I				F									15 T			P	
C			16 S	E	D	A	T	I	V	E			I			N	
S				I									S			O	
			17 A	N	T	I	C	O	N	V	U	L	S	A	N	T	
				E									U			I	
							18 M	I	X	T	U	R	E			C	

Practical Applications

A

1. D
2. C
3. B
4. C
5. A
6. B

B

1. C
2. B

C

1. Nolvadex (tamoxifen)
2. Lasix (furosemide)
3. Motrin (ibuprofen)
4. Benadryl (diphenhydramine)
5. Bactrim (trimethoprim/ sulfamethoxazole)
6. Fosamax (alendronate sodium)
7. BuSpar (buspirone)
8. Prevacid (lansoprazole)
9. Vasotec (enalapril)
10. Lovenox (enoxaparin sodium)

Chapter Twenty-One

Answers to Terminology Section

(textbook pages 901–902)

Terminology	Meaning
aerosol	Particles of drug (in solution) suspended in air.
analgesic	Pertaining to without sensitivity to pain.
bronchodilator	Drug that relaxes the smooth muscle lining bronchial tubes and is used to treat asthma, emphysema, and chronic bronchitis.
chemotherapy	Treatment using drugs.
idiosyncrasy	An unexpected effect of a drug that is peculiar to an individual.
subcutaneous	Pertaining to under the skin.
hypodermic	Pertaining to under the skin.
synergism	Condition of working together; the drug action in which the combination of two drugs causes an effect that is greater than the sum of the individual effects of each drug alone.
anesthesia	Condition of being without nervous sensation.
antihistamine	An agent that acts against histamine production in the body. Histamine is released as a result of an allergic reaction.
hypnotic	Pertaining to a condition of sleep (a trance-like state).
iatrogenic	Pertaining to an adverse condition that is caused or produced by a physician or a specific treatment.
sublingual	Pertaining to under the tongue.
erythromycin	An antibiotic that is produced from a red (erythr/o) mold (myc/o).
narcotic	Pertaining to a substance that produces stupor (has a morphine- or opium-like action).
oral	Pertaining to the mouth.
pharmacology	Study of drugs.
antipruritic	Pertaining to an agent that acts to relieve itching.
antipyretic	Pertaining to an agent that acts to relieve fever.
intrathecal	Pertaining to within the sheath of membranes surrounding the spinal cord.
toxic	Pertaining to poison.
toxicology	Study of poisons and the harmful effects of drugs.
vasodilator	Substance that causes blood vessels to widen.
intravenous	Pertaining to within a vein.
vitamin	A substance in foods that is essential in small quantities for growth and good health (life-giving amines).

Prefixes

anaphylaxis	A hypersensitive state of the body to a foreign protein (antigen) or drug; can produce severe symptoms and shock.
antidote	An agent given to counteract unwanted effect of a drug.
antibiotic	A substance that acts against microorganisms, such as bacteria.
contraindication	Factor in the patient's condition that prevents the use of a drug or treatment.
parenteral	Pertaining to injection of drugs other than through the intestines.
synergistic	Pertaining to synergism (the drug action in which the sum of the effects of giving two drugs together is greater than that of giving each drug alone).

Chapter 22

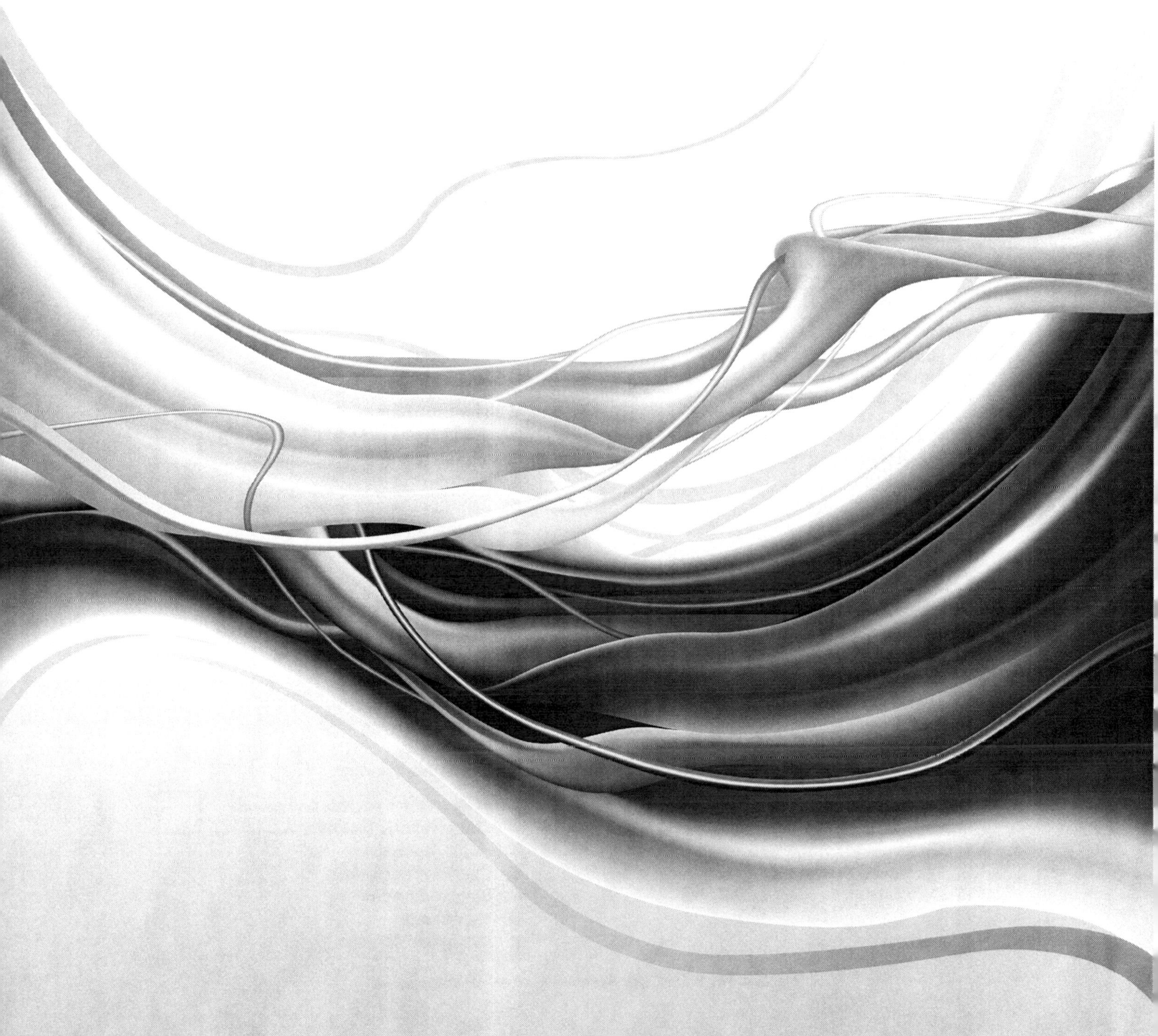

Chapter Twenty-Two

MULTIPLE CHOICE QUIZ

Name: ______________________________

In the box write the letter of the choice that is the definition of the term or best answers the question. There is only one correct answer for each question.

1. A forensic psychiatrist specializes in: ☐

A. Educational psychology
B. Psychoanalysis
C. Child psychiatry
D. Experimental psychiatry
E. Legal aspects of psychiatry

2. Which of the following best describes one of the roles of a clinical psychologist? ☐

A. Uses tests to measure mental health and intelligence
B. Uses drug therapy to treat mental illness
C. Treats only adults
D. Uses electroconvulsive therapy to treat mental illness

3. Which of the following is a mood disorder? ☐

A. Phobia
B. Panic attack
C. Obsessive-compulsive behavior
D. Psychogenic amnesia
E. Manic-depressive illness

4. A term that describes an exaggerated feeling of well-being is: ☐

A. Autism
B. Paranoia
C. Labile
D. Euphoria
E. Delusion

5. An uncontrollable urge to perform an act repeatedly is a(an): ☐

A. Conversion
B. Compulsion
C. Hypochondriasis
D. Mania
E. Paranoia

6. Preoccupation with one's self and lack of responsiveness to others is a characteristic of: ☐

A. Dissociation
B. Dysphoria
C. Delusion
D. Apathy
E. Autism

7. False or unreal sensory perceptions are called: ☐

A. Obsessions
B. Dissociations
C. Hallucinations
D. Phobias
E. Panic disorders

8. What best describes repression? ☐

A. Defense mechanism in which unacceptable thoughts are pushed into the unconscious
B. A mild depression
C. Repetitive acts
D. An involuntary, persistent idea, emotion, or urge
E. Delusions of persecution

9. Fear of leaving one's home is: ☐

A. Acrophobia
B. Agoraphobia
C. Claustrophobia
D. Necrophobia
E. Social phobia

10. Which of the following psychotherapies uses free association and transference? ☐

A. Hypnosis
B. Behavior therapy
C. Psychodrama
D. Psychoanalysis
E. Sex therapy

11. Alternating moods of exalted feelings and excitement with moods of extreme sadness and decreased activity: ☐

A. Major depression
B. Cyclothymic disorder
C. Bipolar disorder
D. Hypomania
E. Dysthymic disorder

12. Short depressive periods and moods with no psychotic features: ☐

A. Major depression
B. Cyclothymic disorder
C. Bipolar disorder
D. Hypomania
E. Dysthymic disorder

13. Numerous periods of mania and depression, but not of long duration; no psychotic features:.......................... ☐
A. Major depression
B. Cyclothymic disorder
C. Bipolar disorder
D. Hypomania
E. Dysthymic disorder

14. Resembling mania, but not as severe:.. ☐
A. Major depression
B. Cyclothymic disorder
C. Bipolar disorder
D. Hypomania
E. Dysthymic disorder

15. Severe dysphoric mood with psychotic features:.. ☐
A. Major depression
B. Cyclothymic disorder
C. Bipolar disorder
D. Hypomania
E. Dysthymic disorder

16. Grandiose sense of self-importance and preoccupation with fantasies of success and power:............................ ☐
A. Antisocial
B. Paranoid
C. Histrionic
D. Narcissistic
E. Schizoid

17. Continually suspicious and mistrustful of other people: .... ☐
A. Antisocial
B. Paranoid
C. Histrionic
D. Narcissistic
E. Schizoid

18. No loyalty or concern for others; without moral standards:.................... ☐
A. Antisocial
B. Paranoid
C. Histrionic
D. Narcissistic
E. Schizoid

19. Emotionally cold and aloof; indifferent to praise or criticism and to the feelings of others:.............................. ☐
A. Antisocial
B. Paranoid
C. Histrionic
D. Narcissistic
E. Schizoid

20. Emotional, immature, and dependent; irrational outbursts and flamboyant behavior: .... ☐
A. Antisocial
B. Paranoid
C. Histrionic
D. Narcissistic
E. Schizoid

21. Mental symptoms such as amnesia hide the pain and anxiety of unconscious conflicts: .... ☐
A. Hypochondriasis
B. Conversion disorder
C. Anorexia nervosa
D. Bulimia nervosa
E. Dissociative disorder

22. Physical symptoms appear as a defense against overwhelming anxiety: .... ☐
A. Hypochondriasis
B. Conversion disorder
C. Anorexia nervosa
D. Bulimia nervosa
E. Dissociative disorder

23. General preoccupation with bodily aches and pains and irrational fear about one's health:.................................... ☐
A. Hypochondriasis
B. Conversion disorder
C. Anorexia nervosa
D. Bulimia nervosa
E. Dissociative disorder

24. Psychological factors such as anxiety, anger, and fear produce unrealistic body image and reluctance to eat:........ ☐
A. Hypochondriasis
B. Conversion disorder
C. Anorexia nervosa
D. Bulimia nervosa
E. Dissociative disorder

25. Fear of obesity in which binge eating is followed by induced vomiting:.. ☐
A. Hypochondriasis
B. Conversion disorder
C. Anorexia nervosa
D. Bulimia nervosa
E. Dissociative disorder

Chapter Twenty-Two
VOCABULARY QUIZ

Name: ______________________

A. Match the following terms with their descriptions below:

affect	autistic thought	cannabis
amnesia	bipolar disorder	conversion disorder
anxiety disorders	bulimia nervosa	compulsion
apathy		

1. A disorder marked by physical symptoms, with no organic basis, appearing as a result of anxiety and unconscious inner conflict ______________________
2. Eating disorder of binge eating followed by vomiting, purging, and depression ______________________
3. Absence of emotions; lack of interest or emotional involvement ______________________
4. External expression of emotion or emotional response ______________________
5. Mood disorder with alternating periods of mania and depression ______________________
6. Thinking is internally stimulated and ideas have a private meaning, fantasy is thought of as reality ______________________
7. Loss of memory ______________________
8. Active substance in marijuana ______________________
9. Characterized by unpleasant tension, distress, and avoidance behavior; phobias, obsessive-compulsive disorder, and post-traumatic stress disorder ______________________
10. Uncontrollable urge to perform an act repeatedly ______________________

B. Match the following terms with their descriptions below:

anorexia nervosa	dementia	ego
defense mechanism	depression	fugue
delirium	dissociative disorder	gender identity disorder
delusion		

1. Major mood disorder with chronic sadness, loss of energy, hopelessness, worry, discouragement ______________________
2. Unconscious technique (coping mechanism) that a person uses to resolve or conceal conflict and anxiety ______________________
3. Chronic or sudden disturbance of memory, identity, or consciousness; multiple-personality disorder is an example ______________________

4. Central coordinating branch of the personality or mind ____________________

5. False sensory perception (hearing "voices" and seeing "things") ____________________

6. Loss of intellectual abilities with impairment of memory, judgment and reasoning ____________________

7. Strong and persistent cross-gender identification with the opposite sex ____________________

8. Flight from customary surroundings ____________________

9. Eating disorder of excessive dieting and refusal to maintain a normal body weight ____________________

10. Confusion in thinking; faulty perceptions and irrational behavior ____________________

C. Match the following terms with their descriptions below:

hallucination	mood disorders	obsessive-compulsive disorder
id	mutism	paranoia
labile	neurosis	paraphilia
mania		

1. Overly suspicious system of thinking with fixed delusions that one is being harassed, persecuted, or unfairly treated ____________________

2. Unstable, undergoing rapid emotional change ____________________

3. Nonreactive state; stupor ____________________

4. Major unconscious part of the personality; instinctual drives and desires ____________________

5. Repressed conflicts leading to mental symptoms such as anxiety and fears; less severe than a psychosis ____________________

6. Extreme excitement; hyperactive elation and agitation ____________________

7. False sensory perception ____________________

8. Anxiety disorder in which recurrent thoughts and repetitive acts dominate behavior ____________________

9. Recurrent intense sexual urge, fantasy, or behavior that involves unusual objects, activities, or situations ____________________

10. Prolonged emotion dominates a person's life; bipolar and depressive disorders ____________________

D. Match the following terms with their meanings below:

personality disorders
pervasive developmental disorders
phobia
post-traumatic stress disorder
projective test
psychiatrist
psychologist
psychosis
reality testing
repression

1. Defense mechanism by which unacceptable thoughts, feelings, and impulses are automatically pushed into the unconscious ____________________
2. Diagnostic, personality test using unstructured stimuli to evoke responses that reflect aspects of an individual's personality ____________________
3. Medical doctor trained in diagnosis, prevention, and treatment of mental disorders ____________________
4. Irrational or disabling fear of an object or situation ____________________
5. Childhood disorders characterized by delays in socialization and communication skills (autism and Asperger syndrome) ____________________
6. Anxiety-related symptoms appear following exposure to personal experience of a distressing event ____________________
7. A PhD or EdD specializing in mental processes and how the brain functions in health and disease ____________________
8. Disorder marked by loss of contact with reality; often with delusions and hallucinations ____________________
9. Ability to perceive fact from fantasy ____________________
10. Lifelong personality patterns marked by inflexibility and impairment of social functioning ____________________

E. Match the following terms with their descriptions below:

amphetamines
benzodiazepines
cognitive behavioral therapy
electroconvulsive therapy
family therapy
free association
schizophrenia
somatoform disorders
substance-related disorders
superego

1. Physical symptoms occur and cannot be explained by actual physical disorders or mental illness ____________________
2. Drugs that lessen anxiety, tension, agitation, and panic attacks ____________________
3. Psychoanalytic technique in which the patient verbalizes, without censorship, the passing contents of his or her mind ____________________

4. CNS stimulants used to treat depression and attention-deficit hyperactivity disorder (ADHD) ______________________________

5. Treatment of an entire family to resolve and understand conflicts ______________________________

6. Psychosis marked by withdrawal from reality into an inner world of disorganized thinking and conflict ______________________________

7. Internalized conscience and moral part of the personality ______________________________

8. Regular overuse of psychoactive materials (alcohol, cannabis, cocaine) that affect the CNS ______________________________

9. Electric current used to produce convulsions in the treatment of depression ______________________________

10. Conditioning is used to relieve anxiety and improve symptoms of mental illness ______________________________

F. *Match the following terms with their descriptions below:*

group therapy	psychodrama	supportive therapy
hypnosis	psychopharmacology	transference
phenothiazines	sedatives	tricyclic antidepressants
psychoanalysis		

1. Antipsychotic drugs (neuroleptics) used to treat severe psychoses, such as schizophrenia ______________________________

2. Treatment of psychiatric disorders with drugs ______________________________

3. Drugs that lessen anxiety ______________________________

4. Trance state is used to increase the pace of psychotherapy ______________________________

5. Treatment that allows the patient to explore inner emotions and conflicts so as to understand and change current behavior ______________________________

6. Offering encouragement and hope to patients facing difficult life transitions and events ______________________________

7. Psychoanalytic process in which the patient relates to the therapist as though the therapist were a prominent childhood figure ______________________________

8. Therapy that allows a patient to express feelings by acting out roles with other patients ______________________________

9. Drugs used to treat severe depression; three-ringed fused structure ______________________________

10. Patients with similar problems gain insight into their personalities through discussion and interaction with each other ______________________________

Chapter Twenty-Two

TERMINOLOGY QUIZ

Name: ______________________________

A. Use the following word parts to create or complete the terms from the definitions below:

anxi/o	hypn/o	neur/o	psych/o
aut/o	iatr/o	phil/o	schiz/o
hallucin/o	ment/o	phren/o	-ia

1. Pertaining to the mind: ______________________ al
2. Condition of sleep: ______________________ osis
3. Pervasive developmental disorder characterized by inhibited social interaction and communication and by restricted, repetitive behavior: ______________ ism
4. Chemical released at the end of nerve cells: ______________ transmitter
5. Specialist in the treatment of the mind: ______________________ ist
6. Drug that relieves anxiety: ______________________ lytic
7. Chronic psychotic disorder that includes hallucinations, disorganized speech and behavior, flat affect and lack of initiation: ______________________ ia
8. Recurrent, intense sexual urge, fantasy or behavior: para ______________
9. Drug that causes a false sensory perception: ______________ ogen
10. Pertaining to a condition caused by treatment: ______________ genic

B. Use the following word parts to create or complete the terms from the definitions below:

klept/o	pyr/o	somat/o	-mania
neur/o	psych/o	-genic	-therapy
pharmac/o	schiz/o	-leptic	

1. Obsessive preoccupation with stealing: ______________________
2. Treatment of the mind: ______________________
3. Withdrawn, introverted personality: ______________________ oid
4. Obsessive preoccupation with fire: ______________________
5. Pertaining to the body and the mind: ______________________ ic
6. Drugs that treat psychotic disorders: ______________________ drugs
7. Pertaining to produced by the mind: ______________________
8. Abnormal condition of the mind: ______________________ osis

9. Disorders with physical symptoms that cannot be explained by an actual physical disorder: ____________________ form disorders
10. Study of drugs that affect the mind: ____________________ logy

C. *Use the following word parts to create or complete the terms from the definitions below:*

chondr/o	-phoria	dys-	hypo-
xen/o	-thymia	cata-	para-
-phobia	a-, an-	eu-	

1. Overly suspicious system of thinking: ____________________ noia
2. Alternating periods of depression and mania: cyclo ____________________
3. Fear of leaving home or a safe place: agora____________________
4. Individual has belief of having a serious disease but physical evaluation does not support a diagnosis: ____________________ iasis
5. Fear of strangers: ____________________
6. Without feeling: ____________________ pathy
7. Depressive symptoms that occur for at least 2 years: ____________________
8. Sadness, hopelessness; depressive mood: ____________________
9. State of psychologically induced immobility and muscular rigidity: ____________________ tonia
10. Exaggerated feeling of well-being: ____________________

Chapter Twenty-Two
ABBREVIATIONS QUIZ

Name: ______________________________

A. On the line provided, give meanings for the following abbreviations, then write each abbreviation next to its explanation below:

1. AD ______________________________
2. ADHD ______________________________
3. ASD ______________________________
4. CBT ______________________________
5. DT ______________________________
6. ECT ______________________________
7. GAD ______________________________
8. LSD ______________________________
9. BZD ______________________________
10. MAOI ______________________________

a. __________ Changes in brain wave patterns are produced to treat depression

b. __________ Therapy focuses on thoughts and gives patients ways to change thoughts and the assumptions behind them

c. __________ Drugs that lessen anxiety, tension, and panic attacks: examples are alprazolam, diazepam, and lorazepam

d. __________ A hallucinogen

e. __________ Characterized by chronic anxiety, exaggerated worry and tension with little or nothing to provoke it

f. __________ Associated with alcohol withdrawal

g. __________ A common form of dementia

h. __________ Pervasive developmental disorder marked by inhibited social interactions and communication

i. __________ Marked by inattentiveness, overactivity, and impulsivity in children

j. __________ Antidepressant drugs

B. On the line provided, give meanings for the following abbreviations, then write each abbreviation next to its explanation below:

1. MDD ______________________________
2. OCD ______________________________
3. PTSD ______________________________
4. SAD ______________________________
5. SSRI ______________________________
6. TD ______________________________
7. TCAs ______________________________
8. ψ Rx ______________________________

a. __________ Type of anxiety disorder; occurs after exposure to a terrifying event

b. __________ Treatment

c. __________ Mood disorder; change of seasons affects mood

d. __________ Drugs used to treat depression; examples are Prozac, Paxil, and Zoloft

e. __________ Type of anxiety disorder; ritualistic behavior occurs

f. __________ Drugs used to treat depression; examples are Elavil, Tofranil, and Aventyl

g. __________ Chronic loss of energy, sadness, hopelessness, worry, discouragement, and often suicidal thoughts and impulses

h. __________ Abnormal movements; side effects of neuroleptic drug treatment

Chapter Twenty-Two
EXERCISE QUIZ

Name: ______________________________

The questions on this quiz have been taken from the exercises at the end of this chapter.

A. Match the following psychiatric symptoms with their meanings below:

anxiety	autism	delusion	mania
amnesia	compulsion	dissociation	mutism
apathy	conversion	hallucination	obsession

1. Loss of memory ______________________
2. State of excessive excitability; agitation ______________________
3. A nonreactive state; stupor ______________________
4. Persistent idea, emotion, or urge ______________________
5. Uncontrollable urge to perform an act repeatedly ______________________
6. Feelings of apprehension, uneasiness, dread ______________________
7. Uncomfortable feelings are separated from their real object and redirected ______________________
8. Anxiety becomes a bodily symptom that has no organic basis ______________________
9. Lack of responsiveness to others; preoccupied with self ______________________
10. Absence of emotions ______________________
11. False or unreal sensory perception ______________________
12. Fixed, false belief that cannot be changed by logical reasoning or evidence ______________________

B. Give meanings for the following terms:

13. dysphoria ______________________
14. euphoria ______________________
15. agoraphobia ______________________
16. labile ______________________
17. affect ______________________
18. paranoia ______________________
19. bipolar disorder ______________________
20. dementia ______________________

C. Select from the following terms to complete the sentences below:

anxiety disorders	eating disorder	somatoform disorders
delirium	mood disorders	substance-related disorders
dementia	personality disorder	
dissociative disorders	sexual disorders	

21. Disorders involving paraphilias are ______________________
22. Mental symptoms (loss of memory and identity) that hide unconscious conflicts are ______________________
23. Troubled feelings, unpleasant tensions, distress, and avoidance behavior are hallmarks of ______________________
24. Illnesses related to regular use of drugs and alcohol are ______________________
25. Bulimia nervosa is an example of a(an) ______________________
26. Illnesses marked by prolonged emotions (mania or depression) are ______________________
27. Mental disorders in which physical symptoms cannot be explained by a known physical problem are ______________________
28. A lifelong personality pattern that is inflexible and causes impairment of social functioning is a ______________________
29. Loss of intellectual abilities with impairment of memory, judgment, and reasoning are known as a(an) ______________________
30. Confusion in thinking with faulty perceptions and irrational behavior is a(an) ______________________

D. Identify the personality disorder from its description below:

31. Fantasies of success and power and grandiose sense of self-importance ______________________
32. Flamboyant, theatrical, emotionally immature ______________________
33. No loyalty or concern for others; does not tolerate frustration and blames others when he or she is at fault ______________________
34. Pervasive, unwarranted suspiciousness and mistrust of people ______________________
35. Emotionally cold, aloof, indifferent to praise or criticism or feelings of others ______________________

E. Identify the psychotherapeutic technique from its description below:

36. An induced trance is used to help the patient recover deeply repressed feelings ______________________
37. Patients express feelings by acting out roles with other patients ______________________
38. Long-term and intense exploration of unconscious feelings, using techniques such as transference and free association ______________________
39. Toys are used to help children express conflict and feelings ______________________
40. Conditioning is used to relieve anxiety and improve symptoms of illness ______________________
41. Neuroleptic substances are used to relieve symptoms of psychiatric disorders ______________________
42. Electric current is applied to the brain to produce convulsions and reverse major depression ______________________
43. Techniques are used to help patients overcome sexual dysfunction ______________________

F. Select from the following terms to complete the sentences below:

agoraphobia	kleptomania	pyromania
amphetamines	MAO inhibitors	tricyclic antidepressants
cyclothymia	minor tranquilizers and sedatives	xenophobia
dysthymia	phenothiazines	

44. Fear of strangers is ______________________
45. Obsessive preoccupation with stealing is ______________________
46. Antidepressant agents that work by blocking the action of a specific enzyme are ______________________
47. A mood disorder marked by depressive periods that are milder than major depression is ______________________
48. Fear of being left alone in unfamiliar surroundings is ______________________
49. Anxiolytic agents used to reduce tension are ______________________
50. Antipsychotic tranquilizers such as Thorazine are ______________________

Chapter Twenty-Two

DICTATION AND COMPREHENSION QUIZ

Name: ______________________________

A. Dictation of Terms

1.	____________________	11.	____________________
2.	____________________	12.	____________________
3.	____________________	13.	____________________
4.	____________________	14.	____________________
5.	____________________	15.	____________________
6.	____________________	16.	____________________
7.	____________________	17.	____________________
8.	____________________	18.	____________________
9.	____________________	19.	____________________
10.	____________________	20.	____________________

B. Comprehension of Terms: Match number of the above term with its meaning below.

______ Confusion in thinking; faulty perceptions and irrational behavior
______ Drug used as a mild tranquilizer
______ Unstable, undergoing rapid emotional change
______ Loss of memory
______ Tranquilizers used to treat psychoses
______ Withdrawal from reality into an inner world of disorganized thinking and conflict; a psychosis
______ Internalized conscience and moral part of the personality
______ Fear of strangers
______ Treatment that allows the patient to explore inner emotions and conflicts; transference, free association, and dream analysis are elements of the therapy
______ Drugs that produce a state of CNS excitement, hyperactivity, and mood change
______ The use of nonliving objects as substitutes for a human sexual love object
______ Sexual gratification is gained by being humiliated, beaten, or made to suffer by another person
______ The outward expression of emotion, or emotional response
______ An anxiety disorder in which recurrent thoughts and repetitive acts dominate behavior
______ Loss of intellectual abilities with impairment of memory, identity, and reasoning
______ Fear of closed places
______ Study of drugs and their effect on the mind and mental illness
______ Sadness, hopelessness, worry, discouragement (literally, "bad feeling")
______ Preoccupation with bodily aches, pains, and discomforts in the absence of real illness
______ Eating disorder marked by refusal to maintain minimally normal body weight

Chapter Twenty-Two
SPELLING QUIZ

Name: ______________________________

A. Circle the term that is spelled correctly and write its meaning in the space provided:

1.	masochism	maschoschism ______________________
2.	dilerium	delirium ______________________
3.	bulemia nervosa	bulimia nervosa ______________________
4.	physchoanalysis	psychoanalysis ______________________
5.	schizophrenia	shizophrenia ______________________
6.	paranoid	paraniod ______________________
7.	dimentia	dementia ______________________
8.	eufouria	euphoria ______________________
9.	narsicissm	narcissism ______________________
10.	bipoler disorder	bipolar disorder ______________________

B. Circle the term that is spelled correctly. The meaning of each term is given.

11.	Troubled feelings, distress, and avoidance behavior	anxeity	anxiety	angsiety
12.	Stimulant drug that causes euphoria and hallucinations	cocaine	cokaine	cociane
13.	External emotion or emotional response of a person	effect	effact	affect
14.	Severe lack of response to other people	autism	aughtism	autoism
15.	Amnesia with fleeing from customary surroundings	feuge	fugue	fugeue
16.	Depressive episodes but not of intensity of major depression	dysthimia	disthymia	dysthymia
17.	Dried leaves and flowers of the hemp plant; causes euphoria	maryjuana	marijana	marijuana
18.	Sexual arousal that requires unusual and bizarre fantasies	paraphilia	paraphillia	parephilia
19.	Absence of emotion	apethy	apathy	apathe
20.	Fear of strangers	xerophobia	xerophobea	xenophobia

Chapter Twenty-Two
PRONUNCIATION QUIZ

Name: ______________________________

A. Underline the accented syllable in the following terms:

1. narcissism
2. opioid
3. agoraphobia
4. dementia
5. catatonic stupor
6. dysthymia
7. voyeurism
8. psychoanalysis
9. autism
10. euphoria

B. Match the term in Column I with its meaning in Column II:

Column I		Column II
1. affect	_______	A. Loss of memory
2. dementia	_______	B. A false belief or idea that cannot be changed by logical reasoning
3. delirium	_______	C. Pervasive lack of responsiveness to other people; stupor
4. delusion	_______	D. Unstable; undergoing rapid emotional change
5. labile	_______	E. The emotional reaction of a patient
6. sadism	_______	F. Pleasure received from inflicting pain on others
7. mutism	_______	G. Loss of higher mental functioning
8. mania	_______	H. A defense mechanism in which anxiety is converted into a bodily symptom
9. amnesia	_______	I. State of excessive excitability and agitation
10. conversion	_______	J. Confusion in thinking; faulty perceptions and irrational behavior

C. Complete the following medical terms from their definitions:

1. ____________________ nervosa	Eating disorder marked by excessive dieting
2. pheno ____________________	Antipsychotic tranquilizers
3. cyclo ____________________	Pertaining to exhibiting cycles of depression and exhilaration
4. ____________________ phrenia	A psychosis involving delusions, hallucinations, bizarre and illogical thinking
5. psycho ____________________	Pertaining to the interrelationship of mind and body
6. ____________________ phobia	Fear of strangers
7. hypo ____________________	Exaggerated concern with one's health
8. ____________________ phobia	Fear of heights

Chapter Twenty-Two
REVIEW SHEET QUIZ

Name: ______________________________

A. Give meanings for the following combining forms:

1. anxi/o ______________________
2. hypn/o ______________________
3. iatr/o ______________________
4. klept/o ______________________
5. ment/o ______________________
6. neur/o ______________________
7. phren/o ______________________
8. psych/o______________________
9. pyr/o______________________
10. schiz/o ______________________

B. Give meanings for the following combining forms and suffixes:

1. somat/o ______________________
2. xen/o ______________________
3. aut/o ______________________
4. phil/o ______________________
5. -genic ______________________
6. -leptic ______________________
7. -mania ______________________
8. -phobia ______________________
9. -thymia ______________________
10. -phoria ______________________

Chapter Twenty-Two

MEDICAL SCRAMBLE

Name: ______________________

Unscramble the letters to form psychiatry terms from the clues. Use the letters in the squares to complete the bonus term.

1. *Clue:* Unstable; undergoing rapid emotional change

   ___ ___ ☐ ___ ___ ☐ L E L A I B

2. *Clue:* Strong impulse (obsessive urge) to set objects on fire

   ☐ ___ ___ ☐ ___ ___ ☐ ___ ___ M Y A I O R A N P

3. *Clue:* Sadness, hopelessness, and depressive mood; feeling "low"

   ___ ___ ___ ___ ☐ ___ ___ ___ ☐ R I Y H S O P D A

4. *Clue:* Drug that relieves anxiety and produces a relaxing effect

   ___ ___ ☐ ___ ☐ ___ ___ ___ ☐ ___ X Y N T A C I L I O

BONUS TERM: *Clue:* Fear of strangers

☐ ☐ ☐ ☐ ☐ ☐ ☐ ☐ ☐ ☐

Chapter Twenty-Two
CROSSWORD PUZZLE

Name: ______________________

Fill in the crossword puzzle below using the clues listed underneath it.

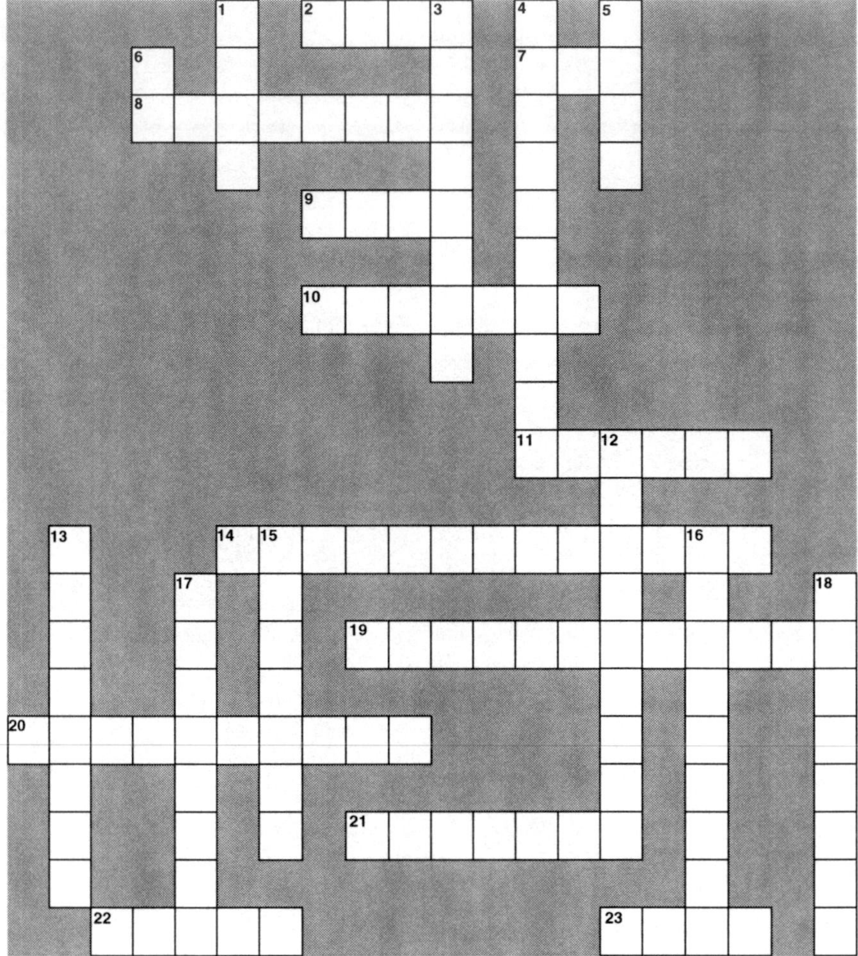

Across Clues

2. Phren/o means ____________.
7. Executive and coordinating aspect of the mind.
8. Confusion in thinking.
9. Cata- means ____________; as in catatonic.
10. Binge eating followed by vomiting and depression.
11. External emotion or emotional response of a person.
14. False sensory perception.
19. Pertaining to grandiose sense of self-importance or uniqueness and preoccupation with fantasies of success or power (a personality type).
20. Uncontrollable urge to perform an act repeatedly.
21. Substance used to treat the manic stage of manic-depressive illness.
22. Extreme excitement, hyperactivity, inflated self-esteem.
23. Psych/o means ____________.

Down Clues

1. Aut/o means ____________.
3. Loss of higher mental functioning and memory.
4. Sexual urges and fantasies involving sexual activity with a prepubescent child.
5. Phil/o means ____________.
6. Major unconscious part of the personality.
12. Use of nonliving objects as substitutes for a human love object.
13. Good feeling; "high".
15. Loss of memory.
16. An involuntary, persistent idea, emotion, or urge.
17. False belief or idea that cannot be changed by logical reasoning or evidence.
18. Personality that is aloof and emotionally cold.

Chapter Twenty-Two
PRACTICAL APPLICATIONS

Name: ______________________

A. The following questions are based on Major Depression: Case Report (page 944)

1. **Postpartum depression is an example of a:** ☐
   A. Personality disorder
   B. Somatoform disorder
   C. Mood disorder
   D. Substance-related disorder

2. **A term that best describes one of Mrs. C's symptoms is:** ☐
   A. Apathy
   B. Labile
   C. Anxiety
   D. Euphoria

3. **Mrs. C's dysphoria meant that she was:** ☐
   A. Agitated
   B. Antisocial
   C. Narcissistic
   D. Depressed

4. **An example of an antidepressant drug is:** ☐
   A. Lithium
   B. Valium
   C. Prozac
   D. Amphetamine

B. The following questions are based on Somatoform Disorder: Case Report (page 944)

1. **An example of a symptom of a somatoform disorder is:** ☐
   A. Obsession
   B. Delusions of persecution
   C. False sensory perception
   D. Conversion

2. **The patient's hypochondriasis was treated successfully with:** ☐
   A. Hypnosis
   B. Neuroleptic therapy
   C. Psychotherapy
   D. ECT

Chapter Twenty-Two
ANSWERS TO THE QUIZZES

Multiple Choice Quiz

1. E
2. A
3. E
4. D
5. B
6. E
7. C
8. A
9. B
10. D
11. C
12. E
13. B
14. D
15. A
16. D
17. B
18. A
19. E
20. C
21. E
22. B
23. A
24. C
25. D

Vocabulary Quiz

A

1. conversion disorder
2. bulimia nervosa
3. apathy
4. affect
5. bipolar disorder
6. autistic thought
7. amnesia
8. cannabis
9. anxiety disorders
10. compulsion

B

1. depression
2. defense mechanism
3. dissociative disorder
4. ego
5. delusion
6. dementia
7. gender identity disorder
8. fugue
9. anorexia nervosa
10. delirium

C

1. paranoia
2. labile
3. mutism
4. id
5. neurosis
6. mania
7. hallucination
8. obsessive-compulsive disorder
9. paraphilia
10. mood disorders

D

1. repression
2. projective test
3. psychiatrist
4. phobia
5. pervasive developmental disorders
6. post-traumatic stress disorder
7. psychologist
8. psychosis
9. reality testing
10. personality disorders

E

1. somatoform disorders
2. benzodiazepines
3. free association
4. amphetamines
5. family therapy
6. schizophrenia
7. superego
8. substance-related disorders
9. electroconvulsive therapy
10. cognitive behavioral therapy

F

1. phenothiazines
2. psychopharmacology
3. sedatives
4. hypnosis
5. psychoanalysis
6. supportive psychotherapy
7. transference
8. psychodrama
9. tricyclic antidepressants
10. group therapy

Terminology Quiz

A

1. mental
2. hypnosis
3. autism
4. neurotransmitter
5. psychiatrist
6. anxiolytic
7. schizophrenia
8. paraphilia
9. hallucinogen
10. iatrogenic

B

1. kleptomania
2. psychotherapy
3. schizoid
4. pyromania
5. psychosomatic
6. neuroleptic drugs
7. psychogenic
8. psychosis
9. somatoform disorder
10. psychopharmacology

C

1. paranoia
2. cyclothymia
3. agoraphobia
4. hypochondriasis
5. xenophobia
6. apathy
7. dysthymia
8. dysphoria
9. catatonia
10. euphoria

Abbreviations Quiz

A

1. Alzheimer disease
2. attention-deficit hyperactivity disorder
3. autism spectrum disorder
4. cognitive behavior therapy
5. delirium tremens
6. electroconvulsive therapy
7. generalized anxiety disorder
8. lysergic acid diethylamide
9. benzodiazepine
10. monoamine oxidase inhibitor

a. ECT
b. CBT
c. BZD
d. LSD
e. GAD
f. DT
g. AD
h. ASD
i. ADHD
j. MAOI

B

1. major depressive disorder
2. obsessive-compulsive disorder
3. post-traumatic stress disorder
4. seasonal affective disorder
5. selective serotonin reuptake inhibitor
6. tardive dyskinesia
7. tricyclic antidepressants
8. psychotherapy treatment

a. PTSD
b. ψRx
c. SAD
d. SSRIs
e. OCD
f. TCAs
g. MDD
h. TD

Exercise Quiz

A

1. amnesia
2. mania
3. mutism
4. obsession
5. compulsion
6. anxiety
7. dissociation
8. conversion
9. autism
10. apathy
11. hallucination
12. delusion

B

13. sadness, hopelessness
14. exaggerated good feeling
15. fear of being alone in open, crowded places
16. unstable, undergoing rapid emotional change
17. external emotion or emotional response of a person
18. delusions of persecution or grandeur
19. intermixed periods of mania and depression
20. loss of higher mental functioning

C

21. sexual disorders
22. dissociative disorders
23. anxiety disorders
24. substance-related disorders
25. eating disorder
26. mood disorders
27. somatoform disorders
28. personality disorder
29. dementia
30. delirium

D

31. narcissistic
32. histrionic
33. antisocial
34. paranoid
35. schizoid

E

36. hypnosis
37. psychodrama
38. psychoanalysis
39. play therapy
40. behavior therapy
41. drug therapy
42. electroconvulsive therapy
43. sex therapy

F

44. xenophobia
45. kleptomania
46. MAO inhibitors
47. dysthymia
48. agoraphobia
49. minor tranquilizers and sedatives
50. phenothiazines

Dictation and Comprehension Quiz

A

1. affect
2. amnesia
3. anorexia nervosa
4. anxiolytic
5. claustrophobia
6. delirium
7. dementia
8. dysphoria
9. fetishism
10. hallucinogens
11. hypochondriasis
12. labile
13. obsessive-compulsive disorder
14. phenothiazines
15. psychoanalysis
16. psychopharmacology
17. schizophrenia
18. sexual masochism
19. superego
20. xenophobia

B

6 Confusion in thinking; faulty perceptions and irrational behavior
4 Drug used as a mild tranquilizer
12 Unstable, undergoing rapid emotional change
2 Loss of memory
14 Tranquilizers used to treat psychoses
17 Withdrawal from reality into an inner world of disorganized thinking and conflict; a psychosis
19 Internalized conscience and moral part of the personality
20 Fear of strangers
15 Treatment that allows the patient to explore inner emotions and conflicts; transference, free association and dream analysis are elements of the therapy
10 Drugs that produce a state of CNS excitement, hyperactivity and mood change
9 The use of nonliving objects as substitutes for a human sexual love object
18 Sexual gratification is gained by being humiliated, beaten, or made to suffer by another person
1 The outward expression of emotion, or emotional response
13 An anxiety disorder in which recurrent thoughts and repetitive acts dominate behavior
7 Loss of intellectual abilities with impairment of memory, identity, and reasoning
5 Fear of closed places
16 Study of drugs and their effect on the mind and mental illness
8 Sadness, hopelessness, worry, discouragement (literally, "bad feeling")
11 Preoccupation with bodily aches, pains, and discomforts in the absence of real illness
3 Eating disorder marked by refusal to maintain minimally normal body weight

Spelling Quiz

A

1. masochism—gratification gained by being humiliated
2. delirium—confusion in thinking; faulty perceptions and irrational behavior
3. bulimia nervosa—binge eating followed by vomiting and depression

4. psychoanalysis—treatment that allows the patient to explore unconscious emotions and conflicts
5. schizophrenia—psychosis involving withdrawal from reality into an inner world of disorganized thinking and conflict
6. paranoid—delusions of persecution or grandeur
7. dementia—loss of higher mental functioning
8. euphoria—exaggerated good feeling; "high"
9. narcissism—pervasive interest in one's self
10. bipolar disorder—alternating periods of mania and depression

B

11. anxiety
12. cocaine
13. affect
14. autism
15. fugue
16. dysthymia
17. marijuana
18. paraphilia
19. apathy
20. xenophobia

Pronunciation Quiz

A

1. narcissism
2. opioid
3. agoraphobia
4. dementia
5. catatonic stupor
6. dysthymia
7. voyeurism
8. psychoanalysis
9. autism
10. euphoria

B

1. E
2. G
3. J
4. B
5. D
6. F
7. C
8. I
9. A
10. H

C

1. anorexia
2. phenothiazines
3. cyclothymia
4. schizophrenia
5. psychosomatic
6. xenophobia
7. hypochondriasis
8. acrophobia

Review Sheet Quiz

A

1. uneasy, anxious, distressed
2. sleep
3. treatment
4. to steal
5. mind
6. nerve
7. mind
8. mind
9. fire
10. split

B

1. body
2. stranger
3. self
4. attraction to, love
5. produced by
6. to seize hold of
7. obsessive preoccupation
8. fear
9. mind
10. feeling, bearing

Medical Scramble

1. LABILE
2. PYROMANIA
3. DYSPHORIA
4. ANXIOLYTIC

BONUS TERM: XENOPHOBIA

Crossword Puzzle

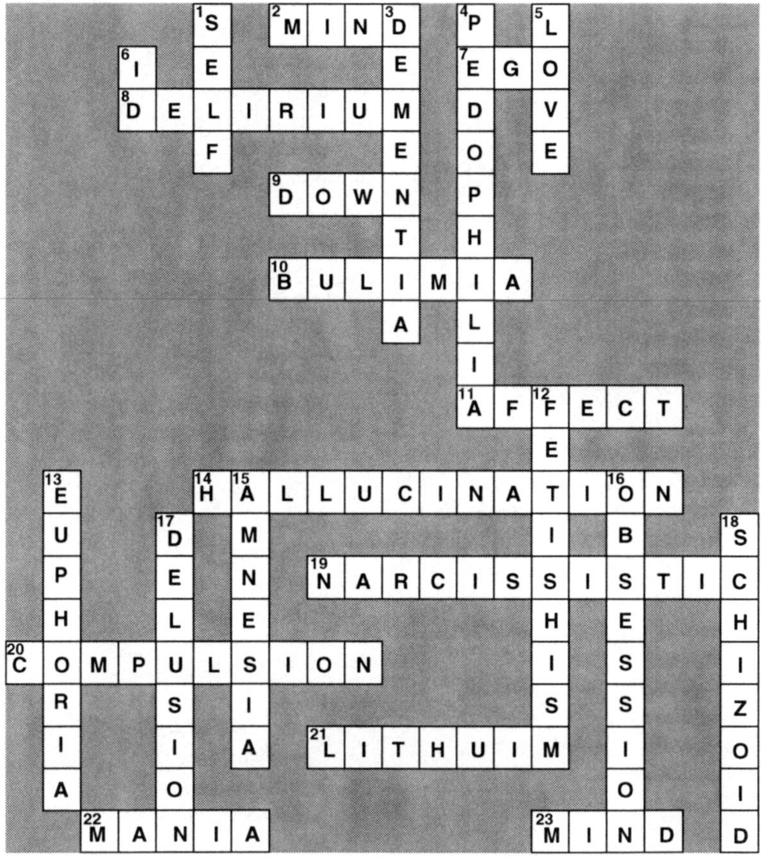

Practical Applications

A

1. C
2. A
3. D
4. C

B

1. D
2. C

Chapter Twenty-Two
Answers to Terminology Section

(textbook pages 939–942)

Terminology	Meaning
anxiolytic	A drug that is used for relief of anxiety; a mild tranquilizer.
autism	Developmental disorder characterized by delays in socialization and communication skills.
hallucinogen	A substance that causes hallucinations (false sensory perceptions).
hypnosis	Condition or state of altered consciousness in which there is increased responsiveness to commands and suggestions.
psychiatrist	One who specializes in the treatment of the mind.
iatrogenic	Pertaining to producing, produced by, or produced in.
mental	Pertaining to the mind.
neurotransmitter	Chemical messenger that stimulates or inhibits another cell.
paraphilia	A psychosexual disorder in which sexual arousal is dependent on bizarre fantasies or acts involving use of a nonhuman object or suffering and humiliation of a human.
schizophrenia	A psychosis involving withdrawal from the external world with a disturbed sense of self; includes delusions, hallucinations, and inappropriate affect. Literally means "split mind".
psychosis	Significant impairment of reality with symptoms such as delusions, hallucinations, and bizarre behavior.
psychopharmacology	Study of the effect of drugs on the mind.
psychotherapy	Treatment of the mind.
schizoid	Traits of shyness, social withdrawal, and introversion that characterize the schizoid personality. Also can refer to schizophrenia-like traits that indicate a predisposition to schizophrenia.
psychosomatic	Pertaining to the effect of the mind on the body in causing illness.
somatoform disorders	Mental disorders that are characterized by symptoms that suggest a physical disorder but can't be explained by an actual physical disorder.

Suffixes

psychogenic	Pertaining to produced by the mind.
neuroleptic drugs	Drugs that modify psychotic behavior and symptoms (phenothiazines are examples).
kleptomania	Madness or compulsion to steal.
pyromania	Madness for setting fires or seeing them.
agoraphobia	Fear of being alone in open or public places.
xenophobia	Fear of strangers.
euphoria	Exaggerated feeling of well-being; "high".
dysphoria	Depressed mood; sadness and hopelessness.
cyclothymia	Mania alternating with depression; mild form of bipolar (manic-depressive) disorder.
dysthymia	Depressed mood that is not as severe as major depression.
euthymic	Feeling well.

Prefixes

anorexia nervosa	Eating disorder characterized by lack of appetite, and refusal to maintain minimally normal body weight.
apathy	Lack of feeling; indifference, without emotion.
catatonia	A state of diminished responsiveness to stimuli associated with.
hypomania	A mood disorder that resembles mania, but is of lesser intensity
hypochondriasis	Condition marked by exaggerated concern for one's physical health and exaggeration of minor complaints and normal sensations.
paranoia	Delusions of grandeur or persecution. Literal meaning is "abnormal mind".

MORE PRACTICAL APPLICATIONS

On the next pages you will find additional examples of medical terminology in context. Here are paragraphs about disease conditions, case reports, research reports, and a wide variety of examples of medical writing. Medical terms are underlined to draw attention to terminology that students may define. I use paragraphs like this for dictation or discussion in class. Sometimes I include a paragraph on a quiz as a bonus question, asking the students to explain the meaning of the sentences in their own words. Many of the paragraphs on diseases were written by me in response to questions that came up in class that were not covered in *The Language of Medicine* or that needed further explanation.

As I have indicated, the possessive of eponyms has been omitted for clarity and consistency. If you are uncomfortable with this change, you may continue to be guided by *Dorland's Medical Dictionary, Mosby's Dental Dictionary,* or other references.

I have noted the chapter in *The Language of Medicine* with which you may choose to use each of the following.

1. Chapter 4

   Reye syndrome. This is an acute disease of childhood, characterized by severe edema of the brain, and increased intracranial pressure, hypoglycemia, and fatty infiltration and dysfunction of the liver.

   The etiology of Reye syndrome is unknown, but it is almost always associated with a previous viral infection. In the United States, the most frequently reported viral diseases present prior to development of Reye syndrome are influenza type B and varicella (chickenpox). There is an association between the administration of aspirin for these illnesses and the subsequent occurrence of Reye syndrome, so children should not be given aspirin for such infections.

   Symptoms of Reye syndrome are persistent emesis, fatigue, increased agitation and delirium, convulsions, and coma. Treatment is aimed at correcting hypoglycemia and reducing intracranial pressure.

2. Chapter 5

   Mr. Smith's hemoglobin was normal and his leukocyte count was 16,000 mm^3, showing slight neutrophilia. Physical examination of the abdomen revealed a mass, and a histological examination disclosed it to be a pancreatic adenocarcinoma. His condition progressively worsened and he died after 23 hospital days. Autopsy revealed carcinoma of the pancreas with metastatic hepatic and peritoneal lesions as well as peritonitis.

3. Chapter 5 or 6

   Colic is acute, paroxysmal abdominal pain. It is marked by spasmodic contractions of the intestine, most commonly during the first 3 months of life. The infant may pull up his or her arms and legs, cry loudly, turn red-faced, and expel gas from the anus or belch it up from the stomach. Etiology is not known, but several factors may contribute to its occurrence. These include excessive aerophagia, too rapid feeding or overfeeding, overexcitement, and occasionally allergy to milk.

4. Chapter 5

   Colonoscopy. The patient had a previous colonoscopic polypectomy and now presents for follow-up interval examination. She has some rectal bleeding that has been attributed to hemorrhoids.

   The scope was introduced without difficulty and advanced through the rectosigmoid. Bowel preparation was adequate, and there was good visualization throughout. Scattered diverticula were seen, particularly in the sigmoid area and around the hepatic flexure. The instrument was advanced through the descending, transverse, and ascending colons to the cecum. There was no evidence for any recurrent mass lesion. On withdrawal of the instrument, small internal hemorrhoids were seen.

5. Chapter 5 or Chapter 16

   Thrush is an infection of the oral mucous membrane by a fungus *(Candida albicans)*. It is characterized by white patches on a red, moist inflamed surface, occurring anywhere in the mouth, including lingual and buccal surfaces. The patches are occasionally accompanied by pain and fever. Thrush is treated with antibiotics and fungicidal drugs. The best preventive measures are good general health, a well-balanced diet, and good oral hygiene.

6. Chapter 6

   Ms. Jones had been taking birth control pills for several years. Lower abdominal pain and non-bloody diarrhea made her seek a doctor's advice after experiencing postprandial nausea and emesis, epigastric pain, and weight loss. Cholecystography and barium swallow were reported as normal. Laparotomy revealed massive gangrene of the sigmoid colon and almost the entire ileum and jejunum. She underwent extensive excision and anastomosis, but she never fully recovered. She finally succumbed to septicemia. On autopsy, it was revealed that her celiac and mesenteric arteries were thrombosed. She had premature atherosclerosis in the common iliac arteries as well.

7. Chapter 6

   The patient, a 53-year-old male, had been well until 3 weeks before hospital admission. At that time he noted anorexia, malaise, and epigastric discomfort. On the day of admission he had hematemesis but had observed no sign of melena or change in bowel habits. He had previously undergone cholecystectomy for calculi and partial colectomy for diverticulitis.

8. Chapter 6

   Barrett esophagus is a premalignant condition that should be suspected in any patient presenting with signs and symptoms of chronic reflux esophagitis. The condition itself is asymptomatic but can be diagnosed by barium swallow, which reveals esophageal strictures or ulcerations with a hiatal hernia.

9. Chapter 6

   Fatigue is often an important symptom of underlying hepatic disease. Intense pruritus and other dermatologic changes in the presence of elevated bilirubin and alkaline phosphatase suggest cholestasis. Transaminase elevations generally signify hepatocellular inflammation or necrosis. Hepatomegaly and elevated alkaline phosphatase may be the only signs of infiltrative disease and mass lesions. Bilirubin exceeding 10 mg/dL is more often associated with carcinoma than with cholecystitis or stones.

10. Chapter 6

    Bilirubin is classified as indirect ("free" or unconjugated) when it is en route to the liver from the spleen, where erythrocytes are destroyed. Bilirubin is classified as direct (bilirubin diglucuronide) after its conjugation (combination) in the liver with glucuronic acid. Elevation of indirect bilirubin means prehepatic jaundice such as in hemolytic jaundice or inability to conjugate bilirubin.

    Elevation of direct bilirubin indicates other types of hepatic jaundice such as in viral or alcoholic hepatitis or posthepatic jaundice as in biliary obstruction.

    Total bilirubin is the sum of direct and indirect bilirubin in blood.

11. Chapter 7

    Persons suffering from nephrotic syndrome have been known to occasionally develop as much as 40 L of excess fluid, and 15 L of this is ascites. In addition, joints swell and pleural and pericardial cavities can become partially filled with fluid. Intravenous infusion of large quantities of plasma proteins can be of only temporary benefit because enough protein can be lost in the urine in a day to return the person to his or her original predicament.

12. Chapter 7

    Peritoneal dialysis versus hemodialysis. Peritoneal dialysis is more quickly initiated because no dialysis machine is needed; anticoagulants are not necessary and there is no need for vascular cannulation (a cannula is a tube or sheath). Also, there is less stress on internal organs because chemicals and fluid exchanges occur more slowly. Hemodialysis is used in cases of severe abdominal trauma, multiple abdominal surgical procedures and adhesions, diffuse peritonitis, and paralytic ileus. It is also used in patients with severe coagulation defects and is more effective in removing toxins from the blood.

13. Chapter 7

    A 65-year-old man with a 2-month history of weakness, gross hematuria, and intermittent hemoptysis was admitted to the hospital. Past history included alcohol abuse, asbestos exposure, and heavy smoking (two packs a day for 42 years). A cystoscopy with retrograde pyelography showed a filling defect in the base of the bladder. Transurethral biopsy of the bladder revealed a transitional-cell carcinoma, grade IV. Chest x-ray showed a right lower lobe lesion, and CT scan confirmed the presence of the abnormality. Biopsy of the lung mass revealed a metastatic bladder carcinoma.

14. Chapter 8

    Much of the focus of neonatology now is on improving survival of premature infants, and nutrition is important for optimum outcome. Total parenteral nutrition (TPN) is used extensively to provide caloric and protein needs to these infants, especially those who have intestinal disease and chronic respiratory distress syndrome. Intrahepatic cholestasis occurring during TPN has surfaced as a major clinical problem and is second only to catheter complications as a reason for discontinuing therapy.

15. Chapter 8

    A 28-year-old premenopausal woman, G0 P0, presented with an upper outer quadrant breast mass of 3 months' duration. Modified radical mastectomy was performed; none of the 33 nodes was positive for metastasis. Tumor size 3.7 cm; pathology report indicated infiltrating ductal carcinoma, grade IV. The tumor is estrogen receptor positive. Bone scan and chest x-ray are negative and liver enzymes are normal.

16. Chapter 8

Ovarian cancer. The ovary is the second most common site of cancer in the female reproductive organs (endometrial carcinoma is the first). Unlike endometrial cancer there is no obvious warning sign (bleeding) and unlike cervical cancer there is no routine diagnostic test (like the Pap smear) that will detect early or occult disease of the ovary.

The common malignancies of the ovary are believed to arise from the surface epithelium of the ovary. The names of the common epithelial tumors are serous, mucinous, endometrioid, clear-cell, and undifferentiated tumors. These tumors can be benign, in which case they are treated by simple excision.

When the ovarian cancer is confined to the ovaries (Stage 1), the patient is usually treated by a total abdominal hysterectomy and bilateral salpingo-oophorectomy. An omentectomy (the omentum is a part of the peritoneum that hangs over the intestines) is performed to be certain that occult disease is not present in the upper abdomen. In addition, any nodules, retroperitoneal or intraperitoneal, are removed and the diaphragm is inspected for metastatic carcinoma. Para-aortic lymph node biopsies are performed and cytologic washings are obtained from the pelvis and paracolic spaces. A bowel resection may be necessary with anastomoses.

The cancer seems to spread by direct extension and not hematogenously, so that debulking surgery is important. Adjuvant therapy for Stage 1 disease may be either cytotoxic chemotherapy or radiation therapy (whole abdominal irradiation using external beam irradiation or intraperitoneal radioactive isotopes).

17. Chapter 8

Kegel exercises, named after Dr. Arnold Kegel, a gynecologist who first developed the exercises to strengthen pelvic-vaginal muscles, are used to control stress incontinence. Patients are taught awareness of the pubococcygeus muscle, a sphincteric muscle that surrounds the vagina, and how to control it. Once the muscle has been strengthened it tends to maintain its strength and is in a state of partial contraction at all times.

18. Chapter 8 or 19

Alpha-fetoprotein (AFP) is a globulin present in the serum of the fetus, infant, and normal pregnant female. High concentrations are often diagnostic of hepatocellular carcinoma in adults. Although they often do not reach the levels found in association with hepatocellular carcinoma, elevated concentrations of AFP are found in association with a variety of malignant neoplasms and inflammatory conditions.

In fetuses with open spina bifida or anencephaly, AFP leaks into the amniotic fluid and maternal serum, and its measurement is of significant diagnostic value.

19. Chapter 9

Chlamydial infections. *Chlamydia* is a type of bacteria. Chlamydia infections have replaced gonorrhea as the most prevalent STD in the United States. Symptoms may be very mild, and those affected may not be aware that they have the disease. Often they do not seek treatment until a serious complication occurs. In males, the symptoms, when they do occur, are dysuria and watery discharge from the penis. Women may suffer pruritus and burning sensation in the genital area; an odorless, thick leukorrhea; dull abdominal pain; and metrorrhagia.

One type of *Chlamydia (trachomatis)* causes about half of all PID. Symptoms can appear from 1 to 5 weeks after exposure to the bacteria, and almost all sexual contacts become infected.

In pregnancy, chlamydial infection can increase the risk of stillbirth or premature birth. The newborns suffer from conjunctivitis that may have serious complications. Chlamydial infection also leads to pneumonia some weeks after birth, probably because of infectious material in the eye draining through the ducts between the eye and the nose and then passing into the lungs.

The infection is treated with an antibiotic such as tetracycline. As in the case of all STDs, both partners should be treated at the same time to prevent reinfection. If left untreated, chlamydial infection can cause scar tissue to form in the fallopian tubes and lead to infertility and ectopic pregnancies. In a man it can lead to epididymitis and sterility.

20. Chapter 9

I saw Mr. John Smith for symptoms of prostatism (lessening of force of urinary flow, hesitancy in initiating voiding, inability to end micturition abruptly, urinary retention) in 1988. At that time he underwent TURP of a clinically benign prostate, and pathology report confirmed benign prostatic hyperplasia. In September of 1992 he was found to have a PSA of 10 ng/mL (elevated). Biopsies were obtained that revealed an adenocarcinoma involving the left lobe of the prostate.

Patient elected to proceed with a radical prostatectomy. Pathology report confirmed the presence of an adenocarcinoma with perineural and left seminal vesicle invasion and transcapsular extension into the left periprostatic fat. Adjuvant radiation therapy was advised.

21. Chapter 10 and Chapter 16

Neurofibromatosis (also called von Recklinghausen disease) is an inherited disorder marked by pigmented skin lesions, multiple tumors of spinal and cranial nerves, tumors of the skin, and brain tumors. There is an increased association with adrenal gland tumors (pheochromocytomas), kidney vascular disease (causing hypertension), fibrous tissue dysplasia, and tumors in the gastrointestinal tract.

The main feature of this disease is the occurrence of many tumors composed of nerve and fibrous tissue (neurofibromas). The tumors can press on nerves, resulting in facial weakness, deafness, and vision loss. Many tumors that appear together can result in elephantiasis (blockage of lymphatic vessels in the lower extremities leads to enlargement of the legs) along with hypertrophy of skin and subcutaneous tissues of the head, neck, and trunk of the body. The spinal cord can become compressed by tumor, and hydrocephalus can develop.

The condition is diagnosed readily by the presence of characteristic neurofibromas and skin-pigmented lesions (light brown marks that are smooth with sharp, regular borders found over the trunk and in the axilla). There is no treatment for neurofibromatosis other than resection of tumors that are causing symptoms and decompression of hydrocephalus if that occurs.

22. Chapter 10 and Chapter 16

Leprosy is a chronic infectious disease caused by a bacillus, which is a rod-shaped bacterium. The bacillus attacks the skin, mucous membranes, and peripheral nerves (nerves that are outside the brain and spinal cord). Transmission occurs most often through infected nasal discharges.

Only about 5% of contacts acquire the disease; others appear to be immune. Leprosy is found mainly around the equator, in Southeast Asia, Africa, and South America. Of the estimated 12 to 20 million cases, about 2000 are in the United States; areas of leprosy occurrence are in Texas, Louisiana, and Hawaii. The disease is also seen in California, Florida, and New York City, primarily among immigrants.

In all forms of leprosy the bacillus invades the peripheral nerves, producing anesthesia of the skin. Paralysis, ulcers, and secondary infections are common. Nasal stuffiness and epistaxis occur early; later, ulceration and necrosis destroy supporting cartilages, causing nasal deformity and collapse. Earlobe enlargement and loss of eyebrows are common. Isolated lesions of the lip, tongue, and palate can occur and must be differentiated from malignancy.

Drug treatment (sulfur drugs) is successful and must be given until 2 years after the disease becomes inactive.

23. Chapter 10

Bacterial meningitis. Common etiologic agents are meningococcus, streptococcus, pneumococcus, and tubercle bacillus.

The streptococcal and pneumococcal types reach the meninges from the middle ear or frontal sinus, but they may be carried by the bloodstream from the lungs as well. The meningococcal type comes from the nose or throat.

Meningococcus is usually the type causing epidemics. The infection is spread by carriers, who harbor the organisms in their throat but do not themselves develop the infection.

Examination of the cerebrospinal fluid by lumbar puncture gives the final diagnosis, including the type of bacterial infection. When normal CSF is removed by LP it is as clear as water, and the pressure is so low that it flows out drop by drop. In meningitis due to pyogenic bacteria, the fluid is turbid because of pus accumulation and the pressure is raised to such a degree that it may spurt from the needle. The fluid contains polymorphonuclear leukocytes and bacteria.

Treatment is with antibiotics; the fatality rate of acute bacterial meningitis is less than 10% if recognized early.

24. Chapter 10

Viral meningitis (encephalitis or aseptic meningitis). In this type of inflammation, no pyogenic organisms can be found in the cerebrospinal fluid. The illness may appear following viral infections such as in chickenpox, measles, smallpox vaccination, and others.

Even desperately ill patients can recover completely. Treatment is supportive and symptomatic (symptoms include fever, headache, stiffness of the neck, and a high lymphocyte count in the CSF), and the disease is self-limiting.

25. Chapter 10

Pain. Receptors for pain stimuli are the dendrites of neurons distributed in the superficial layers of the skin and in certain deeper tissues such as the periosteum, joint surfaces, and arterial walls. The gastrointestinal mucosa is also quite sensitive to irritation and painful stimuli. The parenchymal tissues of the liver and the lung (air sacs) are insensitive to pain, whereas the bile ducts and associated liver tissue, bronchi, and parietal pleura are extremely sensitive.

Some stimuli that excite the pain receptors are mechanical stress of trauma, extremes of heat and cold, and chemical substances such as acids, histamine, and prostaglandins.

A lack of oxygen supply to tissues can also produce pain by causing the release of chemicals from ischemic tissue. Muscle spasm is another cause of pain because it can cause ischemia and stimulate chemosensitive pain receptors.

When superficial pain receptors are excited, the impulses are transmitted to synapses in the gray matter of the spinal cord. They then travel upward through sensory neurons to the thalamus, which is the main sensory relay station of the brain. The thalamus is probably where the conscious perception of pain takes place. Impulses are then transmitted to the cortex of the brain (frontal lobe), where the interpretation of the quality of the pain takes place.

Referred pain occurs in a part of the body distinct from where the cause that produced the pain is situated. Thus, pain originates in a visceral organ but is felt in the skin or another area of the body. Referred pain probably occurs because pain signals from the viscera travel along the same neural pathways used by pain signals from the skin. The person perceives the pain but interprets it as having originated in the skin rather than in a deep-seated visceral organ. An example of this type of pain is radiating pain in the left arm that is felt when a person has heart muscle damage (myocardial infarction) due to ischemia and necrosis.

Analgesics are agents that relieve pain. Aspirin is an example of a non-narcotic analgesic. It relieves pain by blocking the production of prostaglandins.

26. Chapter 10

Migraine. Migraine is a paroxysmal disorder characterized by recurrent attacks of cephalgia, with or without associated visual and GI disturbances.

Etiology is idiopathic, but evidence suggests a disturbance of cranial circulation. Prodromal symptoms (for example, flashes of light, paresthesias, hemianopia) are probably due to intracerebral vasoconstriction, and the actual head pain to dilation of scalp arteries.

Headache may be preceded by a short period of depression, irritability, restlessness, or anorexia. These symptoms may disappear shortly before the headache appears or may merge with it. Pain is either unilateral or generalized. Nausea, emesis, and photophobia are common.

Aspirin or codeine may help in mild attacks. In severe attacks, only codeine or stronger analgesics offer relief and only if taken before the headache has lasted 2 hours.

27. Chapter 11

Angelo Payne, a 70-year-old house painter, noticed chest discomfort in the form of a substernal ache with radiation to the left arm brought on by exertion and relieved by rest. He had undergone repair surgery of an abdominal aortic aneurysm 5 years earlier. His only cardiovascular risk factor was a long history of cigarette smoking; he had no history of diabetes, hypertension, or hyperlipidemia and the family history was not remarkable for premature atherosclerosis.

28. Chapter 11

A 35-year old female with an 8-year history of heroin abuse was admitted to the hospital confused, agitated, and with a right hemiparesis of 2 days' duration. A left common carotid arteriogram demonstrated an aneurysm of the left parietal region involving one of the distal branches of the middle cerebral artery. The patient had subacute bacterial endocarditis and a septic embolus from the heart lodged in this parietal vessel, with the resulting aneurysm brain abscess. The endocarditis was secondary to repeated bouts of septicemia resulting from the unsterile techniques used by the patient for injecting drugs.

29. Chapter 11

Beta-blockers are drugs that block the action of epinephrine at the beta-adrenergic receptors on cells of certain organs. There are two types of these receptors: beta receptors in the myocardium and beta receptors in the bronchial and vascular smooth muscle cells.

Normally if the beta receptors in the myocardium are stimulated by the secretion of epinephrine, they will cause the heart to beat more rapidly. Beta-blockers counter this effect and are used to treat angina pectoris, hypertension, and cardiac arrhythmias. By decreasing the workload of the heart, they are effective in reducing the long-term risk of mortality and reinfarction after recovery from the acute phase of a myocardial infarction.

They are also used as prophylaxis for migraine headaches because they constrict the dilated vessels that are associated with migraines.

Examples of beta-blockers are propranolol (Inderal), nadolol (Corgard), and timolol (Timoptic), an ophthalmic preparation used to treat glaucoma.

30. Chapter 11

An apolipoprotein (apo- is a prefix used in biochemistry to denote the protein portion of a complex molecule) is a protein associated with lipids (such as triglycerides, phospholipids, and cholesterol) to form the various lipoproteins found in plasma and tissues. These proteins transport cholesterol, triglycerides, and phospholipids between tissues, and possess specific binding sites that are recognized by tissues. Apolipoprotein A-I and A-II are components of high-density lipoproteins (HDLs), which transport cholesterol to the liver to be metabolized.

31. Chapter 11

Poisonous chicken soup. A 70-year-old man presented with profound weakness of 3 days' duration. He had a 2-year history of congestive heart failure following a myocardial infarction. His wife had gone out of town and his daughter had been preparing his meals. She made his favorite foods using a salt substitute (the patient was careful to weigh himself daily and watch his salt intake). On the day of admission he had eaten a large bowl of chicken soup to "treat a cold." The patient was found to have hyperkalemia resulting from an overdose of potassium chloride found in the salt substitute. Consumption of a large amount led to depression of the SA node and bradyarrhythmia. A transvenous pacemaker was inserted and hyperkalemia controlled with drugs. Patients with congestive heart failure and renal impairment should be warned about the hazards of using salt substitutes.

32. Chapter 12

Patients with non–small cell lung cancer are candidates for palliative therapy only if they have any one or more of the following:

- Distant metastatic disease
- Supraclavicular adenopathy
- Contralateral pulmonary metastasis
- Recurrent laryngeal nerve paralysis
- Weight loss and anorexia
- Recurrent local disease following surgery or radiotherapy
- Severe coexisting cardiac or pulmonary disease

33. Chapter 12 or Chapter 14

Sarcoidosis is a chronic disorder in which the lymph nodes in many parts of the body are enlarged, and small, fleshy nodules called granulomas develop in the lungs, liver, and spleen. The skin, eyes, nervous system, muscles and bones, and salivary glands also can be affected.

Etiology is unknown, and it is likely that the disease results from an abnormal immune response. In the United States, it is 10 to 20 times more frequent in blacks than in whites, but in Europe it affects mostly whites. Females are slightly more susceptible than males. Most people are between 20 and 40 when they are diagnosed with the illness, but it can occur in children and the elderly.

Symptoms include fever, fatigue, malaise, anorexia, or weight loss. Many people have coughs and discomfort in their chest.

Overall, the prognosis in sarcoidosis is good. Most people recover completely without medication, but others require corticosteroid therapy.

Smoking is harmful because it aggravates impaired lung function, and prolonged exposure to sunlight should be avoided because vitamin D aids absorption of calcium, which can lead to kidney stones.

34. Chapter 12

Tonsils. The tissue usually referred to as tonsils are the palatine tonsils, a pair of oval structures about the size of small almonds, partially embedded in the mucous membrane, one on each side of the oropharynx. Below them, at the base of the tongue, are the lingual tonsils. On the upper rear wall of the mouth cavity are the pharyngeal tonsils, or adenoids, which are of fair size in childhood but usually shrink after puberty.

35. Chapter 12

Chronic obstructive pulmonary disease. This is a term applied to a group of disorders of lung function that share an element of irreversible expiratory airflow obstruction. The three disorders commonly included are emphysema, chronic bronchitis, and chronic asthma in adults.

Emphysema is destruction of alveolar spaces, usually accompanied by the loss of the natural elastic recoil of the lung and weakening of the walls of the bronchiolar airways.

Chronic bronchitis is defined as daily production of sputum for a continuous period of 3 months. Pathologically, there is hypertrophy of mucous glands in the bronchial wall and chronic bronchial inflammation. Emphysema and chronic bronchitis frequently coexist in varying degrees.

Asthma is marked by recurrent attacks of dyspnea with wheezing due to spasmodic constriction of bronchi.

The single most important cause of COPD is smoking, which impairs the lungs' natural defenses against infection. Almost all chronic smokers demonstrate some impairment of pulmonary function. Other causes that frequently coexist with tobacco exposure include exposure to fumes and dust.

In addition to dyspnea, an individual may demonstrate labored breathing, often with halting speech, weight loss, and cyanosis. Rales and rhonchi may be present.

Diagnosis is based on clinical presentation and the results of spirometry, which show reduction in expiratory flow rates and volumes. The main complications of COPD are respiratory failure, overwhelming infections, and right-sided heart failure. When symptoms are present chronically at rest, the prognosis is poor.

36. Chapter 12 or 15

Case Report:

A 29-year-old man with complaints of pain in the low back and mid-epigastrium was found to have vertebral osteomyelitis. Mediastinal abscess was also diagnosed on the basis of findings on chest x-ray film, thoracic ultrasonography, thoracentesis, and cultures of the pleural fluid. Antibiotic therapy was begun, and after 6 weeks of treatment the patient was free of symptoms.

37. Chapter 12

Nosocomial pneumonia accounts for about 10% to 17% of hospital-acquired infections. The rate of acquiring pneumonias in the hospital is 6 to 20 times higher in patients receiving mechanical ventilation, but the disease is most common in elderly intubated patients with chronic underlying disease.

38. Chapter 12

Pleurodesis induces scarring of the pleura to prevent fluid accumulation in the pleural space. An irritant is injected into the pleural space through a thoracotomy or in a more extensive procedure that involves scraping the lungs.

39. Chapter 12

A 67-year-old man had a 10-year history of COPD from heavy cigarette smoking. When he was hospitalized the first time, his major complaints included a 3-year history of increasing cough, SOB, fever, and weight loss. The occurrence of gross hemoptysis set off the alarm for any of several diagnoses: tuberculous pneumonia, pneumonia, acute and chronic bronchitis, bronchiectasis, trauma, pulmonary embolism, and lung cancer.

40. Chapter 13

In summary, this 68-year-old man had diffuse histiocytic lymphoma for 7 years and is currently in clinical remission. His current diagnosis is fungal pneumonitis. His ischemic colitis remains of uncertain etiology, but may result from the presence of numerous intestinal adhesions and recurrent hypotension.

41. Chapter 13

G6PD is glucose-6-phosphate dehydrogenase. It is an enzyme normally found in erythrocytes. Deficiency of this enzyme can lead to hemolysis. Several forms of genetic deficiencies of the enzyme are recognized, affecting some black males, people of Chinese origin, Sephardic (from Spain) Jews, and other persons of Mediterranean origin. Deficiencies of G6PD cause hemolysis when affected people are treated with antimalarial or sulfa drugs or eat certain types of fava beans.

About 10% of black American males suffer from a mild form of G6PD deficiency and only occasionally have symptoms in early infancy. Asians and some groups of Mediterranean origin develop a more severe form, with hemolysis.

42. Chapter 14

Parasitic infections are caused by small plants or animals that live on or within another living organism at whose expense they obtain some advantage. Some examples of these infections are:

acariasis	Infection with mites or ticks. Mange and scabies are examples.
candidiasis	Infection by fungus. Most commonly affects skin, oral mucosa (thrush), respiratory tract and vagina. The most prominent symptom of vaginitis due to *Candida* infection is severe pruritus. Candidiasis is often associated with AIDS infection.
filariasis	Infection with filariae, a type of worm. Most often found in Africa, the South Pacific and Asia, and tropical countries. It is transmitted by a mosquito or by mites (tiny organisms with jointed legs) or flies. Small worms invade lymph tissues and grow to adult worms. Resulting obstruction of the lymphatic vessels causes swelling, lymphadenitis, and pain. Repeated infections with impaired circulation and formation of excess connective tissue may cause enlargement of the affected part of the body (arm, leg, or scrotum), leading to elephantiasis.
giardiasis	Infection with giardia, a type of tiny enteric organism (protozoa), is spread by contaminated food and water or by direct person-to-person contact. Symptoms are diarrhea, nausea, malaise, anorexia, and weight loss.
leishmaniasis	Infection with a type of protozoa (one-celled organism) called leishmania (after Sir William B. Leishman). Disease is transmitted by the sandfly and marked by cutaneous papules that form nodules and break down to form ulcers. The ulcers heal to form scars. Found in the tropics and subtropics; also called Aleppo boil, Delhi sore, Baghdad sore, and oriental sore.

43. Chapter 14

Kaposi sarcoma. Kaposi (named for Morris Kaposi, Austrian dermatologist, 1837-1902) sarcoma (KS) is a rare malignancy that consists of multiple lymph node tumors and angiosarcomas. These lesions appear on the legs or toes as purple or dark brown nodules. It is multifocal and metastasizing, involving chiefly the skin. This is an opportunistic neoplasm associated with AIDS. With metastatic lymphadenopathy, prognosis for a patient with Kaposi sarcoma may not be more than 3 years. Patients often have prodromal symptoms such as fever, diarrhea, weight loss, malaise, thrush (fungal infection), and wasting (cachexia). Lymphadenopathy may occur and then skin lesions characteristic of KS appear. As many as one third of KS patients develop other malignancies such as lymphoma and squamous cell carcinomas.

Treatment of KS is difficult, but chemotherapy is tried and some patients have positive remissions.

44. Chapter 15 or Chapter 16

Systemic lupus erythematosus (SLE) is a chronic inflammatory disease of connective tissue. It also affects the skin and internal organs. Typically there is an erythematous, scaly rash on the face, around the nose and the cheeks, in the shape of a butterfly. Other characteristics of the disease are arthritis and nephropathy.

Although the etiology is unknown, it is thought to be an autoimmune disease and can be diagnosed by the presence of abnormal antibodies in the bloodstream. Another test shows characteristic white blood cells, called LE cells.

Common symptoms of SLE are fatigue, malaise, pyrexia, weight loss, and arthralgias. In addition to arthropathy, myositis can occur as well; alopecia may be present in some patients. Cardiac symptoms include pericarditis and myocarditis.

SLE predominantly afflicts women, 1 in 700 females between the ages of 15 and 64. It also occurs more often in blacks than in whites. Although there is no cure for SLE, treatment involves administration of nonsteroidal anti-inflammatory drugs (NSAIDs) for management of mild symptoms (arthralgias, fever, myalgia) and corticosteroids for life-threatening and severely disabling complications.

45. Chapter 15

Scleroderma. This connective tissue and skin disorder is about four times more common in women than in men; it is rare in children. It may be an autoimmune disorder, meaning that the body produces antibodies against its own good tissue. Common initial complaints are Raynaud phenomenon and swelling of the fingers and toes with gradual thickening of the fingers. Induration (hardening) of the skin is symmetric and may be confined to the fingers or affect most of the body. As the disease progresses, the skin becomes taut, shiny, and hyperpigmented; the face becomes mask-like, and telangiectases appear on the fingers, face, lips, and tongue. Esophageal dysfunction is the most frequent internal disturbance and eventually occurs in the majority of patients. The course of scleroderma is variable and unpredictable. It is often slowly progressive. Most, if not all, patients eventually show evidence of visceral involvement. Prognosis is poor if cardiac, pulmonary, or renal manifestations are present at diagnosis. However, the disease may remain limited in extent and nonprogressive for long periods of time.

Corticosteroids are often helpful in patients with disabling muscle involvement. Immunosuppressive agents are under trial for use in scleroderma. Palliative (relieving symptoms, but not curing) treatment is used for esophageal problems and nephropathy.

46. Chapter 15 or 16

Researchers conducted a study to determine the incidence of bacteremia in association with decubitus ulcers in a general hospital population. The incidence was higher in men, and 46% of the cases of bacteremia in association with decubitus ulcers occurred in paraplegics or in individuals with neurologic defects.

The most common location of decubitus ulcers was the sacrum, followed by the ischial tuberosities, the heels, and the buttocks. Patients with multiple decubitus ulcers were more likely to develop bacteremia.

47. Chapter 16

Hexachlorophene is an antibacterial substance used in soaps and detergents to inhibit bacterial growth. It is contained in pHisoHex. The pH of pHisoHex is slightly acid (5.0 to 6.0). It has a bacteriostatic action against staphylococci and other bacteria.

Infants, especially premature infants or those with dermatoses, are particularly susceptible to absorption of hexachlorophene through the skin. Systemic toxicity may be manifested by signs of stimulation (irritation) of the central nervous system (brain and spinal cord), sometimes with convulsions. Infants have developed dermatitis, irritability, generalized muscle contractions, and rigidity following application of a 6% hexachlorophene powder.

48. Chapter 16 or Chapter 19

Progress Notes

This 50-year-old patient has had a progressively worsening headache for 6 months, and episodic weakness of his R leg for the past several months. These episodes last 5 to 10 minutes and are described as "numbness" or clumsiness of gait, with inability to walk or lift the leg. Has noted a dark mole that progressively enlarged on the upper tip of the R earlobe over the past 3 yr. Suspected a melanoma but did not consult a physician.

FH/SH: denies sun exposure. No fam. hx of cancer. Works as a clerk. No children. Unmarried.

ROS: Smoker (30 pack yr) but not known to have COPD. Heart—no known disease. Had total colectomy for ulcerative colitis at age 12. No Sx since. Has lost about 10 pounds in past few months.

CT and MRI demonstrate R and L cerebral lesions. Chest: multiple 1 cm nodules.

PE: Pale, asthenic, bearded man in NAD (no apparent distress). Conversation appropriate. Large, 1 cm long bluish mole on R earlobe.

No other susp. Lesions. No nodes.

Chest: clear to A&P

Abd: no hepatomegaly or splenomegaly

Extr: no edema, tenderness

Neurol: Oriented and knows president and candidates

No apparent motor defect.

Touch intact

Reflexes good in knees and ankles

Impression: 1. Likely melanoma met. to brain and lung. Bx results pending.

2. COPD

Suggest: 1. RT for brain lesions (no role for surgery)

2. Consult melanoma service

3. Social service evaluation

4. ?HIV status

49. Chapter 18

Cushing syndrome (named for Dr. Harvey Cushing, who first described it in 1932) is a group of symptoms produced by an excess of cortisol from the adrenal gland. This can be caused by hyperplasia of the gland (due to increased stimulation from the pituitary gland and ACTH), ectopic production of ACTH from tumors in the lung or thyroid gland, and iatrogenically by too much administration of corticosteroids by physicians.

Diagnosis is made by laboratory findings indicating a continuous elevation of plasma cortisol. The condition is characterized by increase in adipose tissue (especially between the shoulder blades), moon face, distention of the abdomen, ecchymoses following even minor trauma, acne, hypertension, and amenorrhea and hirsutism in females. If these symptoms are associated with an adenoma of the pituitary gland, the condition is known as Cushing disease.

Treatment of the condition is by surgical removal of any neoplasm or with radiation using cobalt. Drug therapy with adrenocorticolytic agents may be used as an adjunct to surgery and radiation.

50. Chapter 22

Alcoholism. Alcohol is a toxic drug, harmful to all body tissues. Chronic use can lead to pathologic changes in the CNS, liver, heart, kidney, and gastrointestinal tract. Cirrhosis is the most recognized complication of alcoholism, but dementia and brain damage can also occur in the early stages of the disease. Fetal alcohol syndrome with growth deficiency, mental retardation, irritability in infancy, hyperactivity in childhood, and heart defects occurs in newborn infants of mothers who drink heavily throughout their pregnancy.

Alcohol affects the liver by direct hepatotoxic effects as well as from malnutrition associated with chronic alcohol abuse. Gastritis, excessive peristalsis, and esophageal varices are further complications.

Hypertension and coronary artery disease are related to intake of alcohol because alcohol elevates triglycerides in the blood. Alcohol abusers have an increased risk of oral and esophageal carcinoma. Immunosuppression may occur and result in lower resistance to infection. Alcohol has also been associated with sexual impotence by suppressing the production of testosterone.

MEDICAL FORMS

These are a collection of medical forms that I use in class with my students. They contain many terms that are taught in chapters of *The Language of Medicine*. I suggest that you use them because they pertain to the terminology you are teaching. For example, in Chapter 3, when I introduce the different types of blood cells, I hand out a laboratory form and show students the section pertaining to the different types of white blood cells, red cells (cell morphology), and platelets. Students see the terms in their actual context on a laboratory sheet.

You can also use the forms as a quiz by creating questions and asking students to find specific terms or abbreviations on the form that answer the questions. Please let me know (Meddavi@aol.com) if you find these helpful, and please share any interesting ways of using them in your classes. Also, please let me know if you have other forms that you include in your teaching.

The medical forms included here are:

HEALTH LABORATORIES

DATE ____________

PATIENT NAME ____________ ACCESSION # ____________ DOCTOR ____________

CHEMISTRIES

Test	Result	Units	Test	Result	Units
GLUCOSE (65-110)	_____	mg/dl	CALCIUM (8.5-11.0)	_____	mg/dl
BUN (10-25)	_____	mg/dl	PHOSPHATE (2.5-4.5)	_____	mg/dl
CREATININE (0.7-1.4)	_____	mg/dl	CHOLESTEROL (150-300)	_____	mg/dl
NA^+ (135-145)	_____	meq./1	TRIGLYCERIDES (30-200)	_____	mg/dl
K^+ (3.5-5.0)	_____	meq./1	ALK. PHOS. (30-115)	_____	U./1
CI (98-109)	_____	meq./1	AST (SGOT) (0-40)	_____	U./1
CO_2 (24-32)	_____	meq./1	ALT (SGPT) (0-40)	_____	U./1
URIC ACID (2.5-8.0)	_____	mg/dl	LDH (100-225)	_____	U./1
PROTEIN-TOT. (6.0-8.0)	_____	g/dl	BILIRUBIN-TOT. (0.2-1.5)	_____	mg/dl
ALBUMIN (3.5-5.0)	_____	g/dl	IRON (40-150)	_____	mcg/dl
GLOBULIN (2.0-3.6)	_____	g/dl			
A/G (0.9-2.3)	_____				

ORGANISM (S)

				ANTIBIOTICS
				900 AMPICILLIN
				902 CARBENICILLIN
				904 CEPHALOTHIN
				906 CHLOPAMPHENICOL
				908 CLINDAMYCIN
				910 COLISTIN
				912 ERYTHROMYCIN
				914 GENTAMICIN
				916 KANAMYCIN
				918 METHICILLIN
				920 NAFCILLIN
				922 NALIDIXIC ACID
				924 NEOMYCIN
				926 NITROFURANTOIN
				928 PENICILLIN
				930 POLYMYXIN B
				932 SULFONAMIDES
				934 TETRACYCLINE
				936 TOBRAMYCIN

TECHNOLOGIST COMMENTS:

THYROID CHEMISTRIES

T-4 ______ mcg/dl (4.5-13.5)

T-3 ______ % (25-35%)

SYPHILIS SEROLOGY

______ REACTIVE

______ NON REACTIVE

PROTHROMBIN TIME

PATIENT ____ sec ____ %act.

CONTROL ____ sec

DIGOXIN _______ ng/ml (0.8-2.0)

PREGNANCY TEST ______

URINALYSIS

COLOR ____________

APPEARANCE ____________

REACTION ____________

SPEC. GRAVITY ____________

GLUCOSE ____________

PROTEIN ____________

ACETONE ____________

WBC/HPF ____________

RBC/HPF ____________

EPITH. CELLS ____________

BACTERIA ____________

CRYSTALS ____________

CASTS ____________

OTHER: ____________

COMPLETE BLOOD COUNT

Test	Result	Units	MALE	FEMALE
WHITE BLOOD COUNT	_________	$x10^3/mm^3$	4-11	4-11
RED BLOOD COUNT	_________	$x10^6/mm^3$	4.7-6.0	4.0-5.4
HEMOGLOBIN	_________	g/dl	14-18	12-16
HEMATOCRIT	_________	vol. %	42-52	37-47
MCV	_________	cu. microns	80-94	81-91
MCH	_________	pg	27-33	27-33
MCHC	_________	%	31.5-36	31.5-36

Test	Result	Units	MALE	FEMALE
LYMPH	_________	%	20-40	20-40
SEG.	_________	%	50-70	50-70
MONO	_________	%	0-10	0-10
EOSIN	_________	%	0-5	0-5
BASO	_________	%	0-1	0-1
BANDS	_________	%	0-5	0-5
JUVEN	_________	%	0-1	0-1
%ATYP.	_________	%	0	0

CELL MORPHOLOGY: ____________

HYPOCROMIA ____________

ANISOCYTOSIS ____________

POIKILOCYTOSIS ____________

POLYCHROMIA ____________

OTHER: ____________

ADDITIONAL TESTS RESULTS:

Laboratory Diagnostics

PATIENT: SARAH SMITH

FINAL

WBC	RBC	HGB	HCT	MCV	MCH	MCHC	RDW	MPV	PLAT	BAND	NEUT	LYMP	MONO	EOS	BASO	ATYP L	MORPH
4.9	4.27	12.3	37	86	29	34	13.4	9.0	196	0	63	22	13	2	0	0	
3.8-10.8 1000/uL	3.80-5.10 mil/uL	11.7-15.5 g/dL	35-45 %	80-100 fL	27-33 pg	32-36 g/dL	11.0-15.0 %	7.5-11.5 fL	140-400 thou/uL	0-5 %	48-75 %	17-40 %	0-14 %	0-5 %	0-3 %	0-5 %	

Ca	PO4	GLU	BUN	CREAT	BUN/CR	URIC	CHOL	TRIG	HDL	TP	ALB	GLOB	A/G	ALKP	LDH	SGOT	SGPT
8.7		105	24	1.1						7.0	3.9	3.1	1.3	88	161	20	13
8.5-10.4 mg/dL		65-109 mg/dL	7-25 mg/dL	0.5-1.2 mg/dL						6.0-8.3 g/dL	3.2-4.6 g/dL	2.2-4.2 g/dL	0.8-2.0	20-125 U/L	100-250 U/L	2-35 U/L	2-40 U/L

BILI	BILI D	BILI I	Na	K	Cl	CO2	ANION	Fe	TIBC	GGT	T3U	T4	FTI	TSH	T4 F	B12	
0.3	0.1	0.2	146	4.4	104	29				15				17.9 HI			
0.2-1.3 mg/dL	0-0.3 mg/dL	0.0-1.3 mg/dL	135-146 mmol/L	3.5-5.3 mmol/L	98-110 mmol/L	21-33 mmol/L				2-60 U/L				0.3-5.5 uIU/mL			

Urinalysis

COLOR	APP	SPGR	PH	ALB	GLU	KET	BILI	BLOOD	LEU	NIT
Yellow	Clear	1.028	6.0	NEG	NEG	NEG	NEG	NEG	NEG	NEG
Yellow	Clear		5.0-8.0	NEG	NEG	NEG	NEG	NEG	NEG	NEG

Test Name	Result		Reference
Differential (absolute count)			
Absolute Band Count	0		0-500 /uL
Absolute Neutrophil Count	3087		1500-7800 /uL
Absolute Lymphocyte Count	1078		850-3900 /uL
Absolute Monocyte Count	637		200-950 /uL
Absolute Eosinophil Count	98		50-550 /uL
Absolute Basophil Count	0		0-200 /uL
Absolute Atypical Lymphocytes	0		/uL
Cardiac Risk Profile			
Cholesterol	**267**	**HI**	100-199 mg/dL
Triglycerides	**151**	**HI**	30-149 mg/dL
HDL-Cholesterol	56		40-77 mg/dL
LDL-Cholesterol	**181**	**HI**	62-130 mg/dL
Cholesterol/HDL Risk Factor	4.77		
Relative?Risk	**1.2 times average**		1.0 is average risk for CHD

Comments

Risk Category: LDL-Cholesterol Goal
CHD and CHD Risk equivalents: <100
Multiple (2+) factors: <130
Zero to one risk factor: <160

Review of Systems

MR#:____________________
Name: ____________________
Date:____________________

Circle positives, cross out negatives, leave blank items not discussed

GENERAL: fatigue, malaise, chills, fever, night sweats, change in appetite, change in weight, amount of change in weight ________________. History of heat injury; History of radiation therapy.
____
____.

EYES: visual changes. diplopia, scotomata_____
____
last eye exam________________________________

EARS/NOSE/THROAT: tinnitus; hearing loss, epistaxis, sinusitis; post-nasal drip, hay fever, sneezing, nasal stuffiness, sore tongue, gum bleeding, poor dentition; hoarseness __________
____
last dental visit ____________________________

RESPIRATORY: SOB, DOE, wheezing, cough, sputum production, hemoptysis, asthma; exposure to TB or history of TB____________________
____

CARDIOVASCULAR: chest pain, SOB, DOE, orthopnea, edema, palpitations, dizziness, syncope, claudication, heart murmurs, DVT or PE, hypertension, history of heart attack, last cholesterol level__________________________
____

GI: difficulty swallowing, nausea, vomiting, abdominal pain, diarrhea, indigestion, antacid use, constipation, change in stool, melena, rectal bleeding, laxative use; history of polyps; history of ulcerative colitis or Crohn disease____________
last flexible sigmoidoscopy and results:________
____

GENITOURINARY: dysuria, urgency, frequency, polyuria, nocturia, hesitancy, incontinence, foul urine, hematuria, history of STIs: number of sexual partners _________.
Last HIV test date_________Result___________
____.

Male: discharge from penis; lump or skin change of the penis: lump on scrotum, impotence; history of undescended testicle____________________
____

Female: abnormal vaginal bleeding, regular periods, irregular periods, dysmenorrhea, last menstrual period __________________________.
vaginal discharge; age of menarche___________;
last pap smear_______and results ___________.
method of contraception____________________.

MUSCULOSKELETAL: joint pain, redness, swelling, stiffness, muscle pain, muscle weakness, decreased ROM; fracture, sprain, dislocation, history of osteoporosis____________
____

SKIN: color changes, rash, photosensitivity, itching, mole changes; History of skin cancer, history of sun exposure on daily basis or sunburns
____

CNS: headache, seizures, paralysis, incoordination, unsteadiness, abnormal sensations, decreasing mentation, tremor, confusion, pinched nerves; temporary blindness; history of stroke or TIA____________________
____

PSYCHIATRIC: depression. high stress, anxiety, sleep disturbances, suicidal thoughts, homicidal thoughts________________________________

ENDOCRINE: breast masses or discharge, heat or cold intolerance, nervousness, increased thirst, polyphagia; hair changes, last mammogram and result______________________________________

HEMATOLOGY: anemia, bleeding problems, easy bruisability, lymph node enlargement_____
____

SAFETY: guns in home, domestic violence, HIV risk factors, smoke detectors______________

Otolaryngology Associates

S/C	SERVICE	CHG.	S/C	SERVICE	CHG.	S/C	SERVICE	CHG.	S/C	SERVICE	CHG.	S/C	SERVICE	CHG.
1	Comprehen., New Pt.		36	Myringotomy, Bilat.		112	I & D Subling. Abscess		244	Spont. Nystagmus			LABORATORY	
2	Intermed., New Pt.		37	Removal Tube		113	Frenulectomy		245	Posit. Nystagmus		270	Allergy Injection	
3	Limited, New Pt.		38	Removal, Foreign Bdy.		114	Uvulectomy					271	Prist	
4	Consult., Ref. Dr.			NOSE		115	Dilation,Salivary Duct		247	Optokinetic Nystagmus		272	Rast, up to 5 All.	
5	Comprehen., Est. Pt.		60	I&D Intra-Nasal Abscess		116	Steroid Inj. TMJ		248	Oscillating Tracking Tst		273	Rast, 6 or more All.	
6	Intermed., Est. Pt.		61	I&D Septal Abscess			AUDIOLOGY			X-RAY		274	Allergy Serum	
7	Limited, Est. Pt.		62	Excision Polyps, Unila.		230	Air Only		251	Mandible		275	Eosinophil Count	
8	Brief, Est. Pt.		63	Excision Polyps, Bilat.		231	Air and Bone		252	Mastoid		276	Nasal Smear	
9	Consult., Est. Pt.		64	Cautery Nasal Septum		232	Comp. Audiometry		253	Facial Bones		277	CBC	
10	Pre-Op Visit		65	Cautery Turbinates					254	Nasal Bones		278	Mono Spot	
11	Post-Op Visit		66	Antral Punct., Unilat.		237	Speech Audiometry, Threshold only		255	Sinuses		279	Ear Culture	
12	Emerg. Visit, Ext.		67	Antral Punct., Bilat.		235	Ear Mold Fitting		256	Skull		280	Nose Culture	
13	Emerg. Visit, Limited		68	Reduction Nasal Fract.		236	Hearing Aid Consult.		257	Temporal, Mand. Jt.		281	Throat Culture	
	EAR		69	Repair N.S. Perf.					258	Neck, Soft Tissue		282	Sensitivity Studies	
31	I&D Abscess Auricle		70	Inj. Turbinates		239	Tone Decay		259	Sialography				
32	I&D Hematoma Auricle		71	Removal, Foreign Bdy.					260	Int. Auditory Meati				
33	I&D Abscess Ext. Auditory Canal			THROAT		241	Stenger Puretone							
34	Pierce Ears		110	I & D Perit. Abscess		242	Acoustic Reflex					221	Removal of Sutures	
35	Myringotomy, Unilat.		111	Direct Fiberoptic Laryngoscopy								222	Medical Report	

D/C	DIAGNOSIS	D/C	DIAGNOSIS	D/C	DIAGNOSIS	D/C	DIAGNOSIS	D/C	DIAGNOSIS
1	External Otitis	13	Perforated Tymp. Memb.	41	Tonsillitis	48	Sialadenitis	55	Laryngeal Polyps
2	Otitis Media, Acute	20	Rhinitis	42	Laryngitis	49	Dysphagia	56	Foreign Body, Throat
3	Otitis Media, Chronic	21	Allergic Rhinitis	43	Stomatitis	50	Hoarseness	57	Peritonsillar Abscess
4	Serous Otitis Media	22	Sinusitis, Acute	44	Adenitis	51	Cephalgia	58	Meniere Syndrome
5	Sensorineural Hear. Loss	23	Sinusitis, Chronic	45	Cough, Chronic	52	Upper Resp. Infection	59	Bronchitis, Acute
6	Impacted Cerumen	24	Maxillary Sinusitis	46	Adenoiditis	53	T.M. Joint Dysfunction	60	Hypertrophic Tonsils
7	Vertigo	25	Epistaxis	47	Salivary Calculus	54	Vocal Cord Nodules	61	Hypertrophic Adenoids
8	Labyrinthitis	26	Nasal Polyps	DIAGNOSIS					CODE
9	Eustach. Salpingitis	27	Nasal Fracture	1.					
10	Tinnitus	28	Foreign Body, Nose	2.					
11	Otalgia	29	Deviated Nasal Septum	Instructions/Remarks:					
12	Foreign Body, Ear	40	Pharyngitis						
Date of Injury or Illness		Date Dr. First Saw Patient							

GYN Women's Health Encounter Form

Physician________________________
Time____________________________
Date____________________________
Referral #: Yes
Not Needed
Authorized for: ________________

PLAN:

IN OFFICE PROCEDURES

Uterus

	Code	Procedure	CPT
☐	7950058	Endometrial +/or endocervical sampling (biopsy)	58100
			58120

Vaginal-Vulva

	Code	Procedure	CPT
☐	7950140	Bx vaginal mucosa, extensive with suture	57105
☐	7950033	Bx vag.mucosa,simple	57100
☐	7950157	Destr vag lesion(s), ext	57065
☐	7950165	Destr vag lesion(s) simple	57061
☐	7950173	Destr vulvar lesion(s), ext	56515
☐	7950181	Destr vulv lesion(s) simple	56501
☐	7950116	I+D Bartholin's abscess	56420
☐	7950199	I+D vulva or perineal abscess	56405
☐	7950207	Marsup of Barth..gland	56440
☐	7950041	Bx vulva, one lesion	56605
☐	7950371	Bx vulva, each add'l lesion Number of Units ____	56606
☐	7950074	Pessary Insertion	57160
☐		Postcoital Test	89300

Contraception

	Code	Procedure	CPT
☐	7950108	Diaphragm/cervical cap fitting w/ instructions	57170
☐	7950082	IUD Insertion	58300
☐	7950090	IUD removal	58301

Skin

	Code	Procedure	CPT
☐	7950215	Biopsy, skin, single	11100
☐	7950223	Biopsy, skin,each add'l lesion	11101
☐	7950231	Destruct flat warts	17110
☐	795044	Excision Skin Tag <16	11200
☐	795045	Excision Benign Lesion <.5cm	11420
☐	795046	Excision Benign Lesion .6-1 cm	11421
☐	795047	I+D wound infection	10180

Breast

	Code	Procedure	CPT
☐	7950124	Breast Aspiration	19000

Cervix

	Code	Procedure	CPT
☐	7950066	Bx, or local exc of lesions w/wo fulguration	57500
☐	7950322	Colposcopy	57452
☐	7950330	Colpo w/cervical bx +/or endo	57454
☐	7950363	Conization/loop excision	57522
☐	7950025	Cryocautery cervix	57511
☐	7950389	Dilation cervical canal	57800
☐	7950397	Endocervical curettage	57505

Misc/Supplies

	Code	Procedure	CPT
☐		Cath Supplies/Materials	99070
☐		IUD/Paragard	1234Z
☐		IUD/Progestasert	1234Y
☐	7950256	KOH	87220
☐	7950272	Pessary supply	A4560
☐	7950280	Stool Occult Blood	82270
☐	7950264	Urinanalysis dipstick	81002
☐	7950249	Wet Mount	87210
☐	7950413	Breast and Pelvic Screening	G0101
☐	7950421	Pap screening,obtaining, preparing for lab	Q0091
☐		OTHER	

Injections

	Code	Procedure	CPT
☐	7950306	Injection of Med-subQ/IM Substance ____________	90782

Urodynamics

	Code	Procedure	CPT
☐	7950298	Catheterization, simple	53670
☐	795043	Cystometrics - simple	51725
☐	795049	Cystometrogram, complex	51726
☐	795050	Urethral Pressure Profile	51772
☐	795048	Uroflowmetry	51741

37991

ATTENDING PHYSICIAN'S STATEMENT
MEDICAL GROUP LTD.

Patient No.	DR. ______________________			
Account No.	Patient Name		Date of Birth	Sex
Date	Insurance Company	Policy No.–Cert. No.	Soc. Sec. No.	Employer

THIS SUPERBILL IS YOUR INSURANCE CLAIM - SUBMIT DIRECTLY TO YOUR INSURANCE COMPANY FOR PAYMENT OF BENEFITS DUE.

DIAGNOSIS CODES

789.00	Abd Pain	185	Cancer Prostate	250.03	DM, Insul. Dep., Uncont.	729.5	Limb Pain	582.9	Renal Disease Ch
794.8	Abn Liver Funct.	427.9	Cardic Arryth.	787.91	Diarrhea	272.9	Lipid Disorder	398.90	Rheumatic Heart Dis.
790.6	Abn. Blood Chem.	425.4	Cardiomyopathy	562.11	Diverticulitis	710.0	Lupus	V70.0	Routine Med. Exam
042	AIDS	366.9	Cataracts	562.10	Diverticulosis	V58.61	Medication Monitoring Anti Coag	786.05	Shortness of Breath
477.9	Allergic Rhinitis	682.9	Cellulitis	782.3	Edema	V58.69	Medication Monitoring High Risk	427.81	Sick Sinus Syndrome
280.9	Anemia-Iron Def.	437.0	Cerebral Arterio.	530.10	Esophagitis, Unspec.	627.9	Menopausal Syn.	461.9	Sinusitis, Acute
285.9	Anemia Unspec.	786.50	Chest Pain	780.79	Fatigue	346.90	Migraine	848.9	Sprain-Strain
413.9	Angina	428.0	CHF	610.1	Fibrocystic Breast	424.0	Mitral Valve Disorder	780.2	Syncope
424.1	Aortic Valve Disorder	571.5	Cirrhosis	729.1	Fibromyalgia	410.90	Myocardial Infarct.	726.90	Tendinitis
719.40	Arthralgia, Site Unspec.	558.9	Colitis	780.6	Fever	443.9	Occ Peri Vas Dis	435.9	TIA
714.0	Arthritis RH	211.3	Colon Polyps	530.81	GE Reflux	715.90	Osteoarthritis	465.9	URI
414.00	ASHD	564.0	Constipation	578.9	GI Bleed	733.00	Osteoporosis	788.41	Urinary Frequency
493.90	Asthma	496	COPD	241.1	Goiter-M N	785.1	Palpitations	599.0	UTI
427.31	Atrial Fib.	414.9	Coronary Artery Dis.	V72.3	Gynecological Exam	782.0	Paresthesia	454.9	Varicose Veins
300.00	Anxiety	786.2	Cough	784.0	Headache	462.	Pharyngitis	447.6	Vasculitis
724.5	Back Pain	555.9	Crohn's Dis.	455.6	Hemorrhoids	511.9	Pleural Effusion	386.11	Vertigo
600.0	BPH	436	CVA	053.9	Herpes Zoster	486	Pneumonia	079.99	Viral Illness
466.0	Bronchitis Acute	595.0	Cystitis Acute	553.3	Hiatus Hernia	V72.83	Pre-Op Exam, Other Spec.	787.01	Vomiting-Nausea
491.9	Bronchitis Ch	451.11	DVT, Lower Extrem.	272.4	Hyperlipidemia	601.0	Prostatitis, Acute		
727.3	Bursitis	692.9	Dermatitis	401.9	Hypertension	415.19	Pulmonary Emboli		
174.9	Cancer Breast, female	250.00	Diabetes Mellitus	244.9	Hypothyroidism	569.3	Rectal Bleed		
154.0	Cancer Colon	250.02	DM, Uncontrolled	564.1	IBS	530.11	Reflux Esophagitis		
162.9	Cancer-Lung	250.01	Diabetes Insul. Dep.						

PREVIOUS BALANCE	
TODAY'S CHARGES	
PAID	
NEW BALANCE	

This is your Standard Insurance Report Form. Unless so stated, patient's claim is not related to pregnancy or occupation. An additional charge will be made for further information.

Signature of Doctor ______________________

Center for Women's Cancers
Check-Out Sheet

Next Appointment Information

Type		Time Period		Provider Name		
Cancer F/U	☐	PRN	☐	Multi. Session	☐	________
Cancer Post-Op	☐	10+ day post proced.	☐	Med. Onc.	☐	________
Post-Op, Bx	☐	2 mos.	☐	Rad. Onc.	☐	________
Benign F/U	☐	3 mos.	☐	Surg. Onc.	☐	________
		6 mos.	☐	Plastic Surgery	☐	________
		1 year	☐	Nurse Praction.	☐	________
		Other	☐ ________			

Blood	ASAP	Before Next Appt.	Next Appt.	Comments
CBC, Diff	☐	☐	☐	________
Hematocrit	☐	☐	☐	________
Blood cultures	☐	☐	☐	________
Lytes, BUN, Creat.	☐	☐	☐	________
LFT's	☐	☐	☐	________
PT, PTT	☐	☐	☐	________
Sed rate (ESR)	☐	☐	☐	________
Basic Metabolic	☐	☐	☐	________
Cal, Phos, Mg	☐	☐	☐	________
Glucose	☐	☐	☐	________
LDH	☐	☐	☐	________
Total protein	☐	☐	☐	________
Thyroid	☐	☐	☐	________
Ca 125	☐	☐	☐	________
CA 27-29	☐	☐	☐	________
CEA	☐	☐	☐	________
Beta HCG	☐	☐	☐	________
Type and Cross	☐	☐	☐	________
Panels	☐	☐	☐	________
Other	☐	☐	☐	________

Miscellaneous

EKG	________	Urinalysis	________
Beta strep test	________	Urine culture	________
Echocardiogram	________	Port-a-cath P/R	________

Radiology
Breast Imaging:

Mammo. Side: ☐ R ☐ L ☐ B
Sched: ☐ ASAP ☐ 6 mo. ☐ 1 yr ☐ Other ______
Locat: ☐ Zero Emer. ☐ ACC
Mag Views ☐

Ultrasound ☐
U/S guided cyst asp. ☐ Side: ☐ R ☐ L ☐ B
U/S guided core bx ☐
Stereotactic core bx ☐
Breast MRI ☐
Comments: ________________

Radiology		ASAP	Bef. Next Apt.	N. Appt.	Comments
Bone Density		☐	☐	☐	________
Bone Films		☐	☐	☐	________
Bone Scan		☐	☐	☐	________
CT Abd/Pel. +/-		☐	☐	☐	________
CT Chest +/-		☐	☐	☐	________
CT Neck/Head		☐	☐	☐	________
CXR PA/LAT	R/L	☐	☐	☐	________
Gallium scan		☐	☐	☐	________
Gated heart scan		☐	☐	☐	________
MRI ________		☐	☐	☐	________
Pulmonary function test		☐	☐	☐	________
+/- DLCO +/- O2 Sat.					
Vascular Studies		☐	☐	☐	________
Other (please specify)		________			

Surgery	L/R	Comments
Lump + SN Bx	☐	________
Lump ax.	☐	________
Sentinel Node BX	☐	________
ALND	☐	________
Re-excision	☐	________
MRM	☐	________
Simple Mastectomy	☐	________
Reconstruction	☐	________
Open Bx.	☐	________
Needle loc'd Bx.	☐	________
FNA	☐	________
Site-Select	☐	________
Other ________	☐	________

Anesthesia
O Local
O IV Sed
O MAC
O General

Comments:

Chemo scheduling

____ AC	____ CAF	____ CMF
____ Docetaxel	____ Doxorubicin Liposomal	
____ Doxorubicin	____ Doxorubicin High Dose	
____ Gemcitabine	____ Paclitaxel 100	
____ Paclitaxel 175	____ Paclitaxel weekly/Trastuzumb	
____ Trastuzumab	____ Vinorelbine (30)	
____ Paclitaxel/Trastuzumab	____ Vinorelbine/Trastuzumb	

____

XRT scheduling
☐ Yes if yes: 0 ASAP 0 Other ☐ No

Clinician Sign ________

WHITE - OFFICE COPY YELLOW - RECORD TRACKING

REQUEST FOR EKG

DIAGNOSIS CODES *(Check off those that apply)*

Preopertative Exam/Post Op Status
- ___ V72.81 Pre-operative cardiovascular exam
- ___ V42.1 Heart transplant status
- ___ V43.3 Heart valve replacement

Signs and Symptoms
- ___ 786.50 Chest pain NOS
- ___ 786.59 Other chest pain
- ___ 729.5 Pain in limb
- ___ 780.09 Somnolence/Stupor
- ___ 780.2 Syncope and collapse
- ___ 780.4 Dizziness and Giddiness
- ___ 780.79 Malaise and fatigue, other than chronic
- ___ 782.3 Edema
- ___ 785.1 Palpitations
- ___ 785.2 Undiagnosed cardiac mummurs
- ___ 786.09 Respiratory distress/insufficiency
- ___ 789.00 Abdominal pain, unspecified site
- ___ 789.06 Abdominal pain, epigastric
- ___ 789.07 Abdominal pain, generalized
- ___ 799.0 Asphyxia

Coronary Athersclerosis
- ___ 414.00 CAD of unspecified vessel
- ___ 414.01 of native coronary vessel
- ___ 414.02 of autologous vein bypass graft
- ___ 414.03 of nonautologous biological bypass graft
- ___ 414.04 of artery bypass graft (IMA)
- ___ 414.05 of unspecified type of bypass graft
- ___ 440.9 Atherosclerosis, generalized & unspecified

Acute Myocardial Infarction- Initial
- ___ 410.01 Anterolateral wall, initial
- ___ 410.11 Other anterior wall, initial
- ___ 410.21 Inferolateral wall, initial
- ___ 410.31 Inferoposterior wall, initial
- ___ 410.41 Other inferior wall, initial
- ___ 410.51 Other lateral wall, initial
- ___ 410.61 True posterior wall, initial
- ___ 410.71 Subendocardial infarct, initial
- ___ 410.81 Papillary muscle infarct, initial

Acute MI, Subsequent Care Within 8 wks
- ___ 410.02 Anterolateral wall, w/in 8 wks
- ___ 410.12 Other anterior wall, w/in 8 wks
- ___ 410.22 Inferolateral wall, w/in 8 wks
- ___ 410.32 Inferoposterior wall, w/in 8 wks
- ___ 410.42 Other inferior wall, w/in 8 wks
- ___ 410.52 Other Lateral wall, w/in 8 wks
- ___ 410.62 True posterior wall, w/in 8 wks
- ___ 410.72 Subendocardial infarct, w/in 8 wks
- ___ 410.82 Papillary muscle infarct, w/in 8 wks

Acute Myocardial Infarction, Unspecified
- ___ 410.90 Acute myocardial infarct, unspecified site

Digestive Disorders
- ___ 575.0 Acute cholecystitis
- ___ 575.10 Cholecystitis, unspecified
- ___ 575.12 Acute and chronic cholecystitis

IF DIAGNOSIS IS NOT IDENTIFIED EKG WILL NOT BE DONE

Heart Disease
- ___ 411.1 Intermediate coronary syndrome
- ___ 423.9 Pericardial disease, unspecified
- ___ 424.90 Endocarditis, valve unspecified
- ___ 425.9 Secondary cardiomyopathy, unspecified
- ___ 427.0 Paroxysmal supaventricular tachycardia
- ___ 427.2 Paroxysmal tachycardia, unspecified
- ___ 427.31 Atrial fibrillation
- ___ 427.32 Atrial flutter
- ___ 427.41 Ventricular fibrillation
- ___ 427.42 Ventricular flutter
- ___ 427.5 Cardiac arrest
- ___ 427.60 Premature beats, unspecified
- ___ 427.81 Sino-atrial node dysfunction
- ___ 427.89 Other cardiac dysrhythmias NEC
- ___ 427.9 Cardiac dysrhythmias, unspecified
- ___ 428.0 Congestive heart failure
- ___ 428.9 Heart failure, unspecified
- ___ 429.1 Myocardial degeneration
- ___ 429.3 Cardiomegaly
- ___ 429.9 Heart disease, unspecified

Other Circulatory Diseases
- ___ 415.19 Pulmonary embolism and infarction other than iatrogenic
- ___ 416.9 Chronic pulmonary heart disease, unspecified
- ___ 435.9 Transient cerebral ischemia, unspecified
- ___ 436 Acute, but ill-definied CVA
- ___ 441.00 Dissecting aortic aneurysm, unspecified site
- ___ 441.01 Dissecting aortic aneurysm, thoracic
- ___ 441.02 Dissecting aortic aneurysm, abdominal
- ___ 441.1 Thoracic aneurysm, ruptured
- ___ 441.2 Thoracic aneurysm, without mention of rupture
- ___ 441.3 Abdominal aneurysm, ruptured
- ___ 441.4 Abdominal aneurysm, without mention of rupture
- ___ 441.6 Thoracoabdominal aneurysm, ruptured
- ___ 441.7 Thoracoabdominal aneurysm, w/out mention of rupture
- ___ 441.5 Aortic aneurysm of unspecified site, ruptured
- ___ 441.9 Aortic aneurysm of unspecified site w/out mention of ruputre
- ___ 401.9 Essential hypertension, unspecified
- ___ 458.9 Hypotension, unspecified

Respiratory Disorders
- ___ 492.8 Emphysema other than emphysematous bleb
- ___ 493.90 Asthma w/o status asthmaticus
- ___ 511.0 Pleurisy w/out mention of effusion or tuberculous
- ___ 511.9 Pleural effusion, unspecified
- ___ 518.81 Acute respiratory failure
- ___ 518.82 Acute respiratory insufficiency
- ___ 518.83 Chronic respiratory failure
- ___ 518.84 Acute and chronic respiratory failure

Other
- ___ 038.9 Septicemia, unspecified
- ___ 276.1 Hyposmolality and/or hyponatremia
- ___ 276.5 Hypovolemia/dehydration
- ___ 276.7 Hyperpotassemia
- ___ 276.8 Hypopotassemia
- ___ 959.1 Trunk injury, other and unspecified
- ___ V72.85 Other specified exam
- ______ ____________________ (Other)

HAS PATIENT HAD DIGITALIS ☐ YES QUINIDINE ☐ YES ☐ PACEMAKER CHECK WITH, AND WITHOUT MAGNET

SPECIAL BILLING INSTRUCTIONS *(If you checked off "OTHER" at top of form, complete applicable field.)*

BILL TO	FUND NUMBER	COST CENTER	OTHER *(Name of Institution)*

LUNG CANCER STAGING SHEET

Name:___________________ **Hosp #**__________ **JCRT #**________

PAST HISTORY

___ age at dx
y/n Smoking hx; if y, ___ ppd ___ #yrs;
___ yrs since quit (<1yr = 0)
y/n Asbestos exposure
y/n Comorbid lung ds; if y, ___ COPD,
__ emphysema, ___ asthma, __ other:____
y/n History of steroid use;
if y, reason__________, duration ____,
drug __________, date last use_______

SIGNS / SYMPTOMS AT DX

y/n > 10 % Wt loss over 6 mos prior to dx
from ___ to ___ lbs; ___%

check all applicable:

__ no sx __ hoarseness
__ hemoptysis __ cough
__ chest pain __ phrenic n. palsy
__ dysphagia __ recent pneumonia
__ fever __ SVC compromise
__ dyspnea; __ at rest __ w/ min. exertion
__ w/ signif. exertion
__ atelectasis; ___ segmental ___ lobar
___ whole lung
__ pleural effusion

PFTs (pre-treat): date_____, hosp ______
FEV_1 ___l (___ %); FVC ___l (___ %)
___ not done

PATH FINDINGS

Mediastinoscopy

Date :_______, Hosp: _________
Type: ___ cervical, ___ Chamberlain (ant.)
___ med dissection at resection
lymph nodes: [for LN diagram, see over]

station #	pos	neg
______	___	___
______	___	___
______	___	___
______	___	___
______	___	___

Surgery

__ bx only, __wedge, __ segment,
__ lobectomy, __ pneumonectomy

Date surgery:_______, Hosp: _________
Path # _____________
size of primary (max dimension): ____ cm
bronchial margin: __ pos __ ≤ 2mm __neg
other margin: __ pos __ ≤ 2mm __neg
positive nodes at surgery: ____________

Histology: __ adenoca, ___ squamous cell,
___ large cell, ___ non-small cell, NOS,
___ bronchoalveolar, ___ small cell,
___ other, specify: _____________

Differentiation: __ well, __ mod., __ poor
Vessel inv.: __ yes, __ no, __ no comment
Lymphatic inv.: __ y, __ n, __ no comment

STAGING EVALUATIONS

y/n **CXR,** date_______ Hosp _______
__ positve, __ negative, __ equivocal

y/n **Chest CT,** date______ Hosp______
___ (cm) primary tumor size (max diam)
___ solitary ___ multiple lesions
hilar nodes: __ pos __ neg __ equiv
ipsilat med nodes: __ pos __ neg __ equiv
contralat med: __ pos __ neg __ equiv

y/n **liver/adr. CT,** date ____ Hosp ____
__ pos __ neg __ equiv
y/n **bone scan,** date ______ Hosp _____
__ pos __ neg __ equiv
y/n **head CT /MR,**date _____ Hosp ____
__ pos __ neg __ equiv

STAGE [for staging system, see over]

clinical
T ___ **N** ___ **M** ___ **STAGE** ____

pathologic
T ___ **N** ___ **M** ___ **STAGE** ____

If SMALL CELL, ___ limited stage
___ extensive stage

PROPOSED TREATMENT

Local Rx:
___ surgery, specify:______________
___ RT,
___ both, give sequence:___________
Systemic Rx (list agents): _____________
Sequencing: ______________________

PHYSICIAN completing form________ **DATE** ___________

Visit Sheet

Schedule return appointment with Dr. ________________

(and Fellow)________________

Nurse Practitioner ________________

in ____ Day(s) ____ Week(s) ____ Month(s)

Date:

Patient:

DX: ________________ Chemo Regimen: ________________

SCHEDULE:	Today	ASAP	Before Next Appointment	Next Appointment	Clinical Data
CBC, Diff					**CENTRAL VENOUS ACCESS**
Lytes, BUN, Creat					Port: single _____ double _____
Bili total ALK p'tase Bili Direct SGOT Total Protein LDH					PICC: single _____ double _____
ALB/GLOB					
Glucose					Other: ________________
Cal, Phos, Mg					
PT, PTT					Continuous Infusion for Chemo ________
Sed Rate					Consult Dr. ________________
CEA					Reason:
Type & Cross					Procedures:
OrderX-rays					Reason:
CXR					
Chest CT					
Abd CT, Pelvic CT					
Cranial CT					
Neck CT					
Bone Scan					
Gallium Scan					
Gated Heart Scan					
Mammogram Bilateral Unilateral (L, R)					
Vascular Studies					
Ultrasound of:					
MRI (cranial)					
MRI of:					
EKG					
Echocardiogram					
PFT with DLCO with O2 Sat.					

TEACHER TO TEACHER

This section contains selected responses of medical terminology teachers to a questionnaire about methods and activities they use in their classrooms. I hope that this will be a springboard for you to communicate with each other and share ideas about teaching. The questions are listed below, and following is an alphabetical list of teachers who responded and included their name and address. I want to thank all of you who took the time to share. Hopefully, you will continue to send comments and suggestions to me via my e-mail (Daviellenchabner@gmail.com) or our new website for teachers and students (http://evolve.elsevier.com/chabner/language).

Questionnaire

1. What activities or teaching aids have you developed to use in your classroom to make the subject come alive?
2. Have you developed any interesting quiz formats that your students find helpful?
3. Have you developed any supplemental handouts that are helpful to students?
4. What do you do to help students who have poor English skills?
5. What is your method of grading and evaluating students' work, and how do you encourage and praise their efforts?
6. What do you do to help students with pronunciation and spelling of medical terms?
7. Do you have any special hints to teach medical terminology to handicapped (visually- or hearing-impaired) students?
8. What lessons have you developed to teach various sections in *The Language of Medicine*?
9. Can you suggest ways of teaching terminology to a heterogeneous group of students (various backgrounds and abilities)?
10. Do you have any humorous handouts to share with other teachers? (These are included in the next section of the teacher's manual, titled "Medical Terminology Bloopers and Jokes.)"

Teachers

Mary Lu Albee
Biology Department
Lewis & Clark Community College
Godfrey, Illinois

Jeanne Christen
Phoenix College
Phoenix, Arizona

Carol Conti
School of Nursing
Elizabeth General Medical Center
Elizabeth, New Jersey

Brenda Erickson
John A. Logon College
Carterville, Illinois

Peggy G. Fuller
Bossier Parish Community College
Bossier City, Louisiana

Brenda Haueisen
Mason Lake ISD Technical Preparation Partnership
West Shore Community College
Scottville, Michigan

Linda Howe
Roper School of Nursing
Charleston, South Carolina

Trudi James-Parks
Radiologic Technology
Lorain County Community College
Elyria, Ohio

Janet Leitheiser
St. Paul Technical College
St. Paul, Minnesota

Thomas W. Owen
Billings Business College
Billings, Montana

Lu Ann Reicks
Iowa Central Community College
Fort Dodge, Iowa

Joy Renfro
Eastern Kentucky University
Richmond, Kentucky

Connie M. Schoon
Alpena Community College
Alpena, Michigan

Mary Schrader
Southwest Wisconsin Technical College
Fennimore, Wisconsin

Scott Sechrist
Nuclear Medicine
Old Dominion University
Norfolk, Virginia

David Tate
Medical Technology Program
Purdue University School of Health Sciences
West Lafayette, Indiana

Connie Taylor
Department of Biology
Southeastern Oklahoma State University
Durant, Oklahoma

Dottie Tolson
Edgecombe Community College
Tarboro, North Carolina

Susan J. Webb
Victoria, British Columbia
Canada

QUESTION ONE

What activities or teaching aids have you developed to use in your classroom to make the subject come alive?

Albee: I require students to find one article/week with at least 20 medical terms that they define and then summarize the article in common language.

Erickson: (1) Transparencies (color) for some sections; (2) made our own cassette tapes dictating words at the end of each chapter; (3) flash cards.

Fuller: I have included speakers: oncologist, ophthalmologist, physical therapist, x-ray technician, ER physician, and others.

Haueisen: When I teach body planes, positions, and cavities, I use E.L. Fudge cookies and colored toothpicks to help the students see each body area. Each student gets two cookies and one each of red, blue, yellow, and green toothpicks. After using overheads and model torsos to show all the areas, I have the students "put the blue toothpick in the anatomical left lateral portion of the cookie" and "put the yellow toothpick in the anatomical right lateral of the cookie." They are also instructed to "put the green toothpick in the superior aspect and red toothpick in the inferior aspect." Students then compare their toothpick placement to their partner's and if they don't match they check their text to see why not. We continue the activity with "divide the cookie along the coronal plane and break the anterior aspect along the transverse plane." I continue with various instructions until we have covered all body planes and directions. We get a lot of mileage out of two cookies and the students have fun and get a treat. Gummy bears work too and I'm sure some other cookies might be suitable. I have used it with high school and college groups and they all seemed to enjoy it.

Howe: I use A&P films with each unit and play *Jeopardy!* or *Family Feud* as a review.

Leitheiser: Do some lab – microscope work; anatomical models, crossword puzzles, short worksheets to do at the end of each lecture.

Owen: Videotapes of operations. Check with doctors' offices for this type of material.

Schoon: Students are required to make their own flash cards and then with a partner, they flash the cards and test each other. I photocopied the diagram of the heart with the identified parts omitted. This was used to make a transparency, reduced to fit their flash cards, and then became a question on the test. Having the diagram without answers is an excellent study aid for students.

Schrader: I have prepared a telecourse based on *The Language of Medicine*. I also teach a medical terminology course over ITV for students in our district and have prepared TV-ready visuals. I demonstrate the use of flash cards, student-prepared audiotapes, and other teaching tools over the television. Computer-enhanced video has helped emphasize words as I pronounce them.

Sechrist: I use lots of x-rays, scans, other medical images to bring the words "alive." There's nothing like an ultrasound to help demonstrate cholelithiasis! I assign diseases to each student, have another student define the term, and a third student give a second opinion or act as an attorney. I also use history sheets from actual patient files.

Tate: I occasionally break students into small groups. Each group has an MD, lab director/pathologist, and med tech. They are each given a paper with diagnostic requests on it. For example, the MD fills out a lab test and this is run through the pathologist and MT. Each segment requires the student to understand the abbreviation and terminology before moving to the next segment. This helps in that they must explain to me what the tests are asking for. We have fun and results then indicate quality of patient care.

Taylor: Students must make their own flash cards—especially for word parts.

Tolson: I use personal experiences as well as those that have been shared with me by others.

Webb: I encourage students to study with a friend and it works! I also encourage the use of flashcards and tapes, and bring in guest speakers.

Anonymous: Guest speakers, physician speakers, videos, illustrations of procedures (found in physician's library at local hospital).

Anonymous: I use a lot of stories—having worked in health care for 20+ years.

Anonymous: Team *Jeopardy!* for large classes or individual jeopardy for smaller ones. Group discussions of case studies.

Anonymous: For a class on the respiratory system, I take the class outside and ask them to turn their heads upward to the sky to feel the sun and breeze on their faces. Then I ask that they feel air coursing through their air passages. I want them to feel the freedom of exchanging air. Next, I get them to take a finger and close one side of their nose. By closing a naris, the student understands words such as obstruction, anxiety, panic—many of the symptoms that a client with a compromised respiratory system feels. Positive feedback has been given by the students.

Anonymous: Patient records. Approach from a clinical perspective.

Anonymous: I usually write case studies that go along with each chapter—to encourage students to describe in lay terms.

Anonymous: I use CIBA slides.

QUESTION TWO

Have you developed any interesting quiz formats that your students find helpful?

Albee: I select two or three paragraphs containing medical terminology and highlight 10 to 20 terms which the students define. If time permits, they summarize the articles in common language.

James-Parks: My final exam is comprehensive, but it is done by the student outside the classroom. Students are asked to select an article from a medical journal and rewrite a portion of it by changing the medical terms into lay terms. This has proven to be an interesting exercise that takes some thought and skill at interpretation of terms.

Owen: Take selections from source documents and have students write out in common terms to ascertain understanding.

Schoon: Use crosswords and word searches as quizzes.

Sechrist: I give a 50- to 100-question exam every week (course meets for 2-1/2 hours—14 weeks long).

Taylor: I give 100-point tests each week—mostly matching, but they must define word parts as well.

Webb:	Each class begins with 10 minutes to do a crossword puzzle regarding the exam for that night. We then do a 25-word spelling test. Then they do the exam for that night. I use the flow charts and diagrams on the exam if there is one in the chapter.
Anonymous:	I tell my students that I feel that their quiz grades are a grade for me and my abilities as a teacher. Seems to relax them when I stress this.
Anonymous:	The students grade one another in oral quizzes, listening to see if the term is spelled correctly.

QUESTION THREE

Have you developed any supplemental handouts that are helpful to students?

Albee:	I use crosswords or word searches for classroom and homework activities.
Erickson:	(1) Supplemental drug (including new and unusual) and abbreviations handouts, (2) health articles found in local newspapers' health section, (3) handouts made from appendices from health care reference books.
Leitheiser:	I have developed a more in-depth diagram of the kidney, and I use pictures of cells (WBCs and RBCs).
Schrader:	I have prepared a student packet that informs students in all three medical terminology courses as to what and how to cover each unit.
Sechrist:	I have used diagrams, photos, scanned imagesand even myself as a model during class. I also bring in used or discarded equipment to demonstrate medical technology terms (i.e., ophthalmoscope).

QUESTION FOUR

What do you do to help students who have poor English skills?

Christen:	One-on-one tutoring-referral to learning center. It should be noted that medical terminology is approached like learning any second language.
Erickson:	I have prepared cassette tapes in which I dictate the terms at the end of the chapter, pause so students can write the word, then spell the word so students can immediately check their spelling. Some of our adult learners who have difficulty spelling have found this to be very helpful.
Fuller:	I encourage the use of the tape machine—if English is their second language they do very well. If they have non-standard English with no skills, I refer them to the developmental student's office.
Schrader:	We have a special skills department. Students have each and every word pronounced and used on an individual card that has the word written on it. Students can see the word and run it through the machine—one at a time.
Sechrist:	The English as a second language students I have had over the past 7 years have typically done better than the "traditional students." My theory is they work harder at memorization and pronouncing the terms.
Anonymous:	I go down the row (line) and ask each student to give the answer and spell the term.
Anonymous:	We have special tutors for these students. Students must pass an examination for English skills prior to admission to class.
Anonymous:	Emphasize adjectival, adverbial endings, and noun forms of terms.

Anonymous: Individual tutoring if needed. Place in group with students who can assist them.

Anonymous: One-to-one tutoring is offered; all students participate in test reviews and read the questions and answers (reading aloud helps everyone).

QUESTION FIVE

What is your method of grading and evaluating students' work, and how do you encourage and praise their efforts?

Anonymous: Any word misspelled is wrong; every term they get wrong I have them write 5 times correctly and then I give them half of the points they miss.

Albee: 20% of grade is weekly chapter quiz

20% of grade is based on the articles they bring in

40% of grade is 4 unit exams (4 to 6 chapters each)

20% of grade is comprehensive final

Quizzes and exams concentrate on testing knowledge of terms (70%) and anatomy and physiology (30%). Knowing that this will be the format for at least 50% of each quiz instills confidence. I encourage students individually and verbally and on returned papers. Student papers are corrected carefully.

Format for quizzes—5 sections are the core of all quizzes and exams: (1) matching word parts and definitions; (2) defining terms; (3) building terms; (4) defining abbreviations; (5) abbreviating terms.

Christen: Weekly quizzes with quarterly exams and final comprehensive exam. Students may elect to remove one quiz score and "A" students do not have to count the final.

Erickson: Each exam (7) worth from 350 to 500 points. Each exam consists of spelling, roots, suffixes, prefixes, definitions, matching, diagrams and multiple choice. Final is only multiple choice and is comprehensive. Scale: 94 A, 85–93 B, 75–84 C, 69–74 D.

Fuller: 75% of grade comprises chapter examinations, 25% is comprehensive final. Lowest grade is dropped. Final comprehensive exam is not dropped.

James-Parks: Unit exams equal two thirds3 of the final grade, and the final is third of the grade.

Owen: Always put number correct over total number/never use red to correct/believe it or not, hand-drawn comical smiley faces for perfect papers work well.

Schoon: Personal talks and short notes on quizzes. First quiz is a no-brainer—everyone gets 100%—a real morale booster at the beginning of semester.

Schrader: You might enjoy reading "The Teaching Professor." There are often methods shared by other faculty. I try very hard to give feedback. I use a system of name cards to encourage students. As I call on a student with a question, I check the student name card in my hand. If the student had difficulty with several questions over the past week (identified by a mark on my card that only I see), I address an easy, memorization-type question—maybe two or three in a row—and then indicate with another mark if the student is successful. This makes all students comfortable in asking/answering questions. It works.

Sechrist: I keep a seating chart, keep notes on who is up to date and ready to answer each week. Students may elect to "pass" on an oral question twice, then I meet with them one on one.

Taylor: Give 100-point test each week, but drop two grades. Final is comprehensive.

Tolson: I give a test on each chapter and a separate spelling test on each chapter. A comprehensive exam is also given.

Anonymous: I always mark a half point off for spelling and one1 point off for wrong answer.

Anonymous: Much verbal and written praise.

Anonymous: Weekly quiz plus written note on papers; partial credit if term is known. As many of my students are older—"Refrigerator papers" for excellence.

Anonymous: Students are given take-home quizzes and crossword puzzles.

Anonymous: Listen, listen, listen. Most, if not all, students know their weak areas and know what to do about it. For the most part, students want to bounce off their ideas with faculty to see if they are on the right track.

QUESTION SIX

What do you do to help students with pronunciation and spelling of medical terms?

Albee: We go over the word parts and examples together. Students take turns pronouncing and defining the terms to get practice. I point out spelling difficulties with certain terms as they come up.

Christen: Tapes are used, along with verbal sharing in class. Spelling is incorporated in quizzes.

Fuller: Have them listen to tapes and pronounce words in class.

Schoon: Pronounce each term and they repeat after me. Then, divide into groups, have them practice as groups while I stroll among them to make corrections and answer questions. I usually pronounce words for students the class period before they are assigned (e.g., on the last day of Chapter 3, I take a few minutes and pronounce all words for Chapter 4).

Tate: We do group pronunciation and I randomly select students to pronounce words. I also bring in MDs and med techs.

Taylor: We pronounce the terms out loud. I pronounce first and students then pronounce terms. We go through the list at the back of each chapter. Then we go around the room with each student pronouncing a term. They become used to using and saying terms out loud and in front of each other.

Tolson: I pronounce the words and have the students repeat the terms after me. Students are allowed to tape the classes.

Anonymous: Pronunciation drills are a part of each class. Spelling is a part of each weekly quiz. Hints are given to prompt correct spelling as each word is introduced in lecture.

Anonymous: I have taped a total of 60 minutes of words for each section; students may have a copy for their own use.

QUESTION SEVEN

Do you have any special hints to teach medical terminology to handicapped (visually- or hearing-impaired) students?

Chabner: One of my students has multiple sclerosis. I found that if I designed the exams for all matching and multiple choice questions, she could easily circle items or put numbers in answer spaces.

Christen:	Taped lectures for review. I tape quizzes and exams. We have a learning center with special equipment for enlarging type.
Erickson:	Hearing-impaired individuals can easily be accommodated with written materials. If they can read lips, we dictate every term every class. Also, we provide a signer for the hearing-impaired.
Schrader:	I had a visually impaired student in the class and have used single-word audio cards to spell and pronounce the term.
Sechrist:	I allowed the one visually impaired student I had to sit closer to me and to the board.

QUESTION EIGHT

What lessons have you developed to teach various sections in *The Language of Medicine*?

Albee:	I also teach A and P and bring in models and transparencies to illustrate.
Schoon:	We do most of this sort of thing with games, crosswords, word searches, regular classroom drill, use of skeletons and models, group work, etc.
Taylor:	I use overheads and give lectures—mostly work on definitions.
Anonymous:	Hands-on with a skeleton—oral and written questioning pertaining to practical applications boxes. I usually have some form of abbreviations on oral and written questions.
Anonymous:	For practical applications, I use actual history and physicals and let the students decipher them.

QUESTION NINE

Can you suggest ways of teaching terminology to a heterogeneous group of students (various backgrounds and abilities)?

Albee:	I use group work in class—having students work on defining terms in the practical applications section in pairs or in small groups.
Christen:	Utilization of increased student interaction. Increased use of humor and relation to real-life situations.
Howe:	I teach on at least three levels. I reinforce using personal experience or equate to things they know. Also, they work together on teams.
James-Parks:	I have developed a method of teaching medical terminology based on a method called PSI (Personalized System of Instruction). It is a method of mastery learning. Each student progresses through the course (using *The Language of Medicine*) at their own pace and takes exams as they complete each unit. If they are unsuccessful in a unit, they have a second opportunity for mastery. This is one way I have dealt with students of various backgrounds and abilities.
Owen:	Treat them as individuals/Give them immediate success/Relate to their own body—use it as a reference.
Schoon:	This is my regular class population. I usually treat all the same but use those who have had anatomy and physiology as group leaders.
Schrader:	I work hard every semester to be sensitive to individuals.

Anonymous: I have students with less background as leaders in group sessions. Pride makes them try harder!

Anonymous: The more advanced students help the slower ones. Study groups.

Anonymous: I bring the backgrounds of different types of students into the discussion in class.

Anonymous: Give examples of lay terms where the word parts are used. Common words can be identified with and the background of the student doesn't matter.

QUESTION TEN

Do you have any humorous handouts to share with other teachers?

(I have put together some of these handouts and included them in the next sections, Common Usage Terms and Medical Terminology Bloopers and Jokes.)

Erickson: Besides a few assorted cartoons, I have a collection of Frank & Ernest cartoons that make fun of situations in health care. The dry sense of humor is well received with my adult learners.

Schrader: The students get to know me as their teacher and I use jokes—at least one a class period to keep their attention and interest up. Humor works in the standard classroom quite well, but does not work as well on TV.

Anonymous: I use personal experience.

COMMON USAGE TERMS

The following are common terms used by patients to describe symptoms and disorders.

1. "asleep" .... Paresthesias (of an extremity); numbness and tingling.
2. "bad blood"........................ Syphilis or STD.
3. "blackout" .... Syncope (fainting).
4. "bowels" .... Intestines, colon.
5. "bug" .... (1) Insect or spider.
   .... (2) Infectious disease.
6. "charley horse" .... Injury to a leg causing pain and limping; cause is usually pulled muscle or tendon.
7. "clap"................................ Gonorrhea.
8. "clog"................................ Clot of blood.
9. "crabs"............................... Infestation with lice.
10. "crick" .... Painful spasm in a muscle; often in the neck.
11. "dry heaves" .... Retching, gagging without vomiting.
12. "game"............................... Disabled by disease or injury (of an extremity).
13. "gimpy" .... Lame.
14. "goose egg" .... Swelling due to trauma (hematoma).
15. "heaves"............................ Vomiting.
16. "irregularity"..................... Constipation.
17. "mouse"............................ Hematoma around the eye; "black eye."
18. "nature"............................ Male sexual potency.
19. "oyster" .... Mass of mucus coughed up from the lungs.
20. "passage".......................... Defecation.
21. "physic" .... Laxative.
22. "piles"............................... Hemorrhoids.
23. "pins and needles" .... Paresthesias; see "asleep."
24. "plumbing" .... (1) Male or female urinary system.
    .... (2) Penis.
25. "queasy" .... Faint or nauseated.
26. "runs"................................ Diarrhea.
27. "sand"............................... Encrusted secretions around the eye.
28. "shin splints" .... Pain in the anterior muscles of the lower leg caused by running.
29. "shiner" .... Hematoma around the eye; see "mouse."
30. "stitch" .... Sudden, sharp pain.
31. "strain".............................. Urethral discharge in the male.
32. "sugar" .... Diabetes mellitus.
33. "sun poisoning" .... Used to indicate severe form of sunburn.
34. "trick"................................ Unstable (of a joint).

35. "walking pneumonia"....... Viral or other pneumonia that does not cause severe symptoms.
36. "water" .... (1) Urine.
.... (2) Edema.
37. "weak blood"..................... anemia.
38. "zit" .... Blackhead (comedo).

MEDICAL TERMINOLOGY BLOOPERS AND JOKES

Transcription Bloopers

The correct term is in parentheses.

1. "Bilingual" (inguinal) hernias.
2. Marital "discharge" (discord).
3. Bilateral "Cadillacs" (cataracts).
4. "Sick as hell" (sickle cell) anemia.
5. Medication "regime" (regimen).
6. "April" (atrial) fibrillation.
7. There are no other palpable "nerds" (nodes).
8. BuSpar 10 mg, two p.o. b.i.d. #80, no "refunds" (refills).
9. Patient had a "Pabst beer" (Pap smear) today.
10. This was a case of "old timers" disease (Alzheimer's disease).
11. Pelvic ultrasound revealed "firebirds in the Eucharist" (fibroids in the uterus).
12. There was a recent outbreak of chicken "pops" (pox).
13. The colonoscope was passed into the "assending" (ascending) colon.
14. The term visceral means internal "orgasm" (organs).
15. The patient finally had a hysterectomy and "Singapore-roofectomy" (salpingo-oophorectomy).

Patient Malaprops

1. A doctor reported that during an interview with a patient—a middle-aged woman—she reported that she had had her "ovary's sister" (ovarian cyst) removed.
2. A man walked into an ER complaining that he had taken "all six of those explositories" (suppositories) and still wasn't getting any relief.
3. While giving her history, a new patient related that there was a time when she thought she had "hog's skin disease" (Hodgkin's disease), but thankfully was proven wrong.
4. A patient presented at rounds with a complaint of "leakage from the micro-valve" (mitral valve). The doctor thought of recommending a plumber.
5. A patient reported being unable to "decaffeinate" (defecate).
6. Recently a patient appeared in a New York City ER complaining of "toxic sock syndrome" (toxic shock syndrome).

7. A patient informed her doctor that she had diverticulosis and had increased the amount of "fabric" (fiber) in her diet.
8. A man was admitted to the CCU complaining of chest pain. The family history was positive for heart disease, but the physician wasn't sure since the patient reported that his mother had "digestive" (congestive) heart failure.
9. One patient wasn't sure he believed his neurologist when he told him performing a "lumber puncture" (lumbar) wouldn't hurt.
10. One little boy volunteered that he knew his brother had his "independence" (appendix) cut out last year.
11. A patient always refers to her condition as "room of toys" (rheumatoid) arthritis.

Unusual Definitions for Medical Terms

(Humorous definitions of medical terms circulate freely throughout the medical community. This is just a sample of what can be found.)

Aorta .... A statement of something you should do.
Artery .... The study of fine paintings.
Bacteria .... The back door of a cafeteria.
Barium .... What you do when CPR fails.
Benign .... What you are after you are eight.
Bowel .... A letter like A, E, I, O, or U.
Bunion .... Paul's surname.
Carpal .... Someone with whom you drive to work.
Cat scan .... Searching for kitty.
Cauterize .... Made eye contact with her.
Cesarean Section .... A district in Rome.
Chiropractor .... An Egyptian doctor.
Colic .... A sheep dog.
Coma .... A punctuation mark.
Congenital .... Friendly.
Constipation .... Endangered feces.
D & C .... Where Washington is located.
Dilate .... To live long.
Ear .... Where you are now.
Elixir .... What a dog gives to his owner when she gives him a bone.
Enema .... Not a friend; as in "a guy like that is his own worst enema."
Fester .... Quicker.
Fibrillate .... To tell a small lie.
Genital .... Non-Jew.
G.I. series .... Military ball game.
Hangnail .... Coat hook.

Hemorrhoid .... Transportation given to a third person; as, "He didn't have his car so I offered hemorrhoid."
Hernia .... Referring to a female's knee.
Humerus .... Tell us what we want to hear.
Impotent .... Distinguished, well-known.
Inbred .... The best way to eat peanut butter.
Inguinal .... A new type of Italian noodle.
Intubate .... What a fisherman is.
Kidney .... Part of a child's leg.
Labor pain .... Injured at work.
Medical staff .... A doctor's cane.
Migraine .... What a Russian farmer now says about his harvest.
Minor operation .... Coal digging.
Morbid .... A higher offer.
Nitrates .... Cheaper than day rates.
Node .... Was aware of.
Organic .... Church musician.
Outpatient .... A person who has fainted.
Ova .... Finished; done with.
Pap smear .... Fatherhood test; or to slander your father.
Pelvis .... Cousin to Elvis.
Penis .... Someone who plays the piano.
Protein .... In favor of young people.
Post-operative .... A letter carrier.
Recovery room .... A place to do upholstery.
Rectum .... Dang near killed 'em.
Sacrum .... Holy.
Secretion .... Hiding anything.
Seizure .... Roman emperor.
Serology .... A study of English knighthood.
Serum .... What you do when you barbecue steaks.
Sperm .... To reject.
Tablet .... A small table.
Terminal illness .... Getting sick at the airport.
Tumor .... An extra pair.
Urine .... Opposite of you're out.
Urticaria .... Insisting to be manually transported; as "The only reason that child is screaming at his mother is that he wants urticaria."
Varicose .... Nearby.
Vein .... Conceited.
Vitamin .... What you do when friends stop by for a visit.

REFERENCE MATERIAL

The dictionaries, texts, and magazines listed below are materials that I have found helpful in teaching my medical terminology classes. I recommend them to you and your students as sources for study of the medical language as well as related concepts in anatomy and physiology.

I recommend the following two references—iTerms and *Medical Language Instant Translator*—since they correlate directly with *The Language of Medicine*. iTerms is a portable audio study companion providing pronunciations and definitions for all the terms in *The Language of Medicine*. It is available directly at http://iTerms.elsevier.com. *Medical Language Instant Translator* is a handy pocket reference for medical terms and other useful information including medical abbreviations, symbols, acronyms, and more.

Dictionaries

Dorland's Illustrated Medical Dictionary, 32nd edition. Philadelphia, Saunders, 2012.

Dorland's Pocket Medical Dictionary, 29th edition. Philadelphia, Saunders, 2013.

Miller-Keane, O'Toole MT (editor): Miller-Keane Encyclopedia and Dictionary of Medicine, Nursing & Allied Health—Revised Reprint, 7th edition. Philadelphia, Saunders, 2005.

Mosby's Dental Dictionary, 2nd edition, St Louis, Mosby, 2008.

Mosby's Dictionary of Medicine, Nursing & Health Professions, 9th edition. St. Louis, Mosby, 2013.

Texts

Black JM, Hawks J: Medical-Surgical Nursing: Clinical Management for Positive Outcomes, 8th edition. Philadelphia, Saunders, 2009.

Boston Women's Health Book Collective: Our Bodies, Ourselves: A New Edition for a New Era New York, Touchstone Books, 2005.
(Paperback full of readable, accurate information for women and men about many aspects of female health and physiology. Chapters include anatomy and physiology of reproduction and sexuality, venereal disease, birth control, abortion, rape and self-defense, childbearing, menopause, and many others.)

Callen JP, Greer KE, Paller AS, Swinyer LJ: Color Atlas of Dermatology, 2nd edition, Philadelphia, WB Saunders, 2000.

Damjanov I: Pathology for the Health Professions, 4th edition. Philadelphia, Saunders, 2012.

Frazier MS, Drzymkowski J: Essentials of Human Disease and Conditions, 5th edition, Philadelphia, WB Saunders, 2013.

Goldman L, Ausiello DA (editors): Cecil Medicine, 24th edition. Philadelphia, Saunders, 2012.
(Valuable reference source for information about disease processes related to internal medicine.)

Gould BE: Pathophysiology for the Health Professions, 4th edition. Philadelphia, Saunders, 2011.

Guyton AC: Textbook of Medical Physiology, 12th edition. Philadelphia, Saunders, 2011.
(Excellent basic physiology text.)

Haubrich WS (editor): Medical Meanings, A Glossary of Word Origins, 2nd edition. Philadelphia, American College of Physicians, 2003.
(Interesting explanations of medical etymology.)

Hoffbrand A: Color Atlas of Clinical Hematology, Philadelphia, WB Saunders, 2009.

Ignatavicius DD, Workman ML: Medical-Surgical Nursing: Critical Thinking for Collaborative Care, 7th edition. Philadelphia, Saunders, 2013.

Jarvis C: Physical Examination and Health Assessment, 6th edition. Philadelphia, Saunders, 2012.

Kumar V, et al: Robbins Basic Pathology, 9th edition. Philadelphia, Saunders, 2013.
(Easy to read pathology text.)

Lewis SM, et al: Medical-Surgical Nursing: Assessment and Management of Clinical Problems, 8th edition. St. Louis, Mosby, 2011.

Moore KL, Persaud TVN: Before We Are Born, 8th edition. Philadelphia, Saunders, 2012.
(Basic embryology and birth defects.)

Patton KT, Thibodeau GA: Anatomy & Physiology, 8th edition, St. Louis, Mosby, 2013.

Siedel HM et al: Mosby's Guide to Physical Examination, 7th edition. St. Louis, Mosby, 2011.

Silverman, HM: The Pill Book: The Illustrated Guide to the Most Prescribed Drugs in the United States, 14th edition. New York, Bantam Books, 2012.
(Basic information on prescription drugs.)

Solomon EP: Introduction to Human Anatomy and Physiology, 3rd edition, Philadelphia, WB Saunders, 2009.

Swartz MH: Textbook of Physical Diagnosis, 6th edition. Philadelphia, Saunders, 2010.
(Explanations and diagrams of procedures related to patient care.)

Thibodeau GA, Patton KT: Structure & Function of the Body, 14th edition., St. Louis, Mosby, 2012.
(Simplified anatomy and physiology for the student with little or no background in science.)

Townsend CM (et al) (editors): Sabiston Textbook of Surgery, 19th edition. Philadelphia, Saunders, 2012.
(Helpful in describing surgical procedures and related diseases.)

Magazines

The following is a list of magazines I have found helpful in understanding many disease processes. I clip articles, file them by subject, and take them into class for students to read. Although the articles are written for family practitioners and internists, they are written in simple, nontechnical medical language and often include excellent diagrams and illustrations.

American Family Physician. American Academy of Family Physicians, Lisle, Illinois, www.aafp.org.

CA—A Cancer Journal for Clinicians. Lippincott Williams & Wilkins, New York, www.lww.com.

Emergency Medicine. Quadrant HealthCom, Chatham, New Jersey, www.emedmag.com.

Patient Care. Medical Economics Co., Montvale, New Jersey, www.patientcareonline.com/patcare.

Resident and Staff Physician. Ascend Media LLC, Princeton , New Jersey, www.residentandstaff.com.

Publications by R.N. Medical Economics Co., Montvale, New Jersey, (313) 761-4700.

RESOURCES*

Sources for Patient Education Materials

Abbott Laboratories
100 Abbott Park Rd.
Abbott Park, IL 60064-3500
847-937-6100
www.abbott.com

AGC/United Learning
1560 Sherman Ave., Suite 100
Evanston, IL 60201
888-892-3484
www.unitedlearning.com

Alfred Higgins Productions, Inc.
15500 Hamner Dr.
Los Angeles, CA 90077
800-766-5353
www.alfredhigginsprod.com

American Cancer Society
1599 Clifton Rd., NE
Atlanta, GA 30329
800-ACS-2345
www.cancer.org

American Dental Association
211 E. Chicago Ave.
17th Floor
Chicago, IL 60611
312-440-2500
www.ada.org

American Diabetes Association
National Center
1701 N. Beauregard St.
Alexandria, VA 22311
800-342-2383
www.diabetes.org

American Dietetic Association
120 South Riverside Plaza, Suite 2000
Chicago, IL 60606-6995
800-877-1600
www.eatright.org

American Liver Foundation
75 Maiden Lane, Suite 603
New York, NY 10038
800-465-4837
www.liverfoundation.org

American Lung Association
61 Broadway, 6th Floor
New York, NY 10006
212-315-8700
www.lungusa.org

American Red Cross
2025 E Street, NW
Washington, DC 20006
202-303-4498
www.redcross.org

Arthritis Foundation
2970 Peachtree Rd. NW, Suite 200
Atlanta, GA 30305
404-872-7100
www.arthritis.org

Channing Bete Company
One Community Place
South Deerfield, MA 01373-0200
800-477-4776
www.channing-bete.com

**Adapted from O'Toole, M (ed): Miller-Keane Encyclopedia & Dictionary of Medicine, Nursing & Allied Health, 7th ed. Philadelphia, W.B. Saunders Company, 2005.*

Cystic Fibrosis Foundation
6931 Arlington Rd.
Bethesda, MD 20814
1-800-344-4823
www.cff.org

Glaxo SmithKline
One Franklin Plaza
P.O. Box 7929
Philadelphia, PA 19101
888-825-5249
www.gsk.com

Johnson and Johnson
One Johnson and Johnson Plaza
New Brunswick, NJ 08903
732-524-0400
www.jnj.com

Juvenile Diabetes Foundation International
120 Wall Street
New York, NY 10005
800-533-2873
www.jdfcure.org

Eli Lilly and Company
Lilly Corporate Center
Indianapolis, IN 46285
317-276-2000
www.lilly.com

March of Dimes Birth Defect Foundation
1275 Mamaroneck Ave.
White Plains, NY 10605
914-997-4488
www.modimes.org

Maternity Center Association
281 Park Avenue South, 5th Floor
New York, NY 10010
212-777-5000
www.maternity.org

McNeil Laboratories
Consumer Affairs Department
7050 Camp Hill Rd.
Fort Washington, PA 19034-2292
215-233-7171
www.mcneilcampusrecruiting.com

Merck & Co., Inc.
One Merck Drive
P.O. Box 100
Whitehouse Station, NJ 08889-0100
908-423-1000
www.merck.com

Elsevier/Mosby
3251 Riverport Lane
Maryland Heights, MO 63043
800-325-4177
www.elsevier.com

National Council on Alcoholism and Drug Dependence, Inc.
22 Cortlandt St., Suite 801
New York, NY 10007-3128
212-269-7797
www.ncadd.org

National Healthy Mothers, Healthy Babies Coalition
2000 N. Beauregard St., 6th Floor
Alexandria, VA 22311
703-836-6110
www.hmhb.org

National Hydrocephalus Foundation
12413 Centralia Rd.
Lakewood, CA 90715-1623
562-402-3523
www.nhfonline.org

National Institute on Drug Abuse (NIDA)
6001 Executive Blvd., Room 5213
Bethesda, MD 20892
301-443-1124
www.drugabuse.gov

National Kidney Foundation
30 East 33rd St.
New York, NY 10016
800-622-9010
www.kidney.org

National Mental Health Association
2000 N. Beauregard Street, 6th Floor
Alexandria, Virginia 22311
800-969-6642
www.nmha.org

National Multiple Sclerosis Society
733 Third Ave.
New York, NY 10017-3288
1-800-344-4867
www.nmss.org

National Safety Council
1121 Spring Lake Dr.
Itasca, IL 60143
800-621-7619
www.nsc.org

National Scoliosis Foundation
5 Cabot Place
Stoughton, MA 02072
800-673-6922
www.scoliosis.org

National Tay-Sachs and Allied Diseases Association, Inc.
2001 Beacon St., Suite 204
Brighton, MA 02135
800-906-8723
www.ntsad.org

National Women's Health Network
514 10th St., NW, Suite 400
Washington, DC 20004
202-347-1140
www.womenshealthnetwork.org

Novartis Institutes for BioMedical Research, Inc.
250 Massachusetts Ave.
Cambridge, MA 02139
617-871-8000
www.novartis.com

Novo Nordisk Pharmaceuticals
Novo Nordisk Inc.
100 College Rd. West
Princeton, NJ 08540
800-727-6500
www.novo-nordisk.com

Organon Corporation
56 Livingston Ave.
Roseland, NJ 07068
800-241-8812
973-325- 4500
www.organon-usa.com

Ortho Pharmaceutical Corporation
1000 Route 202 S.
Raritan, NJ 08869-0602
800-526-7736
www.ortho-mcneil.com

Pfizer Laboratories
Pfizer, Inc.
235 E. 42nd St.
New York, NY 10017
212-733-2323
www.pfizer.com

Planned Parenthood Federation of America
434 West 33rd St.
New York, NY 10001
212-541-7800
www.plannedparenthood.org

Roche Diagnostics Corporation
9115 Hague Rd.
PO Box 50457
Indianapolis, IN 46256
317-521-2000
www.roche-diagnostics.com

Ross Laboratories
Consumer Relations
625 Cleveland Ave.
Columbus, OH 43215
800-986-8510
www.rosslabs.com

SAMHSA's National Clearinghouse for Alcohol and Drug Information
P.O. Box 2345
Rockville, MD 20847-2345
800-729-6686
www.health.org

Elsevier/WB Saunders
1600 John F. Kennedy Blvd., Suite 1800
Philadelphia, PA 19103-2899
215-239-3900
www.elsevier.com

Skin Cancer Foundation
245 Fifth Ave., Suite 1403
New York, NJ 10016
800-SKIN-490
www.skincancer.org

Spina Bifida Association of America
4590 MacArthur Blvd., NW, Suite 250
Washington, DC 20007
800-621-3141
202-944-3285
www.sbaa.org

United Ostomy Association of America, Inc.
P.O. Box 66
Fairview, TN 37062-0066
800-826-0826
www.uoaa.org

Voluntary Health and Welfare Agencies and Associations

Administration on Aging
Washington, DC 20201
202-619-0724
www.aoa.gov

World Service Office of Alcoholics Anonymous
475 Riverside Dr., Suite 832
New York, NY 10115
212-870-3400
www.alcoholics-anonymous.org

Alzheimer's Association
225 N. Michigan Ave., Floor 1700
Chicago, IL 60601
800-272-3900
www.alz.org

American Academy of Allergy, Asthma, and Immunology
555 East Wells St., Suite 1100
Milwaukee, WI 53202-3823
800-822-2762
414-272-6071
www.aaaai.org

American Anorexia Bulimia Association
418 E. 76th Street
New York, NY 10021
212-734-1114
www.aabainc.org

American Association of Kidney Patients
3505 E Frontage Rd., Suite 315
Tampa, FL 33607
800-749-2257
813-636-8100
www.aakp.org

American Association of Retired Persons (AARP)
601 E Street, NW
Washington, DC 20049
888-687-2277
www.aarp.org

American Association on Mental Retardation
444 N. Capitol Street, NW, Suite 846
Washington, DC 20001-1512
800-424-3688
202-387-1968
www.aamr.org

American Cancer Society
1599 Clifton Rd., NE
Atlanta, GA 30329
800-ACS-2345
www.cancer.org

American Dental Association
211 E. Chicago Ave., 17th Floor
Chicago, IL 60611
312-440-2500
www.ada.org

American Diabetes Association
National Center
1701 N. Beauregard St.
Alexandria, VA 22311
800-342-2383
www.diabetes.org

American Foundation for the Blind
11 Penn Plaza, Suite 300
New York, NY 10001
212-502-7600
www.afb.org

American Liver Foundation
75 Maiden Lane, Suite 603
New York, NY 10038
800-465-4837
www.liverfoundation.org

American Lung Association
61 Broadway, 6th Floor
New York, NY 10006
212-315-8700
www.lungusa.org

American Pain Society
4700 West Lake Ave.
Glenview, IL 60025
847-375-4715
www.ampainsoc.org

American Parkinson Disease Association, Inc.
135 Parkinson Ave.
Staten Island, NY 10305
800-223-2732
718-981-8001
www.apdaparkinson.org

American Speech-Language-Hearing Association
10801 Rockville Pike
Rockville, MD 20852
800-638-8255
www.asha.org

American Tinnitus Association
P.O. Box 5
Portland, OR 97207
800-634-8978
www.ata.org

ARC of the United States
Association for Retarded Citizens
1010 Wayne Ave., Suite 650
Silver Spring, MD 20910
301-565-3842
www.TheArc.org

Arthritis Foundation
2970 Peachtree Rd. NW, Suite 200
Atlanta, GA 30305
404-872-7100
www.arthritis.org

Asthma and Allergy Foundation of America
1233 20th St., NW, Suite 402
Washington, DC 20036
800-727-8462
www.aafa.org

Centers for Disease Control and Prevention
Department of Health and Human Services
U.S. Public Health Service
1600 Clifton Rd.
Atlanta, GA 30333
800-311-3435
www.cdc.gov

Crohn's and Colitis Foundation of America
386 Park Ave. S., 17th Floor
New York, NY 10016-8804
800-932-2423
www.ccfa.org

Cystic Fibrosis Foundation
6931 Arlington Rd.
Bethesda, MD 20814
1-800-344-4823
www.cff.org

Epilepsy Foundation
8301 Professional Place
Landover, MD 20785-7223
800-332-1000
www.efa.org

International Dyslexia Association
Chester Building
8600 LaSalle Rd., Suite 382
Baltimore, MD 21286-2044
800-ABCD-123
410-296-0232
www.interdys.org

La Leche League International
1400 N. Meacham Rd.
Schaumburg, IL 60173-4808
847-519-7730
www.lalecheleague.org

Leukemia & Lymphoma Society
1311 Mamaroneck Ave.
White Plains, NY 10605
800-955-4572
914-949-5213
www.leukemia-lymphoma.org

Muscular Dystrophy Association
3300 E. Sunrise Dr.
Tucson, AZ 85718
800-344-4863
www.mdausa.org

Myasthenia Gravis Foundation
1821 University Avenue W., Suite S256
St. Paul, MN 55104
800-541-5454
www.myasthenia.org

National Center for the American Heart Association
7272 Greenville Ave.
Dallas, TX 75231
800-242-8721
www.americanheart.org

National Easter Seal Society
230 W. Monroe St., Suite 1800
Chicago, IL 60606-4802
800-221-6827
www.easter-seals.org

National Hemophilia Foundation
116 W. 32nd St., 11th Floor
New York, NY 10001
212-328-3700
www.hemophilia.org

National Institute of Allergy and Infectious Diseases
NIAID Office of Communications and Public Liaison
6610 Rockledge Dr., MSC 6612
Bethesda, MD 20892-6612
301-496-5717
www.niaid.nih.gov

National Institutes of Arthritis and Musculoskeletal and Skin Diseases
Information Clearinghouse
1 AMS Circle
Bethesda, MD 20892-3675
301-495-4484
www.niams.nih.gov

National Jewish Medical & Research Center
1400 Jackson St.
Denver, CO 80206
800-222-5864
303-388-4461
www.NationalJewish.org

National Kidney Foundation
30 E. 33rd St.
New York, NY 10016
800-622-9010
www.kidney.org

National Multiple Sclerosis Society
733 Third Ave.
New York, NY 10017-3288
1-800-344-4867
www.nmss.org

National Osteoporosis Foundation
1232 22nd St., NW
Washington, DC 20037-1292
202-223-2226
www.nof.org

National Parkinson's Foundation
1501 NW 9th Ave.
Miami, FL 33136
800-327-4545
www.parkinson.org

National Psoriasis Foundation
6600 SW 92nd Ave., Suite 300
Portland, OR 97223-7195
800-723-9166
www.psoriasis.org

National Safety Council
1121 Spring Lake Dr.
Itasca, IL 60143
800-621-7619
www.nsc.org

National Spinal Cord Injury Association
6701 Democracy Blvd., Suite 300-9
Silver Spring, MD 20817
800-962-9629
www.spinalcord.org

Paget's Foundation for Paget's Disease of Bone & Related Disorders
120 Wall Street, Suite 1602
New York, NY 10005
800-23-PAGET
www.paget.org

Parkinson Disease Foundation
1359 Broadway, Suite 1509
New York, NY 10018
800-457-6676
www.pdf.org

Phoenix Society (assistance following burn injuries)
1835 R W. Berends Dr. SW
Grand Rapids, MI 49519-4955
800-888-2876
www.phoenix-society.org

Prevent Blindness America
211 West Wacker Drive, Suite 1700
Chicago, IL 60606
800-331-2020
www.preventblindness.org

Self Help for Hard of Hearing People (SHHH)
7910 Woodmont Ave., Suite 1200
Bethesda, MD 20814
301-657-2248
www.shhh.org

Sexuality Information and Education Council of the United States (SIECUS)
130 W. 42nd St., Suite 350
New York, NY 10036
212-819-9770
www.siecus.org

Sickle Cell Disease Association of America
231 East Baltimore St., STE 800
Baltimore, MD 21202
800-421-8453
410-528-1555
www.SickleCellDisease.org

SIDS Alliance, Inc.
1314 Bedford Ave., Suite 210
Baltimore, MD 21208
800-221-SIDS
www.sidsalliance.org

United Cerebral Palsy Association (UCPA)
1660 L St., NW, Suite 700
Washington, DC 20036
800-872-5827
www.ucpa.org

United Network for Organ Sharing
P.O. Box 2484
Richmond, VA 23218
888-894-6361
www.unos.org

1-800 Telephone Numbers for Health Care Information, Products, and Services

Alzheimer's Disease and Related Disorders Association 800-272-3900
American Academy of Allergy, Asthma, and Immunology 800-822-2762
American Cancer Society 800-ACS-2345
American Council of the Blind 800-424-8666
American Diabetes Association 800-342-2383
American Dietetic Association 800-877-1600
American Kidney Fund 800-638-8299
American Liver Foundation 800-465-4837
Lupus Foundation Information Line 800-558-0121
American Nurses Association, ... 800-274-4ANA
Asthma and Allergy Foundation of America 800-727-8462
Cystic Fibrosis Foundation 800-344-4823
Drug Abuse Hotline 800-662-HELP
Epilepsy Foundation's National Information Center 800-332-1000
FDA Hotline (for drugs, biologics, and medical devices) 888-463-6332
National Safety Council 800-621-7619
Hearing Impaired AIDS Hotline 800-243-7889
Human Growth Foundation (growth disorders) 800-451-6434
Institute for Limb Preservation @ Presbyterian/St. Luke's Medical Center 800-262-5462
Juvenile Diabetes Foundation International 800-533-2873

Invacare 800-333-6900
The Living Bank International (organ donation) 800-528-2971
Graham Field Inc. 800-347-5678
Medco Instruments .... 800-626-3326 ext. 10
MedicAlert 888-633-4298
Medical Express (traveling health professionals) 800-544-7255
Medicare 800-MEDICARE
CDC National AIDS Hotline 800-HIV-0440
CDC TB & STD Prevention Information Network 800-458-5231
National Cancer Institute, Public Inquiries Office 800-4-CANCER
National Clearinghouse for Alcohol and Drug Information 800-729-6686
National Down Syndrome Society 800-221-4602
National Down Syndrome Congress 800-232-6372
National Health Careers Information Hotline 800-999-4248
Lung Line at National Jewish Medical and Research Center 800-222-LUNG
National Rehabilitation Information Center 800-34-NARIC
National Safety Council Call Center 800-621-7619
CDC Sexually Transmitted Diseases Hotline 800-227-8922
National SIDS Alliance 800-221-SIDS
National Spinal Cord Injury Association Resource Center 800-962-9629
Information Request Line for International Dyslexia Association 800-ABCD-123
Phoenix Society for Burn Survivors 800-888-BURN
Quality Line Health Education Videos 800-356-0986
Simon Foundation for Continence 800-237-4666
SmithKline Glaxo 888-825 5249
Spanish AIDS and STD Hotline 800-344-7432
Spina Bifida Association of America 800-621-3141
United Cerebral Palsy Foundation 800-872-5827
United Ostomy Association 800-826-0826

Professional Organizations, Associations, and Academies

American Academy of Nurse Practitioners
P.O. Box 12846
Austin TX 78711
512-442-4262
www.aanp.org

American Academy of Nursing
555 East Wells St., Suite 1100
Milwaukee, WI 53202-3823
414-287-0289
www.nursingworld.org/aan

American Association for the History of Nursing, Inc.
P.O. Box 175
Lanoka Harbor, NJ 08734
609-693-7250
www.aahn.org

American Association for Medical Transcription
100 Sycamore Ave.
Modesto, CA 95354
800-982-2182
209-527-9620
www.aamt.org

American Association for Respiratory Care
9425 N MacArthur Blvd., Suite 100
Irving, TX 75063
972-243-2272
www.aarc.org

American Association of Blood Banks
8101 Glenbrook Rd.
Bethesda, MD 20814-2749
301-907-6977
www.aabb.org

American Association of Critical-Care Nurses
101 Columbia
Aliso Viejo, CA 92656
800-899-2226
949-362-2000
www.aacn.org

American Association of Medical Assistants
20 N. Wacker Drive, Suite 1575
Chicago, IL 60606
312-899-1500
www.aama-ntl.org

American Association of Neuroscience Nurses
4700 W. Lake Ave.
Glenview, IL 60025
888-557-2266 (US only)
847-375-4733
www.aann.org

American Association of Nurse Anesthetists
222 S. Prospect Ave.
Park Ridge, IL 60068-4001
847-692-7050
www.aana.com

American Association of Nurse Attorneys
P.O. Box 515
Columbus, OH 43216-0515
877-538-2262
www.taana.org

American Association of Occupational Health Nurses
2920 Brandywine Rd., Suite 100
Atlanta, GA 30341
770-455-7757
www.aaohn.org

American Association of Spinal Cord Injury Nurses
75-20 Astoria Blvd.
Jackson Heights, NY 11370-1177
718-803-3782
www.aascin.org

American Clinical Laboratory Association
1250 H Street, NW, Suite 880
Washington, DC 20005
202-637-9466
www.clinical-labs.org

American College of Healthcare Executives
1 North Franklin St., Suite 1700
Chicago, IL 60606-3491
312-424-2800
www.ache.org

American College of Nurse Midwives
8403 Colesville Rd., Suite 1550
Silver Spring, MD 20910
240-485-1800
www.midwife.org

American Dental Association
211 E. Chicago Ave., 17th Floor
Chicago, IL 60611
312-440-2500
www.ada.org

American Dental Hygienists' Association
444 N Michigan Avenue, Suite 3400
Chicago, IL 60611
312-440-8900
www.adha.org

American Dietetic Association
120 South Riverside Plaza, Suite 2000
Chicago, IL 60606-6995
800-877-1600
www.eatright.org

American Health Care Association
1201 L St. NW
Washington, DC 20005-4015
202-842-4444
www.ahca.org

American Health Information Management Association
233 N Michigan Avenue, 21st Floor
Chicago, IL 60601
312-233-1100
www.ahima.org

American Holistic Nurses' Association
P.O. Box 2130
Flagstaff, AZ 86003-2130
800-278-2462
www.ahna.org

American Lung Association
61 Broadway, 6th Floor
New York, NY 10006
212-315-8700
www.lungusa.org

American Massage Therapy Association
500 Davis St.
Evanston, IL 60201
877-905-2700
847-864-0123
www.amtamassage.org

American Medical Association
515 N. State St.
Chicago, IL 60610
800-621-8335
www.ama-assn.org

American Nephrology Nurses' Association
East Holly Ave., Box 56
Pitman, NJ 08071-0056
888-600-ANNA
856-256-2320
www.annanurse.org

American Nurses Association
8515 Georgia Ave., Suite 400
Silver Spring, MD 20910
301-628-5000
800-274-4ANA
www.nursingworld.org

American Nurses Foundation
8515 Georgia Ave., Suite 400 West
Silver Spring, MD 20910
301-628-5227
www.nursingworld.org/anf

American Occupational Therapy Association
4720 Montgomery Lane
P.O. Box 31220
Bethesda, MD 20824-1220
301-652-2682
www.aota.org

American Organization of Nurse Executives
Liberty Place
325 Seventh St., NW
Washington, DC 20004
202-626-2240
www.aone.org

American Pharmacists Association
1100 15th Street NW, Suite 400
Washington, DC 20005-1707
800-237-APHA
202-628-4410
www.aphanet.org

American Physical Therapy Association
1111 N. Fairfax St.
Alexandria, VA 22314-1488
800-999-2782
703-684-2782
www.apta.org

American Psychiatric Nurses Association
1555 Wilson Blvd., Suite 602
Arlington, VA 22209
866-243-2443
www.apna.org

American Public Health Association
800 I Street, NW
Washington, DC 20001
202-777-2742
www.apha.org

American Radiological Nurses Association
7794 Grow Dr.
Pensacola, FL 32514
866-486-2762
850-474-7292
www.arna.net

American Registry of Radiologic Technologists
1255 Northland Dr.
St. Paul, MN 55120
651-687-0048
www.arrt.org

American Society for Clinical Laboratory Science
6701 Democracy Blvd., Suite 300
Bethesda, MD 20817
301-657-2768
www.ascls.org

American Society of Health-System Pharmacists
7272 Wisconsin Ave.
Bethesda, MD 20814
301-657-3000
www.ashp.org

American Speech-Language-Hearing Association
10801 Rockville Pike
Rockville, MD 20852
800-638-8255
www.asha.org

Association for the Care of Children's Health
19 Mantua Rd.
Mt. Royal, NJ 08061
609-224-1742
www.eparent.com/resources/associations/childreshealthassoc.htm

Association of Mental Health Administrators
60 Revere Dr., Suite 500
Northbrook, IL 60062
708-480-9626

Association of Nurses in AIDS Care
3538 Ridgewood Rd.
Akron, OH 44333
800-260-6780
www.anacnet.org

Association of Pediatric Oncology Nurses
4700 West Lake Ave.
Glenview, IL 60025
847-375-4724
www.apon.org

Association of Peri-Operative Registered Nurses
2170 South Parker Rd., Suite 300
Denver, CO 80231
800-755-2676
www.aorn.org

Association of Rehabilitation Nurses
4700 W. Lake Rd.
Glenview, IL 60025-1485
800-229-7530
www.rehabnurse.org

Association of Women's Health, Obstetric and Neonatal Nurses
2000 L Street, NW, Suite 740
Washington, DC 20036
800-673-8499 (toll free U.S.)
800-245-0231 (toll free Canada)
www.awhonn.org

Commission on Graduates of Foreign Nursing Schools (CGFNS)
3600 Market St., Suite 400
Philadelphia, PA 19104
215-349-8767
www.cgfns.org

Dental Assisting National Board
444 N Michigan Ave., Suite 900
Chicago, IL 60611
312-642-3368
www.dentalassisting.com

Development Disabilities Nurses Association
1685 H St PMB 1214
Blaine, WA 98230
800-888-6733
www.ddna.org

Emergency Nurses Association
915 Lee St.
Des Plaines, IL 60016-6569
800-900-9659
www.ena.org

Hospice & Palliative Nurses Association
One Penn Center West, Suite 229
Pittsburgh, PA 15276
412-787-9301
www.hpna.org

Infusion Nurses Society
220 Norwood Park South
Norwood, MA 02062
781-440-9408
www.ins1.org

National Association of Hispanic Nurses
1501 16th St. NW
Washington, DC 20036
202-387-2477
www.thehispanicnurses.org

National Association of Home Care (NAHC)
228 Seventh St., SE
Washington, DC 20003
202-547-7424
www.nahc.org

National Association of Nurse Practitioners in Women's Health
505 C Street, NE
Washington, DC 20002
202-543-9693
www.npwh.org

National Association of Pediatric Nurse Associates and Practitioners
20 Brace Rd., Suite 200
Cherry Hill, NJ 08034-2634
856-857-9700
www.napnap.org

National Association of School Nurses, Inc.
8484 Georgia Ave., Suite 420
Silver Spring, MD 20910
240-821-1130
www.nasn.org

National Athletic Trainers' Association
2952 Stemmons Freeway, #200
Dallas, TX 75247
214-637-6282
www.nata.org

National Black Nurses Association
8630 Fenton St., Suite 330
Silver Spring, MD 20910
800-575-6298
301-589-3200
www.nbna.org

National Board for Respiratory Care
8310 Nieman Rd.
Lenexa, KS 66214
913-599-4200
www.nbrc.org

National Cancer Institute
NCI Public Inquiries Office
6116 Executive Blvd., Room 3036A
Bethesda, MD 20892-8322
800-4-CANCER
www.cancer.gov
www.nci.nih.gov

National Gerontological Nursing Association
7794 Grow Dr.
Pensacola, FL 32514-7072
850-473-1174
www.ngna.org

National League for Nursing
61 Broadway, 33rd Floor
New York, NY 10006
212-363-5555
www.nln.org

National Nurses in Business Association (NNBA)
P.O. Box 561081
Rockledge, FL 32956
877-353-8888
www.nnba.net

International Nurses Society on Addictions
P.O. Box 10752
Raleigh, NC 27605
919-821-1292
http://intnsa.org

National Student Nurses' Association
45 Main St., Suite 606
Brooklyn, NY 11201
718-210-0705
www.nsna.org

North American Nursing Diagnosis Association
100 N. 20th St., 4th Floor
Philadelphia, PA 19103
215-545-8105
800-647-9002
www.nanda.org

Oncology Nursing Society
125 Enterprise Dr.
Pittsburgh, PA 15275
866-257-4ONS
412-859-6100
www.ons.org

Sigma Theta Tau International Honor Society of Nursing
550 W. North St.
Indianapolis, IN 46202
888-634-7575
317-634-8171
www.nursingsociety.org

Society for Vascular Nursing
7794 Grow Dr.
Pensacola, FL 32514
888-536-4786
www.svnnet.org

Society of Gastroenterology Nurses and Associates, Inc.
401 N. Michigan Ave.
Chicago, IL 60611
312-321-5165
800-245-7462 (hotline)
www.sgna.org

Society of Otorhinolaryngology and Head/Neck Nurses
116 Canal St., Suite A
New Smyrna Beach, FL 32168
386-428-1695
www.sohnnurse.com

Transcultural Nursing Society
Madonna University
College of Nursing and Health
36600 Schoolcraft Rd.
Livonia, MI 48150-1173
888-432-5470 (from within the United States)
734-432-5470 (international)
www.tcns.org

CPSIA information can be obtained at www.ICGtesting.com
Printed in the USA
BVOW050937240613

323848BV00002B/1/P